Review for

NCLEX–PN/VN

Third Edition

Sandra F. Smith, RN, MS

Fay Alger O'Brien, RN, MA
Associate Editor

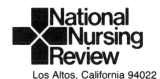

National Nursing Review

Los Altos, California 94022

International Standard Book Number: 0-917010-24-8

Copies of this book may be obtained from:
National Nursing Review, Inc.
342 State St., #6
Los Altos, CA 94022
(415) 941-5784

Contributing Authors

Chapter Contributors

Mary Bierly, R.N., B.S.N.
School of Practical Nursing
Columbus Public Schools, Ohio

Arlene Thorsness Kostoch, R.N., Ph.D.
Del Mar College, Texas

Eva Nunn Gumke, R.N., B.S.N.
Hartnell College, California

Patricia Ann Morrissey, R.N., M.S.
Edna McConnell Clark School of
Nursing, New York

Doris E. Nay, R.N., M.A.
Boulder Valley Health Occupations
Paddock Center
805 Gillaspie Dr.
Boulder, CO 80303

Fay Alger O'Brien, R.N., M.A.
De Anza College, California

Section Contributors

Sharon Matusoff Bell, R.N., M.A.
School of Practical Nursing
Columbus Public Schools, Ohio

Barbara Enderle, R.N.
School of Practical Nursing
Columbus Public Schools, Ohio

Patricia Parr Graves, R.N.
School of Practical Nursing
Columbus Public Schools, Ohio

Judith Hankin, R.N., B.S.
School of Practical Nursing
Presbyterian University of Pennsylvania
Medical Center, Pennsylvania

Sandra Harper, R.N., B.S.N.
Dallas Vocational Nursing Program, Texas

Susan Tamburro Keiser, R.N., B.S.
School of Practical Nursing
Columbus Public Schools, Ohio

Preface

During your practical nursing program, you have studied nursing theory and gained clinical experience. Now you face the important challenge of scoring sufficiently high in the National Council Licensure Examination to qualify for PN/VN licensure. The objective of this book is to provide you with a comprehensive, current, and complete review of practical nursing content.

We are pleased to offer the third edition of our PN/VN review book, written to assist you to prepare for your licensure exam. I am aware of the problems that you may encounter while preparing for these tests. Most candidates for licensure do not know how to review the vast amount of material to which they have been exposed during their nursing education. A key objective of this book is to help you prepare for NCLEX-PN in the most efficient manner.

An effective preparation method is to thoroughly review the material most likely to be covered on the exam and to take practice tests having similar questions. With this program in mind, *Review for PN/VN* is organized into ten chapters. The outline format is designed to help you review quickly, as well as to emphasize significant content.

The question and answer sections serve a dual purpose (1) to acquaint you with the type of questions to expect on the examination and (2) to give you an opportunity to test and improve your knowledge of nurse-patient situations. The answers and rationale sections are intended to discourage rote memorization and to reinforce learning by demonstrating the underlying principle which tells you why the answers are right or wrong. The selection and presentation of content in this book are directed toward minimizing your review time and maximizing your test results.

Acknowledgments

I wish to extend my thanks to all of the contributing authors and to the many other people who helped with the development of this book. I want to thank Fay O'Brien, R.N., M.A. my associate editor, whose dedicated work to organize, edit, and proofread all the material greatly enhanced our efforts. Because of the invaluable assistance of the editors, graphic designers, typesetters, and book manufacturer, this review book is available to help students prepare for the current NCLEX.

Sandra L. Smith

Table of Contents

Introduction

Review for PN/VN is designed to assist the practical/vocational student nurse in reviewing nursing content for the National Council Licensure Examination (NCLEX-PN). The content is planned and the format of the book is designed to help the student utilize review time more effectively. Nursing curriculum varies from school to school, and students may find that they are more knowledgeable in one content area than another.

Review for PN/VN will enable the student to quickly recognize his or her areas of expertise and concentrate on less familiar content. The review questions at the end of each chapter will also assist the student by testing mastery of basic nursing principles and their application to clinical situations.

The NCLEX tests the student's knowledge of practical/vocational nursing. This text includes gross anatomy and physiology as a general review source for students unsure of basic principles. The main emphasis is on basic nursing skills, the vocational nurse's responsibilities, normal growth and development, and major disease processes. The content was selected especially for student nurses to utilize in reviewing for both nursing tests at school and for NCLEX-PN.

The introduction to this book presents general background information on PN/VN licensure and NCLEX, a preview of the contents of *Review for PN/VN,* and helpful techniques for studying and achieving positive test results. The introduction also provides guidelines for the most effective methods in using this review book.

PN/VN Licensure Procedures

The purpose of PN/VN licensure is to establish minimum levels of competency. All the states require that nurses pass a licensing examination to practice as a Licensed Practical or Licensed Vocational Nurse. Current emphasis on consumer protection affects the entire medical field and nearly all of its related professions. The system of licensure provides protection to the general public while at the same time confirming that the qualified candidate can embark on a career with confidence and safety.

The NCLEX-PN is the means by which most states evaluate the applicant's qualifications to practice practical or vocational nursing. This test is given in April and October in all states except California. California administers its own test every other month. A candidate for the examination should contact the licensure authority in the state in which the candidate expects to practice nursing. A complete list of the State Boards of Nursing is included as an appendix to Chapter 10 for your reference. Each state sets its own standards for minimal scores and decides whether to accept test results from another state. Since most states require that the candidate's application be filed at least one month prior to examination, applicants should plan sufficiently ahead to ensure that key dates are not missed.

Licensure examinations may contain several test items that relate to revocation of the PN/VN license. The major reasons for revocation include the following: fraud in securing the license; unprofessional conduct or incompetency on the job; drug addiction; or conviction of a felony. Each state board has the authority to revoke as well as to issue the PN/VN license.

A foreign-trained nurse must have his or her credentials evaluated by the state in which he or she wishes to practice. If the requirements of the State Board of Nursing are met, he or she is then eligible to take the licensure exam.

Organization and Presentation of Review Material

In outline format, this book contains an extensive coverage of nursing content, oriented around eight major subject areas. Nursing theory and practical applications of this theory are presented for each subject area. The nursing theory section for each subject area includes minimal pathophysiology, signs and symptoms of the disease, diagnosis and treatment of medical conditions, and the appropriate nursing care. Practical applications of the nursing theory to clinical situations are made by the student when answering the situational questions that follow each section. The remaining questions are factual and test the student's ability to recall specific data. The tables, appendices, and glossaries throughout the book will assist the student in reviewing this factual material.

The multiple-choice questions are similar in format, subject matter, length, and degree of difficulty to those contained in the NCLEX. The answers to the multiple-choice questions are accompanied by rationale or an identification of the underlying principle. These sections provide the reviewer with an added learning experience; if the student understands the basic principles of nursing content, he or she can transfer them to the clinical situations contained in the NCLEX. Furthermore, the sample tests will provide a basis for understanding the process of selecting the "best" answer to a question.

Finally, the bibliography at the end of the book will serve as an excellent reference if further validation or information is needed to reinforce the student's present level of knowledge. The publications included in this bibliography were selected by the contributing authors both for their clarity of presentation and their coverage of material relevant to NCLEX.

Guidelines for Using This Review Book

The following procedure is recommended for effective utilization of this review text.

Review each of the major outlines, and evaluate your knowledge and understanding of the nursing theories and their clinical applications.

Study carefully the various glossaries, tables, and appendices. These sections contain information essential for mastery of the nursing subject areas.

Take the practice tests at the end of each section, and using the answers provided, correct each question and read the rationale for the correct answer. This procedure will enable you to understand the underlying principle for each answer. These principles will apply to questions on the NCLEX that are similar to the practice questions in this text.

Guidelines for Reviewing and Testing

Since most students have only a few weeks between final examinations at nursing school and the NCLEX, it is most important that the review process be conducted in an efficient manner. The following recommendations suggest an approach that the reviewer can utilize to achieve maximum results for the amount of time invested.

A. Schedule regular periods for your study and review.
1. Arrange to study when mentally alert. Studying during periods of mental and physical fatigue reduces efficiency.
2. Allow short breaks at relatively frequent intervals. Breaks used as rewards for hard study serve as incentives for continued concentrated effort.

B. Analyze your own strengths and weaknesses.
1. Consider past performance on classroom tests and written clinical applications of factual material. Learn from past errors on tests by studying corrected material.
2. Check your past performance tests to identify areas in which knowledge is incomplete and which will require more attention.
3. Allow sufficient time for repeated review of those areas that continue to pose problems.

C. Familiarize yourself with the examination format.
1. Study the format used for NCLEX so you know the different ways in which questions are asked. For example, you must know how to respond to clinical situations and multiple-choice questions.
2. Practice taking tests by answering the questions; taking a test is, in itself, a very valuable intellectual skill. Set time limits for covering a given unit of questions to establish the habit of working within a time frame.

D. Systematically study the material contained in each chapter of this book.
1. First, gain a general impression of the content unit to be reviewed. Skim over the entire section and identify the main ideas.
2. Then, read and study the tables, glossaries, and appendices carefully.
3. Mark key material that is not thoroughly understood.

E. Follow up on your priority areas.
   1. Set priorities on the material that is to be learned or reviewed. Identify the most crucial sections and underline the essential thoughts.
   2. Review what you have read. Think of examples that illustrate the main points you have studied. Recall examples from your own clinical experience or from clinical cases about which you have read.
   3. Solidify newly learned material by writing down the main ideas or by explaining the major points to another person.
F. Test yourself on what you have learned.
   1. Answer practice questions in this review book.
   2. Study answers to practice questions, but more importantly, concentrate on understanding the underlying principles and reasons for the answers.
   3. Acquire the flexibility to answer questions that are phrased in different ways but cover the same wide range of content. Important acquired concepts may be tested repeatedly in exams, but the questions will be phrased differently.

Preparation for Effective Testing

Students who are relaxed and confident while taking tests have a distinct advantage over those who become extremely anxious when facing and taking an important test. Achieving the maximum testing effectiveness involves your mental attitude as well as your knowledge of specific testing techniques.

The following suggestions will help you to maximize your testing effectiveness.

A. Preparation.
   1. The night before the test.
      a. Assemble the materials needed for the test as specified in your instruction booklet.
      b. Get a good night's sleep. Do not stay up all night learning new material.
      c. Avoid the use of stimulants or depressants, either of which may affect your ability to think clearly during the test.

d. Approach the test with confidence and the determination to do your best. Think positively and concentrate on all that you *do* know rather than on what you think you *do not* know.
   2. The day of the test.
      a. Eat a good breakfast. Do not rush.
      b. Allow ample time to travel to the testing site, including time to park, to locate the proper room, etc.
      c. Choose a location in the testing room where you are least likely to be distracted and where you are away from friends.
B. Concurrent readiness.
   1. Carefully read the directions for taking the test so that errors in understanding how to proceed are avoided.
   2. Review the scoring rules. There is no penalty for incorrect answers on NCLEX. You may guess, since you won't be penalized. However, if you can eliminate at least one distractor, your chances of guessing correctly are improved.
   3. To judge how best to use your time, determine the total number of questions, and estimate how much time you have for each question.
   4. Answer the practice questions to initiate the test-taking process.

Test-Taking Strategies

There are several test-taking strategies, each of which can provide you with useful rules of thumb in answering questions. These strategies are not absolute nor fool-proof; they are intended to guide you in choosing the best response for the question.

A. Start at the beginning of the test, check the time periodically, and maintain a good rate of progression throughout the test. Do not spend too much time on any one question. If there is time left over, go back and spend time on questions about which you were uncertain.
B. Carefully read each question. Determine what the question is really asking. Sometimes details are extraneous. Mentally underline important factors; pay attention to key terms

and phrases. For example, do not misread *grams* as *milligrams*.

C. On multiple-choice questions, first eliminate the answers that you know are wrong, and then spend time deciding among the answers that are left. If you are not sure of an answer, pencil in the answer you think is correct, and go back to it later if you have time.

D. Be alert and watch for questions that ask which answers are *not* correct or that say, "All the following are correct except. . . ." Read the question as it is stated, not as you would like it to be stated.

E. A first "hunch" is usually correct. Many students have a first impression, choose an answer, and, upon reflection, go back and change the answer. Sensing that a particular alternative is right has some basis. Simply, your brain has made rapid connections. You came to an immediate conclusion based on your stored knowledge and your experience. The fact that you did not go through the logical steps of arriving at the correct solution does not indicate that your choice is wrong. Research studies have proven that these first impressions are probably correct.

F. Frequently, the most comprehensive answer is the best choice. For example, if two alternatives seem reasonable but one answer includes the other (i.e., it is more detailed, extends the first, or is more comprehensive), then this answer would probably be the best choice.

G. Eliminate answers that focus on medical knowledge or contain nursing actions that would be performed by an RN. Remember, this is a PN/VN test, and the questions are designed to test your competency and safety. It is unlikely that a question would require a medical or RN action for the correct answer; it may, however, offer these actions as distractors.

H. Evaluate the possible answers in relation to the stem (the question), not to other answers. Choose the answer that best fits that question rather than an answer that sounds good in itself.

I. Recognize answers that are obviously different from what is logically right, such as an answer given in grams when other choices are given in milligrams.

J. The answer to a question may be found in the following question. This can be used as validation for your choice of alternative. For example, a condition is described in the first question, and you are asked to label it. If the next question concerns a patient with the same condition, there is a good chance your former answer can be validated against this labeled condition.

K. You may find several questions grouped in sequence, that is, a group of questions that follow one another and are related. When this occurs, watch to see that all of your answers fit together and fall within the framework presented.

L. Do not look for a pattern to the answers. The questions are chosen at random, and the same letter may possibly and correctly answer five or more consecutive questions.

M. Be on guard for answers that contain generalized qualifiers such as *always* and *never*. They rarely fit within a logical framework. Some qualifiers, however, are correct, especially in a negative situation. Some situations may be true only when a qualifier is added.

N. It is important that you do not spend several minutes on any one question because your overall time allotment is approximately one minute per question. If you lose time and become immobilized, this will interfere with your cognitive processes for the rest of the test. Leave the time-consuming questions (those that are excessively long, difficult to comprehend, or those that focus on subject matter with which you are unfamiliar) and come back to them after you have completed the test. Remember, if you skip a question, also leave a blank space on the computer answer sheet or all the succeeding answers will be wrong.

O. When questions are given about a clinical situation, read the situation very carefully. Identify the essential ideas. Be careful of distractors that divert your attention from key ideas. Be careful of distractors that may in themselves be correct, but that are not relevant to the stem of the question or the main idea of the clinical situation.

Summary

In summary, these strategies are guidelines, not absolutes. Always use your own judgment, knowledge, and nursing experience. These assets will serve you well in passing NCLEX. Be confident that you will pass and, in fact, you will.

Anxiety, a forceful deterrent to test-taking success, interferes with your ability to use cognitive processes effectively. Anxiety blocks the search and retrieval process so that the knowledge held in your "memory bank" is inaccessible. Fear of the unknown is a major source of anxiety. This fear can be overcome by diligent review which, as you gain mastery over the nursing content, increases your self-confidence. It is also important to understand test construction and a strategy for taking tests. The chapter section that you have just completed was designed to reduce many of the unknowns associated with NCLEX and to provide you with test-taking strategies and techniques.

Please Note

Throughout this book you will notice a star symbol ☆ opposite content. This symbol identifies a nursing skill. The new PN/VN test plan emphasizes performance of nursing skills. You can expect many NCLEX questions to focus on these skills. Please review them thoroughly.

Nursing Through the Life Cycle

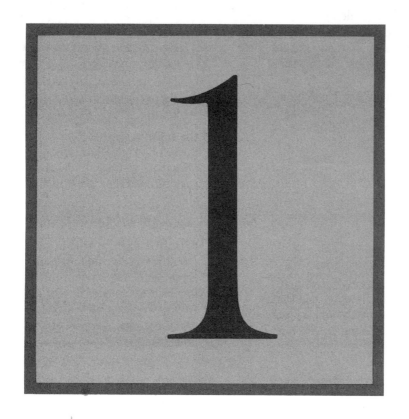

Homeostasis: Stress and Adaptation

Homeostasis

Definition: The maintenance of a constant state in the internal environment through self-regulatory techniques that preserve the organism's ability to adapt to stresses.

A. Dynamics of homeostasis.

1. Danger or its symbols, whether internal or external, result in the activation of the sympathetic nervous system and the adrenal medulla.
2. The organism prepares for flight or fight.

B. Adaptation factors.
1. Age—adaptation is greatest in youth and young middle life, and least at the extremes of life.
2. Environment—adequate supply of required materials is necessary.
3. Adaptation involves the entire organism.
4. The organism can more easily adapt to stress over a period of time than suddenly.
5. Organism flexibility influences survival.
6. The organism usually uses the adaptation mechanism that is most economical in terms of energy.
7. Illness decreases the organism's capacity to adapt to stress.
8. Adaptation responses may be adequate or deficient.
9. Adaptation may cause stress and illness, i.e., ulcers, arthritis, allergy, asthma, and overwhelming infections.

Stress

A. Definitions of stress.

1. A physical, a chemical, or an emotional factor that causes bodily or mental tension and that may be a factor in disease causation; a state resulting from factors that tend to alter an existing equilibrium.
2. Selye's definition of stress
   a. The state manifested by a specific syndrome that consists of all the nonspecifically induced changes within the biologic system.
   b. The body is the common denominator of all adaptive responses.
   c. Stress is manifested by the measureable changes in the body.
   d. Stress causes a multiplicity of changes in the body.

B. General aspects of stress.

1. Body responses to stress are a self-preserving mechanism that automatically and immediately becomes activated in times of danger.

   a. Caused by physical or psychological stress: disease, injury, anger, or frustration.
   b. Caused by changes in internal and/or external environment.

2. There are a limited number of ways an organism can respond to stress (for example, a cornered amoeba cannot fly).

Selye's Theory of Stress

A. General adaptive syndrome (GAS).
1. Alarm stage (call to arms).

   a. Shock: the body translates as sudden injury, and the GAS becomes activated.
   b. Countershock: the organism restored to its pre-injury condition.

2. Stage of resistance: the organism is adapted to the injuring agent.
3. State of exhaustion: if stress continues, the organism loses its adaptive capability and goes into exhaustion, which is comparable to shock.

B. Local adaptive syndrome (LAS).

1. Selective changes within the organism.
2. Local response elicits general response.
3. Example of LAS: a cut, followed by bleeding, followed by coagulation of blood, etc.
4. Ability of parts of the body to respond to a specific injury is impaired if the whole body is under stress.

C. Whether the organism goes through all the phases of adaptation depends both upon its capacity to adapt and the intensity and continuance of the injuring agent.

1. Organism may return to normal.
2. Organism may overreact; stress decreases.
3. Organism may be unable to adapt or maintain adaptation, a condition that may lead to death.

D. Objective of stress response.
1. To maintain stability of the organism during stress.
2. To repair damage.
3. To restore body to normal composition and activity.

Psychological Stress

Definition: All processes that impose a demand or requirement upon the organism, the resolution or accommodation of which necessitates work or activity of the mental apparatus.

Characteristics

A. May involve other structures or systems, but primarily affects mental apparatus.
1. Anxiety is a primary result of psychological stress.
2. Causes mental mechanisms to attempt to reduce or relieve psychological discomfort.
   a. Attack/fight.
   b. Withdrawal/flight.
   c. Play dead/immobility.

B. Causes of psychological stress.
1. Loss of something of value.
2. Injury/pain.
3. Frustrations of needs and drives.
4. Threats to self-concept.
5. Many illnesses cause stress.
   a. Disfigurement.
   b. Venereal disease.
   c. Long-term or chronic diseases.
   d. Cancer.
   e. Heart disease.
6. Conflicting cultural values, i.e., the American values of competition and assertiveness vs. the need to be dependent.

7. Future shock: physiological and psychological stress resulting from an overload of the organism's adaptive systems and decision-making processes brought about by too rapidly changing values and technology.
8. Cultural shock: stress developing in response to transition of the individual from a familiar environment to unfamiliar one.
   a. Involves unfamiliarity with communication, technology, customs, attitudes, and beliefs.
   b. Examples: individual moving to new area from foreign country or individual placed in hospital environment.

Assessment

1. Assess increased anxiety, anger, helplessness, hopelessness, guilt, shame, disgust, fear, frustration, or depression.
2. Evaluate behaviors resulting from stress.
   a. Apathy, regression, withdrawal.
   b. Crying, demanding.
   c. Physical illness.
   d. Hostility, manipulation.
   e. Senseless violence, acting out.

Nursing Care

A. Gather information about patient's internal and external environment.
B. Modify external environment so that adaptation responses are within the capacity of patient.
C. Support the efforts of patient to adapt or to respond.
D. Provide patient with the materials required to maintain constancy of internal environment.
E. Understand body's mechanisms for accommodating stress.
F. Prevent additional stress.
G. Reduce external stimuli.
H. Reduce or increase physical activity depending on the cause of and response to stress.

Growth and Development Milestones

Children

One Month

A. Physical and motor development.
1. Follows with eyes to midline.
2. Follows bright, moving objects with eyes.
3. Lifts head slightly from prone.
4. Lies awake on back with head averted.
5. Keeps fists clenched.
6. Responds to sharp sounds, i.e., bell, etc.
7. Does not grasp objects.

B. Language and social development.
1. Regards face, may smile.
2. Responds to voice.
3. Makes throaty noises.
4. Is alert about one out of every ten hours.

C. Appropriate games and stimulation.
1. Smile and talk to infant.
2. Touch, stroke, cuddle.
3. Talk and sing to infant.
4. Play soft music.
5. Play with infant.
6. Hold infant while feeding.
7. Provide toys such as colorful, hanging mobiles.

Two Months

A. Physical and motor development.
1. Ceases activity to listen for a bell.
2. Follows better vertically and horizontally with jerky eye movements.
3. Moves arms and legs vigorously.
4. Lifts head to 45 degrees when prone on abdomen.
5. Turns from side to back.
6. Grasp becomes voluntary.
7. No longer exhibits crossed extensor reflex.

B. Language and social development.
1. Vocalizes and smiles responsively.
2. Visually follows moving person.
3. Makes single vowel sounds such as "ah," "eh," "uh."
4. Differentiates by crying.
5. Begins social smile.
6. Exhibits tactile and oral stimulation, not social.

C. Appropriate games and stimulation.
1. Smile and talk to infant.
2. Use cradle gym and infant seat.
3. Allow infant the freedom of kicking with clothes off.
4. Place infant in prone position on floor or in bed.
5. Expose infant to different textures.
6. Exercise infant's arms and legs.
7. Provide bright pictures and hanging objects that move.

Three Months

A. Physical and motor development.
1. Lifts head and chest when prone.
2. Brings objects to mouth.
3. Displays nimble and busy fingers.
4. Rotates head from side to side.
5. Improves convergence.
6. Discovers and stares at hands.
7. Briefly holds toy in hand.

B. Language and social development.
1. Babbles, pronounces initial vowels, and coos.
2. Smiles more readily.
3. Ceases to cry when mother enters room or caresses him or her.
4. Enjoys playing during feeding.
5. Stays awake longer without crying.
6. Turns head to follow familiar person.

C. Appropriate games and stimulation.
1. While infant prone on abdomen, move bright object upward to encourage head movement.
2. Bounce infant on bed.
3. Continue to introduce new sounds.
4. Provide social stimulation (important).
5. Play with infant during feeding.
6. Provide rattles, large soft animals.

Four Months

A. Physical and motor development.
1. Infant lifts head and shoulders to a 90-de-

gree angle.

2. Looks ahead while in prone position on abdomen.
3. Can follow object 180 degrees.
4. Can move from side to side; tries to roll over.
5. Grasps for toy with whole hand.
6. Brings hands or toys to mouth.
7. Sucks thumb or fist.
8. Begins teething.

B. Language and social development.
1. Coos, gurgles, and laughs aloud.
2. Begins babbling.
3. Knows mother.
4. Imitates mother.
5. Demands attention by fussing.
6. Begins to respond to "no."
7. Enjoys being placed in sitting position with support.
8. Responds to and enjoys being handled.

C. Appropriate games and stimulation.
1. Show child his or her reflection in mirror.
2. Increase sensory stimulation.
3. Give frequent baths as infant enjoys splashing in tub.
4. Play music as child is quieted by it.
5. Move mobile out of reach; child may grab it and injure self.
6. Repeat child's sounds to him or her.
7. Provide soft, colorful squeeze toys; rattles, mirror; toys whose parts cannot be removed.

Five to Six Months

A. Physical and motor development.
1. Visually pursues lost object.
2. Holds block in each hand.
3. Exhibits hand-eye coordination.
4. Sits for short periods leaning forward on hands.
5. Creeps and rocks.
6. Reaches for objects beyond grasp.
7. Rolls from back to stomach and stomach to back.
8. Weighs twice as much as at birth.

B. Language and social development.
1. Begins to recognize strangers.
2. Shows fear and anger.

3. Vocalizes vowel sounds and well-defined syllables.
4. Shows anticipation; waves and raises arms to be picked up.
5. Expresses protest.
6. Understands name.

C. Appropriate games and stimulation.
1. Play sitting-up games.
2. Encourage reaching for objects.
3. Provide teething toys, soft blocks and squeeze toys, metal cup and wooden spoon for banging.

Seven to Nine Months

A. Physical and motor development.
1. Reaches for objects unilaterally.
2. Can transfer a toy.
3. Exhibits complete thumb opposition.
4. Sits alone steadily with good coordination.
5. Advances from creeping to crawling.
6. Can pull self to feet with assistance.
7. Feeds self a cracker.
8. Develops eye-to-eye contact while talking.
9. Engages in social games.

B. Language and social development.
1. Begins imitative expressions.
2. Shows fear of strangers.
3. Makes polysyllable vowel sounds.
4. Play is self-contained.
5. Laughs out loud.
6. Listens to conversations.

C. Appropriate games and stimulation.
1. Play social games such as peek-a-boo and pat-a-cake.
2. Allow child to drop and retrieve toys.
3. Allow child to play with spoon at feeding.
4. Give child soft finger-foods.
5. Take safety precautions as child puts everything into mouth.
6. Show excitement at child's achievements.
7. Provide squeeze toys in bath, toys that make noise, large nesting toys, crumpled paper.

Ten to Eleven Months

A. Physical and motor development.
1. Sits without support indefinitely.

2. Pulls self to feet.
3. Stands on toes with support.
4. Creeps and cruises very well.
5. Can pick up objects fairly well.
6. Uses index finger and thumb to grasp.
7. Can hold own bottle or cup.
8. Shows interest in tiny objects.

B. Language and social development.
1. Has vocabulary of one to two words ("Mama," "Dada").
2. Recognizes meaning of "no."
3. Shows moods; looks hurt, sad.
4. Is very aware of environment.
5. Responds to own name.
6. Imitates gestures, facial expressions, sounds.
7. Begins to test parental reaction during feeding and at bedtime.
8. Entertains self for long periods of time.

C. Appropriate games and stimulation.
1. Use plastic bottle.
2. Protect child from dangerous objects.
3. Have child with family at mealtime.
4. Allow exploration outdoors.
5. Provide new objects (blocks); toys that stimulate; containers (milk cartons); toys that can be filled, emptied, knocked down, and stacked up; fabric books.

Twelve to Eighteen Months

A. Physical and motor development.
1. Stands and walks alone.
2. Puts objects in and out of containers; can release objects at will.
3. Points to indicate wants.
4. Holds a cup with both hands.
5. Throws a ball.
6. Looks at pictures with interest.
7. Triples birth weight at 12 months; has closed anterior fontanel.
8. Begins to develop fine muscle coordination.
9. Has protruding abdomen.

B. Language and social development.
1. Is aware of expressive function of language; uses jargon, imitates sounds.
2. Cooperates in dressing; removes socks.
3. Likes an audience and will repeat performance.
4. Shows anxiety about strangers.

5. Distinguishes self from others.
6. Has a vocabulary of ten meaningful words.
7. Finds security in a blanket, favorite toy, or thumb sucking.
8. Plays alone but near others (parallel play).
9. Is dependent upon parents but shows first signs of desire for autonomy.

C. Appropriate games and stimulation.
1. Make no attempt to change from use of left to right hand.
2. Provide frequent changes of environment.
3. Allow self-directed play rather than adult-directed play.
4. Continue to expose child to different foods.
5. Show affection and encourage child to reciprocate.
6. Create safe environment (medications locked up and harmful items out of reach).
7. Provide pull and push toys, Teddy bears, pots and pans, musical toys, telephone, sand box and fill toys, cloth picture books with colorful, large pictures.

Eighteen Months to Two Years

A. Physical and motor development.
1. Exhibits well developed eye accommodation.
2. Walks up and down stairs one at a time with pauses.
3. Turns door knobs; climbs on furniture.
4. Chews more effectively.
5. Walks and runs with a stiff gait and wide stance.
6. Uses a spoon without spilling.
7. Builds tower of six cubes.
8. Kicks a ball in front of him or her without support.
9. Has daytime bladder and bowel control; occasional accidents; nighttime control not complete.

B. Language and social development.
1. Displays receptive vocabulary of 200 to 300 words; speaks vowels correctly.
2. Begins to use short sentences.
3. Has fear of parents leaving.
4. Helps to undress; tries to button.
5. Wants to hoard and not share: "snatch and grab stage."
6. Violently resists having toys taken away.

7. Begins to have feelings of autonomy.
8. Begins process of identification; uses "no" as assertion of self.
9. Begins cooperation in toilet training.

C. Appropriate games and stimulation
1. In toilet training, allow child to follow own pattern.
2. Provide peer companionship.
3. Allow child to eat with family.
4. Provide role-modeling for positive behavior (important for child).
5. Provide building blocks, wagons, pull toys, pounding toys like a drum, books with pictures.

Two and One-Half Years

A. Physical and motor development.
1. Pushes and pulls large toys.
2. Jumps; squats to play.
3. Builds tower of eight blocks.
4. Copies horizontal and vertical strokes.
5. Feeds self; uses fork.
6. Pours from pitcher.
7. Can undress.
8. Begins to use scissors.
9. Has full set (20) of baby teeth.

B. Language and social development.
1. Knows full name.
2. Refers to self by pronoun "I."
3. Shows negativism, has temper tantrums, and is ritualistic.
4. Learns power of "yes" and "no."
5. Shows poorly developed judgment.
6. Can tolerate short periods of separation from parents.
7. Begins to identify sex (gender) roles.
8. Explores environment outside the home.
9. Engages in associative play.

C. Appropriate games and stimulation.
1. Allow child his or her preferences.
2. Control temper tantrums.
3. Allow ritualism, especially at night.
4. Be aware that negativism and ritualism is normal behavior at this age.
5. Provide discipline as a way of socializing and educating child. Discipline simply for the sake of establishing authority is counterproductive.

6. Use firmness and consistency.
7. Read simple book to child to help develop language and memory skills.
8. Provide manipulative toys for muscle coodination, crayons and paper, simple games.

Three Years

A. Physical and motor development.
1. Goes up and down stairs, alternating feet.
2. Rides tricycle.
3. Stands momentarily on one foot.
4. Swings, climbs.
5. While running, can stop suddenly or turn corners.

B. Language and social development.
1. Begins to cooperate but is still self-centered.
2. Begins imaginative and make-believe play.
3. Wants to please.
4. Knows own age and sex, and the concept of *one*.
5. Verbalizes toilet needs and goes to toilet by self (needs help wiping).
6. Uses "I," "me," "you" speech.
7. Has vocabulary of 900 words.
8. Begins to understand what it means to take turns.
9. Can remember and repeat three numbers.

C. Appropriate games and stimulation.
1. Encourage and promote social contacts and imaginative outlets.
2. Alternate group activity with solitary play.
3. Listen to child's conversations and narratives.
4. Base expectations within child's limitations.
5. Provide climbing apparatus, keys, tricycle, wagons, dump trucks, simple puzzles, music, record player.

Three to Four Years

A. Physical and motor development.
1. Has 20/20 vision.
2. Races up and down steps.
3. Skips, hops, performs stunts; has good balance.

4. Draws man with two to four parts besides the head.
5. Cuts on line with scissors.
6. Feeds self.
7. Dresses self; laces shoes but cannot tie; buttons.
8. Brushes teeth.

B. Language and social development.
 1. Asks abundant questions: What? Why? How?
 2. Recites nursery rhyme or poem, or sings a song.
 3. Gives full name.
 4. Shows interest in world: nurses, firemen, police, doctors.
 5. Begins to share; seeks peer relationships.
 6. Exhibits excessive imaginative and make-believe play.
 7. Displays less negative behavior.
 8. Can tolerate separation from mother longer.

C. Appropriate games and stimulation.
 1. Encourage widening horizon and exploration of environment, imagination, peer relationships.
 2. Encourage pretending, story telling, expressing.
 3. Give simple explanation as to cause and effect.
 4. Provide alternate periods of active and quiet play.
 5. Provide books, puzzles, drawing materials, puppets.

Four to Five Years

A. Physical and motor development.
 1. Exhibits improved muscle coordination; is more agile and graceful; jumps, hops, skips on alternate feet.
 2. Draws recognizable pictures.
 3. Is quieter and less restless; has greater concentration.
 4. Draws triangle and square from copy.
 5. Names four colors, the heavier of two weights, and the longer of two lines.
 6. Builds steps.
 7. Exhibits good posture; carries arms near body; narrows stance.

8. Transports objects in trucks and cars.
9. Dresses and undresses with skill but still needs some supervision.

B. Language and social development.
 1. Exhibits improved concept and language development.
 2. Asks questions about the meaning of words.
 3. Prints simple words.
 4. Is cooperative, has poise, and controls behavior.
 5. Is creative.
 6. Is capable of longer attention span; completes activities; shows imaginative, dramatic play.
 7. Displays planning, space, depth, expression, and creativity in drawing.
 8. Begins to develop an elementary conscience.
 9. Displays high energy during play.

C. Appropriate games and stimulation.
 1. Give kind but unmistakable discipline.
 2. Build self-confidence.
 3. Provide consistent control.
 4. Encourage responsibility for putting things away.
 5. Widen and vary experiences in reading and music.
 6. Enroll child in kindergarten.
 7. Encourage group play and cooperation and sharing in projects.

Five to Six Years

A. Physical and motor development.
 1. Improves balance.
 2. Begins to ride two-wheel bicycle.
 3. Runs skillfully and plays games at the same time.
 4. Is able to wash without wetting clothing.
 5. Begins to lose baby teeth.
 6. Exhibits good control with small motor movements.
 7. Catches a ball.
 8. Shows little awareness of dangers, but has good motor development.
 9. Uses hands as manipulative tools in cutting, pasting, hammering.

B. Language and social development.

1. Has well-developed vocabulary.
2. Repeats sentence of 10 syllables or more.
3. Talks constantly.
4. Is cooperative.
5. Does simple chores at home.
6. Begins to take responsibility for actions.
7. Understands units such as a week or month.
8. Knows right and left hand.
9. Still requires parental support but pulls away from overt signs of affection.

C. Appropriate games and stimulation.
   1. Provide family atmosphere conducive to child's emotional development.
   2. Give guidance and limits, but avoid humiliating punishment.
   3. Provide sufficient exercise to stimulate motor and psychosocial development.
   4. Include other children for stimulation during play.
   5. Provide books, games, bicycle.

Six to Seven Years

A. Physical and motor development.
   1. Begins growth spurt.
   2. Is very active, impulsive.
   3. Dresses self.

B. Language and social development.
   1. Defines words by use.
   2. Shows more independence in play.
   3. Enjoys group play in small groups.
   4. Begins to accept authority outside home.
   5. Considers ideas of teachers important.
   6. Learns to read.
   7. Knows number combinations to 10.

C. Appropriate games and stimulation.
   1. Provide opportunity for collecting various items.
   2. Provide imaginary dramatic play: "dress up," school, firemen, soldiers; table games (tiddlywinks, marbles); dolls.

Seven to Eight Years

A. Physical and motor development.
   1. Has fully developed eyes.
   2. Is less impulsive and boisterous in activities.

3. Frequently develops nervous habits such as nail-biting.
4. Is more coordinated.
5. Is capable of fine hand movements.

B. Language and social development.
   1. Is more competitive.
   2. Recognizes differences between his or her home and others.
   3. Wishes to be like his or her friends.
   4. Tells time; knows days of the week.
   5. Shows curiosity about sex differences.
   6. May have periods of shyness.

C. Appropriate games and stimulation.
   1. Recognize child's periods of shyness as normal behavior.
   2. Give reassurance and understanding if and when nightmares occur.
   3. Provide table games and card games; magic tricks; games that develop physical and mental skill.

Eight to Nine Years

A. Physical and motor development.
   1. Exhibits long arms in proportion to body.
   2. Shows good coordination of fine muscles.
   3. Engages in active play.
   4. May begin secondary sex characteristics (females).
   5. Learns to use script.

B. Language and social development.
   1. Is more self-assured in environment.
   2. Likes group projects, clubs.
   3. Has increased modesty.
   4. Recognizes property rights.
   5. Needs help accepting defeat in games.
   6. Begins to have sense of humor.
   7. Through play, learns new ideas and independence: competition, compromise, cooperation, and beginning collaboration.

C. Appropriate games and stimulation.
   1. Give child opportunity to obtain adult approval.
   2. Give small household responsibilities.
   3. Answer child's questions regarding sex in simple, honest words.
   4. Do not become overly concerned with common problems such as teasing and quarreling, as they are usually temporary.

5. Provide sports, books (geography and adventure), erector sets, comics and funny papers.

Nine to Ten Years

A. Physical and motor development.
1. Shows skill in manual activities because hand-eye coordination is developed.
2. Exhibits decreased growth in height.
3. Is very active physically.
4. Cares completely for own physical needs.
B. Language and social development.
1. Shows sex differences in play.
2. Likes to have secrets.
3. Displays antagonism between the sexes.
4. Grasps easy multiplication and division.
5. Has special friend to confide in.
C. Appropriate games and stimulation.
1. Determine cause if lying and stealing occur.
2. Provide parental understanding.
3. Provide opportunity to enroll in clubs and organizations.
4. Provide books, musical instruments, TV, records, practical projects.

Ten to Eleven Years

A. Physical and motor development.
1. Shows onset of major secondary sex characteristics (males).
2. Attempts perfection of physical skills.
B. Language and social development.
1. Enjoys companionship more than play.
2. Needs privacy occasionally.
3. Exhibits increased ability to discuss problems.
4. Has growing capacity for thought and conceptual organization.
5. Sees physical qualities as constant despite changes in size, shape, weight, volume.
6. Shows group conformity.
C. Appropriate games and stimulation.
1. Continue sex education and preparation for adolescent body changes.
2. Encourage participation in organized clubs, youth groups.

Eleven to Twelve Years

A. Physical and motor development.
1. Begins puberty; physical changes appear in both males and females.
2. Begins menstruation (females).
3. May require more sleep due to body changes.
B. Social development.
1. Participates in community and school affairs.
2. Tends toward segregation of the sexes.
3. Likes to be alone occasionally.
4. Exhibits interest in world affairs.
5. Comprehends world of possibility and abstraction.
6. Begins to question parental values.
C. Appropriate games and stimulation.
1. Provide help in school and sports to channel energy in proper direction.
2. Provide guidance during dependence/independence conflict.
3. Set realistic limits.
4. Give adequate explanation of body changes.
5. Provide special consideration for child who lags behind in physical development.

Early Adolescence

A. Physical development.
1. Exhibits further development of secondary sex characteristics.
2. Shows poor posture.
3. Exhibits rapid growth and becomes awkward and uncoordinated.
4. Shows changes in body size and development.
B. Social development.
1. Needs social approval of peer group.
2. Strives for independence from family.
3. Has one or two very close friends in peer group.
4. Becomes more interested in opposite sex.
5. Period of upheaval: displays confusion about body image.
6. Must again learn to control strong feelings (love, aggression).
C. Counseling guidelines.

1. Provide adult understanding when adolescent deals with social, intellectual, and moral issues.
2. Allow some financial independence.
3. Provide limits to ensure security.
4. Provide necessary assurance to help adolescent accept changing body image.
5. Show flexibility in adjusting to emotional and erratic mood swings.
6. Be calm and consistent when dealing with an adolescent.

D. Developmental tasks.
  1. Finds identity; moves out of role diffusion.
     a. Integrates childhood identifications with basic drives.
     b. Expands concept of social roles.
  2. Moves toward heterosexuality.
  3. Begins separation from family.
  4. Integrates personality.

Adolescence to Young Adulthood

Developmental Milestones

A. Physical development.
  1. Completes sexual development.
  2. Exhibits signs of slowing down of body growth.
  3. Is capable of reproduction.
  4. Shows more energy after growth spurt tapers off.
  5. Exhibits increased muscular ability and coordination.
  6. Menarche—onset of menstruation—usually occurs between the ages of eleven and fourteen.

B. Social development.
  1. Is less attached to peers.
  2. Shows increased maturity.
  3. Exhibits more interdependence with family.
  4. Begins romantic love affairs.
  5. Increases mastery over biologic drives.
  6. Develops more mature relationship with parents.
  7. Values fidelity, friendship, cooperation.
  8. Begins vocational development.

C. Counseling guidelines.

1. Assist adolescent in vocational choice.
2. Provide safety education, especially regarding driving.
3. Encourage good attitudes toward health in issues of nutrition, drugs, smoking, and drinking.
4. Attempt to understand own (parental) difficulties in accepting transition of adolescent to independence and adulthood.

D. Developmental tasks.
  1. Intimacy and solidarity versus isolation.
     a. Moves from security of self involvement to insecurity of building intimate relationships with others.
     b. Becomes less dependent and more self-sufficient.
  2. Able to form lasting relationships with others.
  3. Learns to be productive and creative.
  4. Handles hormonal changes of developmental period.

Adulthood

Developmental Tasks

A. Achieves goal of generativity versus stagnation or self-absorption.
  1. Shows concern for establishing and guiding next generation.
  2. Exhibits productiveness, creativity, and an attitude of looking forward to the future.
  3. Stagnation results from the refusal to assume power and responsibility of the goals of middle age.
     a. Suffers pervading sense of boredom and impoverishment.
     b. Undergoes but does not resolve midlife crisis.

B. Has relaxed sense of competitiveness.
C. Opens up new interests.
D. Shifts values from physical attractiveness and strength to intellectual abilities.
E. Shows productivity (may be most productive years of one's life).
F. Has more varied and satisfying relationships.
G. Exhibits no significant decline in learning

abilities or sexual interests.

H. Shifts sexual interests from physical performance to the individual's total sexuality and need to be loved and touched.

I. Assists next generation to become happy, responsible adults.

J. Achieves mature social and civic responsibility.

K. Accepts and adjusts to physiological changes of middle life.

L. Uses leisure time satisfactorily.

M. Failure to complete developmental tasks may cause the individual to approach old age with resentment and fear.
 1. Neurotic symptoms may appear.
 2. Increased psychosomatic disorders develop.

Values of Adulthood

A. Becomes more introspective.

B. Shows less concern as to what others think.

C. Identifies self as successful even though all life goals may not be achieved.

D. Shows less concern for outward manifestations of success.

E. Lives more day-to-day and values life more deeply.

F. Has faced one's finiteness and eventual death.

Parenting in Adulthood

A. Characteristics.

 1. Tendency toward smaller families.

 2. Career-oriented women who limit family size or who do not want children.

 3. Early sexual experimentation, necessitating sexual education, contraceptive information.

 4. Tendency toward postponement of children.
  a. To complete education.
  b. Economic factors.

5. High divorce rates.
6. Alternate family designs.
 a. Single parenthood.
 b. Communal family.

B. Family planning.

 1. General concepts.
  a. Dealing with individuals with particular ideas regarding contraception.
  b. No perfect method of birth control.
  c. Method must be suited to individual.
  d. Individuals involved must be thoroughly counseled on all available methods and how they work—including advantages and disadvantages. This includes not only female but also sexual partner (if available).
  e. Once a method is chosen both parties should be thoroughly instructed in its use.
  f. Individuals involved must be motivated to succeed.

 2. Effectiveness depends upon:
  a. Method chosen.
  b. Degree to which couple follows prescribed regimen.
  c. Thorough understanding of method.
  d. Motivation on part of individuals concerned.

Psychosocial Changes

Midlife Crisis

A. A normal stage in the ongoing life cycle in which the middle-aged person reevaluates his or her total life situation in relation to youthful achievements and actual accomplishments.
 1. Struggles to maintain physical attractiveness in relation to younger people.

2. Partner or lover critical self-definition.
3. Feels he or she has peaked in ability.
4. Blames environment or others for failure to succeed.
5. Displays increased interest in sexuality.
6. Exhibits competitiveness in career plans.

B. Unresolved crisis.
1. May result in stagnation, boredom, and decreased self-esteem and depression.
2. Age for crisis varies.
   a. Women pass through it between 35 to 40 years old.
   b. Men experience the crisis between 40 to 45 years old.

Major Causes of Psychological Problems

A. Fears losing job.
B. Competition with younger generation.
C. Loss of job.
D. Loss of nurturing functions.
E. Loss of spouse, particularly females. (Forty-five percent of women over sixty-five are widowed.)
F. Realization that person is not going to accomplish some of the things that he or she wanted to do.
G. Changes in body image.
H. Illness.
I. Role change within and outside of family.
J. Fear of approaching old age.
K. Physiological changes.

The Aged*

Developmental Tasks

A. Maintains ego integrity versus despair.
1. Integrity results when an individual is satisfied with his or her own actions and lifestyle, feels life is meaningful, remains optimistic, and continues to grow.
2. Despair results from the feeling that he or she has failed and that it is too late to change.

For additional focus on the aged, see Chapter 6.

B. Continues a meaningful life after retirement.
C. Adjusts to income level.
D. Makes satisfactory living arrangements with spouse.
E. Adjusts to loss of spouse.
F. Maintains social contact and responsibilities.
G. Faces death realistically.
H. Provides knowledge and wisdom to assist those at other developmental levels to grow and learn.
I. Societal concerns.
1. There are approximately 20 million people over the age of sixty-five in the United States today.
2. Five percent of the aged are currently institutionalized.

Physiological, Psychological and Socioeconomic Implications

A. Physical changes.
1. Decrease in physical strength and endurance.
2. Decrease in muscular coordination.
3. Tendency to gain weight.
4. Loss of pigment in hair and skin.
5. Increased brittleness of the bones.
6. Greater sensitivity to temperature changes with low tolerance to cold.
7. Degenerative changes in the cardiovascular system.
8. Diminution of sensory faculties.
9. Decreased resistance to infection, disease and accidents.

B. Developmental process retrogresses.

1. Increasing dependency.
2. Concerns focus increasingly on self.
3. Interests may narrow.
4. Needs tangible evidence of affection.

C. Major fears of the aged.

1. Physical and economic dependency.
2. Chronic illness.
3. Loneliness.

4. Boredom resulting from not being needed.

D. Major problems of the aged.

1. Economic deprivation.
   a. Increased cost of living on a fixed income.
   b. Increased need for costly medical care.
2. Chronic disease and disability.
3. Social isolation.
4. Blindness.

5. Organic brain changes.
   a. Not all persons become senile.
   b. Most people have memory impairment.
   c. The change is gradual.
6. Nutritional deprivation.

E. Death in the life cycle.

1. In American culture death is very distasteful.
2. The elderly may see death as an end to

Table 1. Erikson's Stages of Personality Development

Stage	Approx. Age	Psychological Crises	Significant Persons	Accomplishments
Infant	0–1	Basic trust vs. mistrust	Mother or maternal figure	Tolerates frustration in small doses Recognizes mother as separate from others and self
Toddler	1–3	Autonomy vs. shame and doubt	Parents	Begins verbal skills Begins acceptance of reality vs. pleasure principle
Preschool	3–6	Initiative vs. guilt	Basic family	Asks many questions Explores own body and environment Differentiates between sexes
School	6–12	Industry vs. inferiority	Neighborhood school	Gains attention by accomplishments Explores things Learns to relate to own sex
Puberty and adolescence	12–?	Identity vs. role diffusion	Peer groups External groups	Moves toward heterosexuality Begins separation from family Integrates personality (altruism, etc.)
Adolescence and young adult	—	Intimacy and solidarity vs. isolation	Partners in friendship, sex	Is able to form lasting relationships with others Learns to be creative and productive

Based on Erikson: *Childhood and Society*

suffering and loneliness.

   3. Death is not feared if the person has lived a long and fulfilled life, having completed all developmental tasks.

   4. Religious beliefs and/or philosophy of life important.

F. The elderly may provide knowledge and wisdom from their vast experiences, which can assist those at other developmental levels to grow and learn.

G. There will be approximately 30 million people over the age of sixty-five in the United States by 1990.

Death, Dying, and Grief Process

The Grief Process

Definition: A process that an individual goes through in response to the loss of a significant or loved person. The grieving process follows certain predictable phases—classic description originally done by Dr. Eric Lindeman. The normal grieving process is described by George Engle, M.D., in "Grief and Grieving," *American Journal of Nursing,* September 1964.

A. First response is shock and refusal to believe that the loved one is dead.
   1. Displays inability to comprehend the meaning of loss.
   2. Attempts to protect self against painful feelings.

B. As awareness increases, the bereaved experiences severe anguish.
   1. Crying is common in this stage.
   2. Anger directed toward those people or circumstances thought to be responsible.

C. Mourning is the next stage where the work of restitution takes place.
   1. Rituals of the funeral help the bereaved accept reality.
   2. Support from friends and spiritual guidance comfort the bereaved.

D. Resolution of the loss occurs as the mourner begins to deal with the void.

E. Idealization of the deceased occurs next where only the pleasant memories are remembered.
   1. Characterized by the mourner's taking on certain qualities of the deceased.
   2. This process takes many months as preoccupation with the deceased diminishes.

F. Outcome of the grief process takes a year or more.
   1. Indications of successful outcome are when the mourner remembers both the pleasant and unpleasant memories.
   2. Eventual outcome influenced by:
      a. Importance of the deceased in the life of mourner.
      b. The degree of dependence in the relationship.
      c. The amount of ambivalence toward the deceased.
      d. The more hostile the feelings that exist, the more guilt that interferes with the grieving process.
      e. Age of both mourner and deceased.
      f. Death of a child is more difficult to resolve than that of an aged loved one.
      g. Number and nature of previous grief experiences.
      h. Degree of preparation for the loss.

Counseling Guidelines

A. Recognize that grief is a syndrome with somatic and psychological symptomatology.
   1. Weeping, complaints of fatigue, digestive disturbance, and insomnia.
   2. Guilt, anger, and irritability.
   3. Restless, but unable to initiate meaningful activity.
   4. Depression and agitation.

B. Be prepared to support the family as they learn of the death.
   1. Know the general response to death by recognizing the stages of the grief process.
   2. Understand that the behavior of the mourner may be unstable and disturbed.

C. Use therapeutic communication techniques.
   1. Encourage the mourner to express feel-

ings, especially tears.

2. Attempt to meet the needs of the mourner for privacy, information, and support.
3. Show respect for the religious and social customs of the family.

Death and Dying

Impact of Dying Process for Adults

A. Physical symptoms of dying.
   1. Cardiovascular collapse.
   2. Renal failure.
   3. Decreased physical and mental capacity.
   4. Gradual loss of consciousness.
B. Stages of dying.
   1. The dying process is ably portrayed in *Death and Dying,* by Elisabeth Kübler-Ross, New York, Macmillan Publishing Company, Inc., 1970.
   2. Individual is stunned at the knowledge he or she is dying and denies it.
   3. Anger and resentment usually follow as the individual questions, "Why me?"
   4. With the beginning of acceptance of impending death comes the bargaining stage, that is, bargaining for time to complete some situation in his or her life.
   5. Full acknowledgment usually brings depression; individual begins to work through feelings and to withdraw from life and relationships.
   6. Final stage is full acceptance and preparation for death.
   7. Throughout the dying process, hope is an important element that should be supported but not reinforced unrealistically.
C. Psychosocial clinical manifestations.
   1. Depression and withdrawal.
   2. Fear and anxiety.
   3. Focus is internal.
   4. Agitation and restlessness.

The Concept of Death in the Aging Population

A. In American culture, death is very distasteful.
B. The elderly may see death as an end to suffering and loneliness.

C. Death is not feared if the person has lived a long and fulfilled life, having completed all developmental tasks.
D. Religious beliefs and/or philosophy of life important.

Death and Children

A. Understanding of death for the young child.
   1. Death is viewed as a temporary separation from parents, sometimes viewed synonymously with sleep.
   2. Child may express fear of pain and wish to avoid it.
   3. Child's awareness is lessened by physical symptoms if death comes acutely.
   4. Gradual terminal illness may simulate the adult process: depression, withdrawal, fearfulness, and anxiety.
B. Older children's concerns.
   1. Death is identified as a "person" to be avoided.
   2. Child may ask directly if he or she is going to die.
   3. Concerns center around fear of pain, fear of being left alone, and fear of leaving parents and friends.
C. Adolescent concerns.
   1. Death is recognized as irreversible and inevitable.
   2. Adolescent often avoids talking about impending death, and staff may enter into this "conspiracy of silence."
   3. Adolescents have more understanding of death than adults tend to realize.

Nursing Management for Dying Patient

A. Nursing management of the adult.
   1. Minimize physical discomfort.
      a. Attend to all physical needs.
      b. Make patient as comfortable as possible.
   2. Recognize crisis situation.
      a. Observe for changes in patient's condition.
      b. Support patient.

3. Be prepared to give the dying patient the emotional support needed.
4. Encourage communication.
    a. Allow patient to express feelings, to talk, or to cry.
    b. Pick up cues that patient wants to talk, especially about fears.
    c. Be available to form a relationship with patient.
    d. Communicate honestly.
5. Prepare and support the family for their impending loss.
6. Understand the grieving process of patient and family.

B. Nursing management for the dying child.
1. Always elicit the child's understanding of death before discussing it.
2. Before discussing death with child, discuss it with parents.
3. Parental reactions include the continuum of grief process and stages of dying.
    a. Reactions depend on previous experience with loss.
    b. Reactions also depend on relationship with the child and circumstances of illness or injury.
    c. Reactions depend on degree of guilt felt by parents.
4. Assist parents in expressing their fears, concerns, and grief so that they may be more supportive to the child.
5. Assist parents in understanding siblings' possible reactions to a terminally ill child.
    a. Guilt: belief that they caused the problem or illness.
    b. Jealousy: demand for equal attention from the parents.
    c. Anger: feelings of being left behind.

Human Sexuality

Overview of Human Sexuality

A. Biological sexuality is determined at conception.
1. Male sperm contributes an X or a Y chromosome.
2. Female ovum has an X chromosome.
3. Fertilization results in either an XX (female) or an XY (male).

B. Preparation for adult sexuality originates in the sexual role development of the child.
1. Significant differences between male and female infants are observable even at birth.
2. Biological changes are minimal during childhood, but parenting strongly influences a child's behavior and sexual role development.
3. Anatomical and physiological changes occur during adolescence which establish biological sexual maturation.

C. Human sexuality pervades the whole of an individual's life.
1. More than a sum of isolated physical acts.
2. Functions as a purposeful influence in human nature and behavior.
3. Observable in everyday life in endless variations.

D. Each society develops a set of normative behaviors, attitudes, and values in respect to sexuality which are considered "right" and "wrong" by individuals.

E. Freud described the bisexual (androgynous) nature of the person.
1. Each person has components of maleness-femaleness, masculinity-femininity, and heterosexuality-homosexuality.
2. These components are physiological and psychological in nature.
3. All components influence an individual's sexuality and sexual behavior.

F. Gender identity (identified at birth) refers to whether a person is male or female.
1. Cases of "ambiguous genitalia" are rare (1/3000 births), and require special care for the infant and parents.
2. Ambiguous genitalia is a clinical label similar to slang term "morphodite," or biological term "hermaphrodite."

G. Sexual object choice is the selection of a mode of outlet for sexual desire, usually with another person.
1. Generally occurs during adolescence and beyond.
2. Includes heterosexuality, homosexuality,

bisexuality, celibacy, and narcissism/onanism.

H. Sexual object choice has strong influence on a person's lifestyle.

1. Individual must establish patterns of intimacy and sexual behavior that are acceptable to self, to significant others, and to society to a certain extent.
2. Psychological demands and expectations throughout life influence an individual's sexual interest, activity, and functional capacity.
3. Sexual object choice can affect a person's choices in life such as whether to be a parent, where to live, and what career to maintain.

Sexual Behavior

A. Sexual behavior is a composite of developed patterns of intimacy, psychological demands and expectations, and sexual object choice.

1. Can be genital (sexual intercourse), intimate (holding, hugging), or social (dating, choice of clothing).
2. Beyond the obvious examples, one never stops "behaving sexually."
3. Dress, communication, and activity are all expressions of sexuality.
4. Every person exhibits sexual behavior continually; no one is sexless.

B. "Transvestite" and "transsexual" are two terms that often cause confusion and need definition and differentiation.

1. Transvestite refers to one who enjoys wearing clothing of the opposite sex; may or may not be homosexual.
2. Transsexual is a person who chooses sexual reassignment: a complex physical (surgical), psychological, and social process of taking on the gender identity, sex role, sexual object choice, and sexual behavior of the opposite sex.

C. Sexuality, although difficult to define, is pervasive from birth to death, and nurses need to look beyond the framework of reproduction and procreation to understand the influence of sexuality on patients' health and illness.

D. Characteristics

1. Difficult to define precisely, human sexuality is considered to be a pervasive life force and includes a person's total feelings, attitudes, and behavior.
2. It is related to gender identity, sex-role identity, and sexual motivation.
3. Touching, intimacy, and companionship are factors that have unique meaning for each person's sexuality.
4. Sex role describes whether a person assumes masculine or feminine behaviors, usually a combination of both.
   a. This role generally considered to be fairly established by age five.
   b. Usually referred to by the concepts boy/girl and man/woman.

Nursing Care Related to Sexual Behavior

A. Assist in providing sex education and counseling.

1. Patients consider nurses to be experts in sexuality.
2. Intervention requires knowledge and skill.
3. Nurses need to know referral sources for interventions beyond their ability.

B. Give patients "permission" or acceptance to maintain sexuality and sexual behavior.

C. Be aware of the effect of medications on patients' sexuality and sexual functioning.

1. Oral contraceptives are considered by some to have played a major role in creating a sense of sexual freedom in contemporary society.
2. Drugs that decrease sexual drive or potency may act directly on the physiological mechanisms or may decrease interest through a depressant effect on the central nervous system.
3. Drugs with an adverse effect on sexual activity include antihypertensive drugs, antidepressants, antihistamines, antispasmodics, sedatives and tranquilizers, ethyl alcohol, and some hormone preparations and steroids.
4. There are no known drugs that specifically increase libido or sexual performance; those

that seem to enhance sexual behavior do so indirectly through transient relaxation of tensions, alleviation of discomfort, or release of inhibitions.

5. Long-term use of any drug or medicine will likely have a negative effect on sexual interest and capability.

D. Be aware of the problems to which nursing personnel should direct themselves in relation to the area of human sexuality.

1. Attitudes.
   a. Nurses should increase their self-awareness of their own attitudes and the effect of these attitudes on the sexual health care of their patients.
   b. Nurses should suppress negative biases and prejudices and/or make appropriate referrals when they cannot give effective sexual health care.

2. Knowledge.
   a. May have to be actively sought although nursing programs are increasing the sexuality content in their curricula.
   b. Also available through books, journal articles, classes and workshops, and preparation for sexuality therapy on the graduate level.

3. Skills.
   a. Primary skills needed are interpersonal techniques such as therapeutic communication, interviewing, and teaching.
   b. As with any skill, practice is needed for proficiency in sexual-history taking, education, and counseling.

Common Problems and Implications for Nursing

A. Masturbation.
   1. A common sexual outlet for many people.
   2. For patients requiring long-term care, masturbation may be only means for gratifying sexual needs.
   3. Nurses frequently react negatively to any type of masturbatory activity, especially by male patients.

4. Patients should be allowed privacy; if nurse walks in on a patient masturbating, he or she should leave with an apology for having intruded on the patient's privacy.

5. Frequent or inappropriate masturbation may be harmful to the patient's health. Limits need to be set to protect patient and other patients if behavior is inappropriate.

B. Homosexuality.
   1. Homosexuality is accepted by many as a viable life style.
   2. Nurses have tended to have negative attitudes and incorrect knowledge about homosexuality.
   3. A patient's homosexual (gay) life style should be accepted and respected.
   4. As with any patient, visitors should be encouraged as appropriate for the health/illness status, and these people should not be embarrassed or ridiculed.
   5. For chronically ill patients, such as in a nursing home, it is essential that sexuality needs be considered in the total care plan and special efforts be made to have these needs met.

C. Inappropriate sexual behavior.
   1. Difficult to precisely define "inappropriate" sexual behavior.
   2. Sometimes sexual behavior is in reaction to unintentional "seductive" behavior of nurses.
   3. Specific nursing interventions.
      a. Set limits to unacceptable behavior immediately.
      b. Interact without rejecting patient.
      c. Help patient express feelings in an appropriate manner.
      d. Teach alternative behaviors that are acceptable.
      e. Provide acceptable outlets to sexual feelings.

D. Rape.
   1. Rape is basically an act of violence and is only secondarily a sex act.
   2. Treatment should consist of both medical and psychological intervention.
   3. Sexual assault can have a long-term impact on the victim.

4. Victims may need encouragement and support to report rape occurrences to authorities.
5. Female nurses especially can play a valuable role in giving assistance and support to female rape victims.
6. Many communities have "hot-lines" that offer telephone information and crisis counseling to victims of sexual assault and to professionals.

E. Child sexual abuse.
1. There is only a beginning awareness of this problem area.
2. Most child sexual abuse involves a male adult and female child, but male children can also be victims of female or male sexual abusers.
3. The child may need special protection or temporary placement outside the home, but often the family unit can be maintained.
4. Child sexual abuse is a form of child abuse, and nurses should know local regulations and procedures for case finding and reporting.

F. Sexuality and disability.
1. Physically and developmentally disabled persons are sexual beings also.
2. Developmentally disabled persons should be given sexuality education and counseling in preparation for responsible sexual expression and behavior.
3. After spinal cord injury, the level of the lesion and degree of interruption of nerve impulses influence sexual functioning; adaptation of previous sexual practices may be needed after the injury.
4. Fertility and the ability to bear children are usually not compromised in women with spinal cord injury.
5. Nurses working with disabled patients must make special effort to include sexuality in total health care and services.

G. Contraception.
1. Nurses are considered experts on forms of birth control.
2. Nurses should be familiar with different methods and relative effectiveness of each one.

3. Patients should be assisted to make their own choices as to whether to use contraception and what method is best for them.
4. More detailed outline of contraception appears in maternity chapter.

H. Therapeutic abortion.
1. Patients need information about resources for and procedures of therapeutic abortions.
2. Patients should be given nonjudgmental assistance and support in decision-making process.
3. If nurse cannot in good conscience assist the patient, referral should be made to someone who can.
4. More detailed outline of abortion appears in maternity chapter.

Venereal Disease

A. Community aspects.
1. Primary objectives are to prevent and control spread of disease.
2. Based on reported cases, the incidence of gonorrhea and syphilis is increasing slowly.

B. Both syphilis and gonorrhea can be cured with appropriate antibiotic therapy.

C. Treatment and care should be given without stigma.

D. Case finding and treatment are still very difficult, especially for adolescents who may need parental consent to obtain health services.

Syphilis

Definition: Chronic infectious disease caused by the *Treponema pallidum* bacterium, a spirochete.

A. Characteristics.
1. Transmitted by intimate physical contact with syphilitic lesions found on the skin or on the mucous membranes of the mouth and genitals; also through the placenta, infected blood and CSF.
2. Caused by spirochetes that enter the body through a skin or membrane break.
3. Incubation period is two to six weeks following exposure.

B. Stages.
1. Primary stage.
   a. Most infectious stage.
   b. Appearance of painless ulcerative lesions (chancres).
2. Secondary stage.
   a. Lesions appear about three weeks after the primary stage and may occur anywhere on the skin or mucous membranes.
   b. Highly infectious through contact with lesions.
   c. Generalized lymphadenopathy.
3. Tertiary stage.
   a. The spirochetes enter the internal organs and cause permanent damage.
   b. Symptoms may occur ten to thirty years following the occurrence of an inadequately or untreated primary lesion.
   c. Invasion of the central nervous system.
      (1) Meningitis.
      (2) Locomotor ataxia—foot slapping and broad-based gait.
      (3) General paresis.
      (4) Progressive mental deterioration leading to loss of mental power.
   d. Most common site of cardiovascular damage is at the aortic valve and the aorta itself.

C. Treatment.
1. Penicillin or drug of choice.
2. Identification of contacts.
3. Usually curable with appropriate antibiotic treatment.
4. Recently there has occurred a strain of syphilis resistant to antibiotic therapy, so prevention is an important teaching concept.

Herpes

Definition: A viral disease caused by herpes virus, hominis types I and II.

A. Characteristics.
1. Herpes I.
   a. Most common type.
   b. Causes burning, tingling, and itching, soon followed by tiny vesicles.
   c. Most frequently occurs on lips, but can occur on the face and around the mouth.
2. Herpes II.
   a. Most often the cause of genital infection.
   b. Transmitted primarily through sexual contact and to baby during birth.
   c. Difficult to treat and to prevent recurrence.

B. Treatment.
1. Herpes I.
   a. Keep area dry and clean; apply ether.
   b. L-lysine: 1 gm daily for 6 months.
2. Herpes II.
   a. Avoidance of sexual contact when lesion is active.
   b. Acyclovir Cream as directed.

Gonorrhea

Definition: Infection of the genitourinary tract caused by the *Neisseria gonorrhoeae* organism.

A. Characteristics.
1. Transmitted almost totally by sexual intercourse.
2. Transmitted to eyes of newborn during vaginal delivery.
3. Incidence currently of epidemic proportions in the United States.

B. Signs and symptoms.
1. In the male.
   a. Painful urination, fever.
   b. Epididymitis with pain, tenderness, and swelling.
2. In the female (usually asymptomatic).
   a. Vaginal discharge.
   b. Urinary frequency and pain.

C. Treatment.
1. Antibiotic therapy frequently cures.
2. Observe for complications.
   a. Female experiences pelvic inflammatory disease (PID) with abdominal pain, fever, nausea, and vomiting; PID can lead to sterility.
   b. Male experiences postgonococcal urethritis and spread of infection to posterior urethra, prostate, and seminal vesicles.
   c. A secondary infection can develop in any organ.

General Nursing Concepts

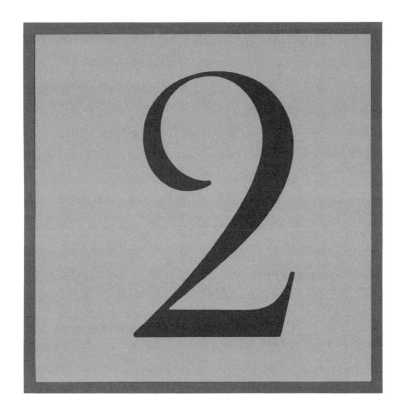

Fundamental Concepts

Environment of the Patient

Safety and Comfort

A. Adequate space.
B. Privacy.
C. Comfortable room temperature.
    1. 66 to 76°F is normal.
    2. Warmer temperature for very young, old, sedentary, or ill patients.
D. Room humidity 30 to 60 percent.
E. Adequate lighting.
    1. Natural light if available; avoid glare.
    2. Use of night lights especially with elderly, very young, very ill.
F. Adequate ventilation.
G. Comfortable sound levels.
H. Pleasing, easy-to-clean decor/furniture.
I. Protection from hazards.
    1. Use of handrails, side rails.
    2. Items placed within reach at the bedside.
J. Identification bands/bracelets.
K. Functional call system within patient's reach.

Assessment

Purpose of Assessment

A. Determine person's current health status.
B. Provide baseline for nursing diagnosis and care planning.
    1. First step in the nursing process.
    2. May not be duty of LVN/LPN but importance should be understood.

Assessment Procedure

A. Collect data by reading chart/care plan.
B. Interview to obtain subjective information/symptoms.
C. Collect cardinal or vital signs.
    1. Temperature.

a. Oral—inappropriate for use with infants, after oral surgery, or with patients who are unconscious or receiving oxygen by mask.
b. Rectal—inappropriate for use with patients who have a rectal disorder or following rectal surgery.
    2. Pulse.
a. Usually palpated over radial artery.
b. Apical—used with babies and irregular heart rates.
c. Pulse deficit—apical rate minus radial rate.
    3. Blood pressure—arterial.
a. Systolic—the pressure in vessel when heart is contracting.
b. Diastolic—the pressure in vessel when heart is at rest.
c. Pulse pressure—the difference between systolic and diastolic.
D. Measure weight and height.
E. Perform a detailed assessment.
    1. May be done from the patient's head-to-toes.
    2. May be done on a system basis.
    3. Used to determine patient's strengths and/or weaknesses. (See specific chapters for outlines.)
    4. Phases.
a. Inspection—overview of patient.
b. Auscultation—use of stethoscope to listen to heart.
c. Palpation—use of entire surface of all five fingers.
d. Percussion—use of middle finger for "tapping."
F. Use data to plan patient care or report the care plan to responsible nurse/team leader for validation, interpretation, or use in planning care.

Recording/Charting

Purpose of Written Records

A. Method of precise communication between staff members.

B. Legal documentation.

C. Provides for continuity of care and documents progress.

D. Research, statistics, and education.

Types of Charting

A. Computer-assisted.

B. Source-oriented.
1. Most common.
2. Organized by sources of information.
3. Types of forms.
   a. Order sheets.
   b. X-ray reports.
   c. Graphs—vital signs.
   d. Flow sheets—intake and output.
   e. Narrative nurses' notes.
      (1) Objective, not interpretive.
      (2) Brief and concise.
      (3) Use of approved symbols and abbreviations.
      (4) Accurate spelling.
      (5) Prepared legibly in ink.
      (6) Signed with name and status.

C. SOAP charting (also called SOAPIER notes).
1. *Subjective:* patient's symptoms and own description of problem.
2. *Objective:* factual data, e.g., intake and output, vital signs, drainage, etc.
3. *Assessment:* your conclusions about the problem.
4. *Plan:* what you decide to do about the problem.
5. *Implementation:* your nursing interventions.
6. *Evaluation:* how the implementation worked.
7. *Revision:* how you plan to change the PCP if improvement is needed.
8. A separate SOAP note is needed for each problem. Do not combine problems.
9. It is not always necessary to include the I, E, and R portions of the note; always include the S, O, A, and P parts, even if the patient does not supply subjective statements.

Nursing Diagnosis

A. A statement of an actual health problem or a potential one.
1. Derived from the assessment phase of the nursing process.
2. Based on both objective and subjective data.
3. As data base is collected, deviations from normal health patterns are identified.

B. Specific problem identified is related to a nursing intervention—not a medical one.

C. There are three major categories.
1. Diagnosis or condition—either potential or actual.
2. Etiology to which condition is related.
3. Defining characteristics that support the etiology.
4. State: Impairment of: *related to*, followed by etiology, if known and the defining characteristics.

Patient Care Plans

A. The two accepted types are: individualized care plan and standard care plan.
1. Individualized care plans have mutually agreed-upon goals set by the patient, family, and health team members.
2. Specific directions are written to define how these goals can be achieved.
3. The usual care plan format contains a problem list, a health team action section, and expected outcomes with deadline dates.
4. Standard care plans provide a guide for patient care.
   a. Identify problem relating to all patients having a specific medical condition.
   b. Health team actions include routine preventive nursing interventions.

B. The information contained in the care plan must be specific.

C. Care plans become a permanent part of the patient's chart.
1. They must be written in ink
2. Resolved problems should be crossed out using a colored felt tip pen.

D. Care plans must be updated on a routine basis (generally every 24 to 48 hours or as the patient's condition changes).

The Nurse-Client Relationship

Definition: The nurse-client relationship is a therapeutic, professional relationship in which interaction occurs between two individuals—the vocational nurse, who possesses the skills, abilities, and resources to relieve another's discomfort; and the client, who is seeking assistance for alleviation of some existing problem.

Characteristics

A. Give the client the feeling of being accepted.
1. Accept the client as having value and worth as an individual.
2. Empathize (feel with the client) but do not sympathize or use platitudes.
3. Offer emotional involvement but maintain objectivity.
4. Protect and promote client's self-esteem.

B. Indicate desire to develop mutual trust.
1. Exhibit verbal and nonverbal behavior that is consistent and congruent.
2. Encourage reality orientation.
3. Interact at client's level of understanding.
4. Understand your own motives and needs.
5. Provide open and honest communication.
6. Communicate with the client using therapeutic communication techniques.

C. Provide a reality-oriented supportive environment.
1. Focus on the total client so as to include all physical needs.
2. Set appropriate behavioral limits.
3. Assist client to identify and cope with feelings.
4. Encourage expression of feelings within a safe limit.
5. Recognize signs of a high anxiety level and seek appropriate help.

Phases of the Relationship.

A. Initiating phase.
1. Identify problems.
2. Get to know each other.
3. Test each other's attitudes.
4. Identify expectations.
5. Plan for the conclusion at the beginning of the relationship.

B. Continuing phase.
1. Accept each other.
2. Use specific therapeutic problem-solving techniques.
3. Work actively on problems.
4. Assess and evaluate problem continually.
5. Encourage client to become more independent and to rely less on the nurse.

C. Terminating phase.
1. Evaluate the initial plan for conclusion.
2. Anticipate problems of termination.
    a. Excessive dependence of client on nurse, who must encourage independence.
    b. Client may have feelings of abandonment, rejection, and/or depression about termination.
    c. Discuss patient's feelings about termination.

Communication Techniques

Definition: Communication is the process of sending and receiving messages by means of symbols, words, signs, gestures, or other actions. It is a multi-level process consisting of the content or information of the message, as well as the part that defines the meaning of the message. Messages sent and received define the relationship between individuals.

Characteristics

A. An individual cannot *not* communicate.
B. Communication is a basic human need.
C. It is both verbal and nonverbal expression (also tone, pace, and manner of dress).

Effective Communication Techniques

Listen	The act of consciously receiving another person's message. Listen eagerly, actively, responsively, and seriously.
Acknowledge	Recognize the person without inserting your own values or judgments. Acknowledgment may be simple and with or without understanding. Example, in the response "I hear what you're saying," the person acknowledges a statement without agreeing with it. Acknowledgment may be verbal or nonverbal.
Give Feedback	The process of the receiver relaying to the sender the effect the message has had. Helps keep the sender on course or alter his course. Involves acknowledging, validating, clarifying, extending, and altering. *Nurse to client:* "You did that well."
Be Congruent (Mutual Fit)	Verbal and nonverbal messages coincide. Example, a client is crying, and the nurse says, "I want to help," and places her hand on the client's shoulder.
Clarify	Checking out or making clear either the intent or hidden meaning of message or determining if the message sent was the message received. *Nurse:* "You said that you felt warm. Would you like to open the window?"
Focus or Refocus	Pick up on central topic or cue given by the client. *Nurse:* "You were telling me how hard it was to talk to your mother."
Validate	The process of verifying the accuracy of the sender's message by paraphrasing thought. *Nurse:* "Yes, it is confusing with so many people around."
Reflect	Identify sender's message and return a message that expresses sender's implied feeling rather than overt idea (conveys acceptance and great understanding). *Nurse:* "You distrust your doctor?"
Ask Open-Ended Questions	Ask questions that cannot be answered "Yes" or "No" or "Maybe" and generally require an answer or several words in order to broaden conversational opportunities and help the patient to communicate. *Nurse:* "What kind of job would you like to do?"
Encourage Nonverbally	Use body language to indicate interest, understanding, support, caring, and/or listening to extract further information. *Nurse:* Nodding appropriately as client talks.
Restate	Echo last few words. This encourages client to elaborate thought. *Nurse:* "You hear voices."
Paraphrase	Reword. This enables sender to hear message meaning in another form. *Nurse:* "You mean you're unhappy."
Respond Neutrally	Show interest and involvement without indicating assent or dissent. *Nurse:* "Yes . . . ." "Uh hm . . . ."
Use Incomplete Sentences	Encourage client to continue. *Nurse:* "Then your life is . . . ."

Minimize Verbalization	Keep your own verbalization at a minimum, and let the patient lead the conversation. *Nurse:* "You feel . . . ?"
Initiate Broad Statements	Open the communication by allowing the patient freedom to talk and focus on himself. *Nurse:* "How have you been feeling?"

Blocks to Effective Communication

Make Assumptions	(Jumping to conclusions.) Suppose or guess meaning of sender's behavior when not validated by sender. The nurse finds the suicidal client smiling and joking, and tells the staff he's in a cheerful mood.
Give Advice	Tell the client what to do, give an opinion, or make a decision that implies sender cannot cope with own self-determination and that receiver will accept responsibility for sender. *Nurse:* "If I were you . . . ."
Change the Subject	Introduce new topics inappropriately, a pattern that may indicate anxiety. The client is crying and discussing her fear of surgery, when the nurse asks, "How many children do you have?"
Use Social Response	Focus attention on receiver of message rather than sender. *Nurse:* "This sunshine is good for my roses. I have a beautiful rose garden."
Invalidate Client	Ignore or deny another's presence, thoughts, or feelngs. *Client:* "Hi, how are you?" *Nurse:* "I can't talk now. I'm on my way to lunch."
Use False Reassurance	Use clichés, pat answers, cheery words, advice, and comforting statements as an attempt to reassure the client. Most of what is called "reassurance" is really false reassurance. *Nurse:* "It's going to be all right."
Overload Conversation	Speak rapidly, change subjects, and give receiver more information than can be absorbed at one time. *Nurse:* "What's your name? I see you're forty-eight years old and that you like sports. Where do you come from?"
Underload Conversation	Remain silent and unresponsive, fail to pick up cues, and fail to give feedback. *Client:* "What's your name?" *Nurse:* Smiles and walks away.
Use Incongruent Messages	Send verbal and nonverbal messages that contradict one another; two or more messages, sent via different levels, seriously *do* contradict one another. The contradiction may be between the content, verbal, nonverbal, and/or content (time, space). This contradiction is a *double message*. *Client:* "I like your dress." *Nurse:* Annoyed, frowns and looks disgusted.
Make Value Judgments	Give one's own opinion, moralize or imply one's own values by using words such as "nice," "good," "bad," "right," "wrong," "should," and "ought." *Nurse:* "I think he's a very good doctor."

D. Effective communication includes:
   1. Feedback.
   2. Appropriateness.
   3. Efficiency.
   4. Flexibility.
E. Communication skills are learned as the individual grows and develops.
F. The foundation of the individual's perception of self and the world is based on communicated messages received from significant others.
G. Factors that affect communication.
   1. The intrapersonal framework of the individual.
   2. The relationship between the participants.
   3. The purpose of the sender.
   4. The content.
   5. The context.
   6. The manner in which the message is sent.
   7. The effect on the receiver.

Interviewing Skills

A. Help the client feel comfortable so that there is no need to be defensive.
B. Use "I" messages, not "you" messages (e.g., "I feel angry," not "you make me angry").
C. Observe carefully and be alert to cues given by the client.
D. Participate in planning a goal- and direction-oriented approach.

Nursing Care

A. Encourage the client to verbalize his or her thoughts and feelings.
B. Assist the client to clarify or make clear what he or she is saying.
C. Focus on the client, not on yourself or others.
D. Help the client understand how he or she affects others.
E. Communicate at the client's level of understanding.
F. Use "how" questions rather than "why" questions.

G. Focus on the present "here and now" rather than on the past "there and then."
H. Help the client learn new ways of problem solving.
I. Give constructive feedback so that the client can self-correct unclear statements.
J. Use nonverbal communication to convey empathy, interest, and encouragement.
K. Send verbal messages that are congruent with your nonverbal messages.
L. Be honest in your answers or statements; say what you mean and mean what you say.
M. Use effective communication techniques (see page 27.)
N. Recognize blocks to effective communication (see page 28.)
O. Make a sustained effort to give and receive a message.

Pain Management

Characteristics

A. Classification of pain fibers.
   1. Class A—large myelinated (fast pain).
   2. Class B—smaller unmyelinated.
   3. Class C—unmyelinated (slow pain).
B. The experience of pain.
   1. Pain source—direct causative factor.
   2. Stimulation of pain receptor—mechanical, chemical, thermal, electrical, ischemic.
   3. Pain pathway.
      a. Sensory pathways through dorsal root, ending on second order neuron in posterior horn.
      b. Afferent fibers cross over to anterolateral pathway, ascend in lateral spinothalamic tract to thalamus.
      c. Fibers then travel to postcentral gyrus in parietal lobe.
C. Types of pain.
   1. Superficial—localized, shorter duration, sharp sensation.

2. Deep pain—long duration, diffuse, dull aching quality; associated autonomic responses, musculoskeletal tension, nausea.
    a. Visceral—internal organs.
    b. Somatic—neuromuscular, segmental distribution.
    c. Referred—area stimulated (deep) and area pain referred to (superficial) are innervated by nerve fibers arising from same segment of spinal cord.
    d. Secondary to skeletal muscle.
3. Central pain— autonomic reflex pain syndrome.
    a. Causalgia—lesion peripheral nerve.
    b. Phantom—after amputation.
    c. Central—lesion in CNS, affecting pain pathway.
4. Psychogenic—due to emotional factors without anatomic or physiological explanation.

D. Gate control theory.
1. Pain impulses can be modulated by a transmission blocking action within CNS.
2. Large diameter cutaneous pain fibers can be stimulated (rubbing, scratching) and may inhibit smaller diameter excitatory fibers and prevent transmission of that impulse.
3. Cerebral cortical mechanisms that influence perception and interpretation may also inhibit transmission.

E. Pain perception—thalamus/awareness and parietal/integration.

F. Pain interpretation—cerebral cortex; delayed response influenced by previous experiences, culture, existing physical/psychological state.

G. Reactions—psychic and/or physiologic.

Assessment

A. Assess type of pain.
1. Acute pain: short duration of a few seconds to six months.
2. Chronic pain: longer duration of six months to years.
3. Intractable pain: severe and constant and resistant to relief measures.

B. Assess location.
1. Ask patient to point to area of the body or verbalize.
2. Ask if pain is superficial or deep.
3. Ask if pain is diffuse or localized.
4. Ask if pain radiates and where it goes.

C. Assess quality.
1. Stabbing, knife-like.
2. Throbbing.
3. Cramping.
4. Vise-like, suffocating.
5. Searing, burning.
6. Other.

D. Assess intensity.
1. Ask patient to indicate intensity of pain on a scale of zero to ten, zero being no pain and ten being the most pain ever experienced.
2. Use this scale to assess relief of pain after intervention.

E. Assess onset and precipitating factors.
1. How movement affects pain.
2. If coughing affects pain.
3. Impact of emotion on pain, e.g., arguing with spouse or receiving disturbing news.

F. Assess aggravating factors.
1. How position affects pain.
2. Environmental stressors.
3. Fatigue.

G. Assess associated factors.
1. Nausea.
2. Vomiting.
3. Bradycardia/tachycardia.
4. Hypotension/hypertension.
5. Profuse perspiration.
6. Apprehension or anxiety.

H. Assess alleviating factors.
1. Position.
2. Elevation of inflamed extremity.
3. Techniques used at home for pain relief.

I. Assess patient's behavioral responses to pain.
1. Depression, withdrawal, or crying.
2. Stoicism or expressive.

Nursing Care

A. Assess pain before treating.

B. Give reassurance, reduce anxiety and fears.

C. Offer distraction.

D. Give comfort measures as ordered: positioning, rest, elevation, heat/cold applications; protect from painful stimuli.

E. Massage—but never massage calf due to danger of emboli.

F. Administer pain medication as ordered: monitor therapeutic, toxic dose, and side effects.
   1. Check physician's orders.
   2. Use a preventive approach to pain management. Give medication before pain becomes severe.
   3. Follow steps outlined in assessment to determine the nature, quality, and extent of pain.
   4. Start with p.o. medications. If ineffective or only mildly effective, give IM medications, or combine p.o. and IM medications.
   5. Evaluate result of pain medication. Was it effective? How long did the effect last? What was the extent of relief?
   6. Evaluate patient for possible side effects of the medication.
   7. Discuss with charge nurse the effects of medication and whether a change of prescription is needed.

G. Monitor alternative methods to control pain.
   1. Dorsal column stimulator: stimulation of electrodes at dorsal column of spinal cord by patient-controlled device to inhibit pain.
   2. Analgesics: alter perception, threshold, and reaction to pain.
   3. Anesthesia: block pain pathway.
   4. Local nerve block.
   5. Neurosurgical procedures: interrupt sensory pathways; usually also affect pressure and temperature pathways.
      a. Neurectomy: interrupt cranial or peripheral nerves.
      b. Sympathectomy: interrupt afferent pathways (ganglia).

H. Nurse's role in pain relief.
   1. Prevent pain from retarding recovery.
   2. Prevent pain from causing nausea and vomiting which could result in fluid and electrolyte imbalance.
   3. Prevent pain from causing undue fatigue.
   4. Prevent pain from inhibiting moving, ambulating, turning and coughing, and thereby increasing possibilities of secondary problems from inactivity (pneumonia, emboli).
   5. Relieve pain or prevent pain from escalating by relaxing muscles (muscle tension increases with pain).
   6. Decrease anxiety that present and future pain relief will not be achieved.
   7. Bring pain relief to a level acceptable to the patient.

Disease Process

Definition: A definite morbid process that affects the body or any of its parts. Symptoms accompany the process; the etiology, course, extent, and prognosis vary.

Etiology
A. Mechanical.
   1. Trauma—accidental injury.
   2. Extremes of heat or cold.
   3. Radioactive elements.
   4. Obstruction of normal body passage.
B. Chemical agents.
   1. Caustic substances.
   2. Drugs.
   3. Insect bites.
   4. GI secretions, or blood that is not in GI tract or in vascular system, etc.
   5. Hormones/electrolytes.
C. Genetic/hereditary factors.
D. Infectious agents.

1. Bacteria.
   a. Cocci—round.
   b. Bacilli—rod-shaped.
   c. Spirochetes—spiral.
2. Virus—very small, must grow on living cells.
3. Rickettsias—small, round or rod-shaped microorganisms, transmitted by bites of fleas, lice, ticks.
4. Fungi—yeasts or molds that thrive in a warm, moist place and feed on living plants or animals and decaying organic material.
5. Protozoa—one-celled microscopic organism that belongs to the animal family.

Inflammation

A. Normal body response/homeostatic mechanism.
B. Common local signs/symptoms.
   1. Heat.
   2. Redness.
   3. Swelling.
   4. Pain.
   5. Loss of motion.

Immunity

A. The body's ability to resist infectious disease.
B. Types.
   1. Natural immunity—"born with"; inborn body characteristic.
   2. Acquired or adaptive immunity.
      a. Develops after exposure to infectious disease or to some form of a particular pathogen or its toxins.
      b. Active—attack of the disease, vaccination, injection of toxoids.
      c. Passive—receive antibodies or antitoxins from mother to unborn fetus or injections of immune serum, gamma globulin, antivenin.
C. Antigens.
   1. Substance that causes an immune response.
   2. Examples: pathogen, toxin, foreign protein.
D. Antibodies—substance that protects the body from antigen.

Fluid and Electrolytes

Fluid Composition of the Body

Body Water

Definition: Total body water represents the largest constituent (45 to 80 percent) of total body weight, depending on the amount of fat present.
A. Intracellular—represents three-fourths of total body water fluid; contained inside the cell; includes the red blood cells.
B. Extracellular—represents one-fourth of total body water; includes remaining fluid not contained within the cell.
   1. Intravascular (plasma)—liquid in which the blood cells are suspended.
   2. Interstitial—liquid surrounding tissue cells.

Electrolytes

Definition: Electrolytes are compounds that dissolve in a solution to form ions. Each ion carries either a positive or negative electrical charge.
A. Types.
   1. Cations—positive charge (Na^+, K^+, Ca^{++}, Mg^{++}).
   2. Anions—negative charge (Cl^-, HCO_3^-, HPO_4^-, SO_4^-).
   3. Equal number of cations and anions (154 each).
B. Concentration in solution is expressed in mEq/L. Total number of cations (mEq) plus total number of anions (mEq) will be the same in both the intracellular fluid and extracellular fluid, thereby rendering the body's fluid composition electrically neutral.
C. Compartment composition.
   1. Extracellular—large quantities of sodium, chloride, and bicarbonate ions.
   2. Intracellular—large quantities of potassium, phosphate, and proteins.

Table A. Major Electrolytes

Cations+		Anions-	
Na^+	Sodium	Cl^-	Chloride
K^+	Potassium	HCO_3^-	Bicarbonate
Ca^{++}	Calcium	HPO_4^{--}	Phosphate
Mg^{++}	Magnesium		

Dynamics of Intercompartmental Fluid Transfer

A. Osmosis—the movement of water molecules across a semipermeable membrane in a direction that equalizes the concentration of water. The flow of water is into a solution that has a high solute concentration.

B. Diffusion—movement of a substance from an area of high concentration to an area of low concentration.

C. Active transport—transport of substances across a membrane from an area of low concentration to an area of high concentration.

D. Filtration—passage of fluids through a semipermeable membrane as a result of a difference in hydrostatic pressures (pressure exerted by a fluid within a closed system).

Balance of Body Fluid

A. Intake.

 1. Ingestion of foodstuff and water.

 2. Oxidation of foodstuff.

B. Output.

 1. Skin and lungs.

  a. Water is lost through vaporization from the skin surface and through expired air from the lungs.

  b. The amount lost increases as metabolism increases.

 2. Gastrointestinal tract.

  a. Routes include saliva, gastric secretions, bile, pancreatic juices, and intestinal mucosa.

  b. A volume in excess of seven liters is transferred from the extracellular fluid (ECF) into the gastrointestinal tract, only to be reabsorbed, excepting some 200 ml which is passed with feces.

 3. Kidneys.

  a. Carry the heaviest load.

  b. Through glomerular filtration and tubular reabsorption, the kidneys maintain homeostatis.

Fluid Imbalance

Dehydration

A. Loss of skin turgor (after being pinched and lightly pulled upward, skin very slowly returns to normal).

B. Thirst.

C. Skin dry and warm.

D. Febrile (usually means there is fluid loss through perspiration).

E. Cracked lips.

F. Decreased urinary output (normal output is 30 cc/hr).

G. Concentrated urine—dark amber color and odorous.

H. Weight loss.

I. Low central venous pressure (CVP).

Circulatory Overload

A. Headache.

B. Flushed skin.

C. Tachycardia.

D. Venous distention, particularly neck veins.

E. Increased blood pressure and CVP.

F. Tachypnea (an increase in respiratory rate), coughing, dyspnea (shortness of breath), cyanosis, and pulmonary edema.

Electrolyte Imbalance

Potassium Imbalance

Definition: Normal serum or plasma level is 3.5 to 5.5 mEq/L. Deficiency or excess of potassium in the blood varies from these levels.

Hyperkalemia (Potassium Excess)

A. Signs and symptoms.
1. Weakness, flaccid paralysis.
2. Hyperreflexia proceeding to paralysis.
3. Bradycardia.
4. Ventricular fibrillation.
5. ECG changes.
6. Nausea.
7. Dizziness.
8. Oliguria.
9. Apprehension.
10. Cardiac arrest.
B. Causes of excess potassium levels.
1. Usually renal disease (cannot excrete potassium).
2. Burns (due to cellular destruction releasing potassium).
3. Crushing injuries (due to cellular breakage releasing potassium from cells).
4. Adrenal insufficiency.
5. Respiratory or metabolic acidosis.
C. Treatment of hyperkalemia.
1. Decrease potassium intake.
2. IV infusion of sodium chloride, providing kidney function is normal.
3. Kayexalate enemas.
4. Dialysis.
5. Observe ECG tracings.
6. Measure intake and output.

Hypokalemia (Potassium Deficiency)

A. Signs and symptoms.
1. Muscle weakness, muscle pain, hyporeflexia.
2. Hypotension.
3. Arrhythmias—PVC's particularly.
4. Anorexia advancing to nausea, vomiting.
5. Apathy, drowsiness leading to coma.
6. ECG changes.
7. Fatigue.
8. Weak pulse.
9. Shortness of breath.
10. Shallow respirations.
B. Causes of hypokalemia.
1. Renal loss most common (usually caused by use of diuretics).
2. Insufficient potassium intake.
3. Loss from vomiting and diarrhea or from gastrointestinal tract via NG tube placement without replacement of electrolyte solution.
C. Treatment of hypokalemia—replacement of potassium, orally or parenterally.

Sodium Imbalance

Definition: Normal serum or plasma level is 135 to 145 mEq/L. Deficiency or excess of sodium varies from these levels.

Hypernatremia (Sodium Excess)

A. Signs and symptoms.
1. The same as for extracellular fluid excesses.
   a. Pitting edema.
   b. Excessive weight gain.
   c. Increased blood pressure.
   d. Dyspnea.
2. If hypernatremia is due to dehydration, in which there is a loss of fluid thereby increasing the number of ions, the signs and symptoms include:
   a. Concentrated urine and oliguria.
   b. Dry mucous membranes.
   c. Thirst.
   d. Flushed skin.
   e. Increased temperature.
   f. Tachycardia.
B. Causes of hypernatremia.
1. Usually from administration of excessive amount of sodium chloride.
2. Dehydration from excessive loss of fluids.

C. Nursing care.
   1. Record intake and output.
   2. Restrict sodium in diet.
   3. Weigh daily.
   4. Observe vital signs.

Hyponatremia (Sodium Deficiency)

A. Signs and symptoms.
   1. The same as those for extracellular fluid deficiency.
      a. Weakness.
      b. Restlessness.
      c. Delirium.
      d. Hyperpnea.
      e. Oliguria.
      f. Increased temperature.
      g. Flushed skin.
      h. Abdominal cramps.
      i. Convulsions.
   2. If sodium is lost but fluid is not, the following signs and symptoms will be present (similar to those of water excess).
      a. Mental confusion.
      b. Headache.
      c. Muscle twitching and weakness.
      d. Coma.
      e. Convulsions.
      f. Oliguria.
B. Causes of hyponatremia.
   1. Excessive perspiration.
   2. Use of diuretics.
   3. Gastrointestinal losses.
   4. Lack of sodium in diet.
   5. Renal disease.
   6. Burns.
C. Nursing care.
   1. Monitor IV fluids with sodium.
   2. Maintain accurate intake and output.

Calcium Imbalance

Definition: Normal serum level is 4.5 to 6.0 mEq/L. Imbalances vary from these levels. 99 percent of all calcium is found in bones and teeth.

Hypocalcemia (Calcium Deficiency)

A. Signs and symptoms.
   1. Abdominal cramps, muscle cramps.
   2. Tetany, carpopedal spasms.
   3. Circumoral tingling, tingling in fingers.
   4. Convulsions.
B. Causes of hypocalcemia.
   1. Acute pancreatitis.
   2. Burns.
   3. Removal of parathyroid glands.
C. Treatment—reestablish normal plasma level and/or treat underlying cause.

Hypercalcemia (Calcium Excess)

A. Signs and symptoms.
   1. Anorexia, nausea.
   2. Lethargy.
   3. Weight loss.
   4. Polydipsia, polyuria.
   5. Flank pain, bone pain.
   6. Decreased muscle tone.
B. Causes of hypercalcemia.
   1. Excessive intake of vitamin D (milk).
   2. Hyperparathyroidism, neoplasm of parathyroids.
   3. Thyrotoxicosis.
   4. Immobilization.
   5. Paget's disease.
C. Treatment—treat the underlying cause and/or reestablish normal plasma level of calcium.

☆ Intravenous Regulation

A. Calculation of drip factor.
   1. Microdrop—60 gtt/cc fluid.
   2. Adult drop factor usually depends on administration set 10–20 gtt/cc fluid.
B. General formula.

$$\frac{\text{Drops/}}{\text{min}} = \frac{\text{Total volume infused} \times \text{drops/cc}}{\text{Total time for infusing in minutes}}$$

Example: Ordered 1000 cc D$_5$W administered over 8-hour period of time.

1. With microdrip, it is easy to remember that the number of drops per minute equals the number of cc's or ml's to be administered per hour.

Example $\dfrac{1000}{8} = 12.5$ cc/hour

Using formula:

$(8 \times 60)\dfrac{1000 \times 60}{480} = \dfrac{60,000}{480} = \dfrac{12.5}{\text{gtt/min}}$

2. With administration set that delivers 10 gtt/min.

$\dfrac{1000 \times 10}{480} = \dfrac{10,000}{480} = 20.8 \text{ or } 21 \text{ gtt/min}$

3. With administration set that delivers 15 gtt/min.

$\dfrac{1000 \times 15}{480} = \dfrac{15,000}{480} = 31 \text{ gtt/min}$

C. Nursing care with IV therapy.
   1. Before infusion, ensure patient is in comfortable position.
   2. Carefully check label against physician's orders.
   3. Check circulation of immobilized extremity.
   4. Frequently check rate of infusion.
   5. Observe for signs of swelling at infusion site.
   6. Take vital signs at least every fifteen minutes for replacement fluid administration.

Acid-Base Balance

Normal Acid-Base Balance

Principles

A. Acid-base balance is the ratio of acids and bases in the body that are necessary to maintain a chemical balance conducive to life.
B. Acid-base ratio is 20 base to 1 acid.

C. Acid-base balance is measured by arterial blood samples and recorded as blood pH. Range is 7.35 to 7.45.
D. Acids are hydrogen ion donors. They release hydrogen ions to neutralize or decrease the strength of the base.
E. Bases are hydrogen ion acceptors. They accept hydrogen ions to convert strong acids to weak acids (for example, hydrochloric acid is converted to carbonic acid.)

Regulatory Mechanisms

A. The body controls the pH balance by use of:
   1. Chemical buffers.
   2. Lungs.
   3. Cells.
   4. Kidneys.
B. The chemical buffer system works fastest, but other regulatory mechanisms provide more reliable protection against acid-base imbalance. The three primary buffer systems are:
   1. Bicarbonate—maintains blood pH at 7.4 with ratio of 20 parts bicarbonate to 1 part carbonic acid.
   2. Plasma proteins—vary the amounts of hydrogen ions in the chemical structure of the protein (along with liver). They can both attract and release hydrogen ions.
   3. Hemoglobin—maintains balance by chloride shift. Chloride shifts in and out of red blood cells according to the level of oxygen in blood plasma. Each chloride ion that leaves the cell is replaced by a bicarbonate ion.
C. Lungs.
   1. Next to react are the lungs.
   2. It takes ten to thirty minutes for lungs to inactivate hydrogen molecules by converting them to water molecules.
   3. Lungs can only inactivate the hydrogen ions carried by carbonic acid. The other ions must be excreted by the kidneys.
D. Cells.
   1. Cells absorb or release extra hydrogen ions.
   2. Cells react in two to four hours.

E. Kidneys.
    1. Kidneys are the mainstay of regulatory mechanisms.
    2. Excretion of excessive acid or base is slow. Compensation takes a few hours to several days, but it is more effective.
    3. Primary function of kidneys is bicarbonate regulation. Kidneys restore bicarbonate by releasing hydrogen ions and holding bicarbonate ions.

Acid-Base Imbalances

Metabolic Acidosis

Definition: Metabolic acidosis occurs when there is a deficit of bases or an accumulation of fixed acids.

A. Changes in pH and serum carbon dioxide.
    1. The pH will become acidic (fall below 7.35).
    2. The serum CO_2 level will be below 22 mEq/L (normal range of CO_2 is 26–28 mEq/L).
B. Compensatory mechanisms.
    1. When compensating for metabolic acidosis, the one clinical manifestation usually observed is the "blowing off" of excessive acids. This is manifested by a respiratory rate increase.
    2. The lungs are the fastest mechanism used to compensate for metabolic acidosis.
C. Causes of metabolic acidosis (seen particularly in the surgical patient).
    1. Diabetes—diabetic ketoacidosis.
    2. Renal insufficiency—kidneys retain the products of protein metabolism, thereby decreasing the bicarbonate that is available to maintain an acid-base balance.
    3. Diarrhea—excessive amounts of base are lost from the intestines and pancreas, resulting in acidosis.
D. Signs and symptoms.
    1. Headache.
    2. Drowsiness.
    3. Nausea, vomiting, diarrhea.
    4. Stupor, coma.
    5. Twitching, convulsions.
    6. Kussmaul's respiration (increased respiratory rate).
    7. Fruity breath (as evidenced in diabetic ketoacidosis as a result of improper fat metabolism).
E. Treatment and nursing care.
    1. These drugs may be given intravenously:
        a. Sodium bicarbonate.
        b. Sodium lactate.
        c. Insulin (in ketoacidosis).
    2. Watch laboratory values closely while treating metabolic acidosis.
    3. Watch for signs of hyperkalemia and dehydration in the patient (oliguria, vital sign changes, etc.).
    4. Record intake and output.

Metabolic Alkalosis

Definition: Metabolic alkalosis is a malfunction of metabolism that causes an increase in blood base or a reduction of available acids in the serum.

A. Changes in pH and serum carbon dioxide.
    1. The pH will become more alkaline (above 7.45).
    2. The CO_2 will increase above 35 mEq/L. Note that this measures the amount of circulating bicarbonate or the base portion of the plasma. (A good way to remember these acid-base values is to recall that as the pH increases, so does the CO_2. The reverse is true for acidosis.)
B. Compensatory mechanisms.
    1. The lungs will attempt to hold on to the carbonic acid in an effort to neutralize the base state.
    2. As a result, the rate of respiration will decrease.
C. Causes of metabolic alkalosis.
    1. Ingestion of excessive soda bicarbonate (used by individuals for acid indigestion).
    2. Excessive vomiting, which results in the loss of hydrochloric acid and potassium.
    3. Placement of NG tube which causes a depletion of both hydrochloric acid and potassium.

4. Use of potent diuretics, particularly by cardiac patients. Not only potassium but also hydrogen and chloride ions are lost, causing an increase in the bicarbonate level of the serum.

D. Signs and symptoms.
1. Nausea, vomiting.
2. Diarrhea.
3. Irritability, agitation.
4. Coma, convulsions.
5. Restlessness.
6. Twitching of extremities.
7. ECG changes.

E. Treatment and nursing care.
1. Maintain diet of foods high in potassium and chloride (bananas, apricots, dried peaches, Brazil nuts, dried figs, oranges).
2. Monitor IV solution of added electrolytes.
3. Give Diamox to promote kidney excretion of bicarbonate.
4. Administer potassium chloride maintenance doses to patients on long-term diuretics.
5. Give ammonium chloride to increase the amount of available hydrogen ions, thereby increasing the availability of acids in the blood.
6. Check laboratory values frequently to watch for electrolyte imbalance.
7. Watch patient for physical signs indicative of hypokalemia or metabolic alkalosis.
8. Keep accurate records of intake and output and vital signs.

Respiratory Acidosis

Definition: Respiratory acidosis refers to increased carbonic acid concentration (accumulated CO_2 which has combined with water) caused by retention of carbon dioxide through hypoventilation. Differs from metabolic acidosis in that it is caused by defective functioning of the lungs.

A. Changes in pH, pCO_2, and pO_2.
1. With an increased acidic state, the pH will fall below 7.35.
2. The pCO_2 will be increased above 50 mm Hg.
3. The pO_2 will be normal (90–100 mm Hg) or it can be decreased as hypoxia increases.
4. The HCO_3 will be normal if respiratory acidosis is uncompensated.

B. Compensatory mechanisms.
1. Because the basic problem in respiratory acidosis is a defect in the lungs, the kidneys must be the major compensatory mechanism.
   a. The kidneys work much slower than the lungs.
   b. As a result, compensation may take from hours to days.
2. The kidneys will retain and return bicarbonate to the extracellular fluid compartment.

C. Causes of respiratory acidosis.
1. Sedatives.
2. Over-sedation with narcotics in postoperative period.
3. A chronic pulmonary disorder, such as emphysema, asthma, bronchitis or pneumonia, leading to
   a. Inability of the lungs to expand and contract adequately.
   b. Difficulty in the expiratory phase of respiration, which causes retention of carbon dioxide.
4. Poor gaseous exchange during surgery.

D. Signs and symptoms.
1. Dyspnea after exertion.
2. Hyperventilation when at rest.
3. Cyanosis.
4. Sensorium changes (drowsiness leading to coma).
5. Carbon dioxide narcosis.
   a. When body has adjusted to higher carbon dioxide levels, the respiratory center loses its sensitivity to elevated carbon dioxide.
   b. Medulla fails to respond to high levels of carbon dioxide.
   c. Patient is forced to depend on anoxia for respiratory stimulus.

    d. If a high level of oxygen is administered, patient will cease breathing.

E. Treatment and nursing care.
1. Turn, cough, and hyperventilate patients at least every two to four hours postoperatively. Use oralpharyngeal suction if necessary.
2. When pulmonary complications present a threat, do postural drainage, percussion, and vibration, followed by suctioning.
3. Keep patient well hydrated to facilitate removal of secretions. If patient is dehydrated, secretions become thick and more difficult to expectorate.
4. Watch vital signs carefully, particularly rate and depth of respirations.
5. Teach pursed-lip breathing to chronic respiratory patients.
6. If oxygen is administered, watch carefully for signs of carbon dioxide narcosis.
7. Place patient on mechanical ventilation if necessary.
8. Administer aerosol medications through IPPB.
    a. Bronchodilators (aminophylline)—relieve bronchospams.
    b. Detergents (tergemist)—liquefy tenacious mucus.
    c. Antibiotics specific to causative agent.
9. Drugs that may be given intravenously:
    a. Sodium bicarbonate.
    b. Sodium lactate.
    c. Ringer's lactate—to replace electrolyte loss.

Respiratory Alkalosis

Definition: Respiratory alkalosis occurs when an excessive amount of carbon dioxide is exhaled, usually caused by hyperventilation. The loss of carbon dioxide results in a decrease in H^+ concentration along with a decrease in pCO_2 and an increase in the ratio of bicarbonate to carbonic acid. The result is an increase in the pH level.

A. Changes in pH, pCO_2, and pO_2.

1. With an increased alkalotic state, the pH will increase above 7.45, indicating there is a decreased amount of carbonic acid in the serum.
2. The pCO_2 will be normal-to-low, as this measures the acid portion of the acid-base system (30 to 45 mm Hg).
3. The pO_2 should be unchanged.
4. The bicarbonate level (HCO_3 or CO_2 content) should be normal unless the patient is compensating.

B. Compensatory mechanisms.
1. Since the basic problem is related to the respiratory system, the kidneys will compensate by excreting more bicarbonate ions and retaining H^+.
2. This process will return the acid-base balance to a normal ratio.

C. Causes of respiratory alkalosis.
1. Hysteria—patient hyperventilates and exhales excessive amounts of carbon dioxide.
2. Hypoxia—stimulates patient to breathe more vigorously.
3. Following head injuries or intracranial surgery.
4. Increased temperature.
5. Salicylate poisoning.
    a. Stimulation of respiration causes alkalosis through hyperventilation.
    b. Acidosis may occur from excessive salicylates in the blood.

D. Signs and symptoms.
1. Hyperreflexia.
2. Muscular twitching.
3. Convulsions.
4. Gasping for breath.

E. Treatment and nursing care.
1. Eliminate cause of hyperventilation.
2. Remain with patient and be supportive to reduce anxiety.
3. Use rebreathing bag to return patient's carbon dioxide to self (paper bag works just as well).

Blood and Blood Factors

Blood Grouping

Major Blood Groups

A. ABO blood group.
  1. A.
  2. AB.
  3. B.
  4. O.
B. Rh blood group.
  1. Positive (85 percent of the population).
  2. Negative (15 percent of the population).

Antigens and Antibodies

A. Blood type based on type of antigens present in red blood cells as well as type of antibodies in the serum.
B. A and B antigens.
  1. Persons with type A blood have antigen A present; persons with type B blood have antigen B present.
  2. Persons with type AB blood have both A and B antigens present.
  3. Persons with type O blood have no antigens present.
C. Anti-A and Anti-B antibodies.
  1. Antibodies develop as a response to exposure. Persons with type A blood have anti-B antibodies. They do not have anti-A antibodies because the blood cells would be destroyed by agglutination.
  2. Persons with type B blood have anti-A antibodies.
  3. Persons with type AB blood have no antibodies.
    a. Considered *universal recipients*.
    b. Cannot destroy donor's red blood cells.
  4. Persons with type O blood have both anti-A and anti-B antibodies.
    a. Considered *universal donors*.
    b. Red blood cells do not contain antigens that could be destroyed by antibodies in recipients' blood.

☆ Transfusion Administration

Procedure

A. Check carefully for correct name and ID number. Double check blood group donor number (have two persons check information).
B. Do not warm blood, as bacteria thrives in this medium.
C. Do not allow blood to be unrefrigerated for more than 30 minutes before administration.
D. Use blood filter to prevent fibrin and other materials from entering the bloodstream.
E. Transfusion will be started with normal saline or another electrolyte solution; blood will agglutinate without the presence of electrolytes.

Table B. Summary of ABO Blood Grouping

Blood Type	Antigen in RBC's	Antibodies in Plasma	Incompatible Donor Blood	Compatible Blood Donor
A	A	Anti-B	AB and B	A and O
B	B	Anti-A	A and AB	B and O
AB	A and B	None	None	All blood groups
O	None	Anti-A and Anti-B	All blood groups	None

Nursing Care

A. Transfusion usually started at 20 to 40 drops per minute. Closely observe transfusion as reaction usually occur during the first fifteen minutes.

B. Take base line vital signs at beginning and five minutes after beginning transfusion.

C. Transfusion is usually completed in no less than two hours and in no more than five hours.

   1. Usually administered at a rate of 60 to 80 drops per minute.

   2. If patient is hypovolemic, blood can be administered at the rate of 500 cc in ten minutes by use of a blood pump. Observe for pulmonary edema and hypervolemia.

Transfusion Reactions

A. Hemolytic or incompatibility reaction.

   1. Most severe complication.

   2. Caused by mismatched blood.

   3. Clinical manifestations.

     a. Increased temperature.

     b. Decreased blood pressure.

     c. Pain across the chest and at the site of needle insertion.

     d. Chills.

     e. Hematuria.

     f. Backache in the kidney region.

     g. Dyspnea and cyanosis.

     h. Jaundice can occur in severe cases.

   4. The reaction is caused by agglutination of the donor's red cells.

     a. The antibodies in the recipient's plasma react with the antigens in the donor's red cells.

     b. The clumping blocks off capillaries and therefore obstructs the flow of blood and oxygen to cells.

   5. Nursing care.

     a. Stop transfusion immediately upon appearance of symptoms.

     b. Return remaining blood and the patient's blood sample to the laboratory for type and cross match.

     c. Keep IV patent after changing blood tubing with either normal saline or preferably D_5W.

     d. Take vital signs every fifteen minutes.

     e. Insert Foley catheter for a urine sample for red blood cells and an accurate output record.

     f. Check for oliguria.

     g. Administer medications such as vasopressors if indicated.

     h. Administer oxygen as necessary.

B. Bacterial contamination.

   1. Check blood for discoloration, cloudiness, and bubbles, which are indicative of contamination.

   2. Signs and symptoms.

     a. Sudden increase in temperature.

     b. Sudden chill.

     c. Headache.

     d. Peripheral vasodilation.

     e. Malaise.

     f. Lumbar pain.

   3. Nursing care.

     a. Do not use blood that is cloudy or discolored or appears to have bubbles present.

     b. If transfusion has been started, discontinue immediately.

     c. Send remaining blood to laboratory for culture and sensitivity. If transfusion has been started, send patient's blood sample as well.

     d. Change IV tubing and keep it patent.

     e. Check vital signs, including temperature, every fifteen minutes.

     f. Insert Foley catheter for accurate output and urine specimen as ordered.

     g. Control hyperthermia, if present, with antipyretics, cooling blankets, or with sponge baths.

C. Allergic reactions.

   1. Allergic response to any type of allergen in the donor's blood.

   2. Common reaction, usually mild in nature.

   3. Signs and symptoms.

     a. Hives.

     b. Urticaria.

     c. Wheezing.

     d. Laryngeal edema.

4. Nursing care.
   a. Administer an antihistamine such as Benadryl to control itching and to relieve edema.
   b. If reaction is severe, discontinue the transfusion; otherwise, decrease the flow rate.

Common Procedures

General Principles

Nursing Actions Prior to Procedures

A. Most procedures require a physician's order.
B. Review written procedure in your hospital's/agency's procedure book; seek help from team leader/head nurse if you do not know method.
C. Explain all procedures to patient; ask patient's cooperation.
D. Wash hands before beginning procedure and maintain medical or surgical asepsis.
E. Provide privacy for patient.

Restraints

A. Uses.
   1. Immobilize a part.
   2. Provide support to a part.
   3. Prevent patient from injuring self or another.
   4. Promote safety while sitting in chair or in bed.
☆B. Procedure.
   1. Check for physician's order.
   2. Explain purpose of restraint to patient and his/her family.
   3. Apply restraint.
   4. Check circulation of extremities distal to restraint.
   5. Chart application and reason.
   6. Intervene every two hours.
      a. Remove restraint.
      b. Observe condition of skin.

c. Check circulation.
d. Reapply restraint.

Infection Control

A. Methods of microorganism transmission.
   1. Direct contact.
   2. Air, droplet.
   3. Fomite (toys, books, etc.).
   4. Food, water.
   5. Animals, insects.
B. Medical asepsis—"clean."
   1. Limits spread of microorganisms.
   2. Handwashing best single technique.
   3. First rinse washable articles in cold water to remove protein; then wash in hot, soapy water.
C. Surgical asepsis—"sterile."
   1. Absence of all forms of microorganisms, including spores.
   2. Method used in surgical procedures/operations.
D. Isolation technique.
   1. Used to confine pathogens (disease-producing microorganisms).
      a. General principles.
         (1) Floors are contaminated.
         (2) Keep doors closed.
         (3) Double bag all items to be removed from room.
         (4) Wash hands immediately after leaving room.
      b. Types of restriction.
         (1) Respiratory.
         (2) Wound and skin.
         (3) Enteric (GI tract).
         (4) Strict—prevents transmission by all methods.
   2. Protective or reverse barrier—used to keep potential pathogens from patient.
      a. Used for patients with increased susceptibility to disease.
      b. All equipment sterile when brought *into* room; no special care necessary to remove equipment from room.
      c. Staff wears "space suits."

☆ Catheterization

A. Procedure involves putting plastic or rubber tube/catheter in bladder via urethra in order to empty bladder or obtain specimen.

B. It is a sterile procedure—use surgical aseptic technique and avoid contaminating equipment.

C. Position for female patient.
1. Dorsal recumbent most common.
2. Sim's or lateral.

D. Make provisions for privacy.

E. Procedure protocol.
1. Screen, position, and drape patient.
2. Place catheter tray for convenience and open it.
3. Put on sterile gloves and arrange equipment.
4. Place sterile drapes.
5. Lubricate catheter.
6. Expose urinary meatus (this gloved hand now considered contaminated). Leave hand in position until procedure completed.
7. Cleanse urinary meatus with provided equipment.
8. Pick up lubricated catheter (do not contaminate it). Insert catheter into urethra until urine flows.
9. When urine stops flowing, pinch and withdraw catheter. (If more than 1000 cc obtained, some facilities suggest clamping catheter for 20 minutes before removing more urine to prevent bladder spasm).
10. Remove gloves.
11. Clean patient and position for comfort.
12. Clean all equipment or discard disposable equipment.
13. Chart time procedure done and amount and character of urine.

F. Retention or Foley catheter (R/C) is inserted in the same manner.
1. When in place, sterile water or sterile air is instilled into a balloon-like structure near the catheter tip. This "balloon" keeps the catheter in the bladder.
2. The catheter is usually attached to a drainage tube and bag.

☆ R/C or Bladder Irrigation

A. Surgical aseptic technique used.

B. Check amount and type of solution ordered.

C. Open method.
1. Cleanse catheter at connection with drainage tube and separate. Protect drainage tube from contamination.
2. Fill sterile irrigating syringe with sterile solution and gently put into catheter.
3. Remove syringe and allow solution to drain into emesis basin—do not contaminate end of catheter.
4. Repeat as necessary until ordered amount is used or desired returns are obtained.
5. Connect catheter to drainage tube.

D. Closed method—most common.
1. Place clamp on catheter immediately above drainage tube connector.
2. Place 22- or 24-gauge sterile needle on sterile syringe. Fill syringe with ordered sterile solution.
3. Cleanse catheter between side arm and clamp with an alcohol swab, and insert needle.
4. Gently inject solution. When ordered amount injected, withdraw needle and remove clamp.

E. Chart method used, amount and type of solution, description of returns, and patient's reaction.

Preoperative and Postoperative Care

Routine Preoperative Care

Psychological Support

A. Reinforce the physician's teaching regarding the surgical procedure.

B. Identify patient's anxieties; notify physician

of extreme anxiety.

C. Listen to patient's verbalization of fears.

D. Provide support to the patient's family (where family can wait during surgery, approximately how long surgery will take, etc.).

Preoperative Teaching

A. Postoperative exercises: leg, coughing, deep breathing, etc.

B. Equipment which will be used during postoperative period: intermittent positive pressure breathing machine (IPPB), NG tube to suction, etc.

C. Pain medication and when to ask for it.

D. Explaination of NPO.

Physical Care

A. Observation and recording of patient's overall condition.
   1. Nutritional status.
   2. Physical defects, such as loss of limb function, skin breakdown.
   3. Hearing or sight difficulties.

B. Chest x-ray, ECG, and blood and urine samples as ordered.

C. Preoperative history and present physical condition.

D. Determination of any drug allergies.

E. Skin prep and shave when necessary; shower with antibacterial soap if ordered.

F. Retention or indwelling catheter, NG tube, or enema if ordered.

G. Have patient void immediately before medicating.

H. Preoperative medications administered.

I. Following preoperative medication, quiet rest with siderails up and curtains drawn.

Nurse's Responsibility

A. Check and report abnormal lab values and vital signs.

B. Complete preoperative check list.
   1. Remove dentures, nail polish, hairpins, artificial eyes, contact lenses, glasses.

2. Give preoperative medicines.

C. Complete ordered preoperative nursing interventions.

D. See that consent form is signed.

E. Check ID band.

F. Perform or check skin prep/shave.

Anesthesia

Preoperative Medications

A. Purpose.
   1. Decrease secretions of the mouth and respiratory tract.
   2. Depress vagal reflexes.
   3. Produce drowsiness and relieve anxiety.
   4. Allow anesthesia to be induced more smoothly and in smaller amounts.

B. Types of drugs administered.
   1. Barbiturates.
      a. Intermediate-acting barbiturate at bedtime.
      b. Short-acting barbiturate one hour preoperatively.
   2. Belladonna alkaloids.
      a. Decrease salivary and bronchial secretions; allow inhalation anesthetics to be administered more easily and prevent postoperative complications.
      b. Scopolamine is used in conjunction with morphine or Demerol to produce amnesic block.
      c. Atropine blocks the vagus nerve response of decreased heart rate which can occur as a reaction to some inhalation anesthetics.
   3. Central nervous system depressants.

General Anesthesia

A. General anesthesia produces a depression of the CNS, amnesia, loss of reflexes, and unconsciousness.
   1. Inhalation agents.
      a. Halothane.
      b. Nitrous oxide.
      c. Cyclopropane.

d. Ethylene.
2. Intravenous anesthesia—thiopental (Pentothal).

B. Stages and planes of general anesthesia.
1. Stage one: early induction—from beginning of inhalation to loss of consciousness.
2. Stage two: delirium or excitement.
    a. No surgery is performed at this point—very dangerous stage.
    b. Breathing is irregular.
3. Stage three: surgical anesthesia.
    a. Begins when patient stops fighting and is breathing regularly.
    b. Four planes, based on respiration, pupillary and eyeball movement, and reflex muscular responses.
4. Stage four: medullary paralysis—respiratory arrest.

C. Anesthetic Agents.
1. Anesthesia produces insensitivity to pain or sensation.
2. Dangers associated with anesthesia depend on overall condition of patient.
    a. High risk if associated cardiovascular, renal, or respiratory conditions.
    b. High risk for unborn fetus and mother.
    c. High risk if stomach full (chance of vomiting and aspiration).
3. Types of anesthesia.
    a. General—administered IV or by inhalation. Produces loss of consciousness and decreases reflex movement.
    b. Local—applied topically or injected regionally. Patient is alert, but pain and sensation are decreased in surgical area.

Routine Postoperative Care

☆ Recovery Room

A. Immediate postoperative care.
1. Maintain patent airway.
2. Administer oxygen by mask or nasal cannula.

3. Check gag reflex.
4. Position patient for adequate ventilation.
5. Observe for adverse signs of general anesthesia or spinal anesthesia.
    a. Level of consciousness.
    b. Movement of limbs.
6. Monitor vital signs.
    a. Check every ten to fifteen minutes.
        (1) Pulse—check rate, quality, and rhythm.
        (2) Blood pressure—check pulse pressure and quality as well as systolic and diastolic pressure.
        (3) Respiration—check rate, rhythm, depth, and type of respiration (abdominal breathing, nasal flaring).
    b. Vital signs are sometimes difficult to obtain due to hypothermia.
    c. Movement from operating room table to guerney can alter vital signs significantly, especially with cardiovascular patients.
    d. Maintain temperature (operating room is usually cold)—apply warm blankets.
7. Check patency of IV; check IV insertion site.
8. Observe dressings and surgical drains.
    a. Mark any drainage on dressings, and note time by drawing a line around the drainage.
    b. Note color and amount of drainage on dressings and in drainage tubes.
    c. Ensure that dressing is secure.
    d. Reinforce dressings as needed.

B. Overall observations of condition.
1. Check skin for warmth, color, and moisture.
2. Check nailbeds and mucous membranes for color (report if cyanotic) and blanching.
3. Observe for return of reflexes.

C. Medications—begin routine drugs and administer all STAT drugs.

D. Assessment for return to room.
1. Be sure vital signs are stable and within normal limits.
2. See if patient is awake and reflexes are present (gag and cough reflex).

3. Take oral airway out (if not out already).

4. Check for movement and sensation in limbs (particularly legs, with spinal anesthesia).

5. Watch for cyanosis.

6. Be sure dressings are intact and there is no excessive drainage.

Surgical Floor

A. Assessment.
   1. Maintain patent airway; administer oxygen as necessary.
   2. Take vital signs—usual orders are VS q 15 minutes until stable; then q ½ hour x 2, q hour x 4; then q 4 hours for 24–48 hours.
   3. Check IV site and patency frequently.
   4. Observe and record urine output.
   5. Keep accurate records of intake and output.
B. Nursing care.
   1. Position patient for comfort and maximum airway ventilation.
   2. Turn q 2 hours and prn.
   3. Give back care at least every four hours.
   4. Encourage coughing and deep breathing every two hours (may use IPPB or blow bottles).
   5. Keep patient comfortable with medications.
   6. Check dressings and drainage tubes q 2–4 hours unless abnormal amount of drainage; then, more frequently.
   7. Give oral hygiene at least q 4 hours; q 2 hours if NG tube, nasal oxygen, or endotracheal tube inserted.
   8. Bathe patient when temperature can be maintained—bathing removes the antiseptic solution and stimulates circulation.
   9. Keep patient warm and avoid chilling, but do not increase temperature above normal.
      a. Increased temperature increases metabolic rate and need for oxygen.
      b. Excessive perspiration causes fluid and electrolyte loss.
   10. Irrigate NG tube q 2 hours and prn with normal saline to keep patent.
   11. Maintain dietary intake—type of diet depends on type and extent of surgical procedure.
      a. Minor surgical conditions—the patient may drink or eat as soon as he or she is awake and desires food or drink.
      b. Major surgical conditions.
         (1) NPO until bowel sounds return.
         (2) Clear liquid advanced to full liquid as tolerated.
         (3) Soft diet advanced to full diet within three to five days (depending on type of surgery and physician's preference).
   12. Place on bedpan two to four hours postoperatively if catheter not inserted.

Postoperative Medications

Narcotic Analgesics

A. Pharmacological action—reduces pain and restlessness.
B. General side effects.
   1. Drowsiness.
   2. Euphoria.
   3. Sleep.
   4. Respiratory depression.
   5. Nausea and vomiting.
C. Types of analgesics.
   1. Opiates.
      a. Morphine sulfate—potent analgesic.
         (1) Specific side effects: miosis (pinpoint pupils); bradycardia.
         (2) Usual dosage: 1/4 to 1/6 gr IM q 3–4 hours prn.
      b. Codeine sulfate—mild analgesic.
         (1) Specific side effects: constipation.
         (2) Usual dosage: 30 mg to 60 mg q 3–4 hours IM
   2. Synthetic opiate-like drugs.
      a. Demerol (meperidine)—potent analgesic.
         (1) Specific side effects: miosis or mydriasis (dilation of pupils); hypotension; tachycardia.

(2) Usual dosage: 25 mg to 100 mg q 3–4 hours IM.
b. Talwin (pentazocine)—potent analgesic.
　(1) Specific side effects: gastrointestinal disturbances, vertigo, headache, and euphoria.
　(2) Usual dosage: 50 mg oral tablets q 3–4 hours; 30 mg IM q 3–4 hours prn.

Antiemetics

A. Pharmacological action.
1. Reduces the hyperactive reflex of the stomach.
2. Makes the chemoreceptor trigger zone of medulla less sensitive to nerve impulses passing through this center to the vomiting center.
B. General side effects.
1. Drowsiness.
2. Dry mouth.
3. Nervous system effects.
C. Common drugs.
1. Phenothiazines.
　a. Compazine (prochlorperazine).
　　(1) Specific side effects: amenorrhea, hypotension, and vertigo.
　　(2) Normal dosage: 5–10 mg q 3–4 hours IM.
　b. Phenergan (promethazine).
　　(1) Specific side effects.
　　　(a) Dryness of mouth.
　　　(b) Blurred vision.
　　(2) Normal dosage: 12.5–50 mg q 4 hours prn.
2. Nonphenothiazines.
　a. Dramamine (dimenhydrinate).
　　(1) Specific side effects: drowsiness.
　　(2) Normal dosage: 50 mg IM q 3–4 hours.
　b. Tigan (trimethobenzamide).
　　(1) Specific side effects (rare).

　　　(a) Hypotension.
　　　(b) Skin rashes.
　　(2) Normal dosage: 200 mg (2 cc) tid or qid IM.

Common Postoperative Complications

Respiratory Complications

Prevention

A. Turn, cough, hyperventilate.
B. Mechanical interventions (provide a means of forced-expiration exercise).
1. Spirometers.
2. Blow bottles.
3. IPPB.
C. Pharmacological therapy (through nebulization or oral route).
1. Antibiotics—to fight infection by causative organism.
2. Bronchodilators—to act on smooth muscle to reduce bronchial spasm.
　a. Sympathomimetics (ephedrine sulfate, Isuprel, adrenalin).
　b. Theophylline (aminophylline).
3. Adrenocorticosteroids—to reduce inflammation (Prednisone).
4. Enzymes—to liquefy thick, purulent secretions through digestion.
　a. Dornavac.
　b. Varidase.
5. Expectorants—to aid in expectoration of secretions.
　a. Mucolytic agents reduce viscosity of secretion (Mucomyst).
　b. Detergents liquefy tenacious mucus (Tergemist, Alevaire).

General Signs and Symptoms

A. Complaint of tightness or fullness in chest.
B. Cough, dypsnea, or shortness of breath.

C. Increased vital signs, particularly temperature and respiratory rate.

D. Restlessness.

Common Respiratory Conditions

A. Pneumonia (see section on respiratory system.)

B. Atelectasis, collapse of pulmonary alveoli, caused by mucous plug or by inadequate ventilation.

C. Signs and symptoms.
   1. Asymmetrical chest movement.
   2. Decreased or absent breath sounds over affected area.
   3. Shortness of breath leading to cyanosis.
   4. Painful respirations.
   5. Increased vital signs: temperature, respiration, pulse.
   6. Anxiety and restlessness.

Nursing Care for Common Respiratory Conditions

A. Encourage coughing and deep breathing exercises; splint incision.

B. Turn frequently and position to facilitate expectoration.

C. Suction as necessary.

D. Instruct in proper use of mechanical measures (blow bottles, etc.).

E. Do clapping, percussion, vibration, postural drainage every four hours.

F. Encourage oral fluid intake to reduce tenacious sputum and to facilitate expectoration.

G. Administer expectorants and other medications as ordered.

H. Place patient in cool room with mist mask or vaporized steam.

I. Administer oxygen if necessary.

J. Mobilize patient as soon as possible.

K. Auscultate breath sounds every two to four hours and report unusual occurrences.

Thrombophlebitis

Definition: Thrombophlebitis is the formation of a clot in a vein. It occurs most often in the femoral vein.

Etiology

A. Dehydration leading to increased cellular components in vessel.

B. Decreased blood flow due to hypothermia and/or decreased metabolic rate during surgery.

C. Injury to vessel during surgery.

D. Incidence most common following abdominal or circulatory surgery.

Signs and Symptoms

A. Red, tender, painful calf.

B. Edema of affected leg.

C. Increased temperature in affected area as well as generalized elevation of temperature.

D. Positive Homan's sign.

Nursing Care

A. Maintain strict bed rest.

B. Do not use knee gatch or pillows under knees.

C. Elevate lower extremities slightly, if ordered; raise entire foot of bed.

D. Administer anticoagulants only after checking lab values.

E. Check for extension of clot.
   1. Check breath sounds for possible emboli.
   2. Check extremity involved for extension of signs (tenderness further up leg, etc.), especially in groin.
   3. Check for circulatory difficulties.

F. Position patient to avoid venous stasis, and turn every two hours.

G. Take vital signs at least every four hours.

H. Apply hot packs if ordered.

I. Use range-of-motion exercises on unaffected limbs only.

J. Do not massage or exercise affected leg unless specified by physician.

K. Apply antiembolic stockings to unaffected leg.
L. Begin exercise gradually with leg-raises to standing briefly every hour, then ambulation.

Patient Instruction

A. Avoid standing in one position for any length of time (when exercise program instituted, patients are told to either walk or to lie flat).
B. Avoid wearing constrictive clothing or garments.
C. Keep extremities at consistent, moderate temperature.
D. Wear support hose consistently.
E. Understand correct use of anticoagulants and the necessity for lab tests.

Wound Infections

Etiology

A. Usual causative agents.
   1. Staphylococcus.
   2. Pseudomonas aeruginosa.
   3. Proteus vulgaris.
   4. Escherichia coli.
B. Usually occur within five to seven days of surgery.

Signs and Symptoms

A. Slowly increasing temperature and tachycardia.
B. Pain and tenderness surrounding surgical site.
C. Edema and erythema surrounding suture site.
D. Increased warmth around suture site.
E. Purulent drainage.
   1. Yellow if staphylococcus.
   2. Green if Pseudomonas.

Nursing Care

A. Administer specific antibiotics for causative agent.
B. Irrigate wound with solution as ordered (usually hydrogen peroxide and normal saline).
C. Keep dressing and skin area dry to prevent skin excoriation and spread of bacteria.
D. Use sterile technique in changing dressings.
E. If excoriation occurs, use karaya powder and drainage bags around area of wound.

Wound Dehiscence and Evisceration

Definition: Dehiscence is the splitting open of wound edges. Evisceration is the extensive loss of pinkish fluid (purulent if infection is present) through a wound and the protrusion of a loop of bowel through an open wound. Patient feels as though "everything is pulling apart."

Etiology

A. Usual causes.
   1. General debilitation.
      a. Poor nutrition.
      b. Chronic illness.
      c. Obesity.
   2. Inadequate wound closure.
   3. Wound infection.
   4. Severe abdominal stretching (by coughing or vomiting).
B. Occurs about seventh postoperative day.

Nursing Care

A. Lay patient in supine position.
B. Cover protruding intestine with moist, sterile, normal saline packs; change packs frequently to keep moist.
C. Notify physician.
D. Take vital signs for baseline data and detection of shock.
E. Apply scultetus binder following dehiscence (preventative measure in obese or debilitated patients).

Shock

Definition: Shock is an abnormal physiological state in which there is insufficient circulating blood volume for the size of the vascular bed, thereby resulting in circulatory failure and tissue anoxia.

Classification of Shock

A. Hematogenic.
 1. Reduced circulating blood volume.
  a. Hemorrhage.
  b. Burns.
  c. Diabetes.
 2. Can be termed hypovolemic shock, referring to decreased fluid volume and other fluid losses from wounds or GI tract.
B. Neurogenic—decreased vasoconstriction leading to vasodilatation.
 1. Insulin shock.
 2. Spinal anesthesia.
C. Vasogenic (septic shock)—vasodilatation and loss of vasomotor stimulation caused by toxic substances (toxic or septic shock, such as gram negative sepsis).
D. Cardiogenic—cardiac pump failure.
 1. Congestive heart failure.
 2. Following left ventriculotomy.

Signs and Symptoms of Early Shock

A. Early stages, regardless of the cause.
 1. Decreased tissue perfusion.
 2. Cellular hypoxia.
 3. Increased sympathetic nervous system activity.
B. Oliguria—usually the first sign of shock.
 1. Decreased blood volume through kidneys.
 2. Decreased urine output; hyperkalemia can be a problem.
C. Hypotension.
 1. Due to compensatory peripheral vasoconstriction (not evident initially, but it does appear in early shock).
 2. Narrowing pulse pressure, due to systolic pressure falling and diastolic pressure being maintained.
D. Tachycardia—due to heart's responding to increased sympathetic activity.
E. Tachypnea.
 1. Medulla is stimulated by buildup in lactic acid through anaerobic metabolism.
 2. As blood pH is lowered, the respiratory rate increases in an effort to blow off excess carbon dioxide and return body to acid-base balance.
F. Cool, dry, or moist skin.
 1. Caused by peripheral vasoconstriction.
 2. Blood is supplied to vital organs rather than to skin.
G. Sensorium changes—due to brain cell hypoxia.
 1. Restlessness.
 2. Apprehension and anxiety.
 3. Lethargy.
 4. Confusion.
 5. Semiconsciousness to coma.
H. Excessive thirst—due to loss of fluids or blood volume as well as peripheral vasoconstriction which decreases salivary secretions.
I. Fatigue and muscle weakness—result of shift from aerobic to anaerobic metabolism leading to lactic acid buildup.

Signs and Symptoms of Severe Shock

A. Blood pressure below 70 mm Hg and narrowing of pulse pressure (body loses ability to compensate and blood pressure drops rapidly).
B. Respirations become shallow and irregular.
C. Tachycardia continues.
D. Unconsciousness to coma occurs as blood supply to brain cells is decreased.
E. Pupils become dilated and fixed, due to decreased oxygen to brain.
F. Anuria is present as blood supply to kidneys is sharply decreased.
G. Skin becomes cyanotic, along with mucous membranes and nailbeds.

Nursing Care

A. Monitor plasma expanders, IV fluids, or blood replacement.
B. Place patient in supine position with feet and/or head slightly elevated (Trendelenburg's position compromises venous return as well as respirations).
C. Insert Foley catheter for hourly urine volumes, if ordered.

1. Record intake and output.
2. Notify physician if urine output is below 30 cc/hour.

D. Take vital signs every fifteen minutes.

E. Place light covering over patient to prevent chilling, but not enough to cause vasodilatation.

F. Provide oxygen via nasal catheter, mask, or cannula.

G. Treat the cause of the shock (stop bleeding, prepare for surgery, etc.).

Pulmonary Embolism

Definition: A type of embolism usually caused by clot lodging in pulmonary artery.

Signs and Symptoms

A. Sudden sharp pain in chest.
B. Shortness of breath.
C. Cyanosis.
D. Increased pulse and respirations.
E. Hypotension—symptoms of shock.
F. Distended neck veins caused by congestive heart failure.
G. Decreased breath sounds.
H. Arrhythmias.
I. Anxiety.

Nursing Care

A. Provide patent airway.
   1. Position in semi- to high-Fowler's position if vital signs allow.
   2. Administer oxygen as needed.
   3. Assist with intubation as needed.
   4. Auscultate breath sounds every one to two hours.
   5. Obtain arterial blood gases to ascertain acid-base imbalance.
   6. Check sputum for presence of blood or blood-tinged mucus.
   7. May administer diuretics or cardiotonics.

B. Administer anticoagulants following initial anticoagulation (check lab values each day

before administering medication).

C. Take vital signs every two to four hours.

D. Turn as directed by physician; do not do percussion or clapping or administer back rubs.

E. Encourage patient to cough and deep breathe every one to two hours.

F. Give emotional support.

G. Observe for possible extension of emboli or occurrence of other emboli.
   1. Check urine for hematuria or oliguria.
   2. Check legs, especially calf.

Fat Embolism

Definition: A type of embolism caused by fat droplets released into the blood stream.

Etiology

A. Embolism occurs after long bone fractures (particularly from mishandling or incorrect splinting of fractures).

B. Fat droplets are released from the marrow and enter circulation. They usually lodge in the lungs. If they lodge in the brain the embolism is severe and sometimes fatal.

C. Fat emboli usually occur within the first twenty-four hours following an injury.

Signs and Symptoms

A. Classical sign: petechiae across chest, shoulders, and axilla; can also involve conjuctiva.

B. Related pulmonary signs: shortness of breath leading to pallor, cyanosis, and hypoxemia.

C. Diaphoresis.

D. Tachycardia without apparent cause.

E. Change in level of consciousness.

F. Shock.

Nursing Care

A. Position patient in high-Fowler's position to allow for respiratory exchange.

B. Administer oxygen to decrease anoxia and to reduce surface tension of fat globules.

C. Obtain arterial blood gases to maintain sufficient pO_2 levels.
D. Intubate and place on respirator if respirations are severely compromised.
E. Institute preventative treatment to avoid further complications such as shock and heart failure.
F. Monitor administration of medications.
   1. Alcohol drip.
   2. Cortisone therapy to reduce inflammation.
   3. Decholin to emulsify fat.
   4. Antihyperlipemic drugs.

Rehabilitative Nursing

Definition: The process of restoring a person's ability to live and work in as normal a manner as possible after a disabling injury.

General Principles

Goals

A. Strive for optimal function.
B. Prevent further injury or complications.
C. Restore normal function.
D. Accept philosophy underlying rehabilitative nursing.
   1. Rehabilitation begins with initial contact.
   2. Every illness has intrinsic threat of disability.
   3. Principles of rehabilitation are basic to care of all patients.

Effects of Disability

A. Impact upon the individual's body image.
   1. Physical appearance.
   2. Bodily sensations.
B. Behavior during reaction period.
   1. Appears confused and disorganized.
   2. Denies disability exists.
   3. Overreacts to situations and physical condition.
   4. Assumes false positive attitude.
   5. Becomes self-centered.
   6. Becomes depressed.
   7. Mourns loss of function or body part.
C. Adaptation and adjustment.
   1. Revises body image by modifying former picture of self.
   2. Reorganizes values.
   3. Accepts degree of dependency.
   4. Accepts limitations imposed by disability.
   5. Begins to develop realistic goals.

Duties of the Rehabilitative Nurse

General Duties

A. Assist in developing nursing care plan to meet patient's needs.
B. Provide direct nursing care.
C. Establish supportive relationship.
D. Teach activities of daily living.
   1. Activities which must be accomplished each day in order for the individual to care for his or her own needs.
   2. Assist in patient evaluation.
      a. Medical condition.
      b. Functional capacity.
      c. Therapeutic goal.
      d. Family background.
      e. Educational background.
   3. Assist in ascertaining best method for patient.
   4. Demonstrate and encourage individual to practice.
   5. Increase activities as individual progresses and is able to assume activity.
   6. Give positive reinforcement for all effort expended.
E. Record and report nursing observations.
F. Evaluate nursing care plan and alter as necessary.
G. Assist in developing discharge plan.

Prevention of Deformities and Complications

A. Specific nursing actions.
   1. Turn and position in good alignment.

a. Prevent contractures.
b. Stimulate circulation.
c. Prevent thrombophlebitis.
d. Prevent decubiti.

2. Prevent edema of extremities.
3. Promote lung expansion.

☆B. Types of exercises.

1. Passive.
   a. Carried out by the therapist or nurse without assistance from patient.
   b. Purpose—retain as much joint range of motion as possible, and maintain circulation.
2. Active assistive.
   a. Carried out by the patient with assistance of therapist or nurse.
   b. Purpose—encourage normal muscle function.
3. Active.
   a. Accomplished by the individual without assistance.
   b. Purpose—increase muscle strength.
4. Resistive.
   a. Active exercise carried out by the individual working against resistance produced by manual or mechanical means.
   b. Purpose—provide resistance in order to increase muscle power.
5. Isometric or muscle setting.
   a. Performed by the individual without assistance.
   b. Purpose—maintain strength in a muscle when a joint is immobilized.
6. Range of Motion (ROM).
   a. Movement of a joint through its full range in all appropriate planes.
   b. Purpose—maintain joint mobility and increase maximal motion of a joint.
   c. Nursing care.
      (1) Assess general condition of patient.
      (2) Establish extent of ROM before present condition.
      (3) Ensure comfortable position.
      (4) Discontinue ROM at point of pain.
   d. Deterrents to ROM exercises: fear and pain.

Proper Use of Aids/Devices

☆A. Cane.

1. Purpose.
   a. Provide greater stability and speed when walking.
   b. Relieve pressure on weight-bearing joints.
   c. Provide force to push or pull body forward.
2. Safety factors.
   a. Handle at level of greater trochanter.
   b. Elbow flexed at 25 to 30 degree angle.
   c. Light-weight material.
   d. Rubber suction tip.
3. Techniques for walking with cane.
   a. Hold cane close to body.
   b. Hold in hand on unaffected side.
   c. Move cane at same time as affected leg.

☆B. Crutches.

1. Purpose—provide support during ambulating when lower extremities unable to support body weight.
2. Safety factors.
   a. Measure 1½ to 2 inches from axillary fold to floor (4 inches in front and 6 inches to side of toes).
   b. Hand piece adjusted to allow 30 degree elbow flexion.
   c. Rubber suction tips on crutches.
   d. Wear well-fitting shoes with nonslip soles.

C. Tilt table.

1. Board or table that can be tilted gradually from a horizontal to a vertical position.
2. Purpose.
   a. Assist individual in gradually adjusting to upright position.
   b. Start weight-bearing activities.
   c. Increase standing tolerance.
   d. Prevent disuse syndrome.
   e. Prevent demineralization of bones.

D. Prosthesis—artificial replacement for a missing body part.

E. Brace—support that protects or supports weakened muscles.

Common Problems from Immobility

Decubitis Ulcers

A. Localized areas of necrosis of skin and subcutaneous tissue due to pressure.

B. Cause—pressure exerted on skin and subcutaneous tissue by bony prominences and the object on which the body rests.

C. Predisposing factors.
1. Malnutrition.
2. Anemia.
3. Hypoproteinemia.
4. Vitamin deficiency.
5. Edema.

D. Common sites: bony prominences of body such as sacrum, greater trochanter, heels, elbows, etc.

E. Prevention.
1. Purpose.
   a. Relieve or remove pressure.
   b. Stimulate circulation.
   c. Keep skin dry.
2. Nursing care.
   a. Encourage patient to keep active.
   b. Change position frequently.
   c. Maintain good skin hygiene.
   d. Provide for active and/or passive exercises.
   e. Ambulate.
   f. Use alternating air pressure mattress, etc.
   g. Use sheepskin padding.
   h. Inspect skin frequently.
   j. Provide for adequate nutritional intake.

External Rotation of Hip

A. Outward rotation of the hip joint.

B. Cause—lying for long periods of time on back without support to hips or incorrect positioning in bed.

C. Prevention.
1. Trochanter roll extending from crest of ilium to midthigh when positioned on back.

2. Frequent change of position.
3. Proper positioning.

Footdrop

A. Tendency for the foot to plantar flex.
B. Causes.
1. Prolonged bed rest.
2. Lack of exercise.
3. Weight of bed clothing forcing toes into plantar flexion.
C. Complications.
1. Individual will walk on his toes without touching heel on ground.
2. Unable to walk.
D. Prevention.
1. Position feet against footboard.
2. Use footcradle to keep weight of top linen off toes.
3. Provide range of motion exercises.

Contractures

A. Abnormal shortening of muscle, tendon, or ligament so joint cannot function properly.
B. Cause—improper alignment, lack of movement.
C. Prevention.
1. Properly align at all times.
   a. Use pillows.
   b. Provide supportive splints.
2. Provide for range of motion exercises.

Bladder Dysfunction

A. Cause.
1. Disease process.
2. Lack of innervation.
3. Lack of motivation.
B. Bladder training.
1. Purpose.
   a. Prevent urinary tract infection and preserve renal function.
   b. Keep individual dry and odor free.
   c. Help individual maintain social acceptance.

⭐2. Nursing care.
   a. Set up specific time to empty bladder.
   b. Give measured amounts of fluids.
   c. Position in normal voiding position.
   d. Instruct to Credé bladder.
   e. Keep record of amount and time of intake and output.
   f. Encourage patient to wear own clothing, particularly underwear.

Bowel Dysfunction

A. Cause.
   1. Disease process.
   2. Inadequate intake.
   3. Poor prior habits.
B. Bowel training.
   1. Purpose.
      a. Develop regular bowel habits.
      b. Prevent fecal incontinence, impaction, and/or irregularity.
⭐2. Nursing care.
   a. Establish specific time.
   b. Provide for adequate roughage and fluid intake.
   c. Use normal posture.
   d. Instruct to bear down and contract abdominal muscles.
   e. Provide privacy and time.
   f. Provide exercise.

Hypostatic Pneumonia.

A. Incidence.
   1. Very young, very old.
   2. Debilitated.
   3. Immobile.
B. Cause—stasis of secretions in lungs.
C. Prevention.
   1. Assess lung function.
   2. Encourage deep breathing, coughing.
   3. Turn every two hours.
   4. Provide for postural drainage, if indicated.
   5. Ensure adequate hydration.

Other Common Problems

A. Muscle atrophy.
B. Venous thrombosis.
C. Psychological deterioration.

Review Questions

1. Which of the following is a normal room temperature for a patient who is aged, sedentary, or ill?

   A. 78°F.
   B. 70°F.
   C. 60°F.
   D. 37°C.

2. Which of these is *not* in the normal range of humidity for a patient's room?

   A. 35 percent.
   B. 45 percent.
   C. 55 percent.
   D. 65 percent.

3. The single best method to maintain medical asepsis is to

   A. Sterilize all equipment.
   B. Wear a mask when caring for a patient.
   C. Use good handwashing technique.
   D. Change all bed linen daily.

4. Surgical asepsis is

   A. Clean technique.
   B. The control of pathogens.
   C. The absence of living pathogens.
   D. The absence of all forms of microorganisms.

5. Which one of the following types of isolation prevents the transmission of microorganisms from the patient by droplet, fomite, direct contact, and food?

   A. Respiratory isolation.
   B. Strict isolation.
   C. Enteric isolation.
   D. Reverse barrier isolation.

6. Which of these is *not* a purpose of basic patient assessment?

   A. To aid in preparing a firm, unchanging patient care plan.
   B. To establish the patient's position on the health/ illness continuum.
   C. To provide a baseline for patient care planning.
   D. To assist in the formation of a nursing diagnosis.

7. Vital signs include

   A. Pulse deficit.
   B. Pulse pressure.
   C. Blood pressure.
   D. Weight.

8. An adult's pulse rate is usually obtained by palpating

   A. The pedal vein.
   B. The heart.
   C. The radial artery.
   D. The temporal artery.

9. During patient assessment chest sounds are usually obtained by

   A. Auscultation.
   B. Palpation.
   C. Inspection.
   D. Observation.

10. Problem-oriented medical records and nurses' notes utilize the SOAP format. Which of the following is *not* true?

    A. "S" denotes specific problems.
    B. "O" denotes objective information.
    C. "A" denotes assessment of status of problem.
    D. "P" denotes plan of care.

11. Information recorded on the patient's chart should include

    A. Mainly subjective, interpretive statements.
    B. Penciled notations to facilitate corrections.
    C. Only approved abbreviations and symbols.
    D. The printed (not written) name of the nurse who made the entry.

12. Trauma is a disease etiology. Trauma is best described as

    A. Bodily injury caused by violence.
    B. Hereditary factors.
    C. Hormones.
    D. An accidental incident.

13. Which of the following will provide an individual with active immunity?

    A. Infectious organism passing across placenta from mother to unborn baby.
    B. Injection of gamma globulin.
    C. Injection of a vaccine.
    D. Injection of antitoxin.

14. Which of these infectious agents is shaped like a spiral or corkscrew?

    A. Bacillus.
    B. Rickettsiae.
    C. Virus.
    D. Spirochete.

15. When bladder training a patient, the nurse should encourage the patient in all the following *except*

    A. Set up a specific time to empty the bladder.
    B. Drink adequate fluids.
    C. Eat adequate roughage.
    D. Wear own clothing.

16. A major cause of urinary incontinence is

A. Improper diet.
B. Lack of opportunity.
C. Lack of activity.
D. Institutional routine.

17. Muscle atrophy can be prevented by providing the patient with

A. Passive range of motion.
B. Active form of exercise.
C. Coughing and deep breathing.
D. Elastic stockings.

18. Rehabilitation is needed today for all the following reasons *except*

A. Approximately 74 million Americans have a chronic or permanent health impairment.
B. Chronic illness increases with advancing age.
C. Jobs in the health care area are needed.
D. Because of increased population, there are increasing numbers of persons impaired in accidents, causing permanent disabilities.

19. The purposes of an exercise program would include all the following *except*

A. Relieve pressure on bony prominences of the body.
B. Maintain muscle strength.
C. Stimulate circulation.
D. Maintain joint function.

20. Which of the following is *not* a rehabilitative nursing function?

A. Make the diagnosis so that therapy can be directed toward realistic goals.
B. Establish a sustained supporting relationship with the patient.
C. Provide health teaching and training that will meet the needs of the individual patient and his family.
D. Provide a nursing care plan that meets the patient's needs.

21. When a bowel training program is developed for a patient, which of the following would *not* be done?

A. Place patient on the bedpan every two hours.
B. Provide diet with adequate roughage.
C. Ensure patient privacy and time.
D. Stimulate anorectal reflex.

22. When teaching a patient how to use a cane, which one of the following is an important principle?

A. The cane is kept close to the body.
B. The cane is used on the affected side.
C. The cane handle should be level with the greater thigh.

D. The cane is moved at the same time the unaffected leg is moved.

23. The most common position in which to place a female patient prior to urinary tract catheterization is

A. Fowler's.
B. Dorsal recumbent.
C. Prone.
D. Trendelenburg's.

24. The chief danger of urinary tract catheterization is in

A. Stimulating bladder spasms.
B. Inaccurately recording output.
C. Developing an infection of the urinary tract.
D. Improperly placing the catheter.

25. During a retention catheter or bladder irrigation the nurse must

A. Use sterile equipment and wear sterile gloves.
B. Use clean equipment and maintain surgical asepsis.
C. Use sterile equipment and maintain medical asepsis.
D. Use clean equipment and technique.

26. A patient receiving atropine preoperatively might expect

A. To hear ringing in his ears.
B. To become drowsy.
C. His mouth to feel dry.
D. His pain to be decreased.

27. Which of these would most likely be used to control postoperative nausea and vomiting?

A. Compazine.
B. Demerol.
C. Talwin.
D. Codeine.

28. In order to prevent postoperative respiratory complications, Mrs. Miller is receiving an enzyme to liquefy her secretions. An example of this type of drug is

A. Isuprel.
B. Prednisone.
C. Mucomist.
D. Varidase.

29. Postoperative patients who develop atelectasis usually have

A. A flushed face.
B. Dyspnea.
C. A decreased temperature.
D. A severe cough.

30. Which of the following would *not* indicate thrombophlebitis?

    A. Pain along a vein.
    B. Severe cramping.
    C. Edema.
    D. Surrounding area cool to touch.

31. Thrombophlebitis may be identified by a positive

    A. Doll's sign.
    B. Kernig's sign.
    C. Hegar's sign.
    D. Homan's sign.

32. Which of the following would indicate a possible wound infection?

    A. Increased temperature within the first 24 hours after surgery.
    B. Serosanguineous drainage on dressing.
    C. Erythema surrounding suture line three to four days after surgery.
    D. Bright red drainage on dressing the night of surgery.

33. Postoperative pain can be controlled by all of the following *except*

    A. Positioning the patient no oftener than every four hours to avoid unnecessary movement.
    B. Medicating the patient for pain at least every four hours for the first 24 hours.
    C. Keeping the bed linens dry and wrinkle free.
    D. Keeping the patient's bladder empty by encouraging him to void at appropriate intervals.

34. The concentration of electrolytes in solution is measured in

    A. mg.
    B. cc/ml.
    C. gr.
    D. mEq/L.

35. Intracellular fluid contains large quantities of

    A. Na, K, PO_4.
    B. K, PO_4, proteins.
    C. K, Cl, HCO_3.
    D. K, Na, HCO_3.

36. The flow of water from a hypotonic to a hypertonic solution across a semipermeable membrane is

    A. Osmosis.
    B. Diffusion.
    C. Active transport.
    D. Filtration.

37. Which of these is a sign/symptom of dehydration?

    A. Increased skin turgor.
    B. Cool skin.
    C. 45 cc/hr. urinary output.
    D. Weight loss.

38. Mr. Randolph complains of shortness of breath and headache. You note his skin is flushed and he has tachycardia and tachypnea. Which of the following fluid and electrolyte imbalances does he most likely have?

    A. Hypokalemia.
    B. Hypercalcemia.
    C. Dehydration.
    D. Circulatory overload.

39. The normal serum potassium level is

    A. 1.010 to 1.030.
    B. 3.5 to 5.5 mEq/L.
    C. 135 to 145 mg.
    D. 22 kg.

40. Potassium excess (hyperkalemia) is often caused by

    A. Excessive diuretic loss.
    B. Cellular destruction of burns.
    C. Respiratory alkalosis.
    D. Adrenal secretion excess.

41. Pitting edema, excessive weight gain, and dyspnea are frequently seen in which fluid and electrolyte imbalance?

    A. Hypernatremia.
    B. Extracellular fluid deficit.
    C. Hypokalemia.
    D. Hypercalcemia.

42. Abdominal cramps, carpopedal spasms, and tetany are often due to

    A. Hyponatremia.
    B. Hypocalcemia.
    C. Hypokalemia.
    D. Fluid excess.

43. Using an administration set that delivers 15 drops per cc, how many drops must be given per minute to give 3,000 cc of IV fluid in 24 hours?

    A. 20 drops/minute.
    B. 31 drops/minute.
    C. 125 drops/minute.
    D. 187 drops/minute.

44. The signs of a third degree burn include all the following *except*

    A. Blisters.
    B. Little or no pain.
    C. Deep tissue destruction.
    D. White or charred appearance.

Answers and Rationale

1. (A) Normal room temperature is 66° to 76°F. The temperature will be higher if the patient is aged, sedentary, very ill, or very young.

2. (D) Normal room humidity is 30 to 60 percent.

3. (C) Medical asepsis is considered the "clean method" and is used to limit the spread of microorganisms. Handwashing is the best single method to accomplish this.

4. (D) Surgical asepsis is "sterile technique" and is used in surgical procedures. It is the absence of all forms of microorganisms, including spores.

5. (B) Respiratory isolation prevents the spread of microorganisms via the respiratory tract by droplet; enteric, via the GI tract. Reverse barrier isolation protects the patient, not the nurse.

6. (A) The nursing care plan should be flexible and altered when necessary to reflect changes in the patient's condition.

7. (C) Vital signs include temperature, pulse, respiration, and blood pressure.

8. (C) The radial artery is usually palpated to determine an adult's pulse rate. Veins are not used.

9. (A) Auscultation is the process of listening, usually using a stethoscope.

10. (A) The "S" stands for subjective information the patient gives you about the problem.

11. (C) Abbreviations that are not approved are frequently misunderstood. Objective data should be charted. The chart is a legal document and all entries must be made in ink and signed by the nurse making the entry.

12. (A) Lasting bodily injury caused by violence is an example of trauma; an accidental incident may or may not cause bodily harm.

13. (C) Vaccination provides for active immunity since the body produces antibodies in response to an injected antigen.

14. (D) A spirochete is shaped like a corkscrew; bacilli are rod-shaped; rickettsiae are round or rod-shaped.

15. (C) Adequate roughage is needed for proper bowel function. Specific time for voiding and adequate fluids are needed in bladder training. Wearing one's own clothing increases one's self-esteem and encourages patient to keep self dry.

16. (B) It is the nurse's responsibility to answer lights promptly and see to it that the patient is offered the opportunity to void at least every two hours.

17. (B) Muscles must be used to prevent atrophy. Passive range of motion prevents joint stiffness; coughing and deep breathing helps prevent hypostatic pneumonia; elastic stockings help prevent thrombophlebitis.

18. (C) Creating jobs is not the primary purpose of rehabilitation.

19. (A) A frequent change of body position will relieve pressure, but this change is *not* part of an exercise program because it is usually passive, not active.

20. (A) The diagnosis of a patient's condition and subsequent therapy is the physician's responsibility. The nurse is responsible for the assessment, development, initiation, and evaluation of a nursing care plan to meet the individual patient's needs.

21. (A) The patient is placed on the bedpan or commode 1/2 hour after meals or at a time regularly established by the patient.

22. (A) The cane is used on the unaffected side, should be kept level with greater trochanter, and the cane is moved at the same time as the affected leg.

23. (B) Dorsal recumbent provides for clear visualization of the female urethral meatus.

24. (C) Bladder spasms rarely occur. Infections are important because pathogens can enter the urinary tract through or with the catheter.

25. (C) To prevent introduction of pathogens into the urinary tract, sterile equipment is used and its sterility maintained.

26. (C) Atropine inhibits parasympathetic stimulation and reduces tracheobronchial secretions; these result in dry mucous membranes.

27. (A) Compazine, in small doses, tends to control nausea and vomiting. The others are central nervous system depressants.

28. (D) Another example is Dornavac. Isuprel is a bronchodilator; prednisone an antiinflammatory; mucomist an expectorant.

29. (B) Patients become short of breath and usually experience severe pain but do not have a severe cough.

30. (D) The surrounding area would be warm to touch and red, indicating an inflammatory response.

31. (D) When the foot is dorsiflexed, the patient feels pain in the calf if a blood clot is present. This is Homan's sign.

32. (C) Erythema is usually one of the first signs of a possible wound infection. An increased temperature the first 24 hours usually indicates dehydration or pulmonary complications.

33. (A) Postoperative patients need to turn, cough, and deep breathe at least every two hours to prevent pulmonary complications.

34. (D) Electrolytes are measured in mEq/L (milliequivalents per liter).

35. (B) Intracellular fluid contains large quantities of potassium, phosphate, and proteins; extracellular fluid contains large quantities of sodium, chloride, and bicarbonate.

36. (A) From hypotonic (low solute concentration) to hypertonic (high solute concentration) is osmosis; diffusion is the opposite.

37. (D) Weight loss; other signs/symptoms are loss of skin turgor, thirst, warm and dry skin, cracked lips, and oliguria.

38. (D) These symptoms indicate circulatory overload.

39. (B) Electrolytes (potassium) are measured in mEq/L. 3.5 to 5.5 is normal serum level.

40. (B) Another cause of potassium excess is cellular destruction from crushing injury.

41. (A) Also same for extracellular fluid excess.

42. (B) Calcium deficiency leads to muscle spasm/convulsion.

43. (B) 31 drops/minute.

    drops/minute =

    $$\frac{\text{total volume infused} \times \text{drops/cc}}{\text{total time for infusing in minutes}}$$

    $$\frac{3000 \times 15}{24 \times 60} = 31.25$$

44. (A) Blisters are signs of second degree burns. Third degree burns show charring due to deep tissue destruction. There is little or no pain because the nerve endings are destroyed.

Pharmacology and Nutrition

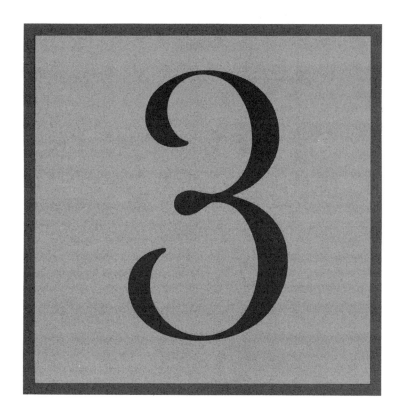

Pharmacology

Pharmacological Concepts

Drug Metabolism

Stages of Metabolism

Definition: Drug metabolism in the human body is accomplished in four basic stages—absorption, transportation, biotransformation, and excretion. In order for a drug to be completely metabolized, it must first be given in sufficient concentration to produce the desired effect on body tissues. When this critical drug concentration level is achieved, body tissues change.

A. Absorption.
   1. The first stage of metabolism refers to the route a drug takes from the time it enters the body until it is absorbed in the circulating fluids.
   2. Drugs are absorbed by the mucous membranes, the gastrointestinal tract, the respiratory tract, and the skin.
      a. The mucous membranes are one of the most rapid and effective routes of absorption because they are highly vascular.
      b. Drugs are absorbed through these membranes.
   3. Drugs given by mouth are absorbed in the gastrointestinal tract.
      a. Portions of these drugs dissolve and absorb in the stomach.
      b. Drugs are enteric coated to prevent absorption in the stomach.
      c. The rate of absorption depends on the pH of the stomach's contents, the food content in the stomach at the time of ingestion, and the presence of disease conditions.
      d. Most of the drug concentrate dissolves in the small intestine where the large vascular surface and moderate pH level enhance the process of dissolution.

   4. Methods of administration include intradermal, subcutaneous, intravenous, and intraarterial injections.
      a. Parenteral methods are the most direct, reliable, and rapid route of absorption.
      b. The actual administration site will depend on type of drug, its action, and the patient.
   5. Another route of administration is inhalation or nebulization through the respiratory system.
      a. This method is not as rapid as parenteral injections but faster than the gastrointestinal tract.
      b. Drugs administered through the respiratory tract must be made up of small particles that can pass through to the alveoli in the lungs.
   6. The final mode of absorption is the skin.
      a. Most drugs, when applied to the skin, produce a local rather than a systemic effect.
      b. The degree of absorption will depend on the strength of the drug as well as where it is applied on the body surface.
B. Transportation.
   1. The second stage of metabolism refers to the way in which a drug is transported from the site of introduction to the site of action.
   2. First, a drug enters or is absorbed by the body.
      a. Drug is transported through circulation to all parts of the body.
      b. If drug binds to plasma protein it is not effective.
   3. As a drug moves from the circulatory system, it crosses cell membranes and enters the body tissues.
      a. Some of the drug is distributed to and stored in fat and muscle.
      b. Greater masses of tissue (such as fat and muscle) attract the drug.
   4. The amount of drug that is distributed to body tissues depends on the permeability of the membranes and the blood supply to the absorption area.
   5. A drug that first accumulates in the brain

may move into fat and muscle tissue and then back to the brain because the drug is still chemically active.

   a. The drug is released in small quantities from the tissues and travels back to the brain.
   b. Equal drug and blood concentration levels in the body are maintained.

C. Biotransformation.

   1. The third stage of metabolism takes place as the drug, a foreign substance in the body, is converted by enzymes into a less active and harmless agent that can be easily excreted.
   2. Most of this conversion occurs in the liver.
      a. Both synthetic and biochemical reactions take place.
      b. Some conversion does take place in the kidney, plasma, and intestinal mucosa.
   3. Synthetic reactions: liver enzymes conjugate the drug with other substances to make it less harmful for the body.
   4. Biochemical reactions: drugs are oxidized, reduced, hydrolyzed, and synthesized so they become less active and more easily eliminated from the body.

D. Excretion.

   1. The final stage in metabolism takes place when the drug is changed into an inactive form or excreted from the body.
   2. The kidneys are the most important route of excretion.
   3. The kidneys eliminate both the pure drug and the metabolites of the parent drug.
      a. During excretion these two substances are filtered through the glomeruli.
      b. They are then secreted by the tubules.
      c. Finally, they are reabsorbed through the tubules or directly excreted.
   4. Other routes of excretion include the lungs (which exhale gaseous drugs), feces, saliva, tears, and mother's milk.

Factors That Affect Drug Metabolism

A. Personal attributes.
   1. Body weight.
   2. Age.
   3. Sex.

B. Physiological factors.
   1. State of health.
   2. Disease processes.
C. Acid-base and fluid and electrolyte balance.
D. Permeability.
E. Diurnal rhythm.
F. Circulatory capability.
G. Genetic and immunologic factors.
H. Drug tolerance.
I. Cumulation effect of drugs.
J. Other factors.
   1. Psychological.
   2. Emotional.
   3. Environmental
K. Responses to drugs vary.
   1. Responses depend on the speed with which the drug is absorbed into the blood or tissues.
   2. Responses depend on the effectiveness of the body's circulatory system.

Origin and Naming of Drugs

Common Sources

A. Plant sources.
   1. Roots, bark, sap, leaves, flowers, and seeds from medicinal plants can be used as drug components.
   2. Component substances.
      a. Alkaloid.
         (1) Alkaline (base) in reaction.
         (2) Bitter in taste.
         (3) Physiologically powerful in activity.
      b. Glycoside: a compound containing a carbohydrate molecule.
      c. Resin: soluble in alcohol; insoluble in water.
      d. Gum.
         (1) Mucilaginous (gelatin-like) excretion.
         (2) Used in bulk laxatives; may absorb water.
         (3) Used in skin preparations as a soothing effect, e.g., Karaya gum.
      e. Oil.

(1) Fixed oil: does not evaporate on warming; occurs as a solid, semi-solid, or liquid, e.g., castor oil.

(2) Volatile oil: evaporates readily; occurs in aromatic plants, e.g., peppermint.

B. Animal sources.
1. Processed from an organ, from organ secretion, or from organ cells.
2. Insulin, as an example, is a derivative from the pancreas of sheep, cattle, or hogs.

C. Mineral sources.
1. Inorganic elements occurring in nature, but not of plant or animal origin; may be metallic or nonmetallic.
2. Usually form a base or acid salt in food.
3. Dilute hydrochloric acid (HCl), as an example, is diluted in water and then taken through a straw to prevent damage to teeth by acid.

D. Synthetic sources.
1. A pure drug made in a laboratory from chemical, not natural, substances.
2. Many drugs, sulfonamides for example, are synthetics.

Methods of Naming Drugs

A. Chemical name.
1. Precise description of chemical constituents with the exact placement of atom groupings.
2. "N-Methyl-4-carbethoxypiperidine hydrochloride" is an example of a chemical name.

B. Generic name.
1. Reflects chemical name to which drug belongs, but is simpler.
2. It is never changed and used commonly in medical terminology.
3. The synthetic narcotic meperidine is an example of a generic name.

C. Trademark name (brand name, proprietary name).
1. Appears in literature with the sign ®, e.g., Demerol ®.
2. The sign indicates the name is registered; use of the name is restricted to the manufacturer who is the legal owner.

3. Trademark name is capitalized or shown in parentheses if generic name stated.

Drug Classification

Classification by Action

A. Anti-infectives.
1. Antiseptics.
   a. Action—inhibit growth of microorganisms (bacteriostatic).
   b. Purpose—application to wounds and skin infections, sterilization of equipment, and hygienic purposes.
2. Disinfectants.
   a. Action—destroy microorganisms (bactericidal).
   b. Purpose—destroy bacteria on inanimate objects (not appropriate for living tissue).

B. Antimicrobials.
1. Sulfonamides.
   a. Action—inhibit the growth of microorganisms.
   b. Reduce or prevent infectious process especially for urinary tract infections.
2. Antibiotics (e.g., penicillin).
   a. Action—interfere with microorganism metabolism.
   b. Usage—reduce or prevent infectious process.
   c. Specific drug and dosage based on culture and sensitivity of organism.

C. Metabolic drugs.
1. Hormones obtained from animal sources, found naturally in foods and plants.
2. Synthetic hormones.

D. Diagnostic materials.
1. Action—dyes and opaque materials ingested or injected to allow visualization of internal organs.
2. Purpose—to analyze organ status and function.

E. Vitamins and minerals.
1. Action—necessary to obtain healthy body function.
2. Found naturally in food or through syn-

thetic food supplements.

F. Vaccines and serums.
1. Action—prevent disease or detect presence of disease.
2. Types.
   a. Antigenics produce active immunity.
      (1) Vaccines—attenuated suspensions of microorganisms.
      (2) Toxoids—products of microorganisms.
   b. Antibodies—stimulated by microorganisms or their products.
      (1) Antitoxins.
      (2) Immune serum globulin.
   c. Allergens—agents for skin immunity tests.
      (1) Extracts of materials known to be allergenic.
      (2) Can be used to relieve allergies.
   d. Antivenins—substances which neutralize venom of certain snakes and spiders.

G. Antifungals—check growth of fungi.

H. Antihistaminics.
1. Action—prevent histamine action.
2. Purpose—relieve symptoms of allergic reaction.

I. Antineoplastics—prevent growth and spread of malignant cells.

Classification by Body Systems

Central Nervous System

A. Drugs affect CNS by either inhibiting or promoting the actions of neural pathways and centers.
1. Action promoting drug groups (stimulants).
   a. Antidepressants—psychic energizers used to treat depression.
   b. Caffeine—increases mental activity and lessens drowsiness.
   c. Ammonia—used as revival from fainting spell (patient smells cap, not contents of bottle).
2. Action inhibiting drug groups (depressants).

   a. Analgesics—reduce pain by interfering with conduction of nerve impulses.
      (1) Narcotic analgesics—opium derivatives may depress respiratory centers; must be used with caution and respiratory rate above 12.
         (a) A narcotic antagonist drug counteracts depressant drugs.
         (b) Such antagonist drugs are Lorfan, Narcan, and Nalline.
      (2) Nonnarcotic antipyretics—reduce fever and relieve pain.
      (3) Antirheumatics—analgesics given to relieve arthritis pain; may reduce joint inflammation.
   b. Alcohol—stimulates appetite when given in small doses but classified as a depressant.
   c. Hypnotics—sedatives that induce sleep; common form is the barbiturates.
   d. Antispasmotics—relieve skeletal muscle spasms; anticonvulsants prevent muscle spasms or convulsions.
   e. Tranquilizers.
      (1) Relieve tension and anxiety, preoperative and postoperative apprehension, headaches, menstrual tension, chronic alcoholism, skeletal muscle spasticity, and other neuromuscular disorders.
      (2) Tranquilizers and analgesics frequently given together (in reduced dosage); the one drug enhances the action of the other (synergy).
   f. Anesthetics—produce the state of unconsciousness painlessly.

B. Precautions to be taken with CNS drugs.
1. Drugs which act on CNS may potentiate other CNS drugs.
2. Patient may be receiving other medications; find out drug name and dosage.
3. Dependence on CNS drugs may occur.

Autonomic Nervous System

A. This system governs several body functions so that drugs that affect the ANS will at the same time affect other system functions.

B. The ANS is made up of two nerve systems—

the sympathetic and parasympathetic.

1. Parasympathetic is the stabilizing system.
2. Sympathetic is the protective emergency system.

C. Each system has a separate basic drug group acting on it.

1. Adrenergics—mimic the actions of sympathetic system.
   a. Vasoconstrictors—stimulants such as Adrenalin.
      (1) Action is to constrict peripheral blood vessels thereby increasing blood pressure.
      (2) Dilate bronchial passages.
      (3) Relax gastrointestinal tract.
   b. Vasodilators—depressants such as nicotinic acid.
      (1) Antagonists of epinephrine and similar drugs.
      (2) Vasodilate blood vessels.
      (3) Increase tone of GI tract.
      (4) Reduce blood pressure.
      (5) Relax smooth muscles.
      (6) *Caution:* If drug is to be stopped, reduce dosage gradually over a period of a week; do not stop it suddenly.
2. Cholinergics—mimic actions of parasympathetic system.
   a. Cholinergic stimulants (e.g., Prostigmin or neostigmine).
      (1) Decrease heart rate.
      (2) Contract smooth muscle.
      (3) Contract pupil in eye.
      (4) Increase peristalsis.
      (5) Increase gland secretions.
   b. Cholinergic inhibiters (anticholinergics).
      (1) Decrease gland secretion.
      (2) Relax smooth muscle.
      (3) Dilate pupil in eye.
      (4) Increase heart action.

Gastrointestinal System

A. Drugs affecting GI system act upon muscular and glandular tissues.
B. Drug groups and actions.

1. Antacids—counteract excess acidity.
   a. Have alkaline base.
   b. Used in the treatment of ulcers.
   c. Neutralize hydrochloric acid in the stomach.
   d. Given frequently (two hour intervals or more often).
   e. May cause constipation, depending on type of medication.
   f. Baking soda is a systemic antacid which disturbs the pH balance in the body. Most other antacids coat the mucous membrane and neutralize hydrochloric acid.
2. Emetics—produce vomiting (emesis).
3. Antiemetics—prevent vomiting or nausea but may cause drowsiness.
4. Digestants—relieve enzyme deficiency by replacing secretions in digestive tract.
5. Antidiarrheics—prevent diarrhea.
6. Cathartics—affect intestine and produce defecation.
   a. Provide temporary relief for constipation.
   b. Rid bowel of contents before surgery, and prepare viscera for diagnostic studies.
   c. Counteract edema.
   d. Treat diseases of GI tract.
   e. Contraindicated when abdominal pain is present.
   f. Classifications.
      (1) By degree of action.
         (a) Laxative—mild action.
         (b) Cathartic—moderate action.
         (c) Purgative—severe action.
      (2) By method of action.
         (a) Increase bulk.
         (b) Lubricate mechanically.
         (c) Irritate chemically.
         (d) Increase or decrease water content with saline.
         (e) Disperse detergent or wetting agent.

Respiratory System

A. Drugs act on respiratory tract, tissues, and

cough center.

B. Action is to suppress, relax, liquefy, and stimulate.
1. Respiratory stimulants stimulate depth and rate of respiration.
2. Bronchodilators relax smooth muscle of trachea.
3. Drug groups that provide cough relief:
   a. Antitussive agents (narcotic, non-narcotic).
      (1) Sedatives prevent cough.
      (2) Not to be accompanied by water.
   b. Demulcents soothe respiratory tract.
   c. Expectorants liquefy bronchial secretions and increase amount of excretions in respiratory tract.

Urinary System

A. Drugs that act on kidneys and urinary tract.
B. Action is to increase urine flow, destroy bacteria, and perform other important body functions.
1. Diuretics.
   a. Rid body of excess fluid and relieve edema.
   b. Some drugs that act on the GI tract and circulatory system also are diuretic in action.
2. Urinary antiseptics.
3. Acidifiers and alkalinizers—certain foods will also increase body acids or alkalies.

Circulatory System

A. Drugs that act on heart, blood, and blood vessels.
B. Action is to change heart rhythm, rate, and force and to dilate or constrict vessels.
1. Cardiotonics used for heart-strengthening.
   a. Direct heart stimulants that speed heart rate, e.g., caffeine, Adrenalin.
   b. Indirect heart stimulants, e.g., digitalis.
      (1) Stimulate vagus nerve.
      (2) Slow heart rate and strengthen it.
      (3) Improve heart action, thereby improving circulation.

      (4) Do not administer if apical pulse below 60.
2. Antiarrhythmic drugs used clinically to convert irregularities to a normal sinus rhythm.
   a. Monitor constantly with ECG when administering these drugs.
   b. Quinidine used for its vasodepressor action.
      (1) Slows impulse of sinoauricular node.
      (2) Slows heart rate.
      (3) Side effects include ringing in ears.
3. Drugs that alter blood flow.
   a. Anticoagulants—inhibit blood clotting action.
   b. Coagulants—maintain blood fluidity.
4. Blood replacement.

Dosage and Preparation Forms

Solids

A. Extract—obtained by dissolving drug in water or alcohol and allowing solution to evaporate; residue is the extract.
B. Powder—finely ground drugs.
C. Pills—common term for tablet; made by rolling drug and binder into a sphere.
D. Suppository.
1. Contains drugs mixed with a firm base.
2. Liquefies at body temperature when inserted into orifice.
3. Releases drug to produce a local or systemic effect.
E. Ointment—semisolid mixture of drugs with a fatty base.
F. Lozenge—flavored flat tablet that releases drug slowly when held in mouth.
G. Capsule.
1. Drugs in small, cylindrical gelatin containers that disguise the taste of the drug.
2. Capsule can be opened and drug mixed with food or jam to mask taste.
H. Tablets
1. Dried, powdered drugs that are com-

pressed into a small disk which easily disintegrates in water.
2. Enteric coated—tablet does not dissolve until reaching intestines, where release of drug occurs.

Liquids

A. Fluidextract.
   1. Concentrated fluid preparation of drugs produced by dissolving crude plant drug in a solvent.
   2. Strength of extract is such that 1 cc (about ¼ teaspoon or 15 to 16 gtt) represents 1 gram of the drug at 100 percent strength.
B. Tincture.
   1. Diluted alcoholic extract of a drug.
   2. Varies in strength from 10 to 20 percent.
C. Spirit—preparation of volatile (easily vaporized) substances dissolved in alcohol.
D. Syrup—drug contained in a concentrated sugar solution.
E. Elixir—solution of drug made with alcohol, sugar, and some aromatic or pleasant-smelling substance.
F. Suspension.
   1. Undissolved, finely divided particles of drug dispersed in a liquid.
   2. Gels and magma are other forms of suspensions.
   3. Shake all bottles of suspension well before giving.
G. Emulsion—suspension of unmixed oils, fats, or petrolatum in water.
H. Liniment and lotion—liquid suspension of medication applied to the skin.

Packaging Methods and Dispensing

A. Unit dosage package method.
   1. Package contains premeasured amount of drug in proper form for administering.
   2. Pharmacy may deliver the daily needs for each patient to the floor.
   3. Procedures for delivery and storage vary from hospital to hospital.

4. Nurse administers the medication to the patient.
B. Traditional method.
   1. Nurse prepares medication on the unit.
   2. Supplies come from stock or bulk on the ward or from a multiple dose bottle of patient's.
C. The nurse is responsible for accuracy of the medication given, regardless of the packaging or dispensing method used.

Routes of Administration

Oral Route

A. Ingested (swallowed).
B. Sublingual (under tongue).
C. Buccal (on mucous membrane of cheek or tongue).

Rectal Route

A. Suppository.
B. Liquid (retention enema).

Parenteral Route

A. Intravenous.
   1. The response is fast and immediate.
   2. Over 5 cc medication can be given.
   3. Drug *must be* given slowly and usually in diluted form.
   4. Check medication leaflets to determine if medication route is IM or IV.
B. Intradermal.
   1. Injected into skin; usual site is inner aspect of forearm or scapular area of back.
   2. A short bevel 26-gauge, 1-cm needle is used.
   3. Needle should be inserted with bevel up.
   4. This route is usually used to inject antigens for skin or tuberculin tests.
   5. Amount injected ranges from 0.01 to 0.1 cc.
C. Subcutaneous.

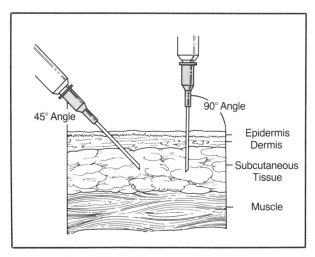

Insert needle at 45- or 90-degree angle for subcutaneous injection.

Insert needle at 15-degree angle under the epidermis for intradermal injection.

1. A 25-gauge, 1.3- to 1.6-cm needle is used.
2. Injection site is the fatty layer under skin.
   a. Abdomen at navel.
   b. Lateral upper arm or thigh.
3. This route usually used for injecting medication that is to be absorbed slowly with a sustained effect.
4. Amount injected ranges from 0.5 to 1.5 cc.
5. If repeated doses are necessary, as with insulin for a diabetic person, rotate the injection sites.

D. Intramuscular.
   1. Needle gauge and length will vary with site.
      a. Deltoid—located by having patient raise arm.
         (1) A 23- to 25-gauge, 1.6- to 2.5-cm needle is used.
         (2) Administer no more than 2 cc.
      b. Thigh and buttock.
         (1) Needle must be long enough to reach muscle; may vary from 2 to 8 cm.
         (2) Needle gauge depends upon substance of medication.
         (3) Oil bases require 20 gauge; water bases require 22 gauge.
   2. Absorption rate of IM medication depen-dent upon circulation of person injected.
   3. This route usually used for systemic effect of an irritating drug.
   4. Amount of medication must not be over 5 cc, as absorption would be difficult and painful.
   5. Techniques for lessening pain for the patient receiving an IM medication:
      a. Encourage relaxation of area to be injected; request patient to lie on side with flexed knee or out flat on abdomen, if giving injection in buttock.
      b. Reduce puncture pain by "darting" needle.
      c. Prevent antiseptic from clinging to needle during insertion by waiting until skin antiseptic is dry.
      d. If medication must be drawn through a rubber stopper, use a new needle for injection.
      e. Avoid sensitive or hardened body areas.
      f. After needle is under skin, aspirate to be certain that needle is not in a blood vessel.
      g. Inject slowly.
      h. Maintain grasp of syringe.
      i. Withdraw needle quickly after injection.
      j. Massage relaxed muscle gently to increase circulation and to distribute medication.

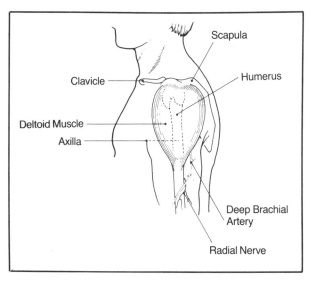

Inject no more than 2cc IM into deltoid muscle.

6. Observe for side effects of medication following injection.

Other Routes

A. Inhalation route.
B. Topical route.

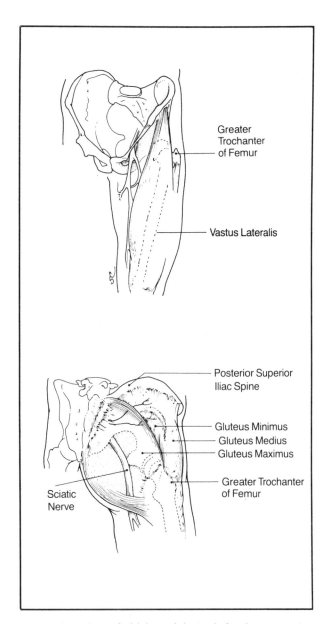

Anatomical view of thigh and buttock for intramuscular injection.

Administration of Medications

Basic Guidelines for Medication Administration

A. Determine the correct dosage, actions, side effects, and contraindications of any medication before administration.
B. Check with head nurse if medications ordered by the physician do not seem appropriate for patient's condition. This is part of the nurse's professional responsibility.
C. Question the physician about any medication orders that are incomplete, illegible, or inappropriate for the patient's condition.
  1. Remember, the nurse may be liable if a medication error is made.
  2. Report every medication error to the head nurse and/or physician.
  3. Complete a medication incident report.
D. Check to determine if the medication ordered is compatible with the patient's condition and with other medications prescribed.
E. Check on what the patient has been eating or drinking before administering a medication.

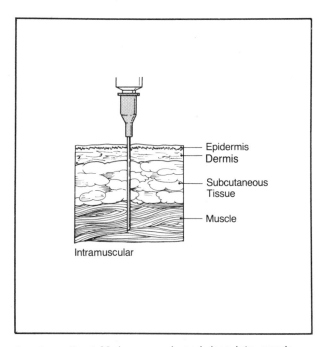

Insert needle at 90-degree angle and deep into muscle tissue for intramuscular injection.

1. Determine what effect the patient's diet has on the medication.
2. Do not administer medication if contraindicated by diet. For example, do not give an MAO inhibitor to a patient who has just ingested cheddar cheese or wine.

F. Check that calculated drug dosage is accurate for young children, elderly people, or for very thin or obese patients. These age and weight groups require smaller or larger dosages.

Safety Rules

A. The five rights.
   1. Right medication.
      a. Compare drug card with drug label three times.
      b. Know general purpose, dosage, method of administration.
      c. Know side effects of drug.
   2. Right patient: check ID band and door number.
   3. Right time.
   4. Right method of administration.
   5. Right amount.
      a. Check all calculations of divided dosages with another nurse.
      b. Check heparin and insulin doses with another nurse.
B. The five rights should be practiced each and every time a medication is given.

Documentation of Medications

Medication Orders

A. Medication administered to patient must have a physician's order or prescription before it can be legally administered.
B. Physician's order is a verbal or written order, recorded in a book or file or in patient's chart.
C. If order is given verbally over the telephone, nurse must write a verbal order in patient's chart for the physician to sign at a later date.

D. Written orders are safer—they leave less room for potential misunderstanding or error.
E. Drug order should consist of seven parts:
   1. Name of the patient.
   2. Date the drug was ordered.
   3. Name of the drug.
   4. Dosage.
   5. Route of administration and any special rules of administration.
   6. Time and frequency the drug should be given.
   7. Signature of the individual who ordered the drug.

Types of Medication Schedules

A. Routine orders.
   1. Administered according to instructions until it is cancelled by another order.
   2. Can also be used for p.r.n. drugs.
      a. Administered when patient needs the medication.
      b. Not given on a routine time schedule.
   3. Continued validity of any routine order should be assessed—physicians occasionally forget to cancel an order when it is no longer appropriate for patient's condition.
B. One-time orders.
   1. Administered as stated, only one time.
   2. Given at a specified time or "stat," which means immediately.

Medication Errors

A. Nurse who prepares a medication must also give it to patient and chart it.
   1. If patient refuses drug, chart that medication was refused—report this information to the physician.
   2. When charting medications, use the correct abbreviations and symbols.
B. If error in a drug order is found, it is nurse's responsibility to question the order.
   1. If order cannot be understood or read, verify with the physician.

2. Do not guess at the order as this constitutes gross negligence.
3. In many hospitals it is the pharmacist's responsibility to contact physicians when medication orders are unclear.

C. Always report medication errors to the physician immediately.
   1. This action minimizes potential danger to the patient.
   2. Measures can be taken immediately to assess and evaluate the patient's status.
   3. A plan of action can be implemented to reverse the effects of the medication.

D. Errors in medication are documented in a medication incident report and on the patient's record.
   1. This action is necessary for both legal reasons and nursing audits.
   2. Nursing audits are conducted to determine problems in medication administration:
      a. A particular source of problems.
      b. A range of problems that seem to have no connection.

Legal Issues in Drug Administration

A. Nurse must not administer a specific drug unless allowed to do so by the particular state's Nurse Practice Act.

B. Nurse is to take every safety precaution in whatever he or she is doing.

C. Nurse is to be certain that employer's policy allows him or her to administer a specific drug.

D. A drug may not lawfully be administered unless all the above items are in effect.

E. General rules.
   1. Never leave tray with prepared medicines unattended.
   2. Always report errors immediately.
   3. Send labeled bottles that are unintelligible back to pharmacist for relabeling.
   4. Store internal and external medicines separately if possible.

Administering Medications

Administering Oral Medications

Preparation

A. Check medication orders for their completeness and accuracy.

B. Assess patient's physical ability to take medication as ordered.
   1. Swallow reflex present.
   2. State of consciousness.
   3. Signs of nausea and vomiting.
   4. Uncooperative behavior.

C. Check to make sure you have the correct medication for the patient.

D. Assess correct dosage when calculation is needed.

☆ E. Preparing the oral medication.
   1. Obtain patient's medication record. Medication record may be a drug card, medication sheet, or drug Kardex,
   2. Compare the medication record with the most *recent* physician's order.
   3. Wash your hands.
   4. Gather necessary equipment.
   5. Remove the medication from the drug box or tray on medication cart.
   6. Compare the label on the bottle or drug package to the medication record.
   7. Correctly calculate dosage if necessary and check the dosage to be administered.
   8. Pour the medication from the bottle into the lid of the container and then into the medicine cup. With unit dosage, take drug package from medication cart tray and place in medication cup. Do not remove drug from drug package.
   9. Check medication label again to ensure correct drug and dosages if drug is not prepackaged.
   10. Place medication cup on a tray, if not using medication cart.
   11. Return the multidose vial bottle to the storage area. If medication to be given is a narcotic, sign out the narcotic record sheet with your name.
   12. Check medication label for third time before returning bottle to storage.

Procedure

☆A. Procedure for administering oral medications to adults.

1. Take medication tray or cart to patient's room; check room number against medication card or sheet.
2. Place patient in sitting position, if not contraindicated by his or her condition.
3. Tell the patient what type of medication you are going to give and explain the actions this medication will produce.
4. Check the patient's Identaband and ask patient to state name so that you are sure you have correctly identified him or her.
5. If prepackaged medication is used, read label, take medication out of package, and put into medication cup.
6. Give the medication cup to the patient.
7. Offer a fresh glass of water or other liquid to aid swallowing, and give assistance with taking medications.
8. Make sure the patient swallows the medication.
9. Discard used medicine cup.
10. Position patient for comfort.
11. Record the medication on the appropriate forms.

☆B. Procedure for administering oral medications to children.

1. Follow the procedures for the previous intervention, keeping the following guidelines in mind:
   a. Play techniques may help to elicit a young child's cooperation.
   b. Remember, the smaller the quantity of dilutent (food or liquid), the greater the ease in eliciting the child's cooperation.
   c. Never use a child's favorite food or drink as an enticement when administering medication because the result may be the child's refusal to eat or drink anything.
   d. Be honest and tell the child that you have medicine, not candy.
2. Assess child for drug action and possible side effects.
3. Explain medication action and side effects to parents.

Administering Parenteral Medications

☆**Preparation**

A. Check that appropriate method for administration of drug:

1. Intradermal (intracutaneous): injection is made below surface of the skin.
2. Subcutaneous: small amount of fluid is injected beneath the skin in the loose connective tissues.
3. Intramuscular: larger amount of fluid is injected into large muscle masses in the body.
4. Intravenous: medication is injected or infused directly into a vein—route used when immediate drug effect is desired.

B. Evaluate condition of administration site for presence of lesions, rash, inflammation, lipid dystrophy, ecchymosis, etc.

C. Assess for tissue damage from previous injections.

D. Assess patient's level of consciousness.

1. For patient in shock: certain methods (subcutaneous) will not be used.
2. For presence of anxiety: make sure patient is allowed to express his or her fear of injections and offer explanations of ways in which injections will be less frightening.

E. Check patient's written and verbal history for past allergic reactions. Do *not* rely solely on patient's chart.

F. Review patient's chart noting previous injection sites, especially insulin and heparin administration sites.

G. Check label on medication bottle to determine if medication can be administered via route ordered.

H. Preparing the medication.

1. Wash your hands.
2. Obtain equipment for injection: needle and syringe, alcohol wipes, medication tray (medication container if needed).
3. Assemble the needle and syringe. Select the appropriate size needle, considering the size of the patient's muscle mass and the viscosity of the medication.

4. Open the alcohol wipe and cleanse the top of the vial or break top of ampule.
5. Remove the needle guard and place on alcohol wipe or medication tray.
6. Pull back on barrel of syringe to markings where medication will be inserted.
7. Pick up vial, insert needle into vial, and inject air in an amount equal to the solution to be withdrawn by pushing barrel of syringe down. If using an ampule, break off top at colored line, insert syringe, but do not inject air into ampule as it causes a break in the vacuum and possible loss of medication through leakage.
8. Extract the desired amount of fluid. Remove needle from container and cover needle with guard. Needle should be changed to prevent tracking medication on skin and subcutaneous tissue.
9. Double-check drug and dosage against drug card or medication sheet and vial or ampule.
10. Place syringe on tray if tray available.
11. Check label and drug card or medication sheet for accuracy before returning multidose vial to correct storage area.
12. Return multidose vial to correct storage area or discard used vial or ampule.

Procedure

☆A. Administering intradermal injections.

1. Take medication to patient's room.
2. Explain the medication's action and the procedure for administration to patient.
3. Check patient's Identaband and ask patient to state name.
4. Wash your hands.
5. Select the site of injection.
6. Cleanse the area with an alcohol wipe, wiping in circular area from inside to outside.
7. Take off needle guard and place on tray.
8. Grasp patient's forearm from underneath and gently pull the skin taut.
9. Insert the needle at 10- to 15-degree angle with the bevel of needle facing up.
10. Inject medication slowly. Observe for wheals and blanching at the site.
11. Withdraw the needle, wiping the area gently with a dry 2×2 bandage to prevent dispersing medication into the subcutaneous tissue.
12. Return the patient to a comfortable position.
13. Discard supplies in appropriate area.
14. Chart the medication and site used.

☆B. Administering subcutaneous (sub q) injections.

1. Take medication to patient's room.
2. Set tray on a clean surface, not the bed.
3. Check patient's Identaband and ask patient to state name.
4. Explain action of medication and procedure of administration.
5. Provide privacy when injection site is other than on the arm.
6. Wash your hands.
7. Select site for injection by identifying anatomical landmarks. Remember to alternate sites each time injections are given.
8. Cleanse area with alcohol wipe. Using a circular motion cleanse from inside outward.

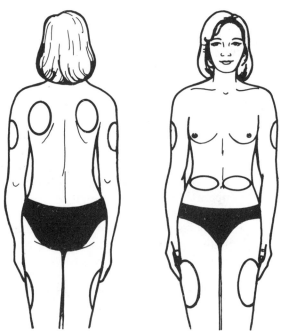

Rotate sites for subcutaneous injections given on a continuing basis.

9. Take off needle guard.
10. Express any air bubbles from syringe.
11. Insert the needle at a 45-degree angle.
12. Pull back on the plunger.
13. Inject the medication slowly.
14. Withdraw needle quickly and massage area with alcohol wipe to aid absorption and lessen bleeding. Put on Bandaid if needed.
15. Return patient to a position of comfort.
16. Discard used supplies in proper areas.
17. Chart the medication and site used.

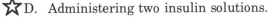C. Administering insulin injections.

1. Gather equipment and check medication orders, injection site, and rotation chart. Insulin does not need to be refrigerated.
2. Wash your hands.
3. Obtain specific insulin syringe for strength of insulin being administered (U100).
4. Rotate insulin bottle between hands to bring solution into suspension.
5. Wipe top of insulin bottle with alcohol.
6. Take off needle guard.
7. Pull plunger of syringe down to desired amount of medication and inject that amount of air into the insulin bottle.
8. Draw up ordered amount of insulin into syringe.
9. Expel air from syringe.
10. Replace needle guard.
11. Check medication card, bottle, and syringe with another RN for accuracy.
12. Take medications to patient's room.
13. Double-check site of last injection with patient.
14. Provide privacy.
15. Wash your hands.
16. Follow protocol for administration of medications by subcutaneous injections.

D. Administering two insulin solutions.

1. Follow steps 1 to 6 above.
2. Inject prescribed amount of air into intermediate acting (NPH, lente) or long acting (PZI, ultralente) bottle.
3. Pull needle out of insulin bottle and withdraw plunger to prescribed regular insulin dosage.
4. Inject air into regular bottle and withdraw medication.
5. Expel all air bubbles.

6. Insert needle into second insulin bottle taking care not to push any regular insulin into bottle. This can be avoided by putting pressure on plunger with your small finger when inserting into bottle.
7. Invert bottle and pull back on plunger to obtain prescribed amount of insulin. Remember the total insulin dose will include the amount of regular insulin already drawn up into syringe.
8. Follow steps 9 to 16 above to complete procedure.

INSULIN TYPES AND ACTION

TYPES	ONSET	PEAK	DURATION
Rapid Acting			
Regular	½ to 1	2 to 4	6 to 8
Semilente	½ to 1	2 to 8	10 to 16
Intermediate Acting			
NPH	1 to 1½	8 to 12	24
Lente	1 to 1½	8 to 12	24
Long Acting			
Protamine zinc (PZI)	4 to 8	14 to 20	24 to 36
Ultralente	4 to 8	16 to 24	36

E. Administering intramuscular (IM) injections.

1. Take medication to patient's room. Check room number against medication card or sheet.
2. Set tray on a clean surface, not the bed.
3. Explain the procedure to patient.
4. Check patient's Identaband and have patient state name.
5. Provide privacy for patient.
6. Wash your hands.
7. Select the site of injection by identifying anatomical landmarks. Remember to alternate sites each time injections are given.
8. Cleanse the area with alcohol wipe. Using a circular motion, cleanse from inside outward.
9. Hold the syringe; take off needle cover.
10. Express air bubbles from syringe. Some clinicians suggest leaving a small air bubble at the tip so that all medicine will be expelled.
11. Insert the needle at 90-degree angle.

12. Pull back on plunger. If blood returns, you know you have entered a blood vessel and need to reposition the needle and aspirate again.
13. Inject the medication slowly.
14. Withdraw the needle and massage the area with an alcohol wipe. Put on a Bandaid, if needed.
15. Return patient to a comfortable position.
16. Discard supplies in appropriate area.
17. Chart the medication and site used.

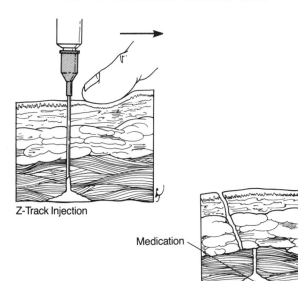

Z-Track Injection

Medication

Z-track is used to prevent tracking of medications on the skin.

☆F. Administering IM Injections Using Z-Track Method
  1. Used for iron injections.
  2. Draw up prescribed medication into syringe.
  3. Draw up 0.3 to 0.5 cc of air into syringe.
  4. Replace needle with 3-inch needle to penetrate deep into muscle.
  5. Pull skin laterally away from injection site.
  6. Cleanse site with alcohol.
  7. Insert needle.
  8. Inject medication slowly—and wait ten seconds keeping skin taut.
  9. Withdraw needle and then release skin.
  10. Discard supplies in appropriate area.
  11. Chart medication and site used.

Administering Medications to the Skin

Preparation

A. Observe skin for open lesions, rashes, or areas of erythema.
B. Check for allergies.

Procedure

☆A. Obtain patient's medication record. Medication record may be a drug card, medication sheet, or drug Kardex, depending on the method of dispensing medications in your facility.
B. Compare the medication record with the most *recent* physician's order.
C. Wash your hands.
D. Gather necessary equipment including gloves or tongue blade as needed.
E. Remove the medication from the drug box or tray on medication cart.
F. Compare the label on the medication tube or jar to the medication record.
G. Place medication tube or jar (include a tongue blade with jar) on a tray if not using medication cart.
H. Take medication to patient's room.
I. Wash your hands.
J. Provide patient privacy.
K. Squeeze medication from a tube or, using a tongue blade, take ointment out of jar.
L. Spread a small, smooth, thin quantity of medication evenly over patient's skin surface using your fingers or a tongue blade.
M. Protect skin surface with a dressing, if needed, so that medication cannot rub off.
N. Cleanse skin surface with soap and water between medication applications, unless contraindicated by patient's condition.
O. Return medication to appropriate storage area.
P. Check to see that patient is comfortable before leaving room.
Q. Wash hands.
R. Chart administration.

Administering a Topical Vasodilator

Procedure

⭐A. Take medication to patient's room.
B. Wash your hands.
C. Provide patient privacy.
D. Put on gloves to prevent absorbing any medication yourself.
E. Obtain premeasured paper, which accompanies medication tube.
F. Place prescribed medication directly on paper (usually one-half to one-inch strip).
G. Apply medicated paper to anterior surface of chest.
H. You may apply medicated paper to any area of the body; however, most patients feel the medication works better if applied to the chest surface.
I. Alternate areas of the chest with each dose of medication.
J. Return medication to appropriate storage area.
K. Check to see that patient is comfortable before leaving room.
L. Wash hands.
M. Chart administration.

Mathematic Conversions

Approximate Equivalents

A. The metric system is the universal system of weights and measures.
B. Apothecary and metric do not use same size units; denominations of one system not compatible with the other.
C. Equivalency tables established to list measurement denominations of one system in terms of another. (See Appendix 1.)
   1. Conversion from one system to another can be computed, but is not equivalent in absolute terms.
   2. If there is occasion to compute, have computations checked by another licensed nurse.
      a. Do not compute unless allowed to do so by your state's Nurse Practice Act.
      b. Check hospital policy for further guidelines.

Computation

A. Drugs are not always labeled clearly as to number of tablets to administer so computation may be necessary. Always have your computation checked by another licensed nurse.
B. Method.
   1. Both desired (ordered) dose and dose on hand must be in same unit of measurement, e.g., grains, grams, milligrams.
   2. If not same, convert so that unit of measure is the same.
      a. Refer to conversion table. (Appendix 1.)
      b. To convert one measure unit to another, basic equivalencies must be memorized.
   3. After converting, divide desired dose by dose on hand to find amount to administer.

Calculation of Dosages

A. Using equivalent tables to calculate drug dosages.
   1. To convert milligrams to grains, use the following formula:

   Example: Convert 180 milligrams to grains.

   $$\frac{1 \text{ gr}}{\text{mg in gr}} = \frac{\text{dose desired}}{\text{dose on hand}}$$

   $$\frac{1}{60} = \frac{x}{180}$$

   $$60x = 180$$

   $$x = 3 \text{ grains}$$

2. You may also make this conversion as a ratio:

1 gr:60 mg: :x gr:180 mg   60x = 180

x = 3 grains

3. Check equivalency tables in the drug supplement.

B. Calculating oral dosages of drugs.

1. To calculate oral dosages, use the following formula:

$$\frac{D}{H} = X$$

where D = dose desired
H = dose on hand
X = dose to be administered

Example: Give 500 mg of ampicillin when the dose on hand is in capsules containing 250 mg.

$$\frac{500 \text{ mg}}{250 \text{ mg}} = 2 \text{ capsules}$$

2. To calculate oral dosages of liquids, use the following formula:

$$\frac{D}{H} \times Q = X$$

where Q = quantity

Example: Give 375 mg of ampicillin when it is supplied as 250 mg/5 ml.

$$\frac{375 \text{ mg}}{250 \text{ mg}} \times 5$$

$$1.5 \times 5 = 7.5 \text{ ml}$$

You can also set up a direct proportion and following the algebraic principle, cross multiply:

$$\frac{375 \text{ mg}}{x} = \frac{250 \text{ mg}}{5 \text{ ml}}$$

$$250x = 1875$$

x = 7.5 ml (of strength 250 mg/ 5 ml)

C. Calculating parenteral dosages of drugs.

1. To calculate parenteral dosages, use the following formula:

$$\frac{D}{H} \times Q = X$$

Example: Give patient 40 mg gentamicin. On hand is a multidose vial with a strength of 80 mg/2 ml.

$$\frac{40}{80} \times 2 = 1 \text{ ml}$$

2. Check your calculations before drawing up medication.

Governing Laws

Federal Food, Drug, and Cosmetic Act of 1938

A. The act is an update of the Food and Drug Act first passed in 1906.

B. It designates *United States Pharmacopeia* and *National Formulary* as official standards.

C. The federal government has the power to enforce standards.

D. Provisions of the act.

1. Drug manufacturer must provide adequate evidence of drug's safety.

2. Correct labeling and packaging of drugs.

E. Amended in 1952 to include control of barbiturates by restricting prescription refills.

F. Amended in 1962 to require substantial investigation of drug and evidence that drug is effective in terms of labeling claims.

Harrison Narcotic Act of 1914

A. Provisions of the act.

1. Regulates manufacture, importation, and sale of opium, cocaine, and their derivatives.

2. Amendments have added addictive synthetic drugs to the regulated drug listing.

B. Applications of the act.

1. Individuals who produce, sell, dispense (pharmacists), and prescribe (dentists, physicians) these drugs must be licensed and registered; prescriptions must be in triplicate.

2. Hospitals order drugs on special blanks that bear hospital registry number. The following information is recorded for each dose:

   a. Name of drug.

   b. Amount of drug.

   c. Date and time drug obtained.

   d. Name of physician prescribing drug.

   e. Name of patient receiving drug.

   f. Nurse's signature and type of license (RN, LVN, or LPN).

The Controlled Substance Act of 1970

A. Provisions of the act.

1. Regulates potentially addictive drugs as to prescription, use, and possession.

   a. Regulations refer to use in hospital, office, research, and emergency situations.

   b. Regulations cover narcotics, cocaine, amphetamines, hallucinogens, barbiturates, and other sedatives.

2. Controlled drugs are placed in five different schedules or categorical listings, each governed by different regulations.

   a. The regulations govern manufacture, transport, and storage of the controlled drugs.

   b. The use of the drugs is controlled as to prescription, authorization, and mode of dispensation, and administration.

B. Application of the act for use of controlled drugs in hospital.

1. The nurse is to keep the stock supply of controlled drugs under lock and key.

   a. Nurse must sign for each dose (tablet, cc) of drug.

   b. Key is held by the nurse responsible for administration of medication.

   c. At the end of each shift, nurse must account for all controlled drugs in the stock supply.

2. Violations of the Controlled Substance Act.

   a. Violations are punishable by fine, imprisonment, or both.

   b. Nurses, upon conviction of violation, are subject to losing their licenses to practice nursing.

Prescription and Medication Orders

A. Prescription is a written order for dispensation of drugs that can be used only under physician's supervision.

B. Prescriptions outside the hospital.

1. Formula to pharmacist for dispensing drugs to patient.

2. Consists of four parts.

   a. Superscription (symbolized by Rx, meaning "take").

     (1) Patient's name.

     (2) Patient's address (required only for controlled drugs).

     (3) Age (required only if age is factor in dose preparation).

     (4) Date (must *always* be included).

   b. Inscription.

     (1) Specifies ingredients and their quantities.

     (2) May specify other ingredients necessary to specific drug form.

   c. Subscription—directions to pharmacist as to method of preparation.

   d. Signature—consists of two parts.

     (1) Accurate instructions to patient as to when, how, and in what quantities to take medication; typed on label.

     (2) Physician's signature and refill instructions.

C. Orders inside the hospital.

1. Physician writes medication order in book, file, or patient's chart; if given over phone, nurse writes verbal order which physician later signs.

2. Order consists of six parts.
   a. Name of drug.
   b. Dosage.
   c. Route of administration with time drug was given.
   d. Reason drug required (not always included).
   e. Length of time patient is to receive drug (not always included).
   f. Signature of individual who ordered drug.
      Example: Aspirin gr xPO q3h for pain for 3 days.

      D. Smith, M.D.

Informational Resources

Official Publications

A. A drug listed in the following publications is designated as official by the Federal Food, Drug, and Cosmetic Act (FDC).
   1. *The United States Pharmacopeia* (USP).
   2. *National Formulary* (NF).
   3. *Homeopathic Pharmacopeia of the United States.*

B. These publications establish standards of purity and other criteria for product acceptability; these standards are binding according to law.
C. Publications contain information on each drug entry.
   1. Source.
   2. Chemical and physical composition.
   3. Method of storage.
   4. General type or category.
   5. Range of dosage and usual therapeutic dosage.

Other Publications

A. *American Hospital Formulary* is a publication indexed by generic and proprietary names.
B. *Physicians' Desk Reference* (PDR).
   1. Annual publication with quarterly supplements.
   2. Handy source of information about dosage and drug precautions.

Miscellaneous Resources

A. Package inserts from manufacturers that accompany the product.
B. Pharmacist.
C. Physician.
D. Nursing journals.
E. Pharmaceutical and medical treatment texts.

Appendix 1. Conversion Tables

Table A. Household Equivalents (Volume)

Metric	Apothecary	Household
0.06 ml	1 minim	1 drop
5 (4) ml	1 fluidram	1 teaspoonful
15 ml	4 fluidrams	1 tablespoonful
30 ml	1 fluidounce	2 tablespoonfuls
180 ml	6 fluidounces	1 teacupful
240 ml	8 fluidounces	1 glassful

Table B. Apothecary Equivalents (Volume)

Metric		Apothecary
1	ml	= 15 minims
1	cc	= 15 minims
0.06	ml	= 1 minim
4	ml	= 1 fluidram
30	ml	= 1 fluidounce
500	ml	= 1 pint
1000	ml (1 L)	= 1 quart

Table C. Apothecary Equivalents (Weight)

Metric			Apothecary
1.0	Gm or	1000 mg	= gr xv
0.6	Gm or	600 mg	= gr x
0.5	Gm or	500 mg	= gr viiss
0.3	Gm or	300 mg	= gr v
0.2	Gm or	200 mg	= gr iii
0.1	Gm or	100 mg	= gr 1½
0.06	Gm or	60 mg	= gr 1
0.05	Gm or	50 mg	= gr ¾
0.03	Gm or	30 mg	= gr ½
0.015	Gm or	15 mg	= gr ¼
0.010	Gm or	10 mg	= gr ⅙
0.008	Gm or	8 mg	= gr ⅛
	4 gm		= 1 dr
	30 gm		= 1 oz
	1 kg		= 2.2 lbs

Appendix 2. Abbreviations and Symbols for Orders, Prescriptions, and Labels

$\overline{aa}$	of each		os	mouth
ac	before meals		oz or $\mathfrak{Z}$	ounce
ad lib	freely, as desired		pc	after meals
Ba	barium		per	by, through
bid	twice each day		prn	whenever necessary
$\overline{c}$	with		qh	every hour
C	carbon		qid	four times each day
Ca	calcium		qs	as much as required
Cl	chlorine		q2h	every two hours
dr or $\mathfrak{z}$	dram		q3h	every three hours
et	and		q4h	every four hours
GI	gastrointestinal		R_X	treatment, "take thou"
gt or gtt	drop(s)		$\overline{s}$	without
H_2O	water		$\overline{ss}$	one-half (½)
H_2O_2	hydrogen peroxide		stat	immediately
IM	intramuscular		tid	three times a day
in	inch		tsp	teaspoon
K	potassium		WBC	white blood cell
lb or #	pound		°	degree
m	minimum (a minim)		−	minus, negative, alkaline reaction
Mg	magnesium		+	plus, positive, acid reaction
N	nitrogen, normal		%	percent
Na	sodium		v	roman numeral five
NPO	nothing by mouth		vii	roman numeral seven
od	everyday		ix	roman numeral nine
oob	out of bed		xiii	roman numeral thirteen

Nutrition

Essential Body Nutrients

Carbohydrates

A. Chief source of energy.
B. Monosaccharides.
   1. Glucose, fructose, galactose.
   2. Easily digested.
C. Disaccharides: sucrose, lactose, maltose.
D. Polysaccharides.
   1. Starch, dextrin, glycogen, cellulose, hemicellulose.
   2. More complex and harder to digest.
E. Convert to glucose.
   1. Appears in body as blood sugar.
   2. Metabolizes in cells.
   3. Converted in liver to glycogen for storage.

Fats

A. Provide energy.
B. Act as carriers for fat-soluble vitamins.
C. Fatty acids are the basic components of fat and comprise two main groups.
   1. Saturated fatty acids usually come from animal sources.
   2. Unsaturated fatty acids primarily come from vegetables, nuts, or seed sources.
      a. This group contains three essential fatty acids.
      b. These acids are called "essential" because they are necessary to prevent a specific deficiency disease.
      c. The body cannot manufacture these acids. They are obtained only from the diet.
      d. These acids are called linoleic acid, arachidonic acid, and linolenic acid.

Proteins

A. Complex organic compounds that contain amino acids.
B. Critical to all aspects of growth and development of body tissues; necessary for the building of muscles, blood, skin, internal organs, hormones, and enzymes.
C. Source of energy.
   1. When there is insufficient carbohydrate or fat in the diet, protein is burned.
   2. When protein is spared, it is either used for tissue repair and maintenance or converted by the liver and stored as fat.
D. When digested and broken down, proteins form 22 amino acids.
   1. Amino acids are absorbed from the intestine into the bloodstream.
   2. They are carried to the liver for synthesis into the tissues and organs of the body.
E. Amino acids are the chemical basis for life, and if just one is missing, protein synthesis will decrease or even stop.
   1. *All* but eight can be produced by the body; these eight must be obtained from the diet.
   2. If all eight are present in a particular food, the food is a "complete protein"; foods that lack one or more are called "incomplete proteins."
   3. Most meat and dairy products are complete proteins; most vegetables and fruits are incomplete proteins.
   4. When several incomplete proteins are ingested, they should be combined carefully so that the result will be a balance yielding complete protein. For example, the combination of beans and rice is a complete protein food.
F. The National Research Council recommends that 0.42 grams of protein be consumed per day per 0.4 kg of body weight.

Water

A. While not specifically a nutrient, water is essential for survival.
   1. Water is involved in every body process from digestion and absorption to excretion.
   2. It is a major portion of circulation and is the transporter of nutrients throughout the body.
B. Body water performs three major functions.
   1. Water gives form to the body, comprising

from 50 to 75 percent of the body mass.

2. It provides the necessary environment for cell metabolism.

3. It maintains a stable body temperature.

C. Almost all foods contain water that is absorbed by the body.

D. The average adult body contains 59 liters of water and loses about 3 liters a day.

1. If a person suffers severe water depletion, dehydration and salt depletion can result and can eventually lead to death.

2. A person can survive longer without food than without water.

Vitamins

A. Vitamins are organic food substances and are essential in small amounts for growth, maintenance, and the functioning of body processes.

B. Vitamins are found only in living things—plants and animals—and usually cannot be synthesized by the human body.

C. Vitamins can be grouped according to the substance in which they are soluble.

D. The fat-soluble group includes vitamins A, D, E, and K.

E. The water-soluble vitamins include B_1, B_2, B_6, B_{12}, niacin, pantothenic acid, folacin, viotin, choline, mesoinositol, para-aminobenzoic acid, and ascorbic acid (vitamin C).

F. Vitamins have no caloric value, but they are as necessary to the body as any other basic nutrient.

1. Currently, there are about 20 substances identified as vitamins.

2. Recent research is concerned with identifying even more of these substances since they are so essential to survival.

G. The most commonly used are the listings of the Recommended Dietary Allowances (RDA), based on standards established by the National Academy of Sciences.

Minerals

A. Minerals are inorganic substances, widely prevalent in nature, and essential for metabolic processes.

B. Minerals are grouped according to the amount found in the body.

C. Major minerals include calcium, magnesium, sodium, potassium, phosphorus, sulfur, and chlorine, all of which have a known function in the body.

D. Trace minerals are iron, copper, iodine, manganese, cobalt, zinc, and molybdenum and their function in the body remains unclear.

E. There remains another group of trace minerals found in scanty amounts in the body and whose function is also unclear.

F. Minerals form 60 to 90 percent of all inorganic material in the body, and are found in bones, teeth, soft tissue, muscle, blood, and nerve cells.

G. Minerals act on organs and in metabolic processes.

1. They serve as catalysts for many reactions such as controlling muscle responses, maintaining the nervous system, and regulating acid-base balance.

2. They assist in transmitting messages, maintaining cardiac stability, and regulating the metabolism and absorption of other nutrients.

H. Even though they are considered separately, all minerals work synergistically with other minerals, and their actions are interrelated.

1. A deficiency in one mineral will affect the action of others in the body.

2. Adequate minerals must be ingested because a mineral deficiency can result in severe illness.

3. Excessive amounts of minerals can throw the body out of balance.

4. Additional information can be found in section on Fluid and Electrolyte Balance.

Essential Body Nutrients

Carbohydrates   Monosaccharides
            Glucose, fructose, galactose
        Disaccharides
            Sucrose, lactose, maltose
        Polysaccharides
            Starch, dextrin, glycogen,
            cellulose, hemicellulose

Fats	Linoleic acid, linolenic acid, arachidonic acid
Proteins	Amino acids Phenylalanine, lysine, isoleucine, leucine, methionine, valine, tryptophan, threonine
Vitamins	Fat-soluble Vitamins A, D, E, and K Water-soluble Vitamins B_1, B_2, B_6, B_{12}, niacin, pantothenic acid, folacin, biotin, choline, mesoinositol, para-aminobenzoic acid, and vitamin C
Minerals	Major elements Calcium, chlorine, iron, magnesium, phosphorus, potassium, sodium, sulfur Trace elements
Water	

Foods Rich in Fat- and Water-Soluble Vitamins

Foods Rich in Fat-Soluble Vitamins

Vitamin A—liver, egg yolk, whole milk, butter, fortified margarine, green and yellow vegetables, fruits

Vitamin D—fortified milk and margarine, fish oils

Vitamin E—vegetable oils and green vegetables

Vitamin K—egg yolk, leafy green vegetables, liver, cheese

Foods Rich in Water-Soluble Vitamins

Vitamin C—citrus fruits, tomatoes, broccoli, cabbage

Thiamine (B_1)—lean meat such as beef, pork, liver; whole grain cereals and legumes

Riboflavin (B_2)—milk, organ meats, enriched grains

Niacin—meat, beans, peas, peanuts, enriched grains

Pyridoxine (B_6)—yeast, wheat, corn, meats, liver, and kidney

Cobalamin (B_{12})—lean meat, liver, kidney

Folic acid—leafy green vegetables, eggs, liver

Assimilation of Nutrients

Gastrointestinal Tract

A. The main functions of the gastrointestinal system consist of the following.
   1. Secretion of enzymes and electrolytes to break down raw materials that are ingested.
   2. Movement of ingested products through the system.
   3. Complete digestion of nutrients.
   4. Absorption of nutrients into the blood.
   5. Storage of nutrients.
   6. Excretion of the end products of digestion.
B. Mechanical digestion.
   1. Begins in the mouth with chewing and swallowing.
   2. Nutrients are churned, and peristaltic waves move the material through the stomach.
   3. At intervals, with relaxation of the pyloric sphincter, they move into the duodenum.
   4. Peristaltic waves move the mass through the small intestines where some absorption occurs.
   5. The large intestine provides for the absorption of nutrients and the elimination of waste products.
      a. Vitamins K and B_{12}, riboflavin, and thiamin are formed.
      b. Water is absorbed from the fecal mass.
C. Chemical digestion relies on the action of digestive enzymes and other substances.
   1. See table of Major Enzymes of Digestion.
   2. Hydrochloric acid is secreted by the stomach. Aids pepsin in its action on protein.

Major Enzymes of Digestion

Enzyme	Source/ Secretion	Substance Acted On
Ptyalin	Oral/Saliva	Starch
Maltose	Oral/Saliva	Maltose
Pepsin	Gastric	Protein
Lipase	Gastric	Fat
Rennin	Gastric	Casein (protein in milk)
Trypsin	Pancreatic	Protein
Steapsin	Pancreatic	Fats
Amylopsin	Pancreatic	Starch
Amylase	Intestinal	Starch
Maltase	Intestinal	Maltose
Lactase	Intestinal	Lactose
Sucrase	Intestinal	Sucrose
Erepsin	Intestinal	Proteins
Enterokinase	Intestinal	Proteins

Accessory Organs

A. The accessory organs of the gastrointestinal tract play an important role in the utilization of nutrients.

B. The liver plays a major role in the metabolism of carbohydrates, fats, and proteins.
   1. Liver converts glucose to glycogen and stores it. It reconverts glycogen to glucose when the body requires higher blood sugar. The process of releasing carbohydrates (end products) into the bloodstream is called glycogenolysis.
   2. Fats are metabolized through the process of oxidation of fatty acids and the formation of acetoacetic acid.
   3. Lipoproteins, cholesterol, and phospholipids are formed, and carbohydrates and protein are converted to fats.
   4. Proteins are metabolized.
   5. The formation of urea and plasma proteins is completed.
   6. Bile is secreted.

C. The gallbladder's primary function is to act as a reservoir for bile.

   1. Bile emulsifies fats through constant secretion.
   2. Secretion rate is 500 to 1000 ml every 24 hours.

D. The pancreas secretes pancreatic juices that contain enzymes for the digestion of carbohydrates, fats, and proteins. These enzymes are activated in the small intestine.

Nutritional Concepts

Normal and Therapeutic Nutrition

A. Normal nutrition.
   1. A guide for determining adequate nutrition is the U.S. Department of Agriculture recommended daily dietary allowances.
      a. The guide is scientifically designed for the maintenance of healthy people in the United States.
      b. The values of the caloric and nutrient requirements given in the guide are used in assessing nutritional states.
      c. Stress periods in the life cycle, which require alterations in the allowances, should be considered during the planning of menus.
   2. The basic four food groups are described in *A Daily Food Guide: the Basic Four* (see Appendix 2).
      a. Choices in four food groups are offered to meet the nutrient recommendations during the life cycle. (Caloric requirement is not included.)
      b. Basic nutrients in each food group should be related to dietary needs during the life cycle when menus are planned for each age group.

B. Therapeutic nutrition.
   1. The therapeutic or prescription diet is a modification of the nutritional needs based on the disease condition and/or the excess or deficit nutrition state.
   2. Combination diets, which include alterations in minerals, vitamins, proteins, carbohydrates, and fats, as well as fluid and texture, are prescribed in therapeutic nutrition.

3. Although not all such diets will be included in this review, study of the selected diet concepts will enable you to combine two or more diets when necessary.

C. Normal and therapeutic nutrition considerations.
   1. Cultural, socioeconomic, and psychological influences, as well as physiological requirements, must be considered for effective nutrition.
   2. In any given situation, the nutrition requirements must be considered within the context of the bio-psycho-social needs of an individual.

Nutritional Problems in the Hospital

A. Nutrition is frequently neglected as an important part of patient care.

B. The nurse must consistently assess the patient (see Appendix 1) to assist in determining needed diet alterations.
   1. Inability to feed self or absence of dentures.
   2. Feelings of depression or fear.
   3. Unpleasant environmental factors prior to meals.
   4. Pain or nausea.

Providing Appropriate Nutrition

1. Verify dietary order.
2. Notify charge nurse and/or physician if patients' needs are not being met.
3. Determine patients' food preferences.
4. Check all diet trays before serving to ensure the diet provided is the one ordered.
5. Ensure that hot food is hot and cold food is cold.
6. Keep food trays attractive. Avoid spilling liquids on tray.
7. Position the patient in a chair or up in bed (unless otherwise ordered) to assist in feeding.
8. Assist the patient with cutting meat and opening milk cartons as needed.
9. Feed the patient if necessary.

Malnutrition Disorders

A. Kwashiorkor—caused by a lack of protein; frequently seen in ages one to three, when high-protein intake is necessary.

B. Nutritional marasmus—a disease caused by a deficiency of food intake. It is a form of starvation.

C. Vitamin A deficiency—night blindness may progress to xerophthalmia and, finally, keratomalacia.

D. Vitamin C deficiency: scurvy—symptoms begin with muscle tenderness as walls of capillaries become fragile. Hemorrhage of vessels results.

E. Vitamin D deficiency: rickets—caused because vitamin D is necessary for adequate calcium absorption by the bones.

F. Thiamine deficiency: beriberi—primarily a disease of rice-eating people; symptoms include numbness in extremities and exhaustion.

G. Niacin deficiency: pellagra—symptoms include dermatitis, diarrhea, dementia, and, finally, death.

H. Iodine deficiency—leads to hyperplasia of the thyroid gland, or goiter.

Recommended Nutrient Requirements

Total Calories

2800 for tissue repair; 6000 for extensive repair

Protein

50 to 75 g/day early in postoperative period 100 to 200 g/day if needed for new tissue synthesis

CHO—sufficient in quantity to meet calorie needs and allow protein to be used for tissue repair

Fat—not excessive as it leads to poor tissue healing and susceptibility to infection

Vitamins

Vitamin C—up to 1 g/day
Vitamin B—increased above normal
Vitamin K—normal amounts

Diabetic Exchange Diets

Food Group	Unit of Exchange	Calories	Foods Allowed
Milk:			
whole	1 cup	170	1 cup whole milk = 1 cup
skim	1 cup	80	Skim milk and 2 fat exchanges
Fruit	Varies according to calories allotted	40	Fresh or canned without sugar or syrup
Vegetables:			
A	1 cup	Vary	Green, leafy vegetables; tomatoes
B	½ cup	35	Vegetables other than green, leafy
Bread	1 slice	70	Can exchange cereals, starch items, some vegetables
Meat	1 ounce	75	Lean meats, egg, cheese, seafood
Fat	1 teaspoon	45	1 teaspoon butter or mayonnaise = bacon, oil, olives, avocado
Unlimited foods:			Coffee, tea, bouillon, spices, flavorings

Tube Feeding for Nutrients

Characteristics

A. Purpose is to maintain adequate food-fluid intake.
B. Reasons for procedure
   1. Patient is unconscious.
   2. Refusal to take in fluids or solid foods (anorexic).
   3. Trauma to upper GI tract.
   4. Patient is unable to chew or swallow.

☆ Nasogastric Tube Insertion

A. Check order for tube feeding.
B. Warm feeding to room temperature.
C. Discuss procedure with the patient.
D. Demonstrate and display items to be used in order to allay the patient's fear and to gain cooperation.
E. Wash your hands.
F. Position the patient at 45-degree angle or higher.
G. Examine nostrils and select the most patent nostril by having the patient breathe through each one.
H. Measure from earlobe to tip of nose to ziphoid process of sternum to determine appropriate length for tube insertion. If tube is to go below stomach, add additional 15 to 25 cm. Mark point on tube with tape.
I. Lubricate first 10 cm of tube with water-soluble lubricant.
J. Insert tube through nostril to back of throat and ask the patient to swallow. Sips of water may aid in advancing tubing past oropharynx.
K. Continue advancing tube until taped mark is reached.
L. Check position of tube.
   1. Inject 10 cc of air through nasogastric tube and listen with the stethoscope over stomach for a rush of air.
   2. Aspirate gastric contents if still unsure (sometimes difficult with small-bore tubes).

3. X-ray confirmation. If nasoduodenal or nasojejunal feedings required, patient should have x-ray to confirm correct placement.

4. Tape tube securely to nose and to cheek.

M. Remain with and talk with the patient until the anxiety level is decreased (tube insertion often raises anxiety).

☆ Tube Feeding Administration

1. Obtain order from the physician for appropriate formula (calories and/or amount).

2. Send requisition for formula to diet kitchen.

3. Check early in shift to ensure adequate formula is available.

4. Warm formula to room temperature using a microwave or set formula in basin of hot water.

5. Assemble feeding equipment. If using bag, fill with ordered amount of formula.

6. Explain procedure to the patient and assure privacy.

7. Place the patient on right side in high-Fowler's position.

8. Aspirate stomach contents to determine amount of residual. Return aspirated contents to stomach to prevent electrolyte imbalance.

9. Check position of tube by injecting 10 cc of air, if gastric contents not available.

10. Pinch the tubing to prevent air from entering stomach.

11. Attach barrel of syringe to nasogastric tube.

12. Fill syringe with formula. (If using feeding bag, adjust drip rate to infuse over 30 minutes.)

13. Hold syringe no more than 39 cm above patient.

14. Allow formula to infuse slowly (between 20 to 35 minutes) through the tubing.

15. Follow tube feeding with water in amount ordered.

16. Clamp end of the tube.

17. Wash tray and return it to client's bedside.

18. Give water in between feedings if tube feeding is the sole source of nutrition.

☆ Nasogastric Tube Irrigation

1. Obtain a disposable irrigation set or emesis basin for irrigation solution, a 20-cc syringe, and a normal saline irrigation solution.

2. Wash your hands.

3. Place patient in a semi-Fowler's position.

4. Check for nasogastric tube placement by instilling air and listening for "woosh" sound.

5. Draw up 20-cc normal saline into the irrigating syringe.

6. Gently instill the normal saline into the nasogastric tube. Do not force the solution.

7. Withdraw the 20-cc irrigation solution and empty into basin.

8. Repeat the procedure twice.

9. Record on I&O sheet the irrigation solution that has not been returned.

☆ Continuous Tube Feedings (Dobhoff, Keofeed Tubes)

1. Insert tube (tubes are weighted at the distal end with mercury or tungsten) or check patency of existing tube.

2. Irrigate feeding tube with sterile water or saline at least every eight hours.

3. Administer formula at prescribed infusion rate. Infusion pumps are used to maintain continuous flow.

4. Avoid keeping formula at room temperature for longer than four hours to prevent spoilage and bacterial contamination.

5. Routinely assess the abdomen for abdominal distention and bowel sounds.

6. Keep patient in semi-Fowler's position.

7. Turn off flow when placing patient supine.

☆ Gastrostomy Feeding

1. Assess gastric contents to determine amount per intermittent feeding. Hold feeding if more than 50–100 cc.

2. Feed slowly for intermittent feeding or keep at prescribed rate for continuous feeding.

3. Observe gastrostomy tube insertion site for signs of dislodging, infection, or skin breakdown.

4. Provide site care; wash area with warm water

and soap.

5. Apply skin protective barrier. Cover area with sterile dressing.

Therapeutic/Prescription Diets

Diets Associated with Carbohydrate Control

A. The source of glucose from food: carbohydrate—100 percent; protein—58 percent; fat—10 percent. The control of glucose in diets is based on these three nutrients.

B. Hypoglycemic diet.
   1. A hypoglycemic diet is utilized to reduce stimulation of excessive insulin by avoiding highly concentrated carbohydrate foods.
      a. Foods prescribed are high protein, high fat. and low carbohydrate.
      b. Foods not allowed are high carbohydrate, for example, sugar, syrup, candy.
   2. A diabetic diet modifies the insulin disorder and controls sugar intake.
      a. Foods prescribed usually use food exchange method
      b. Foods not allowed are refined sugars.

Diets Associated with Protein Control

A. Low protein diet.
   1. Utilized for renal impairments (uremia), hepatic coma, and cirrhosis (according to individual requirements).
   2. Purpose of diet: to control by limiting protein intake the end (breakdown) products of protein metabolism which are disturbing the fluid and electrolytes and/or acid-base balances.
   3. Diet allowances/requirements.
      a. The number of grams of protein allowed is stated for each diet.
      b. Examples of high protein foods to be avoided: eggs, meat, milk and milk products.

B. High protein diet.
   1. Utilized for tissue building conditions, correction of protein deficiencies, burns, liver diseases, malabsorption syndromes, undernutrition, and maternity.

   2. Purpose of diet: to correct protein loss, and/or maintain and rebuild tissues by increasing intake of high quality protein food sources.
   3. Protein supplements are ordered by physician for individual needs. Examples of protein supplements: Sustagen, Meritene, Proteinum.

C. Amino acid metabolism abnormalities diet.
   1. Utilized for phenylketonuria (PKU), galactosemia, and lactose intolerance.
   2. Purpose of diet: to reduce and/or eliminate the offending enzyme in the food intake of protein and utilize substitute nutrient foods.
   3. The main source of enzymes for the three diseases is milk. Milk and milk products must be avoided and substitutes used to meet daily allowances.

Diets Associated with Fat Control

A. Restricted cholesterol diet.
   1. Utilized for cardiovascular diseases, diabetes mellitus, high serum cholesterol levels.
   2. Purpose of diet: to decrease the blood cholesterol level and/or maintain blood cholesterol at a normal level by restricting foods high in cholesterol.
   3. High cholesterol foods to be restricted or avoided (primarily originating from animal sources).
      a. Saturated fats.
      b. Examples: egg yolk, shell fish, organ meats, bacon, pork, avocado, olives.
   4. Low cholesterol foods allowed (primarily originating from plant sources).
      a. Polyunsaturated fats.
      b. Examples: vegetable oils, raw or cooked vegetables, fruits, lean meats, fowl.

B. Modified fat diet.
   1. Utilized according to individual tolerance in malabsorption syndromes, cystic fibrosis, gall bladder disease, obstructive jaundice, and liver diseases.
   2. Purpose of diet: to lower fat content in diet to stop contractions of diseased organs; to reduce fat content where there is inade-

quate absorption of fat.

3. Diet allowances/requirements.

   a. Moderate fat diet.

      (1) Foods to be avoided: gravies, fat meat and fish, cream, fried foods, rich pastries.

      (2) Foods allowed: eggs, lean meat, butter/margarine, cheese.

   b. Low fat diet.

      (1) Foods to be avoided: gravies, fat meat and fish, cream, fried foods, rich pastries, whole milk products, cream soups, salad and cooking oils, nuts, chocolate.

      (2) Foods allowed: eggs (2 to 3 per week), lean meat, butter/margarine.

   c. Fat free diet.

      (1) No fat is allowed in diet; fatty meats are omitted from diet.

      (2) Foods to be avoided; eggs, butter/margarine.

      (3) Foods allowed: vegetables, fruits, lean meats, fowl, fish, bread, cereal.

C. High polyunsaturated fat diet.

1. Utilized for cardiovascular diseases.

2. Purpose of diet: to reduce intake of saturated fats and to increase intake of foods rich in polyunsaturated fats. (Physician usually prescribes caloric level as well as restrictions.)

3. Foods to be avoided: foods originating from animal sources, selected peanuts, olives, avocado, coconuts, chocolate, cashew nuts.

4. Foods allowed: foods originating from vegetable sources (except for those named above); margarine, corn/soybean/safflower oil, fresh ground peanut butter, nuts (except cashews).

5. Frequently used in conjunction with restricted cholesterol diet.

   a. Select foods that are compatible with both diets.

   b. Shellfish is allowed in high polyunsaturated fat diet but is restricted in low cholesterol diet.

Diets Associated with Renal Disease

A. Low protein, essential amino acid diet (modified Giovannetti diet: 20 gm. protein, 1500 mg. potassium).

1. Utilized for renal failure.

2. Purpose of diet: to prevent electrolytes and byproducts of metabolism from accumulating to a fatal level between artificial kidney treatments.

3. Foods allowed:

   a. Eggs (1 daily).

   b. Milk (6 ounces).

   c. Low protein bread.

   d. Fruit (2 to 4 servings): apples, peaches, pears, cherries, pineapple, strawberries, grapefruit, grapes.

   e. Vegetables (2 to 4 servings): usually any vegetable.

   f. Free list: for calories—butter, oil, jelly, candy with chocolate; tea, coffee.

4. Foods restricted or not allowed:

   a. Meat: chicken, roast beef, fish, lamb, veal.

   b. Peanuts; bread other than low protein bread.

B. Low calcium diet.

1. Utilized to prevent formation of renal calculi (96 percent calculi are calcium compounds).

2. Purpose of diet: to decrease the total daily intake of calcium to prevent further stone formation. Total 400 mg. calcium instead of normal 800 mg. calcium per day.

3. Foods allowed:

   a. Milk (1 cup daily).

   b. Fruit juices, tea, coffee.

   c. Eggs (1 daily); fats.

   d. Fresh fruits; vegetables (except dried).

4. Foods restricted:

   a. Rye and whole grain breads and cereals.

   b. Dried fruits and vegetables (peas and beans).

   c. Fish, shellfish, dried and cured meats.

   d. Cheese, chocolate, nuts.

C. Acid ash diet.

1. Utilized to prevent precipitation of stone elements.

2. Purpose of diet: to establish well-balanced diet with total acid ash greater than total alkaline ash daily.
3. Foods allowed:
   a. Breads and cereals of any type.
   b. Fats.
   c. Fruits (1 serving), except those restricted.
   d. Vegetables; potatoes, noodles, rice.
   e. Meat, eggs, cheese, fish, fowl (2 servings).
   f. Spices
4. Foods restricted:
   a. Carbonated beverages.
   b. Foods containing baking powder or soda.
   c. Dried fruits, bananas, figs, raisins.
   d. Dried beans; carrots.
   e. Chocolate candy.
   f. Nuts, olives, pickles.

D. Low purine diet.
1. Utilized to prevent uric acid stones; also utilized for gout patients.
2. Purpose of diet: to restrict purine, which is the precursor of uric acid; 4 percent of urinary stones are composed of uric acid.
3. Foods allowed:
   a. Carbonated beverages, milk, tea, fruit juices.
   b. Breads, cereals.
   c. Cheese, eggs, fat.
   d. Most vegetables.
4. Foods restricted:
   a. Glandular meats, gravies.
   b. Fowl, fish, meat (restricted in amount).

Diets Associated with Vitamin Control

A. Diets adequate in caloric and nutrient requirements usually contain adequate amounts of vitamins.
B. Increased vitamin diet.
1. Utilized for treatment based on specific deficiencies of vitamins.
   a. Dietary increases are needed for patients with burns, healing wounds, raised temperatures, infections, pregnancy.
   b. Water-soluble vitamins may be prescribed for certain diseases such as cystic fibrosis and liver disease.
C. There are no specific diets associated with low vitamin control.

Selected Diets Associated with Mineral Control

A. Restricted sodium diet.
1. Utilized for hypertension, hepatitis, congestive heart failure, renal deficiencies, cirrhosis of liver, adrenal corticoid treatment.
2. Purpose of diet: to correct and/or control the retention of sodium and water in the body by limiting sodium intake. May be done strictly by food restriction or in combination with medications.
3. Restriction varies from eliminating salt in cooking or at the table to strict food restrictions of any product containing sodium such as soda bicarbonate.

B. Increased or high potassium diet.
1. Utilized for diabetic acidosis, extended use of certain diuretic drugs, burns (after first 48 hours), vomiting and fevers.
2. Purpose of diet: to replace potassium loss from the body. (Severe potassium loss is managed with intravenous therapy.)

C. High iron diet.
1. Utilized for anemias (hemorrhagic, nutritional, pernicious), postgastrectomy syndrome, malabsorption syndrome.
2. Purpose of diet: to replace a deficit of iron due to either inadequate intake or chronic blood loss.
3. Foods high in iron content: organ meats (especially liver), meats, egg yolks, whole wheat, seafood, leafy green vegetables, nuts, dried fruit, legumes.

Definitions of Sodium Restrictions

Categories
- Mild: 2 to 3 g sodium
- Moderate: 1000 mg sodium
- Strict: 500 mg sodium
- Severe: 250 mg sodium

Foods High in Sodium

Table salt and all prepared salts, such as
   celery salt
Smoked meats and salted meats
Most frozen or canned vegetables with added
   salt
Butter, margarines, and cheese
Quick-cooking cereals
Shellfish and frozen or salted fish
Seasonings and sauces
Canned soups
Chocolates and cocoa
Beets, celery, and selected greens (spinach)
Foods with salt added, such as potato chips,
   popcorn

Foods High in Potassium

Fruit juices such as orange, grapefruit,
   banana, apple
Instant, dry coffee powder
Egg, legumes, whole grains
Fish, especially fresh halibut and codfish
Pork, beef, lamb, veal, chicken
Milk, skim and whole
Dried dates, prunes
Bouillon and meat broths

Diets Associated with Fiber Control

A. High residue (roughage) diets.
   1. Prescribed for constipation and diverticulosis (prescription varies with physician).
   2. Purpose of diet: to mechanically stimulate the gastrointestinal tract.
   3. Diet allowances/requirements.
      a. Foods high in residue.
         (1) Any meat or fish—fried, canned, or smoked; any poultry with skin.
         (2) Cheese.
         (3) Fat in any form.
         (4) Milk and fruit juices.
         (5) Whole wheat breads, unrefined bran, cereals, shredded wheat.
      b. Foods low in carbohydrates are usually high in residue.
B. Low residue (roughage) diets.

1. Utilized for ulcerative colitis, postoperative colon and rectal surgery, diverticulitis (when inflammation decreases diet may revert to high residue), rheumatic fever, diarrhea and enteritis.
2. Purpose of diet: to soothe and be non-irritating residue in the large intestine.
3. Diet allowances/requirements.
   a. Foods low in residue.
      (1) Ground, tender meat; fresh fish; any boiled, roasted, or broiled poultry without skin or fat.
      (2) Hard-boiled egg.
      (3) Creamed cottage cheese and mild cheeses.
      (4) Limited fat, crisp bacon, plain gravies.
      (5) Warm drinks (not iced); no milk.
      (6) Refined, strained, precooked cereals like pablum; enriched white bread; crackers; toast.
   b. Foods low in carbohydrates usually add high residue.

Bland Food Diets

A. These diets are presented in stages, with gradual addition of specific foods.
B. Frequent, small feedings during active stress periods; then regular meals and patterns should be established.
C. Utilized for duodenal ulcer, gastric ulcers, postoperative stomach surgery.
D. Purpose of diet: to promote the healing of the gastric mucosa by eliminating food sources that are chemically and mechanically irritating.
E. Diet allowances/requirements.
   1. Foods allowed.
      a. Milk, butter, eggs (not fried), custard, vanilla ice cream, cottage cheese.
      b. Cooked refined or strained cereal, enriched white bread.
      c. Jello; homemade creamed, pureed soups.
      d. Baked or broiled potatoes.
   2. Examples of foods that are eliminated.
      a. Spicy and highly seasoned foods.

b. Raw foods.

c. Very hot and very cold foods.

d. Gas-forming foods (varies with individuals).

e. Coffee, alcoholic beverages, carbonated drinks.

f. High fat contents (some butter and margarine allowed).

Diets Associated with Calorie Control

A. Restricted calorie diet.

1. Utilized in obesity, overnutrition in the aged, and specific conditions requiring weight reduction.

2. Purpose of diet: to reduce the caloric intake of food below the energy demands of the body so weight loss will occur. Psychological support and exercise are important components of therapy along with diet.

3. Individual diet plan is based on nutritional requirements for age group. Low caloric intakes may require nutrient supplements.

   a. Food exchange patterns are widely used for weight control diets.

   b. Aging adult requires less calories to maintain normal weight.

4. Foods restricted.

   a. CHO.

   b. Fat.

B. Increased calorie diet.

1. Utilized in burns, pregnancy, aging, childhood, surgery, undernutrition.

2. Purpose of diet: to meet the increased metabolic needs of the body. There is usually an increase in protein and vitamins when increased calories are ordered.

3. Foods allowed:

   a. Any food group.

   b. CHO, particularly high calorie.

Diets Associated with Surgery

A. Preoperative diet.

1. Purpose of diet.

   a. Maintenance of normal serum protein levels.

b. Provide adequate carbohydrate to maintain liver glycogen.

c. Provide adequate amino acids to promote wound healing.

d. Restore nitrogen balance if protein-depleted (burn, elderly, severely debilitated patient).

2. Recommended nutrient requirements.

   a. 0.8 to 1.5 gm of protein/kg body weight/day.

   b. 25 to 50 Kcal/kg/day.

      (1) A calorie is a unit of heat measurement defined as the amount of heat required to raise 1 kg of water 1°C.

      (2) One gram of protein equals 4 kilogram calories (Kcal).

3. Recommended diet.

   a. 2500 Kcal.

   b. A high energy, moderate protein diet.

   c. High protein supplements.

4. Elemental diet.

   a. Low residue diet.

   b. Contains synthetic mixture of CHO, amino acids, essential fatty acids with added minerals and vitamins.

   c. Bulk free, easily assimilated and absorbed.

   d. Replace clear liquid diet for patients with colon surgery.

   e. Diet products: Vivonex and Precision.

B. Postoperative surgical diets.

1. Purpose of diet.

   a. Promote wound healing by adequate protein intake.

   b. Avoid shock from decreased plasma proteins and circulating red blood cells by increasing protein intake.

   c. Prevent edema by adequate protein intake (maintains colloidal osmotic pressure).

   d. Promote bone healing in orthopedic surgery by adequate protein and mineral replacement.

   e. Prevent infection by adequate amino acid replacement (amino acids are involved in body defense mechanisms).

2. Recommended nutrient requirements.

a. Total calories: 2800 for tissue repair; 6000 for extensive repair.

b. Fluid intake.

(1) Uncomplicated surgery: 2000 to 3000/day.

(2) Complicated surgery (sepsis, renal damage): 3000 to 4000/day.

(3) Seriously ill with drainage: 7000/day.

3. Diet progresses from nothing by mouth (NPO) the day of surgery to a general diet. Phases/steps include:

a. A clear-liquid diet is 1000 to 1500 cc/day and is comprised of water, tea, broth, jello, and juices (avoid juices with pulp).

b. A full-liquid diet is clear liquids, milk and milk products, custard, puddings, creamed soups, sherbet, ice cream, and any fruit juice.

c. A soft diet is full liquid and, in addition, pureed vegetables, eggs (not fried), milk, cheese, fish, fowl, tender beef, veal, potatoes, and cooked fruit.

d. General diet, taking into consideration specific alterations necessary for client's health status.

Appendix 1. BASIC NUTRITIONAL ASSESSMENT

Assessment	Normal	Abnormal
Appetite	Remains unchanged	Recently increased or decreased Particular cravings
Weight	Previous weight maintained Normal for patient Appropriate for age and body build	Changed—recently increased or decreased Rapid or slow changes
Nutritional Intake	Adequate foods and fluids to supply body nutrients Nonallergic response to major food groups No pattern of fad diets Absence of drugs, chemicals, or other substances that influence appetite or metabolism	Elimination of certain food categories that results in limited nutrients Emphasis on some food groups (sugar) to the exclusion of others (vegetables) Allergic response to certain foods Constant use of fad diets to lose weight Use of drugs or chemicals that interferes with appetite nutrient assimilation Presence of emotional disorder (depression, anorexia, manic response) that interferes with food ingestion
Meal Patterns	Three to six home-prepared meals per day Adequate time and calm atmosphere for meals	Fast-food or packaged foods Missed meals, constant snacking, or over-eating Eating "on the run" or hurried
Physical Factors	Adequate chewing and swallowing capability Mouth and gums healthy so food can be ingested Physical exercise adequate for calorie intake	Teeth and/or gums in poor condition or ill-fitting dentures Swallowing impairs ingestion Inadequate physical exercise to burn calories

Assessment	Normal	Abnormal
Presence of Disease	No disease process that interferes with nutrient assimilation No congenital condition or postsurgery condition that interferes with nutrient assimilation	Disease present that interferes with ingestion, digestion, assimilation, or excretion Congenital condition, rehabilitation phase, or postsurgery that interferes with food assimilation
Sociocultural-Religious Factors	Ability to afford adequate foods in all food categories Cultural beliefs that do not eliminate whole food groups Religious beliefs that do not eliminate whole food groups Food does not lose all nutrient value in preparation	Economic position that precludes purchase of adequate foods Religious or cultural beliefs that interfere with receiving balanced diet (macrobiotic diets) Inadequate knowledge, experience, or intelligence to prepare healthy meals.
Elimination Schedule	Regular, adequate elimination of foods Absence of constant flatus, discharge, or mucus	Irregular and/or painful elimination Presence of constant flatus Presence of discharge, blood, or mucus

Appendix 2. The Basic Four Food Groups

Milk Group

Foods Included

- ☐ Milk: whole, evaportated, skim, dry, buttermilk
- ☐ Cheese: cottage, cream, cheddar, natural or processed
- ☐ Ice cream

Contribution to Diet Milk is a leading source of calcium, which is needed for bones and teeth. It also provides a high-quality protein, riboflavin, vitamin A (if milk is whole or fortified), and other nutrients.

Amounts Recommended Some milk every day for everyone. Recommended amounts are given below in terms of whole fluid milk.

	237-ml (8-ounce) cups
Children under 9	2 to 3
Children 9 to 12	3 or more
Teenagers	4 or more
Adults	2 or more
Pregnant women	3 or more
Nursing mothers	4 or more

Part or all of the milk may be fluid skim milk, buttermilk, evaporated milk, or dry milk.

Cheese and ice cream may replace part of the milk. To substitute, figure the amount on the basis of calcium content. Common portions of various kinds of cheese and ice cream and their milk equivalents in calcium are:

16 cc (1-inch cube) cheddar-type cheese	= ½ cup milk
½ cup cottage cheese	= ⅓ cup milk
2 tablespoons cream cheese	= 1 tablespoon milk
½ cup ice cream or ice milk	= ⅓ cup milk

Appendix 2 con't.

Meat Group

Foods Included

- ☐ Beef; veal; lamb; pork; variety meats, such as liver, heart, kidney
- ☐ Poultry and eggs
- ☐ Fish and shellfish
- ☐ Alternates: dry beans, dry peas, lentils, nuts, peanuts, peanut butter

Contribution to Diet Foods in this group are valued for their protein, which is needed for growth and repair of body tissues, muscle, organs, blood, skin and hair. These foods also provide iron, thiamin, riboflavin, and niacin.

Amounts Recommended Choose 2 or more servings every day.

Count as a serving: 57 to 85 G (not including bone weight) cooked lean meat, poultry or fish. Count as alternates for ½ serving meat or fish: 1 egg, ½ cup cooked dry beans, dry peas, or lentils, or 2 tablespoons peanut butter.

Vegetable-Fruit Group

Foods Included

All vegetables and fruit. This guide emphasizes those that are valuable as sources of vitamin C and vitamin A.

Sources of Vitamin C

Good Sources: Grapefruit or grapefruit juice, orange or orange juice, cantaloupe, guava, mango, papaya, raw strawberries, brocolli, Brussels sprouts, green pepper, sweet red pepper.

Fair Sources: Honeydew melon, lemon, tangerine or tangerine juice, watermelon, asparagus tips, raw cabbage, cauliflower, collards, garden cress, kale, kohlrabi, mustard greens, potatoes and sweet potatoes cooked in the jacket, rutabagas, spinach, tomatoes or tomato juice, turnip greens.

Sources of Vitamin A

Dark-green and deep-yellow vegetables and a few fruits, namely, apricots, broccoli, cantaloupe, carrots, chard, collards, cress, kale, mango, persimmon, pumpkin, spinach, sweet potatoes, turnip greens and other dark-green leaves, winter squash.

Contribution to Diet Fruits and vegetables are valuable chiefly because of the vitamins and minerals they contain. In this plan, this group is counted on to supply nearly all the vitamin C needed and over half the vitamin A.

Vitamin C is needed for healthy gums and body tissues. Vitamin A is needed for growth, normal vision, and healthy condition of skin and other body surfaces.

Amounts Recommended Choose 4 or more servings every day, including:

- ☐ 1 serving of a good source of vitamin C or 2 servings of a fair source.
- ☐ 1 serving, at least every other day, of a good source of vitamin A. If the food chosen for vitamin C is also a good source of vitamin A, the additional serving of a vitamin A food may be omitted.
- ☐ The remaining 1 to 3 or more servings may be of any vegetable or fruit, including those that are valuable for vitamin C and vitamin A.

Count as 1 serving: ½ cup of vegetable or fruit; or 1 medium apple, banana, orange, or potato, half a medium grapefruit, a slice of cantaloupe, or the juice of 1 lemon.

Bread-Cereal Group

Foods Included

All breads and cereals that are whole grain, enriched, or restored; *check labels to be sure.*

Specifically, this group includes bread, cooked cereal, ready-to-eat cereal, cornmeal, crackers, flour, grits, macaroni and spaghetti, noodles, rice, rolled oats, and quick bread and other baked goods if made with whole-grain or enriched flour. Parboiled rice and wheat also may be included in this group.

Other Foods

To round out meals and meet energy needs, almost everyone will use some foods not specified in the four food groups. Such foods include unenriched, refined bread, cereal, flour; sugar; butter, margarine, other fats. Often these are ingredients in a recipe, or are added to other foods during preparation or at the table. Include some vegetable oil among the fats used.

Review Questions

1. Which one of the following would list only official drugs?

   A. *The Physicians' Desk Reference.*
   B. *The Pharmacopeia of The United States.*
   C. *The American Hospital Formulary.*
   D. Pharmacology texts.

2. Pills are

   A. Drugs shaped in the form of small spheres or balls.
   B. Mixtures of drugs with a firm base, like cocoa butter, and molded into shape for insertion into a body orifice.
   C. Drugs in small gelatin containers.
   D. Dried powdered drugs compressed into small, flat discs, often scored.

3. An enteric coating on a pill or tablet

   A. Prevents the stomach juices from destroying the effect of the drug.
   B. Prolongs the action of the drug over an 8 to 12 hour span.
   C. Speeds the action of the drug when administered rectally.
   D. Reduces toxic effects of the drug.

4. A medication that consists of a suspension of fat globules and water is classified as

   A. An emulsion.
   B. An ointment.
   C. A tincture.
   D. An elixir.

5. All suppositories

   A. Have a base which melts at body temperature.
   B. Are administered rectally.
   C. Are soothing to mucous membranes.
   D. Have a systemic effect.

6. A drug which is absorbed into the bloodstream and carried to specific organs or tissues is said to have

   A. A systemic effect.
   B. A local effect.
   C. Untoward effects.
   D. Therapeutic effects.

7. Capsules are

   A. Sealed glass containers.
   B. Drugs shaped into small balls or spheres.
   C. Dried powdered drugs compressed into small discs.
   D. Drugs contained in small, cylindrical gelatin containers.

8. An example of a tablet might be

   A. Amyl nitrite.
   B. Sodium amytal.
   C. Dulcolax.
   D. Aspirin.

9. One drop is the same as or equal to

   A. 1 minim.
   B. 1 milliliter.
   C. 1 cc.
   D. None of these.

10. Laura is to receive 10 grains of Tylenol. The only Tylenol available is labeled 5 grains. The correct dosage would be

    A. 1/2 tablet.
    B. 1 tablet.
    C. 2 tablets.
    D. 10 tablets.

11. A commonly used analgesic antipyretic is

    A. Phenobarbital.
    B. Demerol.
    C. Aspirin.
    D. Alka-Seltzer.

12. A drug commonly used for the relief of arthritic pain is

    A. Aspirin.
    B. Morphine sulfate.
    C. Phenobarbital.
    D. Empirin with codeine.

13. Adrenalin is classified as a heart stimulant because it

    A. Strengthens the heartbeat.
    B. Speeds up the action of the heart.
    C. Increases the respiratory rate.
    D. Slows the heart rate.

14. Digitalis preparations are called heart tonics because they

    A. Increase the heart rate.
    B. Slow and strengthen the heartbeat.
    C. Raise the blood pressure.
    D. Quicken the action of the heart.

15. Before giving any kind of digitalis preparation, the nurse should

    A. Check the patient's blood pressure.
    B. Count the patient's pulse.
    C. Count the patient's respirations.
    D. Be sure that the patient has had an ECG in the last 24 hours.

16. Nitroglycerin is frequently given to patients who have angina pectoris because this drug

    A. Produces sleep.
    B. Dilates the blood vessels and increases the circulation of blood.
    C. Depresses the pain centers located in the brain.
    D. Relaxes voluntary muscles and relieves muscle spasms.

17. The most common route of administration for nitroglycerin is

    A. Oral.
    B. Subcutaneous.
    C. Intramuscular.
    D. Sublingual.

18. Parenteral administration means

    A. Giving a drug by using a needle.
    B. Rubbing the medication on the skin.
    C. Letting the parents give a child his medicine.
    D. Giving a drug by suppository.

19. Carbon dioxide is

    A. A gas that increases the rate and depth of respiration.
    B. A liquid that stimulates respiration.
    C. A liquid that depresses the respiratory rate.
    D. A gas which makes bronchial secretions thinner and less viscous.

20. A laxative is a substance which

    A. Induces vomiting.
    B. Produces many watery stools.
    C. Produces formed stool with no griping.
    D. Produces many soft stools.

21. The word *analgesic* means

    A. Slowing peristalsis.
    B. Increasing urine output.
    C. Relieving pain.
    D. Producing sleep.

22. An antipyretic is a substance which

    A. Induces vomiting.
    B. Relieves nausea and vomiting.
    C. Makes the heart beat slower and stronger.
    D. Reduces the temperature by causing sweating.

23. Which one of the following is a cause of constipation?

    A. Too much bulk in the diet.
    B. Over-exercise.
    C. Too little fluid intake.
    D. Failure to take any cathartics.

24. Which one of the following is an indication for use of a cathartic?

    A. To remove gas and feces before X-ray.
    B. To prevent initiation of labor.
    C. To keep food soft and avoid the need for straining.
    D. To provide relief from vomiting.

25. Some doctors do not recommend the use of mineral oil because mineral oil

    A. Softens the feces.
    B. Is not absorbed.
    C. Is given in doses of 15 to 30 ml.
    D. Dissolves fat-soluble vitamins.

26. A wetting agent is used to

    A. Increase the flow of urine.
    B. Moisten and soften intestinal waste.
    C. Act as a purgative.
    D. Dissolve other drugs.

27. An example of a wetting agent is

    A. Diuril.
    B. Dioctyl sodium sulfosuccinate (DSS).
    C. Castor oil.
    D. Normal saline.

28. Another example of a wetting agent is

    A. Doxidan.
    B. Psyllium seed.
    C. Milk of magnesia.
    D. Dulcolax.

29. Drugs may be prescribed by a

    A. Physician.
    B. Registered nurse.
    C. Registered pharmacist.
    D. Patient.

30. Which one of the following drugs is potentially dangerous?

    A. Morphine.
    B. Aspirin.
    C. Cortisone.
    D. All the above.

31. Tranquilizers should be taken

    A. When a person feels nervous or is overly anxious.
    B. When a person is in any kind of pain.
    C. Under a doctor's supervision only.
    D. When a person thinks he may be developing mental symptoms.

32. Ethyl alcohol is a

    A. Stimulant of the central nervous system.
    B. Depressant of the central nervous system.
    C. A stimulant to some persons but a depressant to others.
    D. None of the above.

33. When pouring liquid medication

    A. The thumbnail is held on the line on the medicine glass which indicates the correct amount to pour.
    B. The glass is held below the level of the eye so that the mark may be seen through the glass.
    C. The label is read the second time after the drug has been poured.
    D. Any surplus medicine is returned to the bottle if a mistake has been made.

34. How many atropine sulfate gr 1/100 tablets would be needed to give gr 1/200?

    A. 1/2.
    B. 1/6.

C. 5/6.
D. 3/5.

35. The doctor's order reads "give gr $\frac{...}{iii}$," and the label on the bottle reads "gr $\frac{.}{i}$." How many tablets should be given?

    A. 30.
    B. 3.
    C. 1.
    D. 1/3.

36. How many milliliters of drug should be used to give 0.5 gm if the label on the bottle reads 5 gm in 10 ml?

    A. 2.
    B. 1.
    C. 0.5.
    D. 5.0.

37. To be sure that the correct medication is being poured for a patient, it is most important to

    A. Always have the nurse in charge supervise the pouring of medications.
    B. Read the physician's written order three times.
    C. Read the label on the container three times.
    D. Glance at the label on the container just before the medicine is poured.

38. The word *antiseptic* means

    A. Increases body activities.
    B. Inhibits growth of bacteria.
    C. Slows down body activities.
    D. Destroys bacteria.

39. The word *disinfectant* means

    A. Destroys bacteria.
    B. Slows heart action.
    C. Inhibits the growth of bacteria.
    D. Stimulates the bowels.

40. A stimulant is a substance which

    A. Promotes sleep.
    B. Speeds up body activities.
    C. Cures malaria.
    D. Slows body activities.

41. Which of the following drugs is a stimulant?

    A. Thorazine.
    B. Donnagel.
    C. Seconal.
    D. Epinephrine.

42. Which of the following drugs is a depressant?

    A. Diuril.
    B. Hexachlorophene.
    C. Levo-dromoran.
    D. Quinidine.

43. Which of the following drugs is used to treat angina pectoris?

    A. Nitroglycerin.
    B. Ephedrine.
    C. Levarterenol.
    D. Levophed.

44. A drug has a potentiation or synergistic effect when

    A. The drug is absorbed more rapidly than it is excreted.
    B. One drug effect cancels out another drug effect.
    C. The body requires higher and higher dosages to obtain optimum effect.
    D. One drug increases the effect of another drug.

45. The most effective concentration for alcohol when used as an antiseptic is

    A. 100 percent.
    B. 95 percent.
    C. 70 percent.
    D. 50 percent.

46. Sublingual administration may be used

    A. For only a few specific drugs.
    B. When the drug is decomposed in the stomach.
    C. When the patient is too ill to swallow.
    D. When the patient is afraid of injections.

47. Which one of the following symptoms is associated with overdose of digitalis?

    A. Dyspnea.
    B. Arrhythmias.
    C. Tachycardia.
    D. Nausea and vomiting.

48. A drug has an idiosyncrasy effect when

    A. The drug is absorbed into the bloodstream and is carried to all cells.
    B. Psychological and physiological dependence occurs with withdrawal symptoms.
    C. Unusual, unpredictable, unexpected reactions occur.
    D. The metabolic rate of the body is increased when the drug is given.

49. Diphenylhydantoin (Dilantin) is a drug sometimes used to treat cardiac arrhythmias. Its more frequent use, however, is in the control of

    A. Fecal incontinence.
    B. Convulsions.
    C. Hiccoughs.
    D. Renal colic.

50. The "C" in APC stands for

    A. Cascara.
    B. Caffeine.
    C. Codeine.
    D. Cortisone.

51. While using the apothecary system, one-half is indicated by

    A. 0.5.
    B. 1/2.
    C. ss.
    D. None of the above.

52. Which of the following drugs has a diuretic effect?

    A. Reserpine.
    B. Morphine sulfate.
    C. Caffeine.
    D. Papaverine.

53. Which of the following drugs has a constipating side effect?

    A. Metamucil.
    B. Morphine sulphate.
    C. Demerol.
    D. Aspirin.

54. One pint is the same as

    A. 1/4 quart.
    B. 250 ml.
    C. 500 cc.
    D. 1 cup.

55. 15 grains equals

    A. 1/10 gram.
    B. 1/4 gram.
    C. 1/2 gram.
    D. 1 gram.

56. One kilogram is the same as

    A. 10 grams.
    B. 1 pound.
    C. 2.2 pounds.
    D. 1000 milligrams.

57. Jill Montana has a history of hemorrhoids with both of her pregnancies. She is being admitted to the hospital for surgery at this time. Prior to surgical intervention, Mrs. Montana's diet plan will likely include a

    A. Low roughage, low fiber diet.
    B. Low roughage, high fiber diet.
    C. High protein, low roughage diet.
    D. High protein, high fiber diet.

58. Tina Blackburn, a 20-year-old college student, was admitted to the emergency room in a comatose state. She was subsequently diagnosed as having diabetes mellitus. Tina's condition has improved and she is now on a regular diabetic regimen. In teaching her about an ADA diet, you explain the ADA quantitative diet for diabetics consists of a

    A. Caloric distribution of 40% CHO, 40% protein, 20% fats.
    B. Caloric distribution of 50–70% CHO, 30–50% fats, and 12–20% protein.
    C. Diet of no more than 1500–2000 calories/day.

D. Diet with no added sugar and limited starch intake.

59. While Mrs. Young was frying bacon, the grease caught fire and ignited her sleeve. Although her husband was nearby and within a few moments had extinguished the fire by wrapping a blanket about her upper torso, Mrs. Young sustained burns of her right arm, right chest, face, and neck. In promoting adequate nutrition, Mrs. Young's diet after the first week of hospitalization should include

    A. High protein, low sodium, low carbohydrate.
    B. Low fat, low sodium, high calorie.
    C. High protein, high carbohydrate.
    D. High protein, high vitamin B complex, low sodium.

60. Mr. Baxter was admitted to the unit with the diagnosis of rule out M.I. While eating his evening meal Mr. Baxter states that the food is "tasteless." As the nurse caring for Mr. Baxter, you explain that he has been placed on a cardiac diet which is

    A. Low in unsaturated fats.
    B. Usually bland.
    C. Low in salt.
    D. Clear liquid without spices.

61. The next afternoon Mr. Baxter requests a snack. Which of the following foods on the menu would be the most appropriate for him?

    A. Fresh fruit.
    B. Turkey sandwich.
    C. Ice cream.
    D. Seafood salad.

62. After teaching John about an acid ash diet, you should have John repeat to you those foods that are unrestricted in order to determine his retention of knowledge. The foods he should name are

    A. Meat, eggs, whole grains, cheese.
    B. Milk, vegetables, fruits, nuts.
    C. Carbonated beverages, cookies and cakes, milk, vegetables.
    D. Milk, vegetables, cheeses, fruits.

63. The most appropriate breakfast for Mrs. Jamison on the third postop day following a cholecystectomy will include

    A. Cocoa, cereal with half and half, grapefruit, toast and jelly.
    B. Tea, boiled eggs, pork sausage, toast and butter.
    C. Coffee, oatmeal with half and half, scrambled egg, toast and butter.
    D. Tea, banana, boiled egg, toast and jelly.

64. Mr. Apple had a hernia repair this morning. In checking his orders for fluid replacement you need to remember the normal body requirements for fluids per day. The adult body requires how many cc of fluid/day to maintain homeostasis?

    A. 1000 cc/day.
    B. 500–700 cc/day.
    C. 1500 cc/day.
    D. Amount varies according to weather, stress, and individual body needs.

65. The diet for a patient with anemia should include

    A. High carbohydrate, high protein.
    B. Low sodium, high iron, vitamins.
    C. High protein, iron, vitamins.
    D. Low fat, low carbohydrate, high protein.

66. Dietary deficiency of B_{12} alone is rare; however, it has been observed in true vegetarians and their breast-fed infants. Rich food sources of vitamin B_{12} include

    A. Organ meats, especially liver.
    B. Green leafy vegetables.
    C. Fish.
    D. Kidney beans.

67. Mr. Varix has been hospitalized with the diagnosis of cirrhosis of the liver. He has both ascites and jaundice. Mr. Varix's diet teaching should include the information that

    A. He should not eat proteins.
    B. He can have small amounts of proteins.
    C. He must not eat carbohydrates.
    D. He can have very limited amounts of carbohydrates.

68. Mr. Varix says that he likes to snack. He asks for something to eat. Which of the following foods is *not* appropriate for him?

    A. A jelly sandwich.
    B. An apple.
    C. An egg salad sandwich.
    D. Graham crackers and juice.

69. Diet therapy is an integral part of the medical management necessary for dialysis patients. Which one of the following diets will most likely be explained to patients in order to increase their compliance to treatment?

    A. Low calcium, low phosphorous, low iron.
    B. Low potassium, low sodium, low protein.
    C. High protein, low sodium, low potassium.
    D. Low fat, low carbohydrate, high protein, low potassium.

70. Mrs. Hill has been diagnosed as having myxedema. Which of the following diets will most likely be ordered for her and require explanation to ensure compliance to the diet?

    A. Low fat, high protein with limited fluids.
    B. Balanced with limited fluids.
    C. Balanced with limited calories and increased roughage.
    D. Balanced with adequate vitamins and supplemental vitamins.

71. Viola Brown, age 16, suspecting that she is pregnant, comes to the prenatal clinic. It is determined that Viola is three months pregnant. Adequate nutrition is essential during early pregnancy for optimum fetal development. You recommend a daily diet for Viola that would include all of the following *except*

    A. Three grain products.
    B. One fruit or vegetable high in vitamin C.
    C. A total of four fruits and vegetables.
    D. 1500 calories.

72. In helping Viola select the best protein foods from the school cafeteria, you suggest that she choose which of the following for lunch?

    A. A slice of pizza.
    B. Macaroni.
    C. A peanut butter sandwich.
    D. Tomato soup.

73. Which snack would you suggest to increase protein intake?

    A. One-half cup peanuts.
    B. Two apples.
    C. Beef jerky stick.
    D. One cup milk.

74. Mrs. Thomas, a first time mother, asks you about nutrition instructions for breast-feeding mothers. You explain that the diet should include

    A. Four to five glasses of milk a day.
    B. Restricted salt intake.
    C. Low calorie foods.
    D. Restrict fat intake.

75. Vegetarians do not include eggs or any dairy products in their diets. Which vitamins are they most likely to be deficient in?

    A. Vitamin D.
    B. Riboflavin.
    C. Vitamin B_{12}.
    D. Calcium.

76. The daily energy requirements of pregnancy increase the daily calorie requirement of all pregnant women by

    A. 500 calories.
    B. 100 calories.
    C. 250 calories.
    D. 50 calories.

77. Sally More, 3 years old, has been admitted to the pediatric unit with a history of poor weight gain and repeated upper respiratory infections. In talking with Sally's mother you learn that she recently has had large, foul-smelling, bulky stools. The physician has made the tentative diagnosis of cystic fibrosis. In planning for Sally's care, what type of diet would be best?

    A. High caloric, high protein, low fat.
    B. Low carbohydrate, high protein, high fat.
    C. Low caloric, low fat, low protein.
    D. High carbohydrate, high fat, high protein.

78. Which of the following statements about infant nutrition is *not* true?

    A. Egg yolks are a good source of iron and can be introduced at six months.
    B. Solid foods should be introduced in the sixth week of life.
    C. Rice cereal is the least allergenic of the cereals for infants.
    D. Only one new food should be introduced per week.

79. How many calories should a one-month-old infant receive per day?

    A. 35–40 cal/lb/day.
    B. 45–50 cal/lb day.
    C. 50–55 cal/lb/day.
    D. 55–60 cal/lb/day.

80. A low cholesterol diet will include which one of the following foods?

    A. Shell fish.
    B. Avocados.
    C. Cooked vegetables.
    D. Organ meats.

Answers and Rationale

1. (B) The USP and the *American Hospital Formulary* list only official drugs.

2. (A) A pill is a rolled medication with a binder material in the shape of a ball.

3. (A) An enteric coating is a hard coat which prevents dissolving in the stomach and allows absorption in the intestine.

4. (A) An emulsion is a suspension of fat globules and water.

5. (A) The only answer which incorporates the word *all*. Suppositories may be vaginal. Those for bowel evacuation may be irritating in a local reaction. Suppositories generally are not systemic in action though some are, such as Aspirin suppository.

6. (A) Drugs in the bloodstream affect all cells giving a systemic response.

7. (D) Capsules are drugs placed in cylindrical gelatin containers to disguise the taste of the drug.

8. (D) Aspirin is a dried, powdered drug compressed into a small disc.

9. (A) 1 drop equals 1 minim. 1 ml equals 1 cc.

10. (C) Dose desired divided by the dose on hand. 10 grains divided by 5 grains equals 2 tablets.

11. (C) Aspirin is well known to reduce fever and relieve pain. It is an antipyretic and analgesic.

12. (A) Aspirin is also an effective antirheumatic—eases joint pain.

13. (B) Adrenalin is a direct heart stimulant.

14. (B) Digitalis slows and strengthens the heart. It is a heart tonic and an indirect heart stimulant.

15. (B) A safety precaution prior to giving digitalis is to take the pulse and not give the drug if the pulse is below 60. Digitalis slows heart rate and makes it stronger.

16. (B) Nitroglycerin is a smooth muscle relaxant and vasodilator. It dilates the coronary arteries thereby increasing circulation of blood to the heart. Angina pectoris is a spasm and causes vasoconstriction of the coronary arteries.

17. (D) Nitroglycerin enters the bloodstream in about two minutes when absorbed through mucous membranes. It is ineffective if swallowed.

18. (A) Parenteral means treatment by injection with a needle.

19. (A) Carbon dioxide increases rate and depth of respiration.

20. (C) A laxative is a substance which produces a formed stool with no griping. Cathartics produce many soft stools; purgatives produce many watery stools; emetics produce vomiting.

21. (C) Analgesic means reducing pain; hypnotic produces sleep.

22. (D) Pyretic refers to fever; antipyretic reduces fever.

23. (C) Fluid aids in normal evacuation of the bowels by keeping them soft.

24. (A) Abdominal X-rays need to have a clear view with no gas or feces to mask the organs.

25. (D) Mineral oil prevents fat-soluble vitamins from being absorbed. Mineral oil dissolves vitamins A and D.

26. (B) A wetting agent softens fecal matter by lowering surface tension.

27. (B) Only DSS is a wetting agent. Diuril is a diuretic; castor oil is a purgative; normal saline is a parenteral fluid.

28. (A) Doxidan is a wetting agent. Psyllium seed is bulk laxative; milk of magnesia is saline cathartic; Dulcolax is a contact irritant for evacuation of the bowels.

29. (A) Only a doctor may prescribe a drug. Pharmacist makes the prescription; nurse dispenses the medication.

30. (D) All medications are potentially dangerous since they all affect the body and since some people have allergic reactions.

31. (C) Most tranquilizers are controlled by the drug act of 1970 and may be given only under supervision of the physician.

32. (B) Ethyl alcohol is alcohol or ethanol and is a CNS depressant. Contains 92 to 94 percent of alcohol. In a 70 percent solution alcohol is antiseptic. Isopropyl alcohol is not safe for oral ingestion.

33. (A) Only answer which demonstrates safe preparation of medication.

34. (A) Dose desired divided by dose on hand equals 1/200 divided by 1/100, which equals 1/200 multiplied by 100/1, which equals 100/200, which equals 1/2 tablet.

35. (B) 3 divided by 1 equals 3 tablets.

36. (B) Dose on hand is in 10 ml, so multiply answer of dose desired divided by dose on hand by 10 ml. Example: 0.5 divided by 5 multiplied by 10 equals 0.1 multiplied by 10 equals 1 ml.

37. (C) The label on the container states what is in the container. Reading the label three times is a safety measure to ensure the correct medication will be given.

38. (B) Antiseptic inhibits growth of bacteria and is used externally; bactericidal destroys bacteria; stimulant increases body activity; depressant slows body activity.

39. (A) Disinfectant destroys bacteria; a heart tonic slows heart action; bacteriostatic slows growth of bacteria; laxatives stimulate bowel.

40. (B) A stimulant speeds body activities; hypnotic produces sleep; depressant slows body activities; antimalarial drugs cure malaria.

41. (D) Epinephrine is a stimulant; Thorazine is a tranquilizer and antiemetic; Donnagel is an antidiarrheic; Seconal is a barbiturate.

42. (C) Levo-dromoran is an analgesic (CNS depressant); Diuril is a diuretic; hexachlorophene is an antiseptic; quinidine is a heart antiarrhythmitic and heart depressant.

43. (A) Nitroglycerin is a vasodilator; the other three drugs—ephedrine, levarterenol, and Levophed—are all vasoconstrictors.

44. (D) Synergistic means "working together." A drug that is absorbed more rapidly than it is excreted is said to have a *cumulative* effect. A drug that cancels out the effect of another drug is said to be *antagonistic*. A *tolerance* effect occurs when the body requires higher and higher dosages to obtain optimum effect.

45. (C) 70 percent for antiseptic use.

46. (A) Sublingual administration is used for drugs that are readily soluble and quickly absorbed in the capillaries.

47. (D) Nausea and vomiting. Digitalis stimulates the vagus nerve, which increases strength of heart beat and decreases heart rate. Relief of dyspnea, arrhythmias and tachycardia would be expected from digitalis.

48. (C) *Idiosyncrasy* is an unpredictive, unusual, or unexpected reaction. A *systemic* drug is absorbed into the bloodstream and carried to all cells. *Addiction* is psychological and physiological dependence. A *stimulant* increases metabolic rate of the body.

49. (B) Dilantin is an anticonvulsant drug and most frequently is used to control seizures in grand mal epilepsy.

50. (B) "C" stands for caffeine; "P" stands for phenacetin; "A" stands for aspirin.

51. (C) ss is used for 1/2. In all other cases common fractions are used.

52. (C) Caffeine is a general body stimulant and diuretic. Reserpine, morphine sulfate, and papaverine are CNS depressants.

53. (B) Morphine sulfate is a CNS depressant that also slows the peristalsis of the intestine. Metamucil is a bulk laxative; Demerol is a narcotic depressant.

54. (C) 1 pt = 500 cc or 1/2 quart or 500 ml.

55. (D) 15 grains = 1 gram.

56. (C) Approximately 2.2 lbs = 1 kilogram.

57. (B) This diet produces a soft stool without mechanically irritating the hemorrhoidal area.

58. (B) This diet provides sufficient intake of food groups to maintain insulin dose and prevent nutritional complications. Answer (D) describes a

qualitative diet and is prescribed for pre-diabetics or adult-onset diabetics.

59. (C) A diet high in carbohydrates is essential to allow the protein to be spared for tissue regeneration.

60. (C) In order to maintain blood volumes which do not overwork the heart muscle, low sodium diets are recommended. Unsaturated fats are recommended for patients with coronary artery disease as they do not seem to contribute to atherosclerosis formation. Bland diets are used for patients with gastrointestinal diseases who cannot tolerate roughage and spices. A clear liquid diet is used in some centers for patients with myocardial infarctions; this is done to reduce the risk of aspiration and to decrease the workload of the heart.

61. (A) Fresh fruit is the lowest in sodium of the foods listed. Turkey, bread, and mayonnaise contain larger amounts of sodium. Ice cream contains sodium, and seafood salad may contain salty, seasoned sauces.

62. (A) The purpose of the acid ash diet is to provide a well-balanced diet with a greater amount of acid ash than alkaline ash each day.

63. (D) This breakfast has the lowest total grams of fat. The egg will provide some of the daily allotment of protein necessary for tissue building. Fat in the diet should be avoided for at least several weeks postoperatively.

64. (C) Needs do vary according to conditions, but the adult body requires 1500 cc/day at rest for maintenance.

65. (C) A high protein diet with iron and vitamins is needed to form new normal erythrocytes. Vitamin B_{12} is an essential vitamin, which must be administered.

66. (A) Vitamin B_{12} is supplied almost totally by animal foods. The richest sources are liver, kidney, and lean meats. Milk, eggs, and cheese provide B_{12} as well. A natural dietary deficiency is seen with selected true vegetarian groups in England, India, and the United States.

67. (B) Carbohydrates are one of the mainstays of the cirrhotic's diet. His liver can metabolize only very small amounts of protein. Usually he may have only 50 grams of protein per day (the normal diet is 80 grams per day).

68. (C) The most appropriate snack is the one with the least amount of protein and salt. The egg salad sandwich is higher in protein than the other foods. The most appropriate snack would be the apple. Graham crackers contain sodium, and the jelly sandwich contains protein.

69. (B) With kidney failure the body is unable to dispose of unnecessary or even dangerously high levels of electrolytes; therefore, the dietary restriction of sodium and potassium is essential. Protein breakdown byproducts are also not eliminated, so protein must be limited in the diet.

70. (C) Due to the decreased metabolic rate found in myxedema, the patient will require fewer than usual calories to prevent excessive weight gain and increased roughage to prevent constipation.

71. (D) Pregnancy requires the addition of 300 calories a day over regular caloric intake, and 1500 calories a day would be inadequate. The recommended calories for someone aged twenty-eight are 2300 a day.

72. (C) A peanut butter sandwich has 12 gms of protein, more than the other foods.

73. (A) One-half cup of peanuts has twice the protein as one cup of milk or the beef jerky. Apples contain very little protein.

74. (A) Lactating mothers need four to five glasses of milk a day. They should never be advised to restrict any nutrient or attempt to diet during lactation.

75. (C) If animal protein, milk, and eggs are absent in the diet, a vitamin B_{12} deficiency may result.

76. (C) The increased energy and nutritional demands of pregnancy require approximately 250 additional calories a day.

77. (A) The patient should receive a balanced diet including increased carbohydrate and protein and decreased fat. Good nutrition is essential.

78. (B) Not only is solid food not necessary until the child doubles his birth weight, but also the latest research indicates that solid food should not be given until six months. This may prevent allergies later in life, and the infant's digestive system has had time to mature.

79. (C) An infant should receive approximately 50–55 cal/lb/day.

80. (C) Cooked vegetables are allowed on a low cholesterol diet. The remaining three foods are all high in cholesterol and thus need to be avoided when a reduction in cholesterol is necessary.

Medical-Surgical Nursing

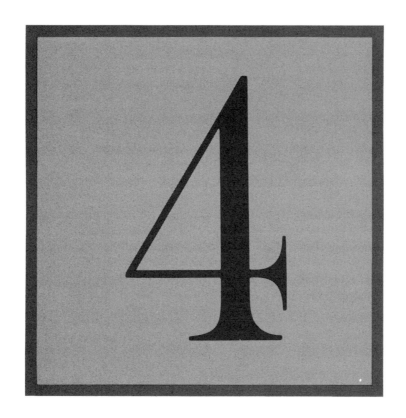

Neurologic System

The nervous system (together with the endocrine system) provides the control functions for the body. It handles thousands of bits of information and stimuli from the sensory organs. This system of nerves and nerve centers coordinates and regulates all of this data and determines the responses of the body.

Anatomy and Physiology of the Nervous System

Structure and Function

Neuron

A. Structure.
  1. Cell body (grey matter).
  2. Processes—dendrites (to cell body) and axon (from cell body).
  3. Synapse—chemical transmission of impulses from axon to dendrites.
  4. Nerve fiber—axon and its myelin sheath (white matter).
     a. Myelin sheath insulates; correlates with function and speed of conduction.
     b. Produced by neurolemma cells in peripheral nerve fibers and neuroglia cells in CNS fibers.
B. Classification by function.
  1. Sensory (afferent)—conduct impulses from end organ to CNS.
  2. Motor (efferent)—conduct impulses from CNS to muscles, glands.
  3. Internuncial (connector)—conducts impulses from sensory to motor neurons.
  4. Somatic—innervate body wall.
  5. Visceral—innervate the viscera.
C. Regeneration of destroyed nerve fibers.
  1. Peripheral nerve—can regenerate, possibly due to neurolemma.

  2. CNS—cannot regenerate as it lacks neurolemma.

D. Reflex arc—basic unit of function.
  1. Involuntary stereotyped response to stimulus.
  2. Components—sensory receptor, sensory neuron, internuncial neuron, motor neuron, and effector.
  3. Classification of reflexes—three types: superficial (cutaneous), deep (tendon), pathological.

Central Nervous System— Brain and Spinal Cord

A. Forebrain.
  1. Cerebrum—highest level of functioning.
     a. Governs all sensory and motor activity, thought, and learning.
     b. Analyzes, associates, integrates, and stores information.
     c. Cerebral cortex (outer grey layer) divided into four major lobes.
        (1) Frontal.
           (a) Motor function.
           (b) Motor speech area.
           (c) Prefrontal lobe—controls morals, values, emotions, judgment.
        (2) Parietal.
           (a) Integrates general sensation.
           (b) Interprets pain, touch, temperature, and pressure.
           (c) Governs discrimination.
        (3) Temporal.
           (a) Auditory center.
           (b) Sensory speech center.
        (4) Occipital—visual area.
  2. Basal ganglia.
     a. Part of extrapyramidal tract.
     b. Controls associated motor movements.
  3. Internal capsule—contains projection fibers connecting cortical areas with other parts of the CNS.

B. Brainstem.
   1. Diencephalon.
      a. Thalamus.
         (1) Screens and relays sensory impulses to cortex.
         (2) Lowest level of crude conscious awareness.
      b. Hypothalamus—regulates autonomic nervous system, stress response, sleep, appetite, body temperature, water balance, emotion.
   2. Midbrain—motor coordination, conjugate eye movements.
   3. Pons.
      a. Contains projection tracts between spinal cord, medulla, and brain.
      b. Controls the involuntary respiratory reflexes.
   4. Medulla oblongata.
      a. Contains all afferent and efferent tracts.
      b. Contains cardiac, respiratory, vomiting, and vasomotor centers.
C. Cerebellum.
   1. Connected by afferent/efferent pathways to all other parts of CNS.
   2. Coordinates muscle movement, posture, equilibrium, and muscle tone.
D. Pyramidal tract.
   1. Initiates skilled voluntary movements.
   2. Originates with cell bodies in motor cortex; fibers form projection tracts which pass through internal capsule and medulla where most decussate; fibers from corticospinal tracts which terminate at anterior horn.
E. Extrapyramidal (outside of pyramidal tract).
   1. Inhibitory or facilitory effect on motor function.
   2. Includes basal ganglia, cerebellum, reticular formation, cortex, and spinal cord.
F. Spinal cord—conveys messages between brain and periphery.
   1. Structure.
      a. Extends from foramen magnum to second lumbar vertebra.
      b. Inner column of H-shaped grey matter which contains the two anterior and two posterior horns.
      c. Posterior horns—contain cell bodies which connect with afferent (sensory) nerve fibers from posterior root ganglia.
      d. Anterior horns—contain cell bodies giving rise to efferent (motor) nerve fibers.
      e. Lateral horns—present in thoracic segments; origin of autonomic fibers of sympathetic nervous system.
   2. Ascending tracts (sensory pathways).
   3. Descending tracts (motor pathways).
G. Protection for CNS.
   1. Skull—rigid chamber with opening at the base (foramen magnum).
   2. Meninges.
      a. Dura mater—tough, outermost, fibrous membrane.
      b. Arachnoid membrane—delicate membrane that contains subarachnoid fluid.
      c. Pia mater—vascular membrane.
   3. Cerebral spinal fluid.
      a. Protective cushion; aids exchange of nutrients, wastes.
      b. Secreted from choroid plexuses in the four ventricles.
      c. Circulates within interconnecting ventricles and subarachnoid space.
   4. Blood-brain barrier.
      a. Prevents damaging substances from entering CSF.
      b. Brain parenchyma.
   5. Blood supply—conductor of oxygen vitally needed by nervous system.
      a. Internal carotids.
      b. Vertebral arteries.
      c. Circle of Willis.

Peripheral Nervous System

A. Carries voluntary and involuntary impulses.
B. Cranial nerves (twelve pairs).
   1. Motor, sensory, or mixed nerve fibers.

2. Names: olfactory, optic, oculomotor, trochlear, trigeminal, abducens, facial, acoustic, glossopharyngeal, vagus, accessory, hypoglossal.

C. Spinal nerves (31 pairs).
  1. All mixed nerve fibers formed by joining of anterior motor and posterior sensory roots.
  2. Anterior root—efferent nerve fibers to glands and voluntary and involuntary muscles.
  3. Posterior root—afferent nerve fibers from sensory receptors. Contains posterior ganglion (cell body of sensory neuron).

Autonomic Nervous System

A. Structure and function.
  1. Part of peripheral nervous system controlling smooth muscle, cardiac muscle, and glands.
  2. Two divisions make involuntary adjustments for integrated balance (homeostasis).
B. Sympathetic nervous system—thoracolumbar division.
  1. Fight, flight, or freeze; diffuse response.
  2. Increases heart rate, blood pressure.
  3. Dilates pupils, bronchi.
C. Parasympathetic nervous system—craniosacral division.
  1. Repair, repose; discrete response.
  2. Decreases heart rate, blood pressure.
  3. Constricts pupils, bronchi.

Basic Neurological Assessment

Signs and Symptoms

A. Numbness, weakness.
B. Dizziness, fainting, loss of consciousness.
C. Headache, pain.
D. Speech disturbances.
E. Visual disturbances.
F. Disturbances in memory, thinking, personality.
G. Nausea, vomiting.

Level of Consciousness

A. Most sensitive, reliable index of cerebral function.
B. Assessment of consciousness.
  1. Orientation of patient as to place, purpose, time.
  2. Response to verbal and tactile stimuli or simple commands.
  3. Response to painful stimuli.
C. Describe behaviors indicating levels of consciousness: clouding, confusion, delirium, stupor, coma.

Pupillary Signs

A. Light reflex—most important sign differentiating structural from metabolic coma.
B. Pupil assessment.
  1. Size—measure in millimeters.
  2. Equality—equal, unequal, fluctuations.
  3. Reactions to light—brisk, slow, fixed.
  4. Unusual eye movements or deviations from midline.
C. Pupillary abnormalities.
  1. Unilateral dilation.
  2. Mid-position, fixed (often unequal).
  3. Pinpoint, fixed.

Motor Function

A. Pattern of motor dysfunction gives information about anatomic location of lesions, independent of level of consciousness.
B. Assessment of face, upper and lower extremities.
  1. Muscle tone, strength, equality.
  2. Voluntary movement.
  3. Involuntary movements.
  4. Reflexes:
    a. Babinski—dorsiflexion ankle and great toe with fanning of other toes.
    b. Corneal—blink reflex.
    c. Gag—gag and vomiting reflex.

C. Patterns of motor function.
   1. Appropriate—spontaneous movement to stimulus or command.
   2. Absent: hemiplegia, paraplegia, quadriplegia.
   3. Inappropriate (nonpurposeful).
      a. Posturing in response to stimuli.
      b. Involuntary: choreiform (jerky, quick); athetoid (twisting, slow); tremors; spasms; or convulsions.

Sensory Function

A. Assess general sensory function in all extremities: touch, pressure, pain.
B. If no motor response to command, may elicit response by sensory stimuli such as supraorbital pressure.
C. Use minimal amount of stimulus necessary to evoke a response.

Vital Signs

A. Monitor for trends—changes often unreliable and occur late with increasing intracranial pressure.
B. Blood pressure and pulse—changes may indicate increasing intracranial pressure.
C. Respiration.
   1. Rate, depth, and rhythm more sensitive indication of intracranial pressure than blood pressure and pulse.
   2. Cheyne-Stokes—respiratory increase and decrease in rate and depth, rhythmically alternating with periods of apnea.
   3. Neurogenic hyperventilation—sustained regular, rapid, and deep.
   4. Ataxic—totally irregular, random rhythm and depth.
D. Temperature (rectal).
   1. Early rise may indicate damage to hypothalamus or brainstem.
   2. Slow rise may indicate infection.
   3. Elevated temperature increases brain's metabolic rate.

Signs of Meningeal Irritation

A. Brudzinski's sign—flexion of head causes flexion of both thighs at the hips and flexion of the knees.
B. Kernig's sign—in supine position, thigh and knee flexed to right angles; extension of leg causes spasm of hamstring, resistance, and pain.

Diagnostic Procedures

Radiologic Procedures

A. Skull series.
   1. Procedure—X-rays of head from different angles.
   2. Purpose—to visualize configuration, density, and vascular markings.
   3. Tomograms—layered vertical or horizontal X-ray exposures.
B. Ventriculography.
   1. Procedure—injection of air directly into lateral ventricles followed by X-rays.
   2. Purpose—to visualize ventricles, localize tumors. May be used if increased intracranial pressure contraindicates pneumoencephalography.
   3. Potential complications—headache, nausea and vomiting, meningitis, increasing intracranial pressure.
   4. Nursing care.
      a. Monitor vital signs.
      b. Check neurological status.
      c. Elevate head.
      d. Administer ice bag and analgesics for headache.
C. Myelography.
   1. Procedure—injection of dye or air into lumbar or cisternal subarachnoid space followed by X-rays of the spinal column.
   2. Purpose—to visualize spinal subarachnoid space for distortions caused by lesions.
   3. Potential complications.
      a. Same as for lumbar puncture.
      b. Cerebral meningeal irritation from dye.

4. Nursing care.
   a. Same as for lumbar puncture.
   b. If dye is used, elevate head and observe for meningeal irritation.
   c. If air is used, keep head lower than trunk.

D. Cerebral angiography.
   1. Procedure—injection of radiopaque dye into carotid and/or vertebral arteries followed by serial X-rays.
   2. Purpose—to visualize cerebral vessels and localize lesions such as aneurysms, occlusions, angiomas, tumors, or abscesses.
   3. Potential complications.
      a. Anaphylactic reaction to dye.
      b. Local hemorrhage.
      c. Vasospasm.
      d. Adverse intracranial pressure.
   4. Nursing care.
      a. Prior to procedure.
         (1) Check allergies.
         (2) Take baseline assessment.
         (3) Measure neck circumference.
      b. During and after procedure.
         (1) Have emergency equipment available.
         (2) Monitor neurological and vital signs for shock, level of consciousness, hemiparesis, hemiplegia, and aphasia.
         (3) Monitor for swelling of neck, difficulty in swallowing or breathing.
         (4) Administer ice collar.

E. Pneumoencephalography (PEG)
   1. Procedure—withdrawal of CSF and introduction of air through lumbar, cisternal puncture, followed by X-rays.
   2. Purpose.
      a. To visualize ventricles, aqueducts, and subarachnoid space.
      b. To demonstrate cerebral atrophy, hydrocephalus, and intracranial lesions.
   3. Potential complications—headache, shock, convulsions, increased intracranial pressure, and herniation of brainstem.

4. Nursing care.
   a. Prior to procedure.
      (1) NPO.
      (2) Take baseline assessment.
      (3) Have emergency equipment available.
   b. During procedure—observe vital signs, hypotension, shock, headache, and level of consciousness.
   c. Post procedure.
      (1) Keep patient in a horizontal position and turn frequently.
      (2) Force fluids.
      (3) Monitor all neurological and vital signs.
      (4) Give ice bag and analgesics for headache.

Brain Scan

A. Procedure—intravenous injection of radioactive isotope substance followed by anterior-posterior and lateral scanning. Concentration of substance is greatest in pathological areas.

B. Purpose—to localize tumors with high degree of accuracy. Accuracy is increased if scanning is combined with arteriography or encephalography.

C. No special preparation or aftercare.

Electroencephalography (EEG)

A. Procedure—graphic recording of brain's electrical activity by electrodes placed on the scalp.

B. Purpose—to detect intracranial lesion and abnormal electrical activity (epilepsy); now used to detect and indicate "brain death."

C. Nursing care.
   1. Wash hair.
   2. Withhold sedatives or stimulants.
   3. Administer fluids as ordered.

Echoencephalogram

A. Procedure—recording of reflected ultrasonic waves from brain structures.

B. Purpose.
   1. To measure position and shifting of midline structures.
   2. To detect subdural hematoma or tumors.

Electromyography (EMG)

A. Procedure—recording of muscle action potential by surface or needle electrodes.
B. Purpose—to diagnose or localize neuromuscular disease.

Lumbar Puncture (LP)

A. Procedure—insertion of spinal needle through L_3-L_4 or L_4-L_5 interspace into lumbar subarachnoid space.
B. Purpose.
   1. To obtain cerebral spinal fluid (CSF).
   2. To measure intracranial pressure.
   3. To instill air, dye, or medications.
C. Potential complications—headache, backache, and herniation with brainstem compression (especially if intracranial pressure is high).
D. Nursing care.
   1. Have patient empty bowel and bladder.
   2. Assist with specimens and pressure measurement.
   3. Maintain strict asepsis.
   4. Monitor vital signs.
   5. Maintain patient in horizontal position.
   6. Encourage fluids if not contraindicated.
   7. Inspect puncture site.
E. Queckenstedt-Stookey test.
   1. Normal if pressure increases with jugular compression and drops to normal ten to thirty seconds after release of compression.
   2. Partial block if slow rise and return to normal.
   3. Complete block if no rise.

Cisternal Puncture

A. Procedure—needle puncture into cisterna magna just below the occipital bone.

B. Purpose—same as for lumbar puncture. May be used if intracranial pressure is high or for infants.
C. Potential complications—respiratory distress.
D. Nursing care.
   1. Same as for lumbar puncture.
   2. Observe for cyanosis, dyspnea, and apnea.

Conditions of the Neurologic System

The Unconscious or Immobilized Patient

Definition: Unconsciousness is the state of depressed cerebral function with altered sensory and motor function. Immobilization is the loss of normal sensory/motor function without loss of consciousness.

Treatment and Nursing Care

A. Maintain open airway and adequate ventilation.
   1. Airway obstruction.
   2. Breath sounds.
   3. Positioning.
      a. Semiprone (to prevent tongue from occluding airway and secretions from pooling in pharynx).
      b. Frequent change of position.
   4. Bronchial hygiene.
      a. Include deep breathing and coughing when possible.
      b. Suctioning.
   5. Assisted ventilation.
B. Maintain adequate circulation.
   1. Positioning.
      a. Avoid Trendelenburg's position with head or neck injuries.
      b. Change position frequently, from horizontal to sitting or standing, as soon as possible.
      c. Passive, active ROM.
      d. Encourage self-help.

114

2. Caution against Valsalva's maneuver (technique of clearing or testing patency of the eustachian tubes).

C. Observe signs and symptoms for potential complications.

1. Neurological (see Basic Neurological Assessment, p. 110).
2. Respiratory function.
   a. Color, chest expansion, deformities.
   b. Rate, depth, and rhythm of respirations.
   c. Movement of air at nose/mouth or intratracheal tube.
   d. Breath sounds.
   e. Accumulation of secretions or blood in the mouth.
   f. Signs of respiratory distress, failure, hypoxemia, hypercapnia, infection, atelectasis.
3. Cardiovascular function.
   a. Blood pressure, pulses.
   b. Skin color, temperature, edema, leg pain.
   c. Heart sounds, arrhythmias.
   d. Signs of shock, hypertension, orthostatic hypotension.
4. Condition of skin.
   a. Inspect entire body, especially susceptible pressure points (heels, malleoli, trochanteric areas, ischium, sacrum).
   b. Note redness, pallor, edema, excoriation, or skin breakdown.
5. Bladder/bowel function.
   a. Bladder distention—urinary stasis, incontinence.
   b. Urinary tract infection.
   c. Urinary calculi—stasis, infection, alkalinity, decreased volume of urine and citric acid.
   d. Abdominal distention—paralytic ileus, constipation, impaction, diarrhea, trauma.
6. Nutrition, fluid, and electrolyte balance.
   a. Intake—NPO, oral, tube feedings, IV.
   b. Output—urinary, feces; unconsciousness, check emesis, nasogastric.
   c. Electrolytes, acid-base.
   d. Dehydration, fluid overload.
   e. Thirst, loss of sensation of thirst.
   f. Swallowing, gag reflex.
7. Musculoskeletal function.
   a. Muscle strength—weakness, paralysis.
   b. Muscle tone or resistance to passive movement—flaccid, atrophied, spastic.
   c. Limitation of function—deformities, contractures.
   d. Osteoporosis.
8. Process of psychological adaptation—patient/family.
   a. Changes in body image; social and family roles.
   b. Sensory deprivation.
   c. Emotional/physiological stress.
   d. Adaptation to loss—anxiety, fear, denial, depression, dependency.

D. Maintain optimal positioning and movement.

1. Prevent further trauma.
   a. Maintain body alignment, support head and limbs when turning, logroll.
   b. Do not flex or twist spine or hyperextend neck if spinal cord injury suspected.
2. Positioning.
   a. Maintain and support joints and limbs in most functional anatomic position.
   b. Avoid improper use of knee gatch or pillows under knee.
3. Avoid complete immobility.
   a. Perform ROM (against resistance if able), weight bearing; provide tilt table.
   b. Encourage self-help.

E. Maintain integrity of the skin.

1. High risk of decubitus ulcers.
   a. Loss of vasomotor tone.
   b. Impaired peripheral circulation.
   c. Paralysis, immobility, and loss of muscle assistance to blood flow.
   d. Hypoproteinemia.
2. Loss of sensation of pressure, pain, or temperature—decreased awareness of developing decubitus ulcers or burns.
3. Skin care.
   a. Clean and dry skin; avoid powder because it may cake.

b. Massage with lotion around and toward bony prominences.

c. Alternate air mattress and sheepskin pad.

d. Keep linen from wrinkling; avoid mechanical friction against linen.

F. Maintain personal hygiene.

1. Eye—loss of corneal reflex may contribute to corneal irritation, keratitis, blindness.

a. Observe for signs of irritation.

b. Irrigate eyes, instill artificial tears or patch.

2. Nose—trauma or infection in nose or nasopharynx may cause meningitis.

a. Observe for drainage of CSF.

b. Clean and lubricate nares; do not clean inside nostrils.

c. Change nasogastric tube at intervals.

3. Mouth—mouth breathing contributes to drying and crusting excoriation of mucous membranes, which may lead to aspiration and respiratory tract infections.

a. Examine the mouth daily with a good light.

b. Clean teeth, gums, mucous membranes, tongue, and uvula to prevent crusting and infection; lubricate lips.

c. Inspect for retained food in the mouth of patients who have facial paralysis; follow with mouth care.

4. Ear—drainage of CSF from the ear indicates damage to the base of the brain and a danger of meningitis.

a. Inspect ear for drainage of CSF.

b. Loosely cover ear with sterile, dry dressing.

G. Promote adequate nutrition, fluid, and electrolyte balance.

1. Intravenous fluids.

a. Electrolyte solutions, hyper-alimentation.

b. Caution with IV rates if intracranial pressure is elevated.

2. Tube feedings—high in proteins and calories.

a. Position patient in semi-Fowler's position, slightly turned to right side.

b. Check position of tube; aspirate and measure gastric contents; usually if greater than 50 to 100 cc, return and subtract that amount from feeding.

c. Give feeding by gravity flow; flush tubing with water; prevent air from entering stomach via tubing.

d. Monitor intake and output, and daily weight.

3. Oral feedings.

a. Check swallowing with ice chips.

b. Put patient in semi-Fowler's position.

c. Have suction equipment available.

d. Give semi-liquid, soft, or blended foods.

H. Promote elimination.

1. Catheter (Foley)—strict asepsis, catheter care.

2. Cathartic—enema on a regular schedule.

3. Bowel/bladder retraining if necessary.

I. Provide psychosocial support for patient and family.

1. Assume that an unconscious patient can hear; frequently reassure and explain procedures to the patient.

2. Encourage family interaction.

Glasgow Coma Scale

A. Comatose state based on three areas associated with level of consciousness.

B. Scoring system.

1. Based on a scale of 1 to 15 points.

2. Any score below 8 indicates coma is present.

C. Eye opening is the most important indicator.

☆D. Coma Scale.

1. Motor response.	Points
Obeys	6
Localizes	5
Withdrawn	4
Abnormal flexion	3
Extensor response	2
Nil	1

2. Verbal response.   Points
  - Oriented   5
  - Confused conversation   4
  - Inappropriate words   3
  - Incomprehensible sounds   2
  - Nil   1
3. Eye opening   Points
  - Spontaneous   4
  - To speech   3
  - To pain   2
  - Nil   1

Increased Intracranial Pressure

Etiology

Trauma, hemorrhage, tumors, abscess, hydrocephalus, edema, or inflammation.

Pathology

A. Cranial cavity is a solid compartment with relatively little room for expansion.
B. Increased intracranial bulk from blood, CSF, or brain tissue will increase intracranial pressure.
C. Increased pressure impedes cerebral circulation, absorption of CSF, and function of the nerve cells.
D. Increasing pressure if transmitted downward toward the brainstem can lead to eventual tentorial herniation, brainstem compression, and death.

Signs and Symptoms

A. See Basic Neurological Assessment, p. 110.
B. Level of consciousness (most sensitive indicator of increasing intracranial pressure) changes from restlessness to confusion to declining level of consciousness and coma.
C. Headache—tension, displacement of brain.
D. Vomiting.
E. Pupillary changes—unilateral dilation of pupil: slow reaction to light; fixed dilated pupil is ominous sign requiring immediate action.
F. Motor function—weakness, hemiplegia, positive Babinski, decerebrate, seizure activity.
G. Vital signs—rise in blood pressure; widening pulse pressure; reflex slowing of pulse; abnormalities in respiration, especially periods of apnea; temperature elevation.

Nursing Care

A. Assess and treat cerebral edema (increased intracranial pressure).
  1. Give medications as ordered—osmotic diuretics, steroids.
  2. Limit fluid intake.
  3. Elevate head of bed; avoid Trendelenburg's position.
B. Prevent further complications.
  1. Monitor neurological dysfunction versus cardiovascular shock.
  2. Prevent hypoxia—avoid morphine.
  3. Monitor fluid-electrolyte and acid-base balance.
  4. Prevent straining by the patient—avoid restraints, prevent coughing and vomiting.
C. Treat underlying cause.

Spinal Cord Injury

Definition: May include cervical injury leading to quadriplegia or respiratory failure; thoracic injury leading to flaccid/spastic paraplegia; or lumbar injury leading to flaccid paraplegia.

Pathophysiology

A. Neurological signs generally due to edema, concussion, compression, hemorrhage, partial or complete transection of cord, and disruption of sensory and motor pathways.
B. Spinal shock—initial flaccid paralysis, loss of sensation and reflexes, urinary and bowel retention, disturbed nerve supply to blood vessels, and hypotension.

C. Autonomic dysfunction—absence of sweating; decreased blood pressure and temperature in affected areas; poor response to reflex stimuli; paralytic ileus often occurs.
D. After spinal shock recedes—spastic paralysis and hyperreflexia; bowel and bladder control may be retained.
E. Lumbar injury (cauda equina)—persisting flaccid paralysis of lower extremities, bladder, and rectum; muscle atrophy.

Nursing Care

A. Direct efforts toward primary nursing goals: prevent further injury or complications and maintain optimal body functioning while patient is immobilized (see section on the unconscious or immobilized patient).
B. Maintain open airway and adequate ventilation—high cervical injuries can cause complete paralysis of muscles for breathing; observe for any signs of respiratory failure.
C. Immobilize patient as ordered, to allow fracture healing and prevent further injury.
   1. Stryker frame permits change of position between prone and supine.
      a. Maintain optimal body alignment.
      b. Place patient in center of frame without flexing or twisting.
      c. Position arm boards, footboards, canvas.
      d. Turn; reassure patient while turning.
      e. Free all tubings; secure bolts and straps.
   2. Regular hospital beds used in many rehabilitation centers.
   3. Halotraction with body cast allows early mobilization.
   4. Soft and hard collars and back braces used about six weeks post-injury.
   5. Maintain skeletal traction if part of treatment.
      a. Cervical tongs for hyperextension (Crutchfield, Gardner-Wells, Vinke).
         (1) Apply traction to vertebral column by attaching weights to pair of tongs.
         (2) Insert tongs into outer layer of parietal area of skull.

   b. Facilitates moving and turning of patient while maintaining spine immobilization.
   c. Observe site of insertion for redness or drainage, alignment and position.
D. Monitor for potential complications. Neurological assessment should include watching for changes in muscle tone, motor movement, sensation, bladder/bowel function, presence/absence of sweating, and temperature.
E. Maintain optimal positioning.
   1. If turning permitted, logroll with firm support to head, neck, spine, and limbs.
   2. Maintain good body alignment with 10 degree flexion of knees, heels off mattress or canvas, and feet in firm dorsiflexion.
   3. Convalescence—cervical collar, tilt table, wheelchair, braces, parallel bars.
F. Maintain integrity of the skin.
   1. Do not administer IM medication below a lesion that is result of impaired circulation and potential skin breakdown.
   2. Provide elastic stockings to improve circulation in legs.
G. Promote adequate nutrition, fluid, and electrolyte balance.
   1. Provide diet high in protein, vitamins, calories.
   2. Avoid all citrus juices, which alkalize the urine and contribute to infection and renal calculi.
   3. Avoid gas-forming and foods with high residue.
   4. Monitor calcium, electrolyte, and hemoglobin levels.
H. Establish optimal bladder function.
   1. During spinal shock—bladder is atonic with urinary retention; danger of overdistention, stretching.
   2. Possible reactions:
      a. Hypotonic—retention with overflow.
      b. Hypertonic—sudden reflex voiding.
   3. Check for bladder distention, voiding, incontinence.
   4. Provide aseptic catheter care.
   5. Prevent urinary tract infection, calculi.
   6. Initiate bladder retraining.

a. Hypertonic—sensation of full bladder, trigger areas, regulation of fluid intake.

b. Hypotonic—the manual expression of urine (Credé).

7. Administer medications to treat incontinence.

a. Hypertonic—propantheline bromide, diazepam.

b. Hypotonic—bethanecol chloride.

I. Establish optimal bowel function.

1. Incontinence and paralytic ileus occur with spinal shock; later, incontinence, constipation, impaction.

2. For severe distention, administer neostigmine methylsulfate and insert rectal tube, which decompresses intestinal tract.

☆ 3. Initiate bowel retraining.

a. Record bowel habits before and after injury.

b. Provide well-balanced diet with bulky foods.

c. Encourage fluid intake.

d. Encourage development of muscle tone, ability to sit in chair.

e. Administer suppository as ordered.

f. Emphasize importance of a regular, consistent routine.

J. Provide psychological support to patient and family.

1. Adjustment to paralysis may be very difficult as patient is usually young; may be inclined toward suicide.

2. Provide nonjudgmental atmosphere, security, sensory input.

3. Provide diversionary activities, socialization, independence, explanations, support.

4. Give encouragement and reassurance but *never* false hope.

K. Encourage optimal physical activity as tolerated by patient.

1. Physical therapy exercises.

2. Independent activity within limitations.

3. Extensive program of rehabilitation and self-care.

Head Injury

Definition: Trauma to the skull by means of compression, tension, and/or shearing force resulting in varying degrees of injury to the brain.

Types

A. Brain concussion—violent jarring of brain within skull; temporary loss of consciousness.

B. Brain contusion—bruising, injury of brain.

C. Skull fracture—linear, depressed, compound, or comminuted.

D. Hemorrhage.

1. Epidural hematoma—most serious; hematoma between dura and skull from tear in meningeal artery; forms rapidly.

2. Subdural hematoma—under dura due to tears in veins crossing subdural space; forms slowly.

3. Subarachnoid hematoma—bleeding into subarachnoid space.

4. Intracerebral hematoma—usually multiple hemorrhages around contused area.

Signs and Symptoms

A. Impaired level of consciousness, unconsciousness, confusion.

B. Headache, nausea, vomiting.

C. Pupillary changes.

D. Changes in vital signs, reflecting increased intracranial pressure or shock.

E. Rhinorrhea, otorrhea, nuchal rigidity.

F. Overt scalp/skull trauma.

Nursing Care

A. Direct efforts toward primary nursing goals: recognize, prevent, and treat complications (see section on the unconscious or immobilized patient, p. 113, for measures to maintain optimal body functioning).

B. Maintain open airway and adequate ventilation.

C. Awaken the patient as completely as possible to assess level of consciousness.

D. Assess and treat convulsions (see Convulsions, p. 122).
E. Control pain and restlessness.
  1. Avoid morphine, which will increase intracranial pressure.
  2. Use codeine or other milder analgesic (use sparingly).
F. Prevent infection.
  1. High risk of meningitis, abscess, osteomyelitis, particularly in presence of rhinorrhea, otorrhea.
  2. Maintain strict asepsis.
G. Assess and treat other complications.
  1. Shock—significant cause of death.
  2. Cranial nerve paralysis.
  3. Rhinorrhea (fracture ethmoid bone) and otorrhea (temporal).
    a. Check discharge—bloody spot surrounded by pale ring; positive testtape reaction for sugar.
    b. Do not attempt to clean nose or ears.
    c. Do not suction nose.
    d. Instruct patient not to blow nose.
  4. Ear—drainage of CSF from the ear indicates damage to the base of the brain and a danger of meningitis.
    a. Inspect ear for drainage of CSF.
    b. Loosely cover ear with sterile, dry dressing.

Encephalitis

Definition: Severe inflammation of the brain caused by arboviruses or enteroviruses.

Signs and Symptoms

A. Fever, headache, vomiting.
B. Signs of meningeal irritation.
C. Neuronal damage, drowsiness, coma, paralysis, ataxia.

Nursing Care

A. Monitor vital signs frequently.
B. Monitor neurological signs for alterations in condition.

C. Administer anticonvulsant medications as ordered: phenytoin.
D. Administer glucocorticoids as ordered: reduces cerebral edema.
E. Administer sedatives to relieve restlessness.
F. Manage fluid and electrolyte balance to prevent fluid overload and dehydration.
G. Position to maintain patent airway and prevent contractures. Provide range-of-motion exercises.
H. Promote adequate nutrition through tube feedings, and parenteral hyperalimentation if necessary.
I. Provide hygienic care, i.e., skin care, oral care, and perineal care.
J. Provide safety measures if patient is confused.

Cerebral Vascular Accident (CVA)

Definition: Impaired blood supply in the brain caused by a hemorrhage or occlusion that results in a sudden focal neurological deficit. It is the most common cause of brain disturbance.

Pathophysiology

A. Causes.
  1. Thrombosis.
  2. Embolism.
  3. Hemorrhage.
  4. Compression or spasm.
B. Risk factors.
  1. Atherosclerosis.
  2. Hypertension.
  3. Anticoagulation therapy.
  4. Cardiac valvular disease.
  5. Synthetic valve and organ replacement.
  6. Atrial arrhythmias.
  7. Diabetes.
C. A transient ischemic attack (TIA) is a precursor symptom or warning of impending CVA.
  1. Rapid onset and short duration (30 minutes to 24 hours); by definition, must be resolved within this time period.

2. Following resolution, no permanent neurological deficit.

3. Most common symptoms: vision loss, diplopia, contralateral hemiparesis, aphasia, confusion, slurred speech, and vertigo.

D. Cerebral anoxia longer than ten minutes to a localized area of brain causes cerebral infarction (irreversible changes).

E. Surrounding edema and congestion cause further dysfunction.

F. Lesion in cerebral hemisphere results in manifestations on the opposite side of the body.

G. Permanent disability unknown until edema subsides. Order in which function may return: facial, swallowing, lower limbs, speech, arms.

Signs and Symptoms

A. Depend on site and size of involved area.
   1. Appear suddenly with embolism.
   2. More gradually with hemorrhage and thrombosis.

B. Generalized symptoms—headache; hypertension; changes in level of consciousness, convulsions; vomiting, nuchal rigidity, slow bounding pulse, Cheyne-Stokes respirations.

C. Focal—hemiparesis, hemiplegia, central facial paralysis, language disorders, cranial dysfunction, conjugate deviation eyes toward lesion, flaccid hyporeflexia (later, spastic hyperreflexia).

D. Residual manifestations.
   1. Lesion left hemisphere.
      a. Right hemiplegia; aphasia, expressive and/or receptive.
      b. Behavior is slow, cautious, disorganized.
   2. Lesion right hemisphere.
      a. Left hemiplegia.
      b. Behavior is impulsive, quick; unaware of deficits; poor judge of abilities, limitations; neglect of paralyzed side.
   3. General.
      a. Memory deficits; reduced memory span; emotional lability.
      b. Visual deficits; loss of half of each visual field.

c. Apraxia (can move but unable to use body part for specific purpose).

Nursing Care

A. Strive for initial nursing goal: support life and prevent complications; long term goal is rehabilitation.

B. See section on the unconscious or immobilized patient, p. 113.

C. Maintain patent airway and ventilation—elevate head of bed 20 degress unless patient is in shock.

D. Monitor clinical status to prevent complications.
   1. Neurological.
      a. Include assessment of recurrent CVA, increased intracranial pressure, bulbar involvement, hyperthermia.
      b. Continued coma is a negative prognostic sign.
   2. Cardiovascular—shock and arrhythmias, hypertension.
   3. Lungs—pulmonary emboli.

E. Maintain optimal positioning.
   1. During acute stages, quiet environment and minimal handling may be necessary to prevent further bleeding.
   2. Upper motor lesion—spastic paralysis, flexion deformities, external rotation of hip.
   3. Positioning schedule—two hours on unaffected side; twenty minutes on affected side; thirty minutes prone, bid-tid.
   4. Complications common with hemiplegia—frozen shoulder, footdrop.

F. Maintain skin integrity.

G. Maintain personal hygiene—encourage self-help.

H. Promote adequate nutrition, fluid, and electrolyte balance.
   1. Encourage self-feeding.
   2. Food should be placed in unparalyzed side of mouth.

I. Promote elimination.
   1. Bladder control may be regained within three to five days.

2. Retention catheter may not be part of treatment regime.
3. Offer urinal or bedpan every two hours day and night.

J. Provide emotional support.
   1. Behavior changes as consciousness is regained—loss of memory, emotional lability, confusion, language disorders.
   2. Reorient, reassure, and establish means of communication.

K. Promote rehabilitation to maximal functioning.
   1. Comprehensive program—begin during acute phase and follow through convalescence.
   2. Guidelines to assist patient with lesion left hemisphere.
      a. Do not underestimate ability to learn.
      b. Assess ability to understand speech.
      c. Act out, pantomime communication; use patient's terms to communicate; speak in normal tone of voice.
      d. Divide tasks into simple steps; give frequent feedback.
   3. Guidelines to assist patient with lesion right hemisphere.
      a. Do not overestimate abilities.
      b. Use verbal cues as demonstrations; pantomimes may confuse.
      c. Use slow, minimal movements and avoid clutter.
      d. Divide tasks into simple steps; elicit return demonstration of skills.
      e. Promote awareness of body and environment on affected side.

Cerebral Aneurysm

Definition: A dilation of the walls of a weakened cerebral artery leading to rupture from arteriosclerosis or trauma.

Signs and Symptoms

A. Diplopia, eye pain, blurred vision, or ptosis.
B. Hemiparesis, nuchal rigidity.
C. Headache, tinnitus, nausea.
D. Irritability, seizure activity.

Nursing Care

A. Establish and maintain a patent airway.
B. Administer oxygen at 6 1/min. unless patient has COPD.
C. Place patient on bedrest in semi-Fowler's or side lying position.
D. Turn, cough, and deep breathe patient every two hours.
E. Suction only with specific order.
F. Provide darkened room without stimulation, i.e., limit visitors and lengthy discussions.
G. Avoid strenuous activity; provide range-of-motion exercises.
H. Provide diet low in stimulants such as caffeine. Restrict fluid intake to prevent increased intracranial pressure.
I. Monitor intake and output.
J. Monitor vital signs for hypertension or cardiac irregularities. Do not take rectal temperature due to vagal stimulation leading to cardiac arrest.
K. Observe for complications indicating rebleeding, clot formation, or increased size of aneurysm.

Hyperthermia

Definition: Increased temperature that has reached 41°C (106°F); associated with increased cerebral metabolism which may increase risk of hypoxia.

Treatment and Nursing Care

A. Induce hypothermia.
   1. External—cool bath, fans, ice bags, hypothermic blanket (most common).
   2. Drugs.
      a. Chlorpromazine—reduces peripheral vasoconstriction, muscle tone, shivering.
      b. Meperidine—relaxes smooth muscle, reduces shivering.
      c. Promethazine—dilates coronary arteries, reduces laryngeal and bronchial irritation.

B. Monitor hypothermia.
   1. Monitor temperature.
      a. Continuous probe or rectal thermometer.
      b. Read and record every 15 minutes.
   2. Prevent shivering.
      a. Shivering increases CSF pressure and oxygen consumption.
      b. Treatment: chlorpromazine.
   3. Prevent trauma to skin and tissue.
      a. Frostbite—crystallization of tissues with white or blue discoloration, hardening of tissue, burning, numbness.
      b. Fat necrosis—solidification of subcutaneous fat creating hard tissue masses.
      c. Initially give complete bath and oil the skin; during procedure, massage skin frequently with lotion or oil to maintain integrity of the skin.
   4. Prevent respiratory complications.
      a. Hypothermia may mask infection and cause respiratory arrest.
      b. Institute measures to maintain open airway and adequate ventilation.
   5. Prevent cardiac complications.
      a. Monitor cardiac status; hypothermia can cause arrhythmias and cardiac arrest.
      b. Have emergency equipment available.
   6. Monitor renal function.
      a. Insert Foley catheter.
      b. Monitor urinary output, BUN; may monitor specific gravity.
   7. Prevent vomiting and possible aspiration; patient may have loss of gag reflex and reduced peristalsis.
   8. Monitor changes in neurological function during hypothermia.
C. Effects of hypothermia.
   1. Reduces cerebral metabolism and demand for oxygen.
   2. Decreases cerebral and systemic blood flow.
   3. Reduces CSF pressure.
   4. Decreases endocrine, liver, and kidney function.
   5. Decreases pulse, blood pressure, and respiration; may affect cardiac pacemaker.

Convulsions

Definition: Forceful involuntary contractions of voluntary muscles; may be one component of a seizure.

Etiology

Cerebral trauma, congenital defects, epilepsy, infection, tumor circulatory defect, anoxia, metabolic abnormalities, excessive hydration.

Classification

A. Tonic convulsion—sustained contraction of muscles.
B. Clonic convulsion—alternating contraction/relaxation of opposing muscle group.
C. Epileptoid—any convulsion with loss of consciousness.

Nursing Care

A. Protect patient from further injury.
B. Observe and record characteristics of seizure activity.
   1. Level of consciousness.
   2. Description of aura, if present.
   3. Description of body position and initial activity.
   4. Monitor activity—initial body part involved, character of movements (tonic/clonic), progression of movement, duration, biting of the tongue.
   5. Respiration, color.
   6. Pupillary changes, eye movements.
   7. Incontinence, vomiting.
   8. Total duration of seizure.
   9. Postictal state—loss of consciousness; sleepiness; impaired speech, motor or thinking; headache; injuries.

10. Post convulsion, neurological and vital signs.

11. Frequency and number of convulsions.

C. Protect patient from trauma.

1. Maintain patent airway.

2. Keep padded tongue blade at bedside; do not force between teeth if they are already clenched.

3. Be sure side rails are padded and there is padding around head.

4. Avoid use of any restraints.

5. Remove any objects from environment that may cause injury.

6. Remain with patient.

D. Care after the seizure.

1. Maintain open airway—positioning, suction.

2. Reorient to environment; give reassurance and support.

3. Monitor clinical status.

4. Administer anticonvulsants.

5. Maintain quiet environment.

Epilepsy

Definition: Paroxysmal disturbance in consciousness, with autonomic, sensory, and/or motor dysfunction; a manifestation of excessive neuronal discharge in the brain.

Etiology

A. Congenital, genetic, trauma, tumors, infections, vascular disorders, ischemia, metabolic disorders, degenerative disorders.

B. Divisions.

1. Symptomatic type—secondary to probable cause.

2. Idiopathic type—primary epilepsy without definite, known cause.

Signs and Symptoms of Common Seizure Types

A. Grand mal.

1. Generalized seizure—symmetrical tonic-clonic movements without focal onset and involving entire body.

2. May be preceded by brief aura which is specific for each patient—visual, olfactory, auditory, gustatory, somatic.

3. Epileptic cry follows aura but precedes loss of consciousness and convulsion.

4. Brief tonic phase—rigid extension, muscle contraction; cessation of respirations; dilated pupils; cyanotic, clenched jaws.

5. Clonic phase follows—alternating forceful contraction and relaxation of muscles creating jerking movements, stertorous respirations, excessive salivation, incontinence; tongue may be bitten.

6. Postictal period after seizure subsides— fatigue, headache, confusion, sleepiness, residual neurological deficit, amnesia.

B. Petit mal.

1. Generalized—frequent episodes of loss of consciousness for a matter of seconds and cessation of motor activity; patient may stop in mid-sentence, stare, and then go on talking.

2. No change in muscle tone; falls seldom occur although patient may stagger in gait or lose bladder control.

3. Most common in children and may affect child's progress in school if attacks are frequent.

C. Jacksonian (focal) seizures.

1. Partial seizure with motor or sensory symptoms.

2. Precipitated by lesion in motor or sensory cortex area; may be identified by characteristics of the seizure.

3. Motor seizures begin with convulsion in particular body part and may progress centrally to other body parts.

4. Loss of consciousness occurs if seizures become generalized.

5. Sensory seizures involve transient numbness, tingling in particular areas.

D. Psychomotor seizures.
  1. Partial seizure with complex symptoms involving the temporal lobe.
  2. Brief lapses of consciousness; mental clouding lasts for a longer period than in petit mal and may continue after attack.
  3. Wide range of automatic, repetitive motor activity occurs which may be inappropriate or asocial.
  4. Psychic phenomena of visual, auditory, or olfactory hallucinations may occur.
  5. Patient has amnesia during and after attack.

Nursing Care

A. Protect patient from injury or complication during seizure (see Convulsions p. 122).

B. Eliminate precipitating factors of seizure.
  1. Accurate observation and recording of seizures.
  2. Possible factors: drugs, alcohol, sleep, nutrition, loud noises, music, flickering lights, hyperventilation.
  3. Treatment of underlying cause—tumor, infection.

C. Promote physical and mental health.
  1. Establish regular routines for activities of daily living.
     a. Diet, sleep, physical activity (activity tends to inhibit seizure activity).
     b. Provide appropriate safeguards during exercise and sports.
  2. Avoid alcohol, stress, exhaustion.
  3. Foster self-esteem and confidence; avoid overprotection of patient.
  4. Provide patient and family with facts regarding epilepsy.
     a. Control of the disorder.
     b. Recognition of impending seizure and care during seizure.
     c. Importance of carrying identification card in case of emergency.
     d. Organizations which provide services, such as the National Epilepsy League and the National Association to Control Epilepsy.

D. Administer and monitor effects of medications.
  1. Medication regime may require periods of adjustments and/or a combination of drugs.
  2. Reinforce necessity for taking medication regularly as prescribed; observe response, any side effects or seizure activity.
  3. Administer anticonvulsants.
     a. Most common drugs: phenobarbital, diphenylhydantoin (Dilantin), mephenytoin (Mesantoin), primidone (Mysoline), paramethadione (Paradione), trimethadione (Tridione), ethosuximide (Zarontin).
     b. Usually used in combination—decreased dosage lessens side effects.
  4. Administer drugs as a preventative measure for further episodes.
     a. Dilantin.
        (1) Prevents seizures through depression of the motor areas of the brain.
        (2) Side effects include GI symptoms, rash, and bleeding gums.
     b. Valium.
        (1) For relief of restlessness.
        (2) To decrease seizure activity.
     c. Phenobarbital.
        (1) Reduces responsiveness of normal neurons to impulses arising in the focal site.
        (2) Side effects are drowsiness, ataxia, nystagmus.
        (3) Toxic effects produce rash but usually no nausea and vomiting.
  5. Monitor toxic side effects of drugs: drowsiness, skin rash, nervousness, nausea, ataxia, gum hyperplasia, blood dyscrasias.
  6. Avoid sudden withdrawal of drugs—may precipitate status epilepticus.

E. Treatment of complicating status epilepticus.
  1. Successive major convulsions without regaining consciousness between attacks are considered a medical emergency which may cause death.
  2. Most frequent cause is sudden withdrawal of anticonvulsants; other factors include insulin, electroshock, acute infections, trauma, and metabolic disorders.

3. Management of complications.
   a. Maintain open airway.
   b. Terminate seizure with IV medications: phenobarbital, diphenylhydantoin, diazepam, paraldehyde.
   c. Monitor patient's condition frequently for complications: cardiac, respiratory, and neurological status; arterial blood gases, glucose, calcium, electrolytes, renal and liver function.

Multiple Sclerosis

Definition: Chronic, slowly progressive, noncontagious, degenerative disease of the CNS.

Etiology

A. Definite cause unknown; autoimmunity or virus likely cause.
B. Incidence is greater in colder climate, equal in the sexes, and usually occurs between ages twenty to forty years.

Pathophysiology

A. Demyelination of nerve fibers within long conducting pathways of spinal cord and brain.
B. Lesions (plaques) are irregularly scattered—disseminated.
C. Destruction of myelin sheath creates patches of sclerotic tissue, degeneration of the nerve fiber, and disturbance in conduction of sensory and motor impulses.
D. Initially the disease is characterized by periods of remission with exacerbation and variable manifestations but is followed by irreversible dysfunction.
E. Clinical course may extend over ten to twenty years.

Signs and Symptoms

A. Highly variable, depending on area of involvement: sensory fibers, motor fibers, brainstem, cerebellum, internal capsule.

B. Weakness, paralysis, incoordination, ataxia, intention tremor, bladder/bowel retention or incontinence, spasticity, numbness, tingling, analgesia, anesthesia, loss of position sense, impaired vision (diplopia, nystagmus), dysphagia, impaired speech, emotional instability, impaired judgment.

Nursing Care

A. Prevent precipitation of exacerbations.
   1. Avoid fatigue, stress, infection, overheating, chilling.
   2. Establish regular program of exercise and rest.
   3. Provide a balanced diet.
B. Administer and assess effects of medications.
   1. Steroids—hasten remission.
   2. Antibiotics, muscle relaxants, mood elevators, vitamin B.
C. Promote optimal activity.
   1. Moderation in activity with rest periods.
   2. Physical and speech therapy.
   3. Diversionary activities, hobbies.
   4. During exacerbation, patient is usually put on bed rest.
D. Promote safety.
   1. Sensory loss—regulate bath water; use caution with heating pads; inspect skin for lesions.
   2. Motor loss—avoid waxed floors, throw rugs; provide rails and walker.
   3. Diplopia—apply eye patch.
E. Encourage regular elimination—bladder/bowel training programs.
F. Provide education and emotional support to patient and family.
   1. Encourage independence and realistic goals; assess personality and behavior changes; observe for signs of depression.
   2. Provide instruction and assistive devices; provide information about services of the National Multiple Sclerosis Society.
G. Assess and prevent potential complications.
   1. Most common: urinary tract infection, calculi, decubitus ulcers.

2. Contracture pain due to spasticity, metabolic or nutritional disorders, regurgitation, depression.

3. Common cause of death: respiratory tract infection, urinary tract infection.

Myasthenia Gravis

Definition: Myasthenia gravis is a neuromuscular disease characterized by marked weakness and abnormal fatigue of voluntary muscles.

Etiology

A. Unknown; question autoimmune reaction.
B. Patients with myasthenia have a high incidence of thymus abnormalities and frequently have systemic lupus erythematosus.

Pathophysiology

A. Basic pathology is a defect in transmission of nerve impulse at the myoneural junction, the junction of motor neuron with muscle.
B. Normally, acetylcholine is stored in synaptic vesicle of motor neurons to skeletal muscles.
C. Defect may be due to:
   1. Deficiency in acetylcholine/excess acetylcholinesterase.
   2. Defective motor-end plate and/or nerve terminals.
   3. Decreased sensitivity to acetylcholine.
D. Generally there is no muscle atrophy or degeneration; there may be periods of exacerbations and remissions.

Signs and Symptoms

A. Symptoms are related to progressive weakness and fatigue of muscles when used; muscles generally are strongest in the morning.
B. Eyes are affected first: ptosis, diplopia, and eye squint.
C. Impaired speech; dysphagia; drooping facies; difficulty chewing, closing mouth, or smiling; breathing difficulty and hoarse voice.
D. Respiratory paralysis and failure.

E. Diagnosis confirmed with Tensilon test.
   1. Positive for myasthenia—improvement in muscle strength.
   2. Negative—no improvement or even deterioration.

Nursing Care

A. Primary goals are to improve neuromuscular transmission and prevent complications.
B. Administer and assess effects of medications.
   1. Anticholinesterase drugs increase levels of acetylcholine at myoneural junction.
      a. Neostigmine, pyridostigmine, ambenonium—main difference is duration of effect.
      b. Edrophonium (Tensilon)—is a rapid, brief-acting anticholinesterase used for testing purposes.
      c. Side effects.
         (1) Related to effects of increased acetylcholine in parasympathetic nervous system: sweating, excessive salivation, nausea, diarrhea, abdominal cramps; possibly bradycardia or hypotension.
         (2) Excessive doses lead to cholinergic crisis—atropine given as cholinergic blocker.
      d. Nursing measures.
         (1) Give medications exactly on time, thirty minutes before meals.
         (2) Give medication with milk and crackers to reduce GI upset.
         (3) Observe therapeutic or any toxic effects; monitor and record muscle strength and vital capacity.
   2. Steroids.
      a. Suppress immune response.
      b. Usually the last resort after anticholinesterase and thymectomy.
   3. The following drugs must be avoided.
      a. Streptomycin, kanamycin, neomycin, gentamicin are drugs that block neuromuscular transmission.
      b. Ether, quinidine, morphine, curare, procainamide, innovar, sedatives—aggravate weakness of myasthenia.

C. Monitor patient's condition for complications.
   1. Vital signs.
   2. Respirations—depth, rate, vital capacity, ability to deep breathe and cough.
   3. Swallowing—ability to eat and handle secretions.
   4. Muscle strength.
   5. Speech—provide method of communication if patient unable to talk.
   6. Bowel and bladder function.
   7. Psychological status.
D. Encourage optimal activity.
   1. Plan short periods of activity and long periods of rest.
   2. Time activity to coincide with maximal muscle strength.
   3. Encourage normal activities of daily living.
   4. Encourage diversionary activities.
E. Provide instruction and emotional support.
   1. Instruct patient about medications and treatment regime and importance of adhering to medication schedule.
   2. Instruct patient to avoid infection, stress, fatigue, and over-the-counter drugs.
   3. Instruct patient to wear identification medal and carry emergency card.
   4. Provide information about services of Myasthenia Gravis Foundation.

Myasthenic or Cholinergic Crisis

A. Myasthenic crisis.
   1. Acute exacerbation of disease may be due to rapid, unrecognized progression of disease; failure of medication; infection; or fatigue or stress.
   2. Myasthenic symptoms—weakness, dyspnea, dysphagia, restlessness, difficulty speaking.
B. Cholinergic crisis.
   1. Cholinergic paralysis with sustained depolarization of motor-end plates is due to over-medication with anticholinesterase.
   2. Symptoms similar to myasthenic state; restlessness, weakness, speaking difficulty, dysphagia, dyspnea.

   3. Cholinergic symptoms—fasciculations, abdominal cramps, diarrhea, nausea, vomiting, salivation, sweating, increased bronchial secretion.
C. Tensilon test to differentiate crises, as symptoms are similar.
   1. Tensilon is given and if strength improves, it is symptomatic of myasthenic crisis and the patient needs more medication; if weakness is more severe, it is symptomatic of cholinergic crisis and overdose has occurred.
   2. Be prepared for emergency with atropine, suction, and other emergency equipment for respiratory arrest.
D. Crisis with respiratory insufficiency; patient cannot swallow secretions and may aspirate.
   1. Bed rest maintained.
   2. Endotracheal or tracheostomy tube to assist with ventilation may be required.
   3. Atropine given and anticholinesterase (cholinergic) may be held.
   4. Anticholinesterase (myasthenic) begun.

Parkinson's Disease

Definition: Degenerative disease of the brain resulting in dysfunction of the extrapyramidal system.

Etiology

A. Idiopathic.
B. Other possible causes: atherosclerosis, drug induction, postencephalitis.

Pathophysiology

A. Degeneration of basal ganglia due to depleted concentration of dopamine.
B. Depletion of dopamine correlated with degeneration of substantia nigra (midbrain structures which are closely related functionally to basal ganglia).

C. Loss of inhibitory modulation of dopamine to counterbalance cholinergic system and interruption of balance-coordinating extrapyramidal system.

D. Slowly progressive disease with high incidence of crippling disability; mental deterioration occurs very late.

Signs and Symptoms

A. Appears in five stages: unilateral, bilateral, impaired balance, fully developed severe disease, and confinement to bed or wheelchair.

B. Symptoms.
 1. Tremor at rest—especially in hands and fingers (pill-rolling).
    a. Increases when stressed or fatigued.
    b. May decrease with purposeful activity or sleep.
 2. Rigidity—blank facial expression (mask-like).
    a. Drooling, difficulty with swallowing or speaking.
    b. Short, shuffling steps with stooped posture.
    c. Propulsive gait.
    d. Immobility of muscles in flexed position, creating jerky cogwheel motions.
    e. Loss of coordinated and associated automatic movement and balance.
 3. Akinesia—difficulty initiating voluntary movement.
 4. Autonomic dysfunction—lacrimation, incontinence, decreased sexual function, constipation.

Nursing Care

A. Strive for primary goals: reduce muscle tremor and rigidity and prevent complications.

B. Administer and assess effects of medications.
 1. Amantadine: used to treat patients with mild symptoms but no disability; side effects uncommon with usual dose.
 2. Anticholinergic drugs: most effective is Ethopropazine; used to treat tremors and rigidity, and inhibit action of acetylcholine; side

effects include dry mouth, dry skin, blurring vision, urinary retention, and tachycardia.
 3. Levodopa (converted in body to dopamine).
    a. Reduces akinesia, tremor, and rigidity.
    b. Passes through blood-brain barrier.
    c. Effectiveness may decline after 2–3 years.
    d. Side effects.
       (1) Anorexia, nausea, and vomiting (administer drug with meals or snack; avoid coffee, which seems to increase nausea).
       (2) Postural hypotension, dizziness, tachycardia, and arrhythmias (monitor vital signs; caution patient to sit up or stand up slowly; have patient wear support stockings).
    e. Contraindicated in patients with closed-angle glaucoma, psychotic illness, and peptic ulcer disease.
 4. Sinemet—combination of carbidopa and levodopa; has fewer side effects than levodopa.
 5. Antihistamines: reduce tremor and anxiety; side effect is drowsiness.
 6. Antispasmodics (Artane, Kemadrin): improve rigidity but not tremor.
 7. Bromocriptine (drug often used to replace levodopa when it loses effectiveness).
    a. Acts on dopamine receptors.
    b. Side effects: anorexia, nausea, vomiting, constipation, postural hypotension, cardiac arrhythmias, headache.
    c. Contraindicated in patients with mental illness, myocardial infarction, peptic ulcers, peripheral vascular disease.
 8. Avoid the following drugs:
    a. Phenothiazines, reserpine, pyridoxine (vitamin B_6)—block desired action of levodopa.
    b. Monamine oxidase inhibitors—precipitate hypertensive crisis.
    c. Methyldopa—potentiates parkinsonian effects.

C. Provide appropriate nursing care following surgery.
 1. Stereotaxic surgery to reduce tremor.
 2. Implantation of electrodes through burr

holes into target area of brain; creation of lesion with high frequency of coagulation probe.

D. Maintain regular patterns of elimination.
   1. Constipation is often a problem due to side effects of medications, reduced physical activity, and muscle weakness.
   2. Provide stool softeners, suppositories, mild cathartics.

E. Promote physical therapy and rehabilitation.
   1. Provide preventive, corrective, and postural exercises.
   2. Institute massage and stretching exercises, stressing extension of limbs.
   3. Encourage daily ambulation; have patient lift feet up when walking and avoid prolonged sitting.
   4. Facilitate adaptation for activities of daily living and self-care; encourage rhythmic patterns to attain timing; foster independence; utilize special aids and devices.
   5. Remove hazards that might cause falls.

F. Provide education and emotional support to patient and family.
   1. Remember, intellect is usually not impaired.
   2. Assess changes in self-consciousness, body image, sexuality, moods.
   3. Instruct patient to avoid emotional stress and fatigue, which aggravate symptoms.
   4. Instruct patient to avoid foods high in vitamin B_6 and monamine oxidase.

Meningitis

Definition: Acute infection of the pia-arachnoid membrane.

Etiology

Organisms: meningococcus, staphylococcus, streptococcus, pneumococcus, Haemophilus influenzae, tuberculous.

Signs and Symptoms

A. Painful, stiff neck—nuchal rigidity, Kernig's and Brudzinski's signs.
B. Severe headache, photophobia.
C. Fever.
D. Irritability, stupor, coma.

Nursing Care

A. Maintain open airway.
B. Treat the infective organism—antimicrobic therapy, intravenously.
C. Assess and treat increased intracranial pressure or seizures.
D. Control body temperature.
E. Provide adequate fluid and electrolyte balance.
F. Provide quiet environment.

Cranial Nerve Disorders

Trigeminal Neuralgia (Tic Douloureux)

Definition: Sensory disorder of the fifth cranial nerve, resulting in severe, recurrent paroxysms of sharp facial pain along the distribution of the trigeminal nerve. Etiology and pathology are unknown; incidence is higher in older women.

Signs and Symptoms

A. Trigger points on the lips, gums, nose, or cheek.
B. May be stimulated by a cold breeze, washing, chewing, food/fluids of extreme temperatures.

Treatment and Nursing Care

A. Observe characteristics of attack and ways patient protects face from stimulus.
B. Avoid extremes of heat or cold; give small feedings of semiliquid or soft food.

C. Medical treatment.
  1. Massive doses of B_{12}.
  2. Inhalation: 10–15 drops of trichloroethylene on cotton.
  3. Anticonvulsants: Dilantin and Tegretol.
  4. Alcohol injections to produce anesthesia of the nerve.
D. Surgical treatment.
  1. Peripheral—avulsion of supraorbital, infraorbital, or mandibular division.
  2. Intracranial.
      a. Division of the sensory nerve root for permanent anesthesia.
      b. Patient may experience numbness, stiffness or burning after surgery.
      c. Microsurgery allows for selective sectioning of the fifth nerve.
      d. Pain and temperature fibers are destroyed, and sensation of touch and corneal reflex are preserved.
E. Assess and treat complications after surgery.
  1. Facial paralysis.
  2. Irritation or ulceration of cornea due to loss of sensation.
  3. Local trauma to inside of mouth.

Bell's Palsy (Facial Paralysis)

Definition: Lower motor neuron lesion of the seventh cranial nerve, resulting in paralysis of one side of the face.

Signs and Symptoms

A. Flaccid muscles.
B. Shallow nasolabial fold.
C. Inability to raise eyebrows, frown, smile, close eyelids, or puff out cheeks.
D. Upward movement of eye when attempting to close eyelid.
E. Loss of taste in anterior tongue.

Nursing Care

A. Palliative.

B. Analgesics, steroids, physiotherapy, support of facial muscles, protection of cornea.
C. Promote active facial exercises to prevent loss of muscle tone.
D. Instruct patient to chew food on unaffected side.
E. Present attractive, easy-to-eat foods to prevent anorexia and weight loss.
F. Provide special eye care to prevent keratitis.
G. Reassure and support.

Meniere's Disease

Definition: Dilatation of the endolymphatic system causing degeneration of the vestibular and cochlear hair cells.

Etiology

A. Etiology is unknown.
B. Possible causes may include allergies, toxicity, localized ischemia, hemorrhage, viral infection, and edema.

Treatment and Nursing Care

A. Direct care toward alleviating obstruction and reducing the pressure.
B. Surgical division of vestibular portion of the nerve or destruction of the labyrinth may be necessary for severe cases.
C. Maintain bedrest during acute attack.
  1. Prevent injury during attack.
  2. Provide side rails if necessary.
  3. Keep room dark when photophobia present.
D. Provide drug therapy.
  1. Vasodilators (nicotinic acid).
  2. Diuretics, antihistamines (Benadryl).
  3. Sedatives.
E. Monitor diet therapy.
  1. Low sodium.
  2. Lipoflavonoid vitamin supplement.
  3. Restricted fluid intake.
F. Assist with ambulation if necessary.

Guillain-Barré Syndrome

Definition: An acute infectious neuronitis of cranial and peripheral nerves. Immune system overreacts to an infection destroying the myelin sheath.

Characteristics

A. Etiology is unknown.
B. Occurs at any age but increased incidence between thirty and fifty years of age.
C. Both sexes equally affected.
D. Recovery is a slow process, taking 2 months to 2 years.
E. Diagnostic test results: CSF contains high protein, abnormal EEG.

Signs and Symptoms

A. First report may be of a mild upper respiratory infection or gastroenteritis.
B. Initial symptom of weakness of lower extremities.
C. Gradual progressive weakness of upper extremities and facial muscles (24–72 hours); paresthesias may precede weakness.
D. Respiratory failure may occur.
E. Sensory changes—usually minor, but in some cases severe impairment of sensory information occurs.
F. Cardiac arrhythmias.

Nursing Care

A. No specific treatment available; supportive treatment includes monitoring for complications (respiratory, circulatory).
B. Carefully observe for respiratory paralysis and inability to handle secretions.
C. Provide chest physiotherapy and pulmonary toilet.
D. Maintain cardiovascular function.
   1. Monitor vital signs and cardiac rhythm.
   2. Vasopressors and volume replacement.
E. Prevent complications of immobility.
   1. Turn frequently.
   2. Provide skin care.
F. Provide appropriate diversion.
G. Reassure patient, especially during paralysis period.
H. Previous treatment included corticosteroids; this is now considered controversial.

Amyotrophic Lateral Sclerosis (Lou Gehrig's Disease)

Definition: The most common motor neuron disease of muscular atrophy. It is a rapidly fatal, upper and lower motor neuron deficit affecting the limbs.

Characteristics

A. May result from several causes.
   1. Nutritional deficiency related to disturbance in enzyme metabolism.
   2. Vitamin E deficiency resulting in damage to cell membranes.
   3. Metabolic interference in nucleic acid production by nerve fibers.
   4. Autoimmune disorders.
B. Inherited in 10 percent of the cases.
C. Occurs after age 40; most common in men.
D. Is fatal within 3–10 years after onset.
E. Diagnostic tests: EMG and muscle biopsy; increased protein in CSF.

Signs and Symptoms

A. Atrophy and weakness of upper extremities.
B. Difficulty swallowing and chewing.
C. Respiratory excursion and breathing patterns.
D. Impaired speech.
E. Secondary depression.

Nursing Care

A. Assist with rehabilitation program to promote independence.
B. Monitor for complications.
   1. Prevent skin breakdown: reposition regularly, provide back care, and utilize pressure-relieving devices.

2. Prevent aspiration of food or fluids: offer soft foods and keep patient in upright position during meals.
3. Promote bowel and bladder function.

C. Provide emotional support.

Intracranial Surgery

Preoperative and Postoperative Care

Preoperative Care

A. Observe and record neurological symptoms.
   1. Paralysis.
   2. Seizure foci.
   3. Pupillary response.
B. Prepare patient physically and psychologically for surgery.
   1. Prep and shave cranial hair (save hair).
   2. Apply scrub solution to scalp, as ordered.
   3. Avoid using enemas unless specifically ordered; the strain of defecation can lead to increased intracranial pressure.
   4. Explain postoperative routine orders such as neurological checks and headaches.
   5. Administer steroids or mecurial diuretics, as ordered, to decrease cerebral edema.
   6. Insert NG tube and/or Foley catheter as ordered.

General Postoperative Care

A. Observe neurological signs.
   1. Evaluate level of consciousness.
      a. Orientation to time and place.
      b. Response to painful stimuli.
      c. Ability to follow verbal command.
   2. Evaluate pupil size and reactions to light.
      a. Are pupils equal, not constricted or dilated.
      b. Do pupils react to light
      c. Do pupils react sluggishly or are they fixed.

3. Evaluate strength and motion of extremities.
   a. Are handgrips present and equal.
   b. Are handgrips strong or weak.
   c. Can patient move all extremities on command.
   d. Are movements purposeful or involuntary.
   e. Do the extremities have twitching, flaccid, or spastic movements (indicative of a neurological problem).
4. Observe vital signs (TRP and BP).
   a. Keep patient normothermic to decrease metabolic needs of the brain.
   b. Observe respirations for depth and rate to prevent respiratory acidosis from anoxia.
   c. Observe blood pressure and pulse for signs of shock or increased intracranial pressure.
5. Evaluate reflexes.
   a. Babinski—positive Babinski is illicited by stroking the lateral aspect of the sole of the foot, backward flexion of the great toe or spreading of other toes.

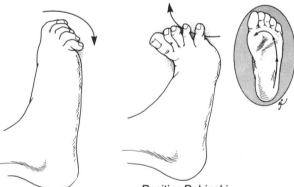

Negative Babinski   Positive Babinski

   b. Romberg—when patient stands with feet close together, he or she falls off balance. If positive, may have cerebellar, proprioceptive, or vestibular difficulties.
   c. Kernig—patient is lying down with thigh flexed at a right angle; extension of the leg upward results in spasm of hamstring muscle, pain, and resis-

tance to additional extension of leg at the knee (indicative of meningitis).

6. Watch for headache, double vision, nausea, or vomiting.

B. Provide for special needs.

1. Maintain patent airway—oxygen deprivation and an increase of carbon dioxide may produce cerebral hypoxia and cause cerebral edema.

2. Suction as necessary, but not through nose without specific order.

3. Maintain adequate oxygenation and humidification.

4. Place patient in semi-prone or semi-Fowler's position (or totally on side). Turn every two hours, side to side.

5. Maintain fluid and electrolytes.
   a. Do not give fluid by mouth to semi-conscious or unconscious patient.
   b. Weigh to determine fluid loss.
   c. Monitor IV fluids; overhydration leads to cerebral edema.

6. Record accurate intake and output.

7. Take seizure precautions.

8. Provide hygienic care, including oral hygiene.

9. Observe dressing for unusual drainage (bleeding, cerebral spinal fluid).

10. Prevent straining with bowel movements.

Medications

A. Steroids.
   1. Decrease cerebral edema by their anti-inflammatory effect.
   2. Decrease capillary permeability in inflammatory process, thus decreasing leakage of fluid into tissue.

B. Mannitol.
   1. Decrease cerebral edema.
   2. Diuretic action by carrying out large volume of water through the nephron.

C. Dilantin.
   1. Prevents seizures through depression of the motor areas of the brain.
   2. Side effects include gastrointestinal symptoms and rash.

D. Valium.
   1. Relieves restlessness.
   2. Decreases seizure activity.

E. Phenobarbital.
   1. Reduces responsiveness of normal neurons to the nervous impulses arising in the focal site.
   2. Side effects are drowsiness, ataxia, nystagmus.
   3. Toxic effects produce rash but usually no nausea and vomiting.

Precautions for Care of Neurosurgical Patient

A. Do not lower head in Trendelenburg position or place in supine position.

B. Do not suction through nose without specific order.

C. Be careful when administering sedations and narcotics.
   1. Cannot evaluate neurological status.
   2. May cause respiratory embarrassment.

D. Do not give oral fluids unless patient fully awake.

E. Do not administer enemas or cathartics (may cause straining, therefore increasing intracranial pressure).

F. Do not place on operative side if large tumor or bone removed.

Neurosurgical Postoperative Complications

Increased Intracranial Pressure

A. Signs and symptoms.
   1. Brain becomes compressed as intracranial pressure increases.

2. Change in level of consciousness.
3. Lethargy, slurring speech, and slow responses.
4. Changes in condition (often rapid).
   a. Patient becomes restless.
   b. Patient becomes confused.
   c. Increased drowsiness.
   d. Stupor to coma.
5. Changes in vital signs.
   a. Pulse changes—may decrease to 60 or occasionally increase above 100.
   b. Respiratory irregularities—progresses to Cheyne-Stokes and apnea can result.
   c. Blood pressure increases with wide pulse pressure (difference between systolic and diastolic).
   d. Moderately elevated temperature.
6. Headache.
7. Vomiting.
8. Pupil changes—increasing pressure or an expanding clot can displace the brain against the oculomotor or optic nerve.

B. Nursing care.
1. Inform physician of any vital sign changes or sensorium changes.
2. Observe intake and output for possible fluid overload leading to cerebral edema.
3. Observe surgical incision site for signs of edema.
4. Administer diuretics or steroids to decrease edema as ordered.
5. Administer anticonvulsant drugs as ordered.
6. Have spinal or ventricular puncture tray available to drain off cerebral spinal fluid as necessary.
7. Observe for level of consciousness—lethargy, slurred speech, slowed responses.

C. Precautions for care of neurosurgical patient.
1. Do not lower head in Trendelenburg's position or place in supine position.
2. Do not suction through nose without specific order.
3. Be careful when administering sedations and narcotics.
   a. Cannot evaluate neurological status.
   b. May cause respiratory embarrassment.
4. Do not give oral fluids unless patient fully awake.
5. Do not administer enemas or cathartics (may cause straining, therefore increasing intracranial pressure).
6. Do not place on operative side.

Seizures

A. Grand mal (see p. 123).
B. Petit mal (usually not seen in neurosurgical patients).
C. Treatment and nursing care.
1. Administer drugs as ordered (Dilantin, phenobarbital and other related drugs).
2. Provide safe environment.
   a. Pad side rails.
   b. Do not restrain during seizure.
   c. Use tongue blade to prevent tongue from falling back into throat.
3. Observe and record.
   a. Activities preceding the seizure (aura, movements, etc.).
   b. Type of movements and area of body involved.
   c. Incontinence.
   d. Presence of unconsciousness during seizure.
   e. Length of seizure.
   f. Conditions following seizure.
      (1) Somnolent.
      (2) Continuation of previous activities.
      (3) Awareness of seizure activity.
4. Provide privacy during seizure.

Hemorrhage

Symptoms are the same as for increased intracranial pressure or seizures, depending on cause and area involved.

Brain Abscess or Wound Infection

A. Signs and symptoms.
1. Increased temperature unless abscess walled off, in which case temperature can be subnormal.

2. Headache.
3. Neurological deficits relative to area involved (focal seizures, blurred vision, etc.).
4. Increased intracranial pressure.

B. Nursing care.
   1. Observe neurological signs.
   2. Decrease temperature.
      a. Sponge bath.
      b. Antipyretic drugs (Tylenol).
      c. Cooling blanket.
   3. Administer appropriate antibiotics for causative agent.

Eye and Ear Surgery

Cataracts of the Eye

Definition: Clouding or opacity of the lens that leads to blurring vision and eventual loss of sight.

Etiology

A. Opacity is due to chemical changes in the protein of the lens.
B. Condition is the result of slow degenerative changes of age or from injury, poison, or intraocular infection.

Surgical Procedure

A. Usually based on individual needs, that is, how well the patient can see out of the other eye.
   1. If any inflammation is present, surgery is not performed.
   2. Cataracts are removed under local anesthesia.
   3. Some simple cataracts are removed by use of alpha-chymotrypsin, which loosens the zonular fibers that hold the lens in position.
   4. Surgery is performed on one eye at a time.
B. Removal techniques.
   1. Intracapsular: the lens is removed within its capsule.

2. Extracapsular: an opening is made in the capsule, and the lens is lifted out without disturbing the membrane.
3. Cryoextraction: the lens is frozen with a probe—cooled to a temperature of −35°C or lower—and then lifted from its position in the eye.

C. All surgeries are preceded by an iridectomy, which creates an opening for the flow of aqueous humor.

Postoperative Nursing Care

A. Prevent nausea and vomiting, restlessness, or coughing.
B. Observe for shock, hemorrhage from the eye, and sudden pain in the eye.
C. Apply dressing and shield to prevent injury to the operated eye. The unoperated eye is usually left uncovered.
D. Dressing is changed by the physician on the first to third postoperative day; the dressing is removed on the seventh to tenth day.
E. Keep patient flat or in low-Fowler's position the day of surgery.
F. Get patient out of bed the first postoperative day.
G. Turn patient on unoperated side if ordered; if patient cannot be turned, use sandbags to position head.
H. Temporary glasses are prescribed, one to four weeks postoperatively.

Specific Adjustment Problems

A. Once the lens is removed, the eye can no longer accommodate, and glasses must be worn at all times.
B. Glasses prescribed for cataract magnify so that everything appears to be one-fourth closer than it is; hence, the patient must be taught to accommodate to this situation.
   1. It takes time to learn to judge distance and climb stairs.
   2. Color, as seen by the eye from which a cataract has been removed, is slightly changed.

3. If the lens has been removed from one eye only, the patient will use only one eye at a time and not both together unless a contact lens is fitted for the operated eye.

C. The patient should wait three months before getting permanent glasses.

Retinal Detachment

Definition: The retina is the part of the eye that perceives light; it coordinates and transmits impulses from its seeing nerve cells to the optic nerve. As the detachment extends and becomes complete, blindness occurs.

Signs and Symptoms

A. Opacity of the eyes.
B. Flashes of light.
C. Floating spots—blood and retinal cells that are freed at the time of the tear and that cast shadows on the retina as they drift about the eye.
D. Progressive constriction of vision in one area.
   1. The area of visual loss depends on the location of detachment.
   2. When the detachment is extensive and rapid, the patient feels as if a curtain has been pulled over his eyes.

Preoperative Care

A. Keep patient on bed rest.
B. Cover both eyes with patches to prevent further detachment.
C. Position patient's head so the retinal hole is in the lowest part of the eye.

Surgical Procedure

A. Immediate surgery with drainage of fluid from subretinal space so that retina returns to normal position.
B. Retinal breaks are sealed by various methods that produce inflammatory reactions (chorioretinitis).

1. Adhesions will form between the edges of the break and the underlying choroid to obliterate the opening.
2. Laser beam can also be used to produce the chorioretinitis.

Postoperative Nursing Care

A. Maintain safe environment.
   1. Keep side rails up.
   2. Feed patient.
   3. Maintain bedrest for 1 or 2 days.
   4. Keep bed flat or in low-Fowler's position.
B. Prevent complications.
   1. Observe for hemorrhage, which is a common complication. Notify physician immediately of any sudden, sharp eye pain.
   2. Cover both eyes.
   3. Position so area of detachment is in dependent position. (If air bubble is present, position on abdomen.)
   4. Prevent clinical manifestations which can cause hemorrhage.
      a. Nausea and vomiting.
      b. Restlessness.
   5. Encourage patient to do deep breathing but to avoid coughing.
   6. Administer good skin care to prevent breakdown.
   7. Avoid external eye pressure.
C. Provide emotional support.
   1. Provide audible stimulation.
   2. Warn patient as you enter the room and always speak before touching.
   3. Orient to surroundings.
D. Provide patient instruction.
   1. During convalescent period.
      a. Wear patch at night to prevent rubbing of eyes.
      b. Wear dark glasses.
      c. Avoid squinting.
   2. During postconvalescent period.
      a. Avoid straining and constipation.
      b. Avoid lifting heavy objects for six to eight weeks.
      c. Avoid bending from the waist.

Glaucoma

Definition: Abnormally increased intraocular pressure, which may produce serious visual defects.

Characteristics

A. Chronic open-angle glaucoma.
  1. Results from an overproduction or obstruction to the outflow of aqueous humor.
  2. Ninety percent of all glaucoma cases are of this type.
B. Chronic closed-angle glaucoma follows an untreated attack of acute closed-angle glaucoma.
C. Acute closed-angle (narrow-angle) glaucoma.
  1. Results from an obstruction to the outflow of aqueous humor.
  2. Caused by trauma, drugs, or inflammation.
D. Evaluate risk conditions.
  1. Over forty years of age.
  2. Diabetic.
  3. Black patient.
  4. Hypertensive.
  5. Familial history of glaucoma.
  6. "Large-eyed" children.
  7. History of eye injury.

Signs and Symptoms

A. Schoitz Tonometer Test (7 to 21 mm Hg is normal).
B. Chronic open-angle.
  1. Loss of peripheral vision and eventual loss of central vision.
  2. Mild aching in the eyes.
  3. Halos around lights.
C. Acute closed-angle glaucoma.
  1. Unilateral inflammation.
  2. Pain.
  3. Pressure over eye.
  4. Moderate pupil dilation, nonreactive to light.
  5. Cloudy cornea.
  6. Blurring and decreased visual acuity.
  7. Photophobia.
  8. Halos around light.
  9. Nausea and vomiting.
D. Chronic closed-angle glaucoma.
  1. Usually no symptoms.
  2. Halos around lights may occur.
  3. Progresses to blindness.

Treatment and Nursing Care

A. For chronic open-angle glaucoma.
  1. Aqueous humor production decreased through beta blockers.
  2. Intraocular pressure lowered with epinephrine or diuretics.
  3. Miotic eyedrops, such as pilocarpine, facilitate the outflow of aqueous humor.
  4. Patient is prepared for surgical intervention.
B. For acute closed-angle glaucoma.
  1. Treated as an emergency problem.
  2. Drugs administered to lower intraocular pressure.
  3. Patient is prepared for peripheral iridectomy.
    a. Part of iris is excised to reestablish aqueous humor outflow.
    b. Acetazolamide, mannitol administered.
    c. Pilocarpine given to constrict pupil and force iris away from trabecular, allowing fluid to escape.
C. For chronic closed-angle glaucoma.
  1. Pilocarpine administered.
  2. Patient is prepared for bilateral peripheral iridectomy.
D. Postoperative care.
  1. Cycloplegic eyedrops to affected eye to relax the ciliary muscle and decrease inflammation.
  2. Early ambulation.
  3. Observe unaffected eye for symptoms of acute closed-angle glaucoma if cycloplegic drops are given by mistake.

☆ Instilling Eye Drops

A. Take medication to patient's room, and check room number against medication card or sheet.

B. Check patient's identaband and ask patient to state name.

C. Wash your hands.

D. Explain procedure to patient.

E. Tilt patient's head slightly backward.

F. Squeeze the prescribed amount of medication into eye dropper. Hold dropper with bulb in uppermost position.

G. Give tissue to patient for wiping off excess medication.

H. Expose lower conjunctival sac.

I. Drop prescribed medication into center of sac. (Do *not* place medication directly on cornea, since medication can cause injury to cornea.)

J. Ask patient to close eyelids and move eyes to distribute solution over conjunctival surface and anterior eyeball.

K. Remove excess medication from surrounding tissue.

☆Removal of Foreign Body From Eye

A. Have patient look upward.

B. Expose and evert lower lid to expose conjunctival sac.

C. Wet cotton applicator with sterile normal saline and gently twist swab over particle and remove it.

D. If particle cannot be found, have patient look downward. Place cotton applicator horizontally on outer surface of upper lid.

E. Grasp eyelashes with fingers and pull upper lid outward and upward over cotton stick.

F. With twisting motion upward, loosen particle and remove.

Ear Surgery

Stapedectomy

Definition: Surgery performed to correct otosclerosis; otosclerosis is a condition in which the normal bone of the middle ear is replaced by abnormal osseous tissue.

Surgical Procedure

A. An incision is made deep within the ear canal, close to the eardrum, so that the drum can be turned back and the middle ear exposed.

B. The surgeon frees and removes the stapes and the attached footplate, leaving an opening in the oval window.

C. The patient can usually hear as soon as this procedure has been completed.

D. The opening in the oval window is closed with a plug of fat or Gelfoam, which the body eventually replaces with mucous membrane cells.

E. A steel wire or a Teflon piston is inserted to replace the stapes.

   1. The wire is attached to the incus at one end and to the graft or plug at the other end.

   2. The wire transmits sound to the inner ear.

Postoperative Nursing Care

A. Keep patient in supine position or as ordered by physician.

B. Do not turn the patient.

C. Put side rails up.

D. Have patient deep breathe every two hours until ambulatory, but do not allow coughing.

E. Check for drainage; report excessive bleeding.

F. Prevent vomiting.

G. Give antibiotics as ordered.

H. Patient may have vertigo when ambulatory; stay with the patient and avoid quick movements.

I. Advise patient not to smoke.

☆Irrigation of External Auditory Canal

A. Remove any discharge on outer ear.

B. Place emesis basin under ear.

C. Gently pull outer ear upward and backward for adult, or downward and backward for child.

D. Place tip of syringe or irrigating catheter at opening of ear.

E. Gently irrigate with solution at 95° to 105°F, directing flow toward the sides of the canal.

F. Dry external ear.

G. If irrigation does not dislodge wax, instillation of drops will need to be carried out.

Cardiovascular System

The heart and the circulatory system, both systemic and pulmonary, comprise one of the most essential parts of the body. Failure of the heart to function results in death of the organism. Blood, composed of cells and plasma, circulates through the body and is the means by which oxygen and nutritive materials are transported to the tissues and carbon dioxide and metabolic end products are removed from the tissues for excretion.

Cardiovascular Anatomy

Gross Structure of the Heart

A. Muscular organ that functions as a pump.
B. Separated by a septum into a right, or venous, chamber and into a left, or arterial, chamber.

Layers

A. Pericardium.
   1. Fibrous pericardium—fibrous sac.
   2. Serous pericardium—allows for free cardiac motion.
B. Epicardium—covers surface of heart, extends onto great vessels, and becomes continuous with the inner lining of the pericardium.
C. Myocardium—muscular portion of heart.
D. Endocardium—thin, delicate inner layer of tissue which lines cardiac chambers and covers surface of heart valves.

Chambers

A. Right chambers.
   1. Right atrium (RA)—thin walled, distensible, low-pressure collecting chamber for systemic venous return (receives blood from superior vena cava, interior vena cava, and coronary sinus).
   2. Right ventricle (RV)—thin walled, low pressure receiving chamber for blood from right atrium (pumps blood into low resistance pulmonary system).
B. Left chambers.
   1. Left atrium (LA)—thin-walled, low pressure collecting chamber for pulmonary venous system (receives oxygenated blood via the four pulmonary veins).
   2. Left ventricle (LV)—thick-walled, high-pressure chamber that propels blood into the high resistance systemic circuit (pumps oxygenated blood via aorta to all body tissues).

Valves

A. Strong membranous openings that operate to permit flow of blood only in one direction.
B. Classifications of valves.
   1. Atrioventricular valves, located as heart-guard openings between atria and ventricles, prevent backflow of blood from ventricles to atria during systole.
      a. Tricuspid—right heart valve.
         (1) Three cusps, or leaflets.
         (2) Free edges anchored to papillary muscles in right ventricle by chordae tendineae which contract when the ventricular walls contract.
      b. Mitral—left heart valve.
         (1) Two cusps, or leaflets.
         (2) Free edges anchored to papillary muscles in left ventricle by chordae tendineae which contract when the ventricular walls contract.
   2. Semilunar valves, located at blood's exit points inside pulmonary artery and aorta, prevent backflow from the aorta and pulmonary artery into the ventricles during diastole.
      a. Pulmonic—three cusps, or leaflets.
      b. Aortic—three cusps, or leaflets.

Coronary Blood Supply

A. Arteries.
   1. Two arteries provide the myocardium with its own blood supply.

a. Right coronary artery supplies mainly the right ventricle but also part of the left ventricle.

b. Left coronary artery divides into two branches (left anterior descending artery and circumflex artery) and supplies mainly the left ventricle.

2. Coronary blood flow is regulated by oxygen needs of the myocardium.

3. Aortic pressure determines perfusion of myocardium.

B. Veins.

1. Principle coronary veins empty into coronary sinus.

2. Coronary sinus veins drain into right atrium.

Conduction System

A. Composed of specialized tissue that initiates rapid transmission of electrical impulses for orderly sequence of cardiac contraction.

B. Sinoatrial (SA) node.

1. Main pacemaker of heart in which normal, rhythmic, self-excitatory impulse is generated.

2. Normal heart elicits 60 to 100 electrical impulses/minute.

3. External control is through autonomic nervous system.

a. Sympathetic—speeds rate and increases force of contraction.

b. Parasympathetic—slows rate and decreases force of contraction; has predominant control.

C. Internodal tracts—transmits electrical impulses through atria from sinoatrial node to atrioventricular node.

D. Atrioventricular (AV) node—contains delay tissue to allow atrial contraction to eject blood into ventricle before ventricular contraction.

E. Bundle of His—conducts the electrical impulse from the atria into ventricles.

F. Left and right bundles to Purkinje fibers—conduct impulses to all parts of the ventricles.

Gross Structure of Vasculature

Arteries

A. Arteries are elastic, muscular tubes that transport blood from the heart to the capillaries in the body tissue.

B. Strong, muscular walls of the arteries force blood onward to all parts of the body.

C. Blood flows rapidly to the tissues.

D. Factors influencing arterial flow.

1. An adequate volume of blood (cardiac output).

2. A closed system of unobstructive tubes.

3. Set of heart valves to ensure flow of blood in one direction only.

4. Resistance to flow, i.e., an increased thickness of blood causes slowing of blood flow.

Capillaries

A. Capillaries are minute passageways in which the exchange of blood and tissue fluid take place.

B. Capillary walls are thin and permeable to small substances.

C. Blood flow varies depending on type of tissue.

D. Capillaries permit rapid exchange of water and solutes.

Veins

A. Veins are thin-walled tubes that transport blood from tissues back to the heart.

B. Venous system.

1. Pressure is low.

2. Walls able to contract or expand, which permits storing of small or large amounts of blood.

3. Many veins, particularly in the extremities, have valves which help to prevent backflow of blood.

C. Factors influencing venous return.

1. Decrease in volume of circulating blood decreases venous return.

2. Resistance in the venous system (such as occurs in CHF) decreases venous return.

3. Muscle contraction increases venous return.
4. Gravity.
5. Respiration.
   a. Inspiration increases venous return.
   b. Expiration decreases venous return.
6. Ability of right heart to handle venous return.

Cardiovascular Physiology

Function of Heart and Vessels

A. Heart supplies sufficient amounts of blood to meet the metabolic demands of body tissues.
B. Vessels provide the means of transporting blood to every part and organ of the body.

Regulation of Cardiac Activity

A. Properties of cardiac cells.
   1. Automaticity—ability to initiate an electrical impulse without external stimuli. Conduction of the impulse: SA node→AV node→bundle of His→Purkinje system.
   2. Conductivity—ability to transmit electrical impulses.
   3. Contractility—ability of muscle to shorten with electrical stimulation.
   4. Excitability—ability to be stimulated.
B. Cardiac cycle—cycle is one complete heart beat.
   1. Contraction (systole).
      a. Atria contract, A-V valves close, ventricles pump out blood.
      b. "Lub" sound heard through stethoscope.
   2. Relaxation (diastole).
      a. Closure of semi-lunar valves, relaxation of atria and ventricles (volume of blood is constant in chambers).
      b. "Dub" sound heard through stethoscope.

C. Cardiac output (CO)—equals the volume of blood ejected from each ventricle in one minute.
   1. Stroke volume (SV) is the volume of blood ejected from each ventricle with each contraction.
   2. Calculation of cardiac output: stroke volume × heart rate = cardiac output.
      Example: Stroke volume (SV) = 90 cc.
      Heart rate (HR) = 60 beats/minute.
      Then, 90 cc (SV) × 60 (HR) = 5400 cc (CO).

Cardiac Muscle Principles

A. Frank-Starling law states that, within physiological limits, the more the heart muscle is stretched by blood flow, the greater is the force of contraction.
   1. The heart can pump a large or a small amount of blood depending on the amount that flows into it from the veins.
   2. The heart can adapt to whatever the required load may be within the physiological limits of the total amount the heart can pump.
B. All or none principle states that cardiac muscle either contracts or does not contract when stimulated.

Compensatory Cardiac Mechanisms

A. Cardiac reserve—the difference between actual work being done and the maximum effort of which the heart is capable; a normal heart can increase its output four to six times.
B. Alterations in heart rate—a normal heart will increase its rate in response to increased oxygen need.
C. Dilatation—an increase in the *length* of the muscle fibers of the heart.
   1. Characterized by an increase in the *volume* of the heart chambers.
   2. There are physiological limits to dilatation.

D. Hypertrophy—an increase in the *diameter* of the muscle fibers of the heart.
   1. Characterized by *thickening* of the walls of the heart chambers.
   2. There are physiological limits to hypertrophy.

Pulse

A. Rhythmic dilation of an artery caused by contraction of the heart.
B. Palpated over any large surface artery.
C. Pulse deficit—difference between apical and radial pulse, which is due to weakened or ineffective contraction of the heart.

Blood Pressure

A. Pulse pressure—difference between systolic and diastolic pressure.
B. Factors influencing blood pressure.
   1. Force of heart contractions.
   2. Volume of blood (hemorrhage, for example, will cause decrease in blood pressure).
   3. Diameter and elasticity of blood vessels (arteriosclerosis, for example, will increase blood pressure).
   4. Viscosity of blood (polycythemia vera, for example, will increase blood pressure).

Nervous System Control

A. Control of the heart—impulses from the autonomic nervous system can modify the rate and strength of cardiac contractions.
   1. Sympathetic nervous system (adrenergic).
      a. Secretes epinephrine and norepinephrine.
      b. Increases heart rate.
      c. Increases force of contraction.
   2. Parasympathetic nervous system (cholinergic).
      a. Secretes acetylcholine.
      b. Exerts constant control as the "brake of heart."
      c. Slows heart rate.
      d. Decreases force of contraction.

B. Control of blood vessels.
   1. Sympathetic nervous system.
      a. Causes vasoconstriction of blood vessels.
      b. Causes *vasodilation* of coronary arteries.
   2. Parasympathetic nervous system.
      a. Causes vasodilation.
      b. Has little direct effect on coronary arteries.

Blood Components

A. Plasma.
   1. Accounts for 55 percent of the total volume of blood.
   2. Plasma composition.
      a. Consists of 92 percent water and 7 percent proteins (proteins include serum, fibrinogen, albumin, gamma globulin).
      b. Less than one percent organic salts, dissolved gases, hormones, antibodies, and enzymes.
B. Solid particles (blood cells and platelets).
   1. Comprise 45 percent of the total blood volume.
   2. Blood cells.
      a. Erythrocytes (red blood cells).
         (1) Normal count in an adult male is 4.6 million to 6.2 million cells, adult female is 4.2 million to 5.4 million cells/cu mm of blood.
         (2) Contain hemoglobin which carries oxygen to cells and carbon dioxide from cells to lungs.
         (3) Originate in bone marrow and are stored in the spleen.
         (4) Average life span is 10 to 120 days.
      b. Leukocytes (white blood cells).
         (1) Normal count in an adult is 4500 to 11,000 cells per cu mm of blood.
         (2) Primary defense against infection.
         (3) Leukocyte types.
            (a) Neutrophils play an active role in the acute inflammatory process and are phagocytic (able to destroy bacteria).

(b) Lymphocytes play an important role in immunologic responses.

(c) Monocytes are the largest of the leukocytes.

c. Platelets (thrombocytes).

(1) Normal count in an adult is 250,000 to 500,000 per cu mm of blood.

(2) Necessary for normal blood coagulation.

(3) Decreased platelet count leads to bleeding problems.

Spleen

A. Gland-like organ located in the left upper quadrant of the abdominal cavity.

B. Functions.

1. Stores blood.

2. Purifies blood by removing waste and infectious organisms.

3. Provides the primary source of antibodies in infants and children.

4. Produces lymphocytes, plasma cells, and antibodies in adults.

5. Produces erythrocytes in fetus.

6. Destroys erythrocytes when they reach the end of their life span.

Cardiovascular System Assessment

Patient History

A. Check for relevant signs and symptoms.

1. Pain.

a. Character.

b. Location.

c. Duration.

d. Intensity.

e. Precipitating, aggravating factors.

f. Relieving factors.

2. Respiratory problems.

a. Dyspnea—shortness of breath, feeling of inability to get enough air.

(1) Exertional dyspnea (DOE)—occurs while exercising.

(2) Paroxysmal nocturnal dyspnea (PND)—has sudden onset and interrupts patient's sleep.

b. Orthopnea—occurs while in recumbent position.

3. Fatigue.

4. Palpitations (heart feels like it's pounding).

5. Cerebral anoxia.

a. Irritability.

b. Restlessness.

c. Confusion.

d. Apprehension.

e. Syncope.

6. Hemoptysis—coughing and spitting up of blood.

7. Edema—collection of fluid in interstitial spaces.

a. Rales present in lungs.

b. Ascites (abdominal cavity).

c. Dependent (pedal).

8. Condition of extremities.

a. Color.

b. Temperature.

c. Skin integrity.

d. Presence of petechiae.

9. Syncope—transient loss of consciousness due to inadequate cerebral blood flow.

10. Neck vein distention.

11. Peripheral pulses.

a. Presence or absence.

b. Character.

c. Rate.

12. Pulse deficit.

13. Blood pressure—lying, sitting and standing.

14. Lung sounds.

a. Rales: fine, medium, coarse.

b. Rhonchi: sibilant, sonorous.

B. Check for predisposing factors.

1. Hypertension.

2. Obesity.

3. Diabetes mellitus.

4. Hypercholesterolemia.

5. Smoking.

6. Sedentary life style.

7. Emotional stress.

Diagnostic Procedures

A. Electrocardiogram—record of the heart's electrical activity as reflected by changes in electrical potential at skin level.
   1. Purpose is to determine types and extent of heart damage, cardiac irregularities, and electrolyte imbalance.
   2. Noninvasive and nonpainful, but procedure should be explained to patient.
   3. Requires relaxation so as to reduce electrical interference from muscle movement.
B. Stress test—an electrocardiogram that is taken while the patient is exercising on a stationary bike or treadmill.
   1. Purpose is to determine possible cardiac irregularities that may occur during exercise.
   2. Test is monitored by physician.
   3. Test is discontinued if electrocardiogram records change, if blood pressure increases, or if patient complains of angina.
C. Cardiac catheterization—insertion of a catheter into the heart and vessels surrounding the heart to examine one or both sides of the heart.
   1. Purpose is to collect data such as pressure measurements of various chambers, blood oxygen measurement, cardiac output determination, and confirmation of the presence of coronary vessel disease.
   2. Catheterization pathways.
      a. Right catheterization: venous system → superior vena cava → right atrium → right ventricle → pulmonary artery.
      b. Left catheterization: femoral artery → aorta → left atrium → left ventricle.
   3. Possible complications/consequences.
      a. Fatigue, backache.
      b. Pain, bleeding, ecchymosis, swelling at insertion site.
      c. Thrombosis at insertion site.
         (1) Numbness, tingling, or coldness of extremity.
         (2) Loss of peripheral pulse.
      d. Arrhythmias with passage of catheters through ventricles, especially premature ventricular contraction and ventricular fibrillation.
      e. Perforation of heart (rare).
   4. Nursing care.
      a. Prior to procedure.
         (1) Give no food and fluids as ordered.
         (2) Prep skin in areas of insertion site.
         (3) Have patient rest quietly for three or more hours.
         (4) Inform patient that there will be little or no pain, but that a fluttery sensation may be felt around heart as catheter is passed through vessels into heart.
      b. After the procedure.
         (1) Provide bed rest for 12–24 hours as ordered.
         (2) Take vital signs same as for any post-op patient. Report blood pressure decreases of more than 10 percent or pulse increases of 10 percent.
         (3) Check peripheral pulses distal to catheter insertion site (radial or pedal).
         (4) Observe insertion sites for bleeding, swelling, infection, or thrombosis (pressure dressing may be in place).
         (5) Elevate extremity if bleeding occurs.
         (6) Instruct patient not to bend limb used for insertion site.
         (7) Force fluids if not contraindicated.
         (8) Observe for and report arrhythmias.
D. Routine chest films—for observation of silhouette of heart, chambers, and great vessels.
E. Fluoroscopy—examination of heart, lungs, and vessel movement as viewed on fluorescent screen in darkened room.
F. Coronary artery angiography—taking pictures of coronary circulation after injection of radiopaque dye.
G. Phonocardiogram—record produced by registering sounds produced by action of heart;

sounds translated into electrical energy by a microphone.

H. Tests for serum enzymes levels.
   1. Elevated following myocardial damage.
   2. Serum enzyme studies include serum glutamic pyruvic transaminase (SGPT), lactic dehydrogenase (LDH), and creatine phosphokinase (CPK), which is most definitive.

I. Echocardiography—records high frequency sound vibrations; assists in evaluating structures of the heart, dimensions of the chambers, and thickness of septum and walls.

J. Holter monitor—tape-recorded ambulatory electrocardiogram. Monitors cardiac cycle for 24 hours.

Common Cardiovascular Drugs

Digitalis

A. Therapeutic effects.
   1. Increases force of cardiac contraction.
   2. Slows heart rate.
   3. Slows conduction through AV node.
   4. Increases automaticity which may cause many arrhythmias.

B. Used in congestive heart failure.
   1. Increases contractility which reduces oxygen need.
   2. Increases cardiac efficiency.
   3. Reduces heart size.

C. Dosage individualized to patient and clinical situation.

D. Precautions.
   1. Used with caution for patients with impaired renal or hepatic function.
   2. Used with caution for patients with hypokalemia, which predisposes them to digitalis toxicity.

E. Nontherapeutic effects.
   1. All types of cardiac arrhythmias.
   2. Gastrointestinal effects.
      a. Anorexia.
      b. Nausea and vomiting.
      c. Diarrhea and/or constipation.
      d. Abdominal pain.
   3. Central nervous system effects.
      a. Fatigue.
      b. Depression.
      c. Lethargy.
      d. Headache.
      e. Confusion, agitation.
   4. Ophthalmic effects.
      a. Disturbed color perception.
      b. Halos circling dark objects.
   5. Hypersensitivity.
      a. Pruritus.
      b. Urticaria.

F. Implications for nursing care.
   1. Take apical pulse for one full minute; notify physician if above 120 or below 60.
   2. Administer digitalis after meals to avoid gastric distress.
   3. Monitor for toxicity in the elderly as they are more sensitive to digitalis.
   4. Assist in designing instructional plan for patient.
      a. Drug action.
      b. Dosage.
      c. Keeping records.
      d. Method and timing for taking pulse.
   5. Store in tightly covered, light-resistant containers.

Calcium Blocking Agents

A. Therapeutic effects.
   1. Inhibits the influx of calcium ions across cell membrane.
   2. Decreases heart rate as conduction is slowed through SA and AV nodes.
   3. Increases myocardial oxygenation by causing coronary vasodilation.
   4. Decreases peripheral vascular resistance by causing vasodilation of peripheral arteries.

B. Used for angina, usually when beta blocker and nitrate therapy are not effective.

C. Drugs.
   1. Cardizem (diltiazem hydrochloride)—nausea, edema, arrhythmia, headache.

2. Procardia (nifedipine)—vertigo, nausea, peripheral edema, headache, and flushing.
3. Calan, Isoptin (verapamil hydrochloride)—hypotension, peripheral edema, vertigo. (Verapamil is also being used to treat supraventricular arrhythmias.)

Coronary Vasodilators

A. Therapeutic effects.
   1. Dilates vascular smooth vessels.
   2. Decreases peripheral arterial vascular resistance (afterload).
   3. Decreases venous blood return to heart (pre-load).
   4. Reduces myocardial oxygen consumption.
B. Used for angina.
C. Side effects.
   1. Flushed face.
   2. Headache.
   3. Vertigo and faintness.
   4. Postural hypotension.
D. Drugs.
   1. Short acting.
      a. IV—Tridil, Nitrobid, Nitrostat.
      b. Sublingual—nitroglycerin.
      c. Topical—Nitrol.
      d. Oral—Nitrobid.
   2. Long acting.
      a. Sublingual—Cardilate, Isordil.
      b. Oral—Peritrate, Sorbitrate.
      c. Topical disk—Nitrodisk, Nitro-Dur, Trans-derm.

Antihypertensive Drugs

A. Therapeutic use—reduce blood pressure to normal or near normal without side effects.
B. Drugs.
   1. Thiazides—potentiates second drug when used in combination with other antihypertensive drugs.
   2. Hydralazine (Apresoline).
      a. Effect—adrenergic blocker.
      b. Side effects—headache, tachycardia, and postural hypotension.
   3. Methyldopa (Aldomet).
      a. Effect—decreases blood pressure.
      b. Side effects—postural hypotension.
C. Implications for nursing care.
   1. May need to monitor blood pressure in lying, sitting, and standing position during dosage adjustment.
   2. Observe for postural hypotension.
      a. Change patient's position slowly.
      b. Dangle patient's legs a few minutes before standing.
   3. Monitor intake and output.
   4. Weigh daily.
   5. Encourage regular medical check-ups.

Diuretics

A. Therapeutic use—most diuretics block sodium and chloride reabsorption in ascending loop of Henle and distal tubule of the kidney and decrease ionic exchange of sodium in distal tubule, thereby excreting water.
B. Drugs.
   1. Thiazides.
      a. Common drugs—chlorothiazide (Diuril), hydrochlorothiazide (Hydrodiuril), chlorthalidone (Hygroton).
      b. Administration—oral and parenteral.
      c. Advantages—potent by mouth; effective antihypertensives.
      d. Disadvantages or side effects—electrolyte imbalance; loss of potassium.
   2. Potassium-sparing agents.
      a. Common drugs—spironolactone (Aldactone), triamterene (Dyrenium).
      b. Administration—oral only.
      c. Advantages—conserve potassium.
      d. Disadvantages—usually not effective when used alone (best used with thiazides), and electrolyte imbalance.
   3. Potent diuretics.
      a. Common preparations—furosemide (Lasix), ethacrynic acid (Edecrin).
      b. Administration—oral and parenteral.
      c. Advantages—rapid, potent action useful in cases of severe pulmonary edema

and refractory edema.

   d. Disadvantages—allergic reactions, severe electrolyte imbalance (potassium and chloride loss), and hypovolemia.

C. Implications for nursing care.
1. Time administration to avoid nocturia and sleep interruption.
2. Monitor intake and output.
3. Weigh daily.
4. Observe for postural hypotension.
5. Reduce potassium depletion by providing foods high in potassium (bananas, oranges).
6. Monitor for signs of fluid and electrolyte imbalance.

Anticoagulant Drugs

A. Heparin.
1. Therapeutic effects.
   a. Blocks conversion of prothrombin to thrombin and fibrinogen to fibrin.
   b. Prolongs clotting time.
2. Uses.
   a. Prophylaxis.
   b. Treatment of thrombi and emboli.
3. Dosage individualized according to patient's partial thromboplastin time.
4. Contraindications.
   a. Bleeding tendency.
   b. Severe liver or kidney disease.
   c. Following brain surgery.
5. Nontherapeutic effects.
   a. Spontaneous bleeding.
   b. Injection site reactions.
6. Nursing care.
   a. Administer dosage ordered by physician according to patient's partial thromboplastin time.
   b. Observe for any signs of bleeding in stools or urine or in emesis; report immediately.
   c. Utilize subcutaneous injection for administration.
     (1) Use lower abdominal skin area.
     (2) Do not pull back on plunger.
     (3) Do not rub area following injection.

   d. Observe for signs of toxicity.
     (1) Bruises or skin discoloration.
     (2) Frequent nosebleeds.
     (3) Hematuria.
   e. Instruct patient of precautions to take and observations to make when discharged.

B. Coumadin.
1. Uses.
   a. Decreases prothrombin activity.
   b. Depresses hepatic synthesis of several clotting factors.
   c. Prevents utilization of vitamin K by liver.
   d. Takes 24 to 72 hours for action to develop and continues for 24 to 72 hours after last dose.
   e. Pro time kept at 18 to 30 seconds (normal is 12 to 14 seconds).
2. Antagonist.
   a. Vitamin K—aqua Mephyton IM or IV.
   b. Returns to hemostasis within six hours.
   c. Blocks action of Coumadin for one week.
3. Nursing care.
   a. Check pro time before giving.
   b. Give at same time each day.
   c. Teach patient to avoid foods high in vitamin K (cabbage, cauliflower, spinach, and leafy vegetables).

Antiarrhythmic Drugs

A. Therapeutic effects.
1. Increases recovery time of atrial and ventricular muscle.
2. Decreases myocardial excitability.
3. Increases conduction in cardiac muscle, Purkinje's fibers, and AV junction (exception: lidocaine).
4. Decreases contractility (exception: lidocaine).
5. Decreases automaticity.

B. Quinidine.
1. Uses—atrial fibrillation, atrial flutter, supraventricular and ventricular tachycardia, premature systoles.

2. Side effects.
   a. Hypersensitivity, thrombocytopenia.
   b. Cinchonism—nausea, vomiting, diarrhea, tinnitus, vertigo, visual disturbances.
   c. Sudden death from ventricular fibrillation.
   d. Congestive heart failure due to negative inotropism.
   e. Conduction disturbances.

C. Procainamide hydrochloride (Pronestyl).
   1. Uses—premature ventricular systoles.
   2. Side effects.
      a. Anorexia, nausea, vomiting, diarrhea.
      b. Systemic lupus erythematosus and agranulocytosis.
      c. Cardiac AV block.

D. Norpace.
   1. Uses—premature ventricular contractions.
   2. Side effects.
      a. CNS—vertigo, syncope, fatigue.
      b. CV—hypotension, edema, weight gain, SOB.
      c. GI—nausea, vomiting, diarrhea.
      d. GU—urinary retention.

E. Xylocaine (lidocaine).
   1. Uses—ventricular tachyarrhythmias.
   2. Side effects.
      a. CNS disturbances—drowsiness, paresthesias, slurred speech, blurred vision, seizures, coma.
      b. Cautious use in patients with liver disease or low cardiac output (metabolism of drug slowed).

F. Epinephrine (Adrenalin).
   1. Effect: beta stimulation—increases heart rate and contractility.
   2. Use: cardiac arrest most common.

G. Propranolol (Inderal).
   1. Effect: blocks beta stimulation.
      a. Decreases heart rate and contractility; that is, it decreases oxygen consumption.
      b. Depresses automaticity of pacemakers and AV conduction.
      c. Produces bronchoconstriction.
   2. Uses.
      a. Decreases ventricular rate from atrial flutter, fibrillation, and tachycardia.
      b. Suppresses ectopic arrhythmias, especially ventricular arrhythmias.
      c. Angina.
   3. Side effects—should not be used in AV block, bradycardia, congestive heart failure, or lung disease (bronchospasm).

H. Atropine.
   1. Effects: anticholinergic.
      a. Increases rate of SA node.
      b. Increases conduction through AV node.
   2. Uses.
      a. Symptomatic sinus bradycardia.
      b. Partial AV block.
   3. Side effects.
      a. Inability to void, especially with prostate enlargement.
      b. Dry mouth, skin, flushing, dilation of pupil.
      c. Decrease in bronchial secretions.

Heart Disorders

Coronary Artery Disease

Definition: Occurs as the result of accumulation of fatty materials (lipids, cholesterol being primary one), which narrows the lumen of coronary arteries. Clinical manifestations of disease reflect ischemia to myocardium, resulting from inadequate blood supply to meet metabolic demands.

Risk Factors

A. Diet—increased intake of cholesterol and saturated fats.
B. Hypertension—aggravates atherosclerotic process.
C. Cigarette smoking.
D. Diabetes mellitus—accelerates atherosclerotic process.

E. Lack of exercise; sedentary living.

F. Psychosocial tensions—may precipitate acute events.

G. Obesity—susceptibility to hypertension, diabetes mellitus, hyperlipidemia.

Signs and Symptoms

A. Chest pain.
   1. Angina, burning, squeezing, crushing tightness substernally or over precordial area.
   2. May radiate down arms.

B. Nausea, vomiting.

C. Increased perspiration and cool extremities.

Treatment and Nursing Care

A. Monitor vital signs, particularly blood pressure and pulse.

B. Assist with EKG.

C. Administer nitrates if chest pain present (as ordered).

D. Evaluate chest pain—type, duration, relieved with medication.

E. Monitor breath sounds and signs of peripheral edema to detect early complications.

Angina

Definition: Severe chest pain due to temporary inability of coronary arteries to meet metabolic needs of myocardium. Pathophysiology involves narrowing of lumen of coronary artery, usually by atherosclerotic process. There is an interference with supply of oxygen to the heart.

Precipitating Factors

A. Exertion and effort.

B. Emotional upsets.

C. Tachyarrhythmias.

D. Overeating.

E. Extremes of temperature, especially cold.

F. Smoking.

Signs and Symptoms

A. Pain.
   1. Location—precordial, substernal.
   2. Character—compressing, choking, burning, squeezing, crushing and heaviness.
   3. Radiation—left or right arm, jaw, neck, back.
   4. Duration—usually five to ten minutes; relieved by rest or nitroglycerin.

B. Dyspnea.

C. ECG changes; may not be evident at rest.

D. There are no physical signs 90 percent of the time.

Nursing Care

A. Instruct patient how to reduce frequency of attacks.
   1. Learn to live with moderation; physical activity should be sufficient to maintain general physical state, but short of causing angina.
   2. Avoid stress and emotional upset.
   3. Reduce caloric intake if overweight.
   4. Refrain from smoking.
   5. Decrease use of stimulants, e.g., coffee, tea, cola.
   6. Avoid heavy meals.
   7. Avoid extremes of temperature, especially cold.

B. Primary medication—nitroglycerin.
   1. Drug action.
      a. Dilates coronary arteries that are not atherosclerotic.
      b. Enhances blood flow to myocardium without increasing oxygen consumption.
   2. Use of drug is to relieve pain from myocardia ischemia.
   3. Side effects—hypotension, headache.
   4. Important considerations.
      a. Effective only sublingually.
      b. Dosage of one to two tablets may be repeated at five-minute intervals.
      c. Physician should be called if no relief

in fifteen minutes.

d. No limit to number that may be taken in twenty-four hour period.

e. Is not addictive.

f. May be used prophylactically before engaging in activity known to precipitate angina.

g. Avoid alcohol consumption with drug.

h. Must be stored in closed, dark glass container to avoid light, heat, and moisture. Has only six-month shelf-life.

☆C. Instruct patient in use of nitroglycerin ointment.

1. Apply directly to skin.

2. Wash off remaining ointment before new application.

3. Change skin placement with each application.

D. Other medications used.

1. Long-acting nitrites (Isordil, Cardilate).

2. Beta-blocker: propranolol (Inderal).

3. Calcium blocking agents (Calan, Cardizena).

E. If medications ineffective, may require coronary artery bypass surgery.

Myocardial Infarction

Definition: Formation of destroyed tissue in cardiac muscle due to interruption of or insufficient blood supply for a prolonged period, resulting in sustained oxygen deprivation.

Etiology

A. Atherosclerotic heart disease.

B. Coronary artery embolism.

C. Decreased blood flow with shock and/or hemorrhage.

D. Direct trauma.

Signs and Symptoms

A. Pain that is similar to angina but is usually more intense and has longer duration (thirty minutes or longer).

1. Location—left precordial, substernal.

2. Character—crushing, vise-like, tightening and burning.

3. Radiation—jaw, back, arms.

B. Feeling of apprehension or doom.

C. Dyspnea or orthopnea.

D. Nausea and vomiting.

E. Diaphoresis.

F. Pallor or cyanosis.

G. Arrhythmias.

H. Signs of congestive heart failure.

Diagnosis

A. History (very important).

B. ECG changes.

C. Laboratory studies—serum enzymes (SGPT, LDH, CPK) released with death of tissue.

D. Increase of white cell count.

E. Increased sedimentation rate.

Treatment and Nursing Care

A. Death-producing arrhythmias treated immediately with lidocaine.

B. IV or IM narcotic analgesics, as ordered, to relieve pain and anxiety.

C. Cardiac rhythm monitored continuously.

D. Lidocaine drip monitored.

E. Oxygen via cannula.

F. Monitored closely for signs of CHF (seen within first 24 hours).

G. IV nitroglycerin drip.

H. Swan-Ganz catheter with PAWP and CO readings.

I. Nursing care.

1. Administer narcotic analgesics to relieve pain and anxiety.

2. Administer oxygen with cannula.

3. Observe for arrhythmias.

4. Monitor vital signs, urine output.

5. Observe for signs of congestive heart failure.

6. Provide physical rest and emotional support.

a. Sedation, graduated activity.

b. Use of commode and self-feed.

7. Maintain patient on stool softeners and soft diet to prevent increased workload on heart and prevent Valsalva maneuver.
8. Provide low-fat, low-cholesterol, low-sodium diet.
9. Rehabilitate patient to enable him to return to physical level according to cardiac capability.
   a. Plan exercise program.
   b. Provide psychological support.
   c. Avoid stressful environment.
   d. Consider possible change of life style.
J. Rehabilitation: encourage patient to participate in organized cardiac rehabilitation program. Program usually consists of:
   1. Monitored exercise program based on METs.
   2. Stress reduction classes.
   3. Alterations in nutrition.
   4. Sex counseling.

Complications

A. Arrhythmias.
B. Congestive heart failure.
C. Cardiogenic shock.
D. Thrombophlebitis.
E. Pericarditis.
F. Ventricular aneurysm or rupture (late complication) due to weakened area of myocardium as result of myocardial infarction.

Heart Valve Stenosis

Definition: A progressive thickening of the valve cusps that results in the narrowing of the lumen of the valve opening.

Signs and Symptoms

A. Predisposing factors.
   1. History of congenital heart disease.
   2. Rheumatic heart disease.
   3. Arteriosclerosis.
B. May be asymptomatic.
C. May evidence mild symptoms.
   1. Decreased cardiac output—tired and lethargic.
   2. Dizziness and syncope.
   3. Angina.

Nursing Care

A. Treat heart failure and arrhythmias.
B. Decrease cardiac workload.
C. Prevent and/or treat infections.
D. Monitor administration of anticoagulants for treatment and/or prevention of thrombi.
E. Provide emotional support.
F. Prepare patient for valvotomy if no calcification of valve or for surgical replacement of the valve.
G. Complications.
   1. Atrial fibrillation.
   2. Subacute bacterial endocarditis.
   3. Thrombi formation.
   4. Heart failure.

Congestive Heart Failure

Definition: A group of symptoms, not a disease, which results from decreased pumping effectiveness of the heart. Circulatory congestion occurs in response to the decreased or inadequate cardiac output.

Types of Heart Failure

A. Left heart failure—congestion occurs mainly in the lungs due to inadequate ejection of the blood into the systemic circulation.
B. Right heart failure—congestion occurs systemically due to inadequate pumping of the blood from the systemic circulation into the lungs.

Pathophysiology

A. Left heart failure.
   1. Damage to myocardium of the left ventricle.
   2. Left ventricle unable to pump adequate

amount of blood; pressure increases in pulmonary vessels.

3. Backflow of blood into the lungs causes pulmonary congestion.
4. Symptoms are pulmonic in nature.

B. Right heart failure.
   1. Increased pulmonary pressure.
   2. Right ventricle unable to effectively pump blood to lungs.
   3. Right side of heart becomes congested with blood.
   4. Venous blood returning to right heart cannot be pumped quickly and efficiently.
   5. Congestion of blood develops in the large veins leading to the right heart and, eventually, in the organs and tissues of the body.
   6. Symptoms are systemic in nature.

Signs and Symptoms of Left Heart Failure

A. Fatigue.
B. Dyspnea—orthopnea, PND, DOE.
C. Anxiety, apprehension, irritability, confusion, restlessness.
D. Cough—may be associated with blood-tinged, frothy sputum.
E. Wheezing.
F. Rales.
G. Cyanosis or pallor.
H. Arrhythmias.
I. Diaphoresis.

Signs and Symptoms of Right Heart Failure

A. Peripheral edema in dependent parts—feet and legs; sacrum, back, buttocks.
B. Ascites.
C. Nausea, vomiting, anorexia.
D. Weight gain.
E. Hepatomegaly, liver congestion.
F. Oliguria during day; polyuria at night.
G. Arrhythmias.
H. Increased central venous pressure.
I. Jugular vein distention.

Nursing Care

A. Treat underlying cause.
B. Reduce pain and anxiety.
   1. Morphine sulfate.
   2. Physical and emotional rest.
C. Administer oxygen therapy as ordered; use cannula rather than mask because patient already feels he or she cannot breathe.
D. Reduce water and sodium retention.
   1. Diuretics.
   2. Restrict fluid intake.
   3. Restrict sodium intake.
   4. Bed rest in Fowler's position.
   5. Intake and output measure.
   6. Weigh daily.
   7. Special skin care to edematous areas.
E. Administer digitalis—increases strength of contraction and decreases rate.
F. Observe for arrhythmias.
G. Provide emotional support.
H. Instruct patient in principles of care.

Complications

A. Digitalis toxicity.
B. Electrolyte imbalance (especially hypokalemia) from diuretics.
C. Pulmonary embolism from bed rest.
D. Oxygen toxicity, especially with COPD patients.
E. Acute pulmonary edema.

Acute Pulmonary Edema

Definition: An excessive quantity of fluid in the pulmonary interstitial spaces or in the alveoli usually following severe left ventricular decompensation.

Characteristics

A. The most common cause is greatly elevated capillary pressure resulting from failure of left heart and damming of blood in lungs.

B. Alveoli filled with fluid and bronchioles congested.

C. Retention of fluid resulting from reduced renal function.

Signs and Symptoms

A. Moist rales and frothy sputum.

B. Severe anxiety, feelings of impending doom.

C. Marked dyspnea.

D. Stertorous breathing.

E. Marked cyanosis.

F. Profuse diaphoresis—cold and clammy.

G. Blood pressure and pulse changes.

Nursing Care

A. Administer oxygen at 6 1/min if patient does not have COPD.

B. Administer medications (diuretics and digitalis) to improve myocardial contractility and reduce pulmonary and systemic blood volume.

C. Place in semi-or high-Fowler's position.

D. Instruct patient in deep breathing and coughing exercises.

E. Monitor fluid intake and output, weigh daily.

F. Monitor vital signs.

G. Provide sedation with ordered medication. Observe respiratory rate and depth.

H. Administer drug therapy as ordered.

I. Assist with rotating tourniquets on patient's extremities.
1. Purpose.
   a. Reduce venous return to heart.
   b. Pool blood temporarily in extremities.
   c. Treatment for pulmonary edema.
   ☆ 2. Complete procedure.
   a. Take blood pressure to determine midway between systolic and diastolic reading.
   b. Apply four pressure cuffs high up on all four extremities.
   c. Inflate three cuffs to pressure midway between systolic and diastolic pressure.

d. Rotate the tourniquets every 15 minutes, using clockwise rotation.

e. Release one tourniquet and then inflate the next tourniquet.

f. Observe for presence of arterial blood flow by checking peripheral pulses. Arterial pulses should be present, venous pulses absent.

g. Take frequent blood pressure readings to readjust cuff pressure.

h. Continue treatment for prescribed time, usually when diuretic has adequately functioned and signs of pulmonary edema lessened.

i. Discontinue tourniquets one at a time, continuing the cuff deflation in clockwise manner, and every 15 minutes.

Pacemaker Insertion

Definition: A temporary or permanent device to initiate and maintain heart rate when patient's pacemaker is nonfunctioning.

Conditions Requiring Pacemakers

A. Conduction defect following open heart surgery.

B. Heart block (usually third degree).

C. Tachyarrhythmias.

D. Stokes-Adams syndrome.

E. Bradyarrhythmias.

Types of Pacemakers

A. Demand—functions only if patient's own pacemaker fails to discharge.
1. The pacemaker is set at a fixed rate and will discharge only if patient's own rate falls below it.
2. Used mainly in Adams-Stokes or bradyarrhythmias or following cardiac surgery.

B. Asynchronous.
1. Fixed rate—the pacemaker is set at a fixed rate and will fire regardless of patient's own rhythm.
2. Variable rate—rate can be varied.

Pacemaker Placement

A. Epicardial.
   1. Electrodes are implanted on outside of left ventricle, and they barely penetrate myocardium.
   2. Battery pack is placed subcutaneously in a skin pocket.
B. Endocardial implantation—pacing electrode inserted through neck vein and placed near the apex of right ventricle.
   1. Permanent—battery is implanted beneath skin.
   2. Temporary—battery is located outside of skin.

Nursing Care

A. Preplacement.
   1. Assess vital signs for baseline data.
   2. Evaluate heart sounds to determine arrhythmias for baseline data.
   3. Assess lung sounds.
B. Postplacement.
   1. Observe for battery failure (pacemaker not firing as set).
      a. Faints easily.
      b. Hiccoughs.
      c. Rhythm change.
   2. Observe for hematoma at site of insertion.
   3. Observe for arrhythmias.
   4. Monitor vital signs.
   5. Observe for pacemaker failure.
      a. Decreased urine output.
      b. EKG pattern changes.
      c. Decreased blood pressure.
      d. Cyanosis.
      e. Shortness of breath.
   6. Check for complications.
      a. Hemorrhage and shock.
      b. Infection.

Inflammatory Diseases of the Heart

Definition: Conditions in which various microorganisms cause infection and inflammation of the structures of the heart. Damage to the valves of the heart is among the most serious consequences of inflammatory heart disease.

Types

A. Bacterial endocarditis—an infection of the lining of the heart.
B. Pericarditis—inflammation of the pericardium.
C. Myocarditis—inflammation of the muscle of the heart walls.
D. Rheumatic fever—a systemic disease of connective tissue which may involve the endocardium, myocardium, and pericardium.
E. Rheumatic heart disease—a chronic cardiac condition which usually follows one or more episodes of rheumatic fever with valvular damage.

Signs and Symptoms

A. Signs of infection.
   1. Fever.
   2. Chills.
   3. Diaphoresis.
   4. Lassitude.
   5. Anorexia.
B. Tachycardia.
C. Chest pain.
D. Dyspnea.

Nursing Care

A. Administer specific antibiotic therapy as ordered.
B. Provide bed rest.
C. Administer salicylates.
D. Provide adequate nutrition.

Complications

A. Mitral stenosis—progressive thickening of the valve cusps which results in the narrowing of lumen of mitral valve.
B. Mitral insufficiency—distortion of the valve that allows backward flow of blood from ventricle to atrium.

C. Aortic stenosis—narrowing of the aortic valve opening due to fibrosis and calcification.

D. Aortic insufficiency—occurrence of blood flow back into the ventricle from aorta.

E. Tricuspid stenosis—progressive narrowing of tricuspid valve lumen.

F. Tricuspid insufficiency—occurrence of blood flow back into atrium from ventricle.

Peripheral Vascular Disorders

Hypertension

Definition: Sustained elevation of arterial pressure with systolic pressure greater than 140 mm Hg and diastolic pressure greater than 90 mm Hg.

Types

A. Primary (essential)—no known etiology.

B. Secondary hypertension—etiology.
   1. Renal disease.
   2. Endocrine disorders.
      a. Pheochromocytoma (adrenal tumor).
      b. Adrenal cortex lesions—aldosteronism, Cushing's syndrome.
   3. Toxemia of pregnancy.
   4. Increased intracranial pressure.
   5. Congenital heart disease.
   6. Increased workload of the heart.
      a. Congestive heart failure.
      b. Myocardial infarction.

Signs and Symptoms

A. Asymptomatic in early stage.

B. Headache, dizziness, tinnitus.

C. Fatigue, insomnia.

D. Epistaxis, blurred vision, spots before eyes.

E. Identify if target organ involvement is present.
   1. Eyes—narrowing of arteries, papilledema (malignant hypertension), visual disturbances.
   2. Brain—mental and neurologic abnormalities, encephalopathy, CVA.
   3. Cardiovascular system—left ventricular hypertrophy and failure, angina, aggravation and acceleration of atherosclerotic process in coronary arteries and peripheral vessels.
   4. Kidneys—renal failure.

Nursing Care

A. Treat causes of secondary hypertension.

B. Diet.
   1. Decrease sodium intake.
   2. Decrease calorie intake if overweight.

C. Drug therapy.
   1. Diuretics.
      a. Thiazides (Diuril, Esidrix, Enduron).
      b. Potassium sparing (Aldactone).
      c. Loop—potent diuretics (Lasix, Edecrin).
   2. Antihypertensives (Inderal, Aldomet, Catapres, Ismelin).
   3. Vasodilators—(Apresoline, Vasodilan).

D. Exercise—moderate; may increase when weight is reduced.

E. Help to relieve patient's environmental stress and anxiety.

F. Emphasize to patient the importance of following medical treatment regime.
   1. Weight control.
   2. Low-sodium diet.
   3. Change in life style.
   4. Periodic medical checkups.

Thromboangitis Obliterans (Buerger's Disease)

Definition: Chronic inflammation of arteries and veins, and, secondarily, inflammation of nerves.

Signs and Symptoms

A. Pain, temperature, and color changes (cyanosis); alterations in skin of lower extremities at rest and especially after exercise.

B. Intermittent calf claudication—severe calf cramping following exercise; relieved upon resting.
C. Decreased pulse rates.
D. Complications of swelling, ulceration, gangrene.

Treatment and Nursing Care

A. Cessation of smoking.
B. Bilateral sympathectomy.
C. Reduction of pain.

Raynaud's Disease

Definition: A vasospastic condition of arteries that occurs with exposure to cold or to strong emotion and affects fingers, toes, ears, nose, and cheeks.

Signs and Symptoms

A. Blanching or cyanosis of extremities.
B. Numbness.
C. Pulses present and normal.
D. Gradual onset.

Treatment

A. Conservative treatment.
B. Sympathectomy.

Thrombophlebitis

Definition: Inflammation of wall of vein resulting in venous thrombi obstruction.

Precipitating Causes

A. Stagnation of blood flow such as occurs from bed rest.
B. Change in clotting of blood.
C. Change in lining of blood vessel (trauma).

Signs and Symptoms

A. In superficial vein.
  1. Vein hard to the touch.
  2. Skin reddened, hot, tender.
B. In deep vein.
  1. Affected area swollen, tender.
  2. Increased temperature, pulse, and white blood count.

Nursing Care

A. Take preventive measures.
  1. Exercise.
  2. Nonconstrictive clothing.
  3. Foot-board walking.
  4. No "gatching" of bed.
  5. No pillow under knees.
  6. No calf massage.
  7. Adequate hydration.
B. Ensure proper fitting of elastic stockings.
C. Elevate affected limb.
D. Administer anticoagulant drug therapy as ordered.
E. Apply heat to affected area.

Varicose Veins

Definition: A condition in which the veins are dilated because of incompetent valves.

Precipitating Causes

A. Pregnancy.
B. Standing for long periods of time.
C. Poor venous return.
D. Heredity.
E. Obesity.
F. Poor posture.

Signs and Symptoms

A. Aching of legs.
B. Swelling of ankles.
C. Browning of skin from blood which has escaped from overloaded veins.
D. Ulceration.

Treatment

A. Prevention.
B. Elevation of legs; wearing of nonconstrictive clothing and elastic stockings.
C. Surgery—vein ligation, stripping.

Nursing Care for Peripheral Vascular Problems

A. Limit disease and prevent complications.
B. Maintain adequate blood supply to affected areas.
   1. Warmth.
   2. Cleanliness.
   3. Infection control.
   4. Avoidance of heat and cold extremes.
C. Encourage patient to stop smoking.
D. Have patient wear nonconstrictive clothing and use body positions which protect affected areas from pressure.
E. Avoid emotional stress.
F. Teach patient to recognize an increase or extension of symptoms.
   1. Increase of pain in extremities.
   2. Changes in skin color.
   3. Ulceration.
   4. Change of temperature in extremities.
G. Lead patient to recognize limitations caused by disease.

Vein Stripping and Ligation

Definition: The ligation and removal of affected veins in the legs. Usually affects greater and lesser saphenous veins.

Preparation

A. Have patient scrub legs and lower abdomen once a day for three days prior to surgery.
B. Instruct on ambulation postoperatively.
C. Check that completion of preoperative scrub is done.
D. Observe for physician's marks on veins.
E. Take pulses for baseline data.

Postoperative Nursing Care

A. Observe feet for edema, warmth, color (tight elastic bandages applied following surgery can impede circulation).
B. Take peripheral pulses.
C. Elevate feet above level of heart.
D. Position flat in bed or have patient walk. Do not allow to dangle legs or sit in a chair for at least one week.
E. Ambulate early—five minutes every hour.
F. Following bandage removal, utilize elastic stockings.

Diseases of the Blood and Blood Forming Organs

Pernicious Anemia

Definition: A chronic and, if untreated, progressive anemia caused by the failure of gastric mucosa to provide an intrinsic factor essential for absorption of vitamin B_{12}.

Characteristics

A. Causes
   1. Total gastrectomy.
   2. Surgical resection of small intestine.
   3. Atrophy of gastric mucosa.
   4. Malabsorption disease—sprue.
   5. Bacterial or parasitic infections.
B. May be autoimmune difficulty.
C. Genetic predisposition (especially in northern Europe).
D. Diagnostic tests.
   1. RBC count megaloblastic maturation.
   2. Bone marrow aspiration.
   3. Upper GI series.
   4. Schilling test (maintain npo for 12 hours; collect 24-hour urine).
   5. Gastric analysis—insertion of nasogastric tube, collection of aspirant, injection of histamine.

Signs and Symptoms

A. Weakness, unsteady gait.
B. Dyspnea.
C. Palpitation, tachycardia.
D. Anorexia, dyspepsia.
E. Diarrhea.
F. Numbness and tingling of extremities.
G. Pallor, slight jaundice.
H. Glossitis.
I. Mild hepatomegaly (enlarged liver).
J. Splenomegaly (enlarged spleen).

Treatment and Nursing Care

A. Provide safety measures if neurological deficit is present—assist with ambulation.
B. Avoid pressure on lower extremities due to circulation deficit (foot cradle, etc).
C. Avoid extremes of heat and cold.
D. Administer B_{12} deep IM, as ordered.
E. Instruct in administration of B_{12}. This is a lifelong therapy.
F. Provide support and explain behavior changes to patient and family.

Aplastic Anemia

Definition: Deficiency of circulating RBCs resulting from bone marrow suppression.

Characteristics

A. Causes.
   1. Toxic action of drugs (Chloromycetin, sulfonamides, Dilantin, alkylating agents, and antimetabolites).
   2. Exposure to radiation.
   3. Diseases that suppress bone marrow activity (leukemia and metastic cancer).
B. Pancytopenia frequently accompanies RBC deficiency.

Signs and Symptoms

A. Increased fatigue.
B. Lethargy.
C. Dyspnea.
D. Cutaneous bleeding.
E. Low platelet and leukocyte count.

Treatment and Nursing Care

A. Medical treatment.
   1. Bone marrow transplant and WBC transfusion are becoming more prevalent.
   1. Splenectomy (especially in severe thrombocytopenia).
B. Administer androgens and/or corticosteroids as ordered.
C. Monitor transfusion of fresh platelets (RBC transfusion may be introduced also).
D. Administer antibiotics when infection occurs.
E. Carry out reverse isolation procedure.
F. Protect from infections.
G. Provide for adequate rest periods.
H. Observe for complications.
I. Provide physical comfort measures.
J. Provide emotional support for patient and family, especially while in isolation.
K. Educate public in use of toxic pesticides and chemicals.

Purpuras

Definition: The extravasation of blood into the tissues and mucous membranes.

Characteristics

A. Idiopathic thrombocytopenic purpura is characterized by platelet deficiency.
B. Vascular purpura is characterized by weak, damaged vessels, which rupture easily.

Signs and Symptoms

A. Petechiae.
B. Postsurgical bleeding.
C. Increased bleeding time.
D. Abnormal platelet count.
E. Ecchymosis.

Treatment and Nursing Care

A. Identify underlying cause if possible.
B. Complete steps to control bleeding.
C. Monitor transfusion of platelets.
D. Monitor administration of corticosteroids.

Agranulocytosis

Definition: An acute, potentially fatal blood disorder characterized by profound neutropenia and most commonly caused by drug toxicity or hypersensitivity.

Signs and Symptoms

A. Chills and fever.
B. Sore throat.
C. Exhaustion and depletion of energy.
D. Ulceration of oral mucosa and throat.

Nursing Care

A. Discontinue suspected chemical agents or drugs.
B. Isolate to reduce exposure to infections.
C. Administer corticosteroids if ordered.

Polycythemia Vera

Definition: A chronic disease of unknown etiology characterized by overactivity of bone marrow with overproduction of red cells and hemoglobin.

Signs and Symptoms

A. Reddish-purple hue to the skin.
B. Increased blood volume.
C. Capillary engorgement.
D. Hemorrhage.
E. Venous thrombosis.
F. Arterial hypertension.
G. Hepatomegaly and splenomegaly.

Treatment

A. Radiophosphorus in dosages based on body weight; initially IV, then orally.
B. Phlebotomy to remove 500–2000 ml of blood per week until hematocrit reaches 50 percent; repeated when hematocrit rises.

Leukemia: Acute and Chronic

Definition: A disorder of blood-forming tissue characterized by proliferation of one type of white blood cell (granulocyte, lymphocyte, or monocyte), occurring in all races and developing at any age.

Signs and Symptoms

A. Generalized discomfort.
B. Poor appetite.
C. Ulceration of the mouth and pharynx.
D. High fever.
E. Diarrhea.
F. Severe infection, e.g., pneumonia and septicemia.
G. Anemia with fatigue, lethargy, weakness, hypoxia, and pallor.
H. Bleeding gums, ecchymosis, and petechiae.
I. Splenomegaly, hepatomegaly, and lymphadenopathy.
J. Headache, disorientation, and convulsions.

Treatment and Nursing Care

A. Chemotherapeutic drugs, e.g., Methotrexate, Cytoxan, Lukeran.
B. Blood transfusions as required.
C. Steroids, such as prednisone, to decrease symptoms.

Hodgkin's Disease

Definition: A chronic, progressive, neoplastic, invariably fatal disease of unknown etiology, involving the lymphoid tissues of the body. It is most common between the ages of twenty and forty.

Signs and Symptoms

A. Painless enlargement of the lymph nodes.
B. Severe pruritus.
C. Irregular fever.
D. Splenomegaly and hepatomegaly.
E. Jaundice.
F. Edema and cyanosis of the face and neck.
G. Pulmonary symptoms including dyspnea, cough, chest pain, cyanosis, and pleural effusion.
H. Progressive anemia with resultant fatigue, malaise, and anorexia.
I. Bone pain and vertebral compression.
J. Nerve pain and paraplegia.
K. Laryngeal paralysis.
L. Increased susceptibility to infection.
M. Progresses in stages.
1. Stage I: disease is restricted to single anatomic site, or is localized in a group of lymph nodes; asymptomatic.
2. Stage II(a): two or three adjacent lymph nodes in the area on the same side of the diaphragm are affected.
3. Stage II(b): symptoms appear.
4. Stage III: disease is widely disseminated on both sides of diaphragm into the lymph areas and organs.
5. Stage IV: involvement of bone, bone marrow, pleura, liver, skin, gastrointestinal tract, central nervous system, and gradually the entire body.

Treatment and Nursing Care

A. Radiation is used for stages I, II, and III in an effort to eradicate the disease.
B. Wide-field megavoltage radiation with doses of 3500 to 4000 roentgens over a four- to six-week period.
C. Chemotherapy with Cytoxan, nitrogen mustard, thiotepa, TEM, Velban, Oncovin, prednisone, and Matulane.
D. Diagnostic laparotomy.
E. Nursing care is supportive.
1. Provide supportive relief from effects of radia-

tion and chemotherapy.
a. Side effects include nausea and vomiting.
b. Controlled by premedication of sedatives and antiemetic agents.
2. Assist patient to maintain as normal a life as possible during course and treatment of disease.
3. Prevent infection as body's resistance is lowered.
4. Continually observe for complications: pressure from enlargement of lymph glands on vital organs.

Autoimmune Disorders

Acquired Immunodeficiency Syndrome (AIDS)

Definition: Acquired disease linked to human T cell leukemia-lymphoma virus (HTLV).

Characteristics

A. Specific etiology is unknown.
B. Risk factors.
1. IV drug abusers.
2. Homosexual males with multiple sexual partners.
3. Hemophiliacs.
C. Incubation period may be as long as five years.
D. Individuals may have antibodies and be carriers but not exhibit AIDS.
E. Some individuals exhibit a mild version of immune system depression.
F. Disease is known to be spread through semen and blood products; other body fluids are not yet determined to be a source of communicability.
G. Disease is known to be lethal in a high proportion of persons, especially those with Kaposi's sarcoma.

Signs and Symptoms

A. Initial symptoms indicative of syndrome onset.
   1. Weight loss, anorexia.
   2. Elevated temperature.
   3. Lymphadenopathy.
   4. Malaise.
   5. Dry, productive cough.
   6. Acute onset presents with overwhelming infection.
B. Lungs exhibit adventitious sounds (pneumocystis carinii).
C. Purple lesions on skin (Kaposi's sarcoma).
D. Mucous membranes of mouth have fungus from candida albicans and ulcerating infections.

Nursing Care

A. Treatment is symptomatic.
B. Provide good skin care to prevent breakdown.
C. Provide respiratory care: turn, cough and deep breathe.
D. Place on secretion precaution.
E. Provide pain control.
F. Provide supportive care for patient who develops Pneumocystosis (an acute pneumonia caused by pneumocystis carinii).
   1. Disease occurs in about 60 percent of AIDS patients and is a major cause of death.
   2. There is an abrupt onset with fever, tachycardia, severe hypoxemia, and uncompensated respiratory alkalosis.

Nursing Care for Blood Disorders

Infections

A. Institute reverse isolation and meticulous medical asepsis.
B. Provide bed rest.
C. Provide protein, high vitamin, and high caloric diet.
D. Administer antibiotics as ordered.

Fatigue and Weakness

A. Conserve the patient's strength.
B. Provide frequent rest periods.
C. Institute ambulation activities as tolerated.
D. Decrease disturbing activities and noise.
E. Provide optimal nutrition.

Ulcerative Lesions

A. Provide nonirritating foods and beverages.
B. Provide frequent oral hygiene with mild, cool mouthwash and solutions.
C. Use applicators or soft-bristled toothbrush.
D. Lubricate the lips.
E. Give mouth care both before and after meals.

Dyspnea

A. Elevate the head of the bed.
B. Support the patient in the orthopneic position.
C. Administer oxygen when indicated.
D. Prevent unnecessary exertion.
E. Avoid gas-forming foods.

Bone and Joint Pains

A. Use cradle to relieve pressure of bedding.
B. Apply hot or cold compresses as ordered.
C. Immobilize joints when ordered.

Fever

A. Apply cool sponges.
B. Administer antipyretic drugs as ordered.
C. Encourage fluid intake unless contraindicated.
D. Maintain a cool environmental temperature.

Pruritus and/or Skin Eruptions

A. Keep patient's fingernails short.
B. Use soap sparingly, if at all.
C. Apply emollient lotions in skin care.

Anxiety

A. Explain the nature, the discomforts, and the limitations of activity associated with the diagnostic procedures and treatments.
B. Listen to the patient.
C. Treat the patient as an individual.
D. Allow the family to participate in the patient's care.
E. Encourage the family to visit with the patient; provide privacy for the family and patient.

Rupture of the Spleen

Definition: Traumatic bursting following violent blow or trauma to the spleen.

Signs and Symptoms

A. Weakness due to blood loss.
B. Abdominal pain and muscle spasm particularly in the left upper quadrant.
C. Depression of abdominal bleeding.
D. Rebound tenderness.
E. Referred pain to left shoulder.
F. Palpable tenderness.
G. Leukocytosis well over twelve thousand.
H. Progressive shock with rapid, thready pulse; drop in blood pressure; and pallor.

Treatment

Splenectomy.

Respiratory System

The respiratory system is a group of related organs that together perform pulmonary ventilation. The act of breathing involves an osmotic and chemical process by which the body takes in oxygen from the atmosphere and gives off end products, mainly carbon dioxide, formed by oxidation in the alveolar tissues.

Anatomy and Physiology

Ventilation Tract

Nose

A. Structure.
   1. Septum divides nose into two cavities.
   2. Ciliated mucous membrane lines the cavities.
   3. Four pairs of sinuses drain into nose.
B. Function.
   1. Serves as passage for air.
      a. Filters.
      b. Warms.
      c. Moistens.
   2. Serves as organ of smell.
   3. Aids in phonation.

Pharynx

A. Structure.
   1. Tube-like structure.
   2. Composed of muscle.
   3. Ciliated mucous membrane lines the cavity.
   4. Divides into three areas.
      a. Nasopharynx—contains adenoids.
      b. Oropharynx—contains tonsils.
      c. Laryngopharynx.
B. Function.
   1. Serves as passage for air and food.
   2. Aids in phonation.

Larynx

A. Structure.
   1. Composed largely of cartilage held together by muscles.
   2. Major cartilages.
      a. Thyroid (forms Adam's apple).
      b. Epiglottis.
      c. Cricoid.
   3. Ciliated mucous membrane lines the structure.
   4. Contains vocal cords.
B. Function.
   1. Passage for air.
   2. Produces sound.

Trachea

A. Structure.
   1. Cylindrical structure.
   2. Walls consist of smooth muscle and C-shaped rings of cartilage.
   3. Divides at lower end into two primary bronchi.
B. Function—passage for air.

Pulmonic Organs

Lungs

A. Structure.
   1. Medial surface is roughly concave to allow room for mediastinal structures.
   2. Bronchi enter through slits (hili) in each lung.
   3. Left lung is partially divided by fissures into two lobes (upper and lower).
   4. Right lung is partially divided by fissures into three lobes (upper, middle, and lower).
   5. Visceral pleura covers outer surfaces.
   6. Interior consists of bronchial tree.
B. Function.
   1. Distribute air to alveoli.
   2. Exchange gas between air and blood.

Bronchi

A. Structure.
   1. Right mainstem bronchus (RMSB)—slightly larger and more vertical than left bronchus; most frequent route for aspirated materials.
   2. Left mainstem bronchus (LMSB)—branches off the trachea at a 45 degree angle.
   3. Walls contain incomplete cartilaginous rings at site where they enter lungs.
   4. Ciliated mucous membrane lines the structures.
   5. Primary bronchi divide into smaller branches (secondary bronchi) just past site of lung entry.
   6. Secondary bronchi continue to branch, forming small bronchioles.
   7. Bronchioles subdivide into smaller and smaller tubes and terminate into alveolar ducts and their several alveolar sacs.
B. Function—distribute air to lung's interior.

Alveoli

A. Structure—makes up the walls of alveolar sacs composed of single layer of tissue.
B. Function—gas exchange between air and blood.

Thorax

A. Structure.
   1. The thorax (chest) is divided into three divisions, separated by partitions of pleura.
      a. Pleural divisions—each division occupied by a lung.
      b. Mediastinum—occupied by esophagus, trachea, large blood vessels, and heart.
   2. Pleura.
      a. Parietal layer lines entire thoracic cavity.
         (1) Adheres to internal surface of ribs, superior surface of diaphragm.
         (2) Partitions off mediastinum.
      b. Visceral layer covers outer surface of each lung.
      c. The two layers, separated only by a potential space (pleural space), contain just enough pleural fluid for lubrication.
B. Function—pleura allows for changes in chest size required for inspiration and expiration.

Principles of Pulmonary Ventilation

Respiratory Cycle Mechanics

A. Inspiration—active process.
   1. Diaphragm descends, external intercostal muscles contract.
   2. Chest expands, allowing air volume into the lungs as alveolar pressure decreases.
B. Expiration—passive process.
   1. Diaphragm ascends, external intercostal muscles relax.
   2. Chest becomes smaller, air moves out of lungs.
C. Atmospheric pressure—intrapulmonic pressure.
   1. Air moves into and out of the lungs because of the differences in air pressure inside and outside of the lung. (Atmospheric pressure—760 mm Hg.)
   2. During inspiration, air moves into the lungs. Intrapulmonic pressure (pressure within the lungs) is lower than atmospheric pressure.
   3. During expiration intrapulmonic pressure is higher than atmospheric pressure.

Exchanged Air Volumes

A. Total lung capacity (TLC)—total volume of air that is present in the lungs after maximum inspiration.
B. Vital capacity (VC)—volume of air that can be expelled following a maximum inspiration.
C. Tidal volume (TV)—volume of air exhaled after a normal inspiration.

D. Expiratory reserve volume (ERV)—largest additional volume of air that can be forcibly expired after tidal air expiration.
E. Inspiratory reserve volume (IRV)—amount of air that can be forcibly inspired over and above a normal inspiration.
F. Residual volume (RV)—amount of air remaining in lung following maximal expiration.

Exchange of Gases

A. In lungs.
  1. Air and blood exchange gases through membrane of capillaries around alveoli.
  2. Oxygen enters blood from the alveolar air.
  3. Carbon dioxide enters alveolar air from the blood.
B. In tissues.
  1. Takes place between arterial blood flowing through tissue capillaries and cells.
  2. Oxygen diffuses out of the arterial blood into the cells.
  3. Carbon dioxide diffuses out of the cells into the blood.

Transportation of Gases in Blood

A. Oxygen combines with hemoglobin, the means of transportation, in blood to form oxyhemoglobin.
B. Half of the carbon dioxide is carried in the plasma as bicarbonate ions.
C. About one third of blood carbon dioxide combines with the hemoglobin to form carbominohemoglobin.

Regulation of Respiration

A. Chemoreceptors—cells sensitive to changes in carbon dioxide concentrations in arterial blood.
  1. Above normal range (35–45 mm Hg) concentrations of carbon dioxide stimulate respirations.
  2. Below normal concentrations of carbon dioxide slow respirations.
  3. A decrease in arterial blood pH stimulates respirations.
B. Arterial blood pressure.
  1. A sudden rise in arterial blood pressure results in reflexive slowing of respirations.
  2. A sudden drop in arterial blood pressure results in reflexive increase in rate and depth of respirations.
C. Conditions that decrease lung compliance.
  1. Atelectasis—collapse of the alveoli as a result of obstruction or hypoventilation.
  2. Pneumonia—inflammatory process involving the lung tissue.
  3. Pulmonary edema—accumulation of fluid in the alveoli.
  4. Pleural effusion—accumulation of pleural fluid in the pleural space compressing lung on the affected side.
  5. Pulmonary fibrosis—scar tissue replacing necrosed lung tissue as a result of infection.
  6. Pneumothorax—air present in the pleural cavity; lung is collapsed as volume of air increases.

Surfactant

A. Surface-active material that lines the alveoli and changes the surface tension, depending on the area over which it is spread.
B. Surfactant in the lungs allows the smaller alveoli to have lower surface tension than the larger alveoli.
  1. Results in equal pressures within both and prevents collapse.
  2. Production of surfactant depends on adequate blood supply.
C. Conditions that decrease surfactant.
  1. Hypoxia.
  2. Oxygen toxicity.
  3. Aspiration.
  4. Atelectasis.
  5. Pulmonary edema.
  6. Pulmonary embolus.
  7. Mucolytic agents.
  8. Hyaline membrane disease.

Compliance

A. Relationship between pressure and volume:

elastic resistance. This is determined by dividing the tidal volume by peak airway pressure (V_t PAP). Total compliance equals chest wall compliance plus lung compliance.

B. Conditions that decrease chest wall compliance.
1. Obesity—excess fatty tissue over chest wall and abdomen.
2. Kyphoscoliosis—marked resistance to expansion of the chest wall.
3. Scleroderma—expansion of the chest wall limited when the involved skin over the chest wall becomes stiff.
4. Chest wall injury—as in crushing chest wall injuries.
5. Diaphragmatic paralysis—as a result of surgical damage to the phrenic nerve, or disease process involving the diaphragm itself.

Diagnostic Procedures

A. Pulmonary function tests.
1. Measurement of blood gases.
   a. An effective way to evaluate lung function and lung adequacy.
   b. Measure oxygen tension (arterial) (PaO_2) and carbon dioxide tension (arterial) ($PaCO_2$).
2. Measurement of lung air.
   a. Analyzes physical phenomena involved with the movement of the air in and out of the chest.
      (1) Vital capacity—measurement of the maximum amount of air that can be expired following a maximal inspiration.
      (2) Maximum breathing capacity—measurement of airway resistance within the lungs.
      (3) Timed vital capacity—the pattern of vital capacity as related to time.
   b. Measures the effectiveness of the mechanical processes and blood gases.
B. Chest x-ray.
1. Necessary in the assessment of respiratory disorders.

2. The view may be taken back to front (posteroanterior), side (lateral), or at an angle (oblique).
3. No specific preparation is necessary.
C. Bronchoscopy.
1. A direct visual examination of the trachea, two major bronchi, and multiple smaller bronchi.
2. A hollow instrument (bronchoscope) is passed into the trachea, under local anesthesia.
3. A biopsy of tissue or sample of secretions can be obtained.
4. Preparation of patient.
   a. NPO 8 to 12 hours before procedure.
   b. Remove dentures.
   c. Provide mouth care.
   d. Explain process to patient so that he or she can relax and cooperate during procedure.
   e. Administer sedative for relaxation.
5. Post-procedural care.
   a. NPO for several hours, until gag reflex returns.
   b. Encourage patient to expectorate.
   c. Advise patient to smoke and talk as little as possible; procedure may cause throat irritation.
D. Bronchography.
1. Specialized x-rays of the bronchi and bronchioles.
2. Catheter introduced into the trachea and positioned above the bifurcation, under local anesthesia.
3. Radio-opaque oil injected by catheter into the trachea, and patient is tilted in various positions so that the dye flows throughout the bronchial tree.
4. Preparation of patient.
   a. Same as for a bronchoscopy.
   b. May require postural drainage to remove thick bronchial secretions.
5. Post-procedural care.
   a. Same as for a bronchoscopy.
   b. May require postural drainage to remove excess oil.
E. Sputum examination.

1. A microscopic examination of the cells of the sputum.
2. Sputum should be raised from deep within the bronchi such as sputum first expectorated in the morning.
3. If culture is to be grown, specimens need to be collected in a sterile container.
4. May require a 24-hour specimen.
5. Patient's mouth should be first washed out to remove food particles.
6. Note color, consistency, odor and quantity of sputum.

F. Gastric analysis.
   1. Laboratory examination of stomach contents may include bronchial secretion the patient previously swallowed.
   2. A gastric tube is inserted and stomach contents are aspirated.
   3. Patient is NPO 8 to 12 hours prior to the procedure.

G. Thoracentesis.
   1. Removal of fluid from chest cavity.
   2. Under local anesthesia an aspiration needle inserted into the pleura.
   3. Purpose is both diagnostic and therapeutic.
   4. Nursing care.
      a. Assist patient to proper position.
      b. During procedure, observe patient for change of skin color and for changes in pulse and/or respiratory rate.
      c. After procedure, observe patient for change in respiratory rate and for coughing, expectoration of blood, or blood-tinged sputum.

H. Lung scintigraphy: measures concentration of gamma rays from lung after intake of isotope.

I. Perfusion studies: outline pulmonary vascular structures after intake of radioactive isotopes IV.

J. Biopsy of respiratory tissue
   1. May be done by needle, via bronchoscope, or an open lung procedure biopsy.
   2. Nursing care: observe for hemothorax and/or pneumothorax.

K. Tuberculin skin test
   1. Mantoux intradermal test (more reliable).
      a. Tuberculin injected intradermal, inter-

mediate PPD.
      b. Test read 48 to 72 hours postintradermal wheal production.
      c. Erythema not important.
      d. Area of induration more than 10 mm: indicates positive reaction (client has had contact with the tubercle bacillus).
      e. Reactions of 5 to 9 mm require retest.
   2. Tine test.
      a. Not recommended for diagnosis.
      b. Test read on third day.
      c. Mantoux test if induration more than 2 mm.

Respiratory System Assessment

A. Check for airway patency.
   1. Clear out secretions.
   2. Insert oral airway if necessary.
   3. Position patient on side if there is no cervical spine injury.

B. Listen to lung sounds.
   1. Absence of breath sounds: indicates lungs not expanding, due either to obstruction or deflation.
   2. Rales (crackling sounds): indicate vibrations of fluid in lungs.
   3. Rhonchi (coarse sounds): indicate partial obstruction of airway.
   4. Decreased breath sounds: indicate poorly ventilated lungs.
   5. Detection of bronchial sounds that are deviated from normal position: indicates mediastinal shift due to collapse of lung.

C. Determine level of consciousness; decreased sensorium can indicate hypoxia.

D. Observe sputum or tracheal secretions; bloody sputum can indicate contusions of lung or injury to trachea and other anatomical structures.

E. Evaluate vital signs for temperature, respiratory rate, pulse, and changes in skin color.

F. Evaluate for tightness or fullness in chest.

G. Determine degree of pain patient is experiencing.

H. Assess for respiratory complications.
   1. Assess for abnormal breathing patterns.

a. Dyspnea—labored or difficult breathing.
b. Hyperpnea—abnormal deep breathing.
c. Hypopnea—reduced depth of breathing.
d. Orthopnea—difficulty breathing in other than upright position.
e. Tachypnea—rapid breathing.
f. Stridor—noisy respirations as air is forced through a partially obstructed airway.

2. Evaluate cough.
a. Normally a protective mechanism utilized to keep the tracheobronchial tree free of secretions.
b. Common symptom of respiratory disease.

3. Assess bronchospasm.
a. Bronchi narrow and secretions may be retained.
b. Condition may lead to infection.

4. Observe for hemoptysis—expectoration of blood or blood-tinged sputum.

5. Assess for cyanosis—late sign of hypoxia, due to large amounts of reduced hemoglobin in the blood (PaO$_2$ of about 50 mm Hg).

6. Observe for hypoxia (anoxia)—a deficiency of oxygen in body tissues.

7. Evaluate for hypercapnia.
a. Occurs when carbon dioxide is retained.
b. High levels of oxygen depress and/or paralyze the medullary respiratory center.
c. Peripheral chemoreceptors (sensitive to oxygen) become the stimuli for breathing.

8. Assess for presence of respiratory alkalosis or acidosis.

I. Assess for other system complications.
1. Evaluate for polycythemia—increase in RBCs as a compensatory response to hypoxemia.
2. Observe for clubbing of fingers. Pathogenesis is not well understood.
3. Evaluate for cor pulmonale—enlargement of the right ventricle as a result of pulmonary arterial hypertension following respiratory pathology.

4. Evaluate for chest pain.
5. Assess for atelectasis.
6. Check for abdominal distention.
7. Assess for hypertension.

Chronic Pulmonary Diseases

Bronchial Asthma

Definition: Recurrent paroxysms of dyspnea with a characteristic wheezing due to an inherited allergic tendency.

Signs and Symptoms

A. Dyspnea, orthopnea.
B. Sense of tightness in the chest; feeling of impending suffocation.
C. Wheezing.
D. A slight dry cough.
E. Anxious expression.
F. Perspires freely.

Treatment and Nursing Care

A. Administer bronchodilators, sedatives, and/or tranquilizers.
B. Humidify inspired air.
C. Provide oxygen therapy only after a long attack and occurrence of cyanosis.
D. Manage environment so that it is as free as possible from contributive factors to respiratory infection.
E. Protect patient from feeling closed in.
F. Provide rest.
G. Encourage fluids.
H. Watch for toxic effects of drugs.

Bronchitis

Definition: The hypersecretion of mucus by the bronchial glands; a chronic or a recurrent respiratory infection often following a long history of bronchial asthma or an acute respiratory infection.

Signs and Symptoms

A. Cough is usually the earliest symptom; most marked on arising in the morning and just prior to going to bed.

B. Expectoration of thick, white, stringy mucus.

C. As the disease progresses, the sputum may become purulent, copious, and occasionally streaked with blood.

D. Possible sensation of heaviness in the chest.

E. Characteristic appearance is drawn, anxious, pale, and markedly dyspneic.

F. Speech characterized by short, jerky sentences.

G. Upright position often leaning slightly forward.

H. Distention of veins in neck during expiration.

Treatment and Nursing Care

A. Provide prompt and effective treatment of predisposing factors; good treatment directly related to the control of cigarette smoking and air pollution.

B. Increase pulmonary ventilation by reducing bronchospasms.

C. Administer expectorants, intermittent antibiotic therapy.

D. Control humidity.

E. Postural drainage.

F. Control infection.

G. Provide intermittent positive pressure breathing (IPPB).

H. Maintain mouth care.

Emphysema

Definition: The permanent overdistention of the alveoli with resulting destruction of the alveolar walls. (Emphysema is a Greek word meaning "overinflated.")

Signs and Symptoms

A. Cough—may be present many years before dyspnea.

B. Dyspnea.

C. Increased sputum production.

D. Weight loss.

E. Hypoxia, hypercapnia.

F. Barrel chest.

G. Prolonged expiratory phase.

H. Wheezes, forced expiratory rhonchi.

I. Complications.

    1. Pulmonary hypertension.

    2. Right-sided heart failure.

    3. Spontaneous pneumothorax.

Nursing Care

A. Monitor for signs of impending hypoxia.

B. Monitor for alterations in lung sounds.

C. Teach pursed lip breathing exercises.

D. Administer low concentration oxygen. Usually 2 l/min.

E. Monitor for signs of carbon dioxide narcosis.

F. Provide hydration.

    1. Necessary to liquefy secretions present, or to prevent formation of thick, tenacious secretions.

        a. Oral intake of fluids.

        b. IV administration of fluids.

        c. Humidification via face mask or aerosol mask.

G. Provide chest physiotherapy.

Specialized Nursing Care
Chronic Pulmonary Disease

A. When progress is slow, be patient, give attention to detail, and maintain interest and hope.

B. Give instruction for general health care.

    1. Principles of optimum nutrition for patient and family.

    2. A plan for adequate rest, recreation, and suitable work.

    3. The value of treatment program.

    4. Instructions concerning medications, breathing exercises, and avoidance of infection.

C. Observe and record symptoms.
   1. Amount of coughing, amount and character of sputum, degree of dyspnea and/or wheezing.
   2. Color, weight, and appetite of patient.
   3. Attitudes and sense of well-being.
   4. Complications and progression of illness.
D. Help adjust activities for the patient within the framework of his or her tolerance.
☆ E. Positions for Chest Physiotherapy.
   1. To affect RUL and LUL, place patient upright.
   2. To affect RML, position patient on left side with head slanted down, right shoulder one-quarter turn onto pillow. Cup anteriorly over left nipple.
   3. To affect lingula LL, position patient on right side with head slanted down, left shoulder one-quarter turn onto pillow. Cup anteriorly over left nipple.
   4. To affect RLL and LLL, place patient in Trendelenburg's position, alternating sides, or prone.

Administration of Oxygen

A. Conditions requiring oxygen therapy
   1. Atmosphere hypoxia: oxygen therapy will correct depressed level of oxygen.
   2. Hypoventilation hypoxia: 100% oxygen will yield five times more oxygen into the alveoli than normal air.
B. Conditions where oxygen therapy is not corrective
   1. Hypoxia caused by anemia, carbon monoxide poisoning, or abnormality of hemoglobin transport.
   2. Inadequate tissue use of oxygen (cyanide poisoning).
   3. Chronic obstructive lung disease requires that oxygen be used with caution since oxygen could suppress respiratory drive and result in respiratory arrest.
C. Symptoms of Hypoxia
   1. Early symptoms
      a. Restlessness
      b. Headache
      c. Visual disturbances
      d. Slight confusion
      e. Hyperventilation
      f. Tachycardia
      g. Hypertension
      h. Dyspnea
   2. Advanced symptoms
      a. Hypotension
      b. Bradycardia
      c. Metabolic acidosis (production of lactic acid)
      d. Cyanosis
   3. Chronic hypoxia
      a. Polycythemia
      b. Clubbing of fingers and toes
      c. Thrombosis

D. Properties of oxygen.
   1. Colorless, odorless, and tasteless gas.
   2. Supports combustion.

E. Methods of administration.
   1. Nasal catheter (used infrequently)—produces oxygen concentration of 30–50 percent.
      a. Insert so tip of catheter is visible immediately behind the uvula.
      b. Change every 8–12 hours.
      c. Apply nonoily lubricant to irritated or dry nasal mucous membrane.
   2. Face mask—produces oxygen concentration of 30 to 65 percent.
      a. May cover nose only, or nose and mouth.
      b. May have rebreathing bag so patient inhales part of the air previously exhaled.
   3. Cannula—produces oxygen concentration of 35–40 percent.
      a. Fit small prongs into each nostril.
      b. Remove and clean every eight hours.
   4. Tent—produces oxygen concentration of 50–60 percent.
      a. Cover either entire or upper third of the bed.
      b. Used infrequently.

Nursing Care

A. Check equipment
1. Eliminate kinks in tubing.
2. Maintain proper positioning.
3. Check water supply in humidification bottle.
4. Adjust to proper liter flow.

B. Maintain safety measures.
1. No smoking or fire of any kind.
2. No materials that produce static electricity.
3. No electrical equipment; however, some hospital equipment may be safely used.

☆C. Monitoring a patient with oxygen
1. Check order for type of therapy, use of catheter or cannula, and desired liter flow.
2. Place patient in semi- or high-Fowler's position to ensure adequate lung expansion.
3. Turn and reposition patient frequently to prevent skin decubiti.
4. Encourage deep breathing and coughing exercises unless directed otherwise.
5. Ensure adequate hydration, especially if secretions are thick and tenacious.
6. Assess patient's progress by frequently checking vital signs, color, and level of consciousness.
7. Remain with patients who are frightened or anxious until they feel secure.
8. Use oxygen very conservatively on anyone with chronic lung disease—high levels of oxygen will knock out carbon dioxide center and lead to respiratory arrest.

☆D. Using an Oxygen Analyzer
1. Calibrate analyzer with room atmosphere prior to each reading.
2. Open tubing to the air, and compress two full times to fill analyzer.
3. Depress button. Analyzer should read 20% for room air. Adjust dial as necessary to obtain this reading.
4. Place tubing close to patient's nose.
5. Compress bulb 3 to 6 times, depress button, and read findings.
6. Based on reading, adjust oxygen flow.
7. Check analyzer with 100% oxygen at least one time per day.

Acute Pulmonary Diseases

Common Cold (Coryza)

Definition: An infectious viral disease of the upper respiratory tract. It has a duration of 4–14 days and is endemic throughout the world.

Signs and Symptoms

A. Sneezing.
B. Chills and slight fever.
C. Headache.
D. Watery eyes.
E. Dry, scratchy, sore throat.
F. Copious nasal discharge.

Treatment and Nursing Care

A. Encourage bed rest or extra sleep.
B. Advise avoidance of contact with others.
C. Force fluids.
D. ASA (aspirin) to relieve discomforts.
E. Instruct patient in proper use of tissues and preventive measures for spread of infection.

Pneumonia

Definition: Inflammation of the lungs due to infection caused by virus, bacteria, or fungus. Inflammation leads to replacement of air in the alveolar sacs by fluid or tissue.

Signs and Symptoms

A. Complaint of tightness or fullness in chest.
B. Cough, dypsnea, or shortness of breath.
C. Increased vital signs, particularly temperature and respiratory rate.
D. Restlessness.

Treatment and Nursing Care

A. Administer antibiotics.
B. Administer oxygen therapy (see section on administration of oxygen, p. 154).
C. Monitor IV's or force fluids.
D. Elevate head of bed.
E. Monitor vital signs.
F. Encourage bed rest with frequent position change.
G. Monitor urinary output.
H. Check frequency of bowel movement.
I. Isolate patient if required.
J. Encourage expectoration.

Atelectasis

A. Collapse of pulmonary alveoli, caused by mucous plug or inadequate ventilation.
B. Signs and symptoms.
   1. Asymmetrical chest movement.
   2. Decreased or absent breath sounds over affected area.
   3. Shortness of breath leading to cyanosis.
   4. Painful respirations.
   5. Increased vital signs: temperature, respiration, pulse.
   6. Anxiety and restlessness.

Pleurisy

Definition: Inflammation of the pleura that is usually a complication of pulmonary diseases.

Types

A. Acute fibrinous (dry pleurisy)—only small amounts of exudate are formed during the inflammatory process.
B. Pleurisy with effusion—large amounts of fluid are secreted and collect in the space between the pleural layers.

Signs and Symptoms

A. Very sharp pain during respiration.
B. Pain gradually subsides as fluid is formed in pleural space.

C. Dry cough.

D. Fatigue.

E. Possible shortness of breath.

Treatment and Nursing Care

A. Thoracentesis performed to remove fluid if condition is severe.

B. Encourage bed rest.

C. Ventilate room well but maintain warmth.

D. Encourage coughing.

E. Position patient on side of the effusion.

F. Apply heat to painful area.

Influenza

Definition: Infectious epidemic disease of short duration that is caused by a virus.

Signs and Symptoms

A. Sudden onset with variable individual symptoms.

B. Chills, high fever.

C. Severe headache, muscular aches.

D. Anorexia, weakness, apathy.

E. Sneezing, dry cough.

F. Sore throat, nasal discharge.

Treatment and Nursing Care

A. Administer ASA for muscle aches and headache, and codeine to control cough.

B. Cool vapor steam inhalation.

C. Encourage bed rest.

D. Ventilate room well.

E. Take TPR every four hours during temperature elevation.

F. Provide large amounts of fluid.

Pulmonary Tuberculosis (TB)

Definition: An infectious disease of the parenchyma of the lung, bronchi, bronchioles, alveoli, pleurae, and bronchopulmonary lymph nodes that is characterized by the formation of tubercles. It is caused by the organism *Mycobacterium tuberculosis* (Koch's bacillus). It is acquired by inhalation of disseminated air droplets of excretions from the nose, mouth, throat, and lungs of infected individuals.

Signs and Symptoms

A. Insidious onset, early symptoms mild and nonspecific.

B. Fatigue.

C. Anorexia, weight loss.

D. Elevated temperature, particularly in the late afternoon and the evening.

E. Night sweats.

F. Initial nonproductive cough that later becomes productive of mucopurulent and blood-streaked sputum.

G. Hemoptysis (expectoration of blood from respiratory tract or lungs).

Chemotherapeutic Treatment

A. Maintain respiratory isolation.
   1. Strict isolation for 2–4 weeks or coughing has ceased or negative sputum.
   2. Masks necessary only for uncooperative patient.

B. Administer medications on time.

C. Treatment long-term; may be life-long for some people.

D. Drugs are more effective when administered in a single daily dose.

E. Most common drugs.
   1. Isoniazid—300 mg daily.
   2. Ethambutol—15 mg/kg daily.
   3. Streptomycin—500 mg daily.
   4. Rifampin—600 mg daily.
   5. Para-aminosalicylic acid—8 to 15 grams.

F. Usually INH, ethambutol, rifampin, or streptomycin used in combination, once daily.

G. Chemoprophylaxis; Isoniazid and vitamin B_6 therapy for one year.

Chest Injuries

Emergency Assessment of Respiratory Function

A. Check for airway patency and ventilation.

B. Inspect thoracic cage for injury.

1. Inspect for contusions, abrasions, and deep open wounds.

2. Watch for movement of chest; asymmetrical movement indicates tension pneumothorax, hemothorax, fractured ribs, and/or flail chest.

C. Observe color; cyanosis indicates decreased oxygenation.

D. Observe type of breathing; stertorous breathing usually indicates obstructed respiration.

E. Listen to lung sounds.

1. Absence of breath sounds indicates lungs not expanding, due to either obstruction or deflation.

2. Rales (crackling sounds) are produced by vibrations of fluid and indicate fluid in lungs.

3. Rhonchi (coarse rattlings) indicate partial obstruction of airway.

4. Decreased breath sounds indicate poorly ventilated lungs.

5. Bronchial sounds, deviated from normal position, indicate mediastinal shift due to collapse of lung.

F. Determine level of consciousness; decreased sensorium may indicate hypoxia.

G. Observe sputum or tracheal secretions; bloody sputum may indicate contusions of lung or injury to trachea and other anatomical structures.

Emergency Nursing Care

A. Take brief history from patient (or individual accompanying patient) to aid in total evaluation of his or her condition.

B. Assist with electrocardiogram to establish if there is associated cardiac damage.

C. Maintain patent airway.

1. Place hand over nose and mouth to detect breathing; maintain adequate ventilation.

2. Clear out secretions; suction.

3. Insert either oral airway or endotracheal tube as necessary.

D. Position patient on side if no spinal injury.

E. Seal off open chest wound immediately with pressure dressing to prevent air from entering thoracic cavity.

F. Maintain fluid and electrolyte balance.

1. When replacing blood and fluid loss, watch carefully for fluid overload as it can lead to pulmonary edema.

2. Record intake and output.

G. Maintain acid-base balance; assist with frequent blood gas determination as acid-base imbalances occur readily with compromised respirations or with mechanical ventilation.

H. Provide for relief of pain.

1. Use analgesics with caution as they depress respirations. (Demerol is drug of choice.)

2. Avoid atropine or morphine sulfate and barbiturates.

3. Nerve block used as necessary.

Open Wounds of the Chest

Pathophysiology

A. Air that enters the pleural cavity from the atmosphere causes collapse of lung.

B. Air entering and leaving the wound during inspiration and expiration can be detected.

C. Intrapleural negative pressure is lost, thereby embarrassing respirations. If not corrected promptly, this leads to hypoxia and death.

Nursing Care

A. Apply vaseline gauze to wound with pressure dressing.

B. Place patient on assisted ventilation if necessary.

C. Prepare for insertion of chest tubes.

D. Place patient in high-Fowler's position (unless contraindicated) to help provide adequate ventilation.

Hemothorax or Pneumothorax

Definition: Hemothorax is an accumulation of blood within the pleural space. Pneumothorax is an accumulation of air within the pleural space. The blood or air accumulation builds up positive pressure in the pleural space and collapses the lung.

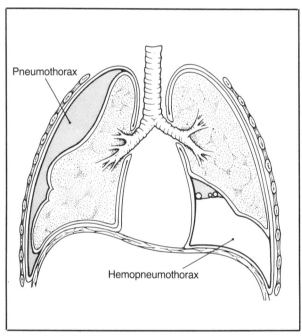

Anatomical View of Lungs

Signs and Symptoms

A. Pain.
B. Decreased breath sounds.
C. Tracheal shift to unaffected side.
D. Dyspnea and respiratory embarrassment.

Treatment and Nursing Care

A. A number 18 needle may be inserted into the second intercostal space, midclavicular line, followed by aspiration of the fluid or air by means of a thoracentesis (emergency treatment).
B. Chest tubes may be inserted and connected to closed-chest drainage.
C. Observe vital signs continuously for shock and cardiac failure complications.

Fractured Ribs

Definition: Fracture varies from simple to severe multiple breaks with flail chest and internal injuries; rib fracture is the most common chest injury.

Signs and Symptoms

A. Pain and tenderness over fracture area.
B. Bruises at injury site.
C. Respiratory distress resulting from bone splinters that have punctured lung, causing pneumothorax.
D. Shallow respirations, from splinting of chest, can cause a reduction in lung compliance as well as respiratory acidosis.

Treatment and Nursing Care

A. Administer mild analgesic (small dose of Demerol) for relief of pain. (*Caution:* Narcotics can depress respiration and the cough reflex.)
B. Encourage deep breathing and coughing to prevent respiratory complications such as atelectasis and pneumonia.
C. Observe for signs of hemorrhage and shock.
D. Intercostal nerve block is administered, if necessary, to decrease pain.

Flail Chest

Definition: Unstable chest wall with respiratory impairment resulting from multiple rib fractures.

Signs and Symptoms

A. Pain.
B. Dyspnea leading to cyanosis.

C. Detached position of flail chest moving in opposition to other areas of chest cage and lung.
   1. On inspiration, the affected chest area is depressed; on expiration, it is bulging outward.
   2. Opposing chest movement causes poor expansion of lungs and leads to carbon dioxide retention and respiratory acidosis.
D. Inability to cough effectively, which leads to accumulation of fluids and respiratory complications such as pneumonia and atelectasis.
E. Cardiac failure due to impaired filling of blood to the right side of the heart caused by the high venous pressure built up by paradoxical breathing.
F. Rapid, shallow, and noisy respirations.

Treatment and Nursing Care

A. Prepare for tracheostomy with a cuffed tracheostomy tube.
B. Place patient on volume-controlled respirator (MA-I), which delivers the same amount of tidal volume with each breath independent of patient's respirations.
C. Suction frequently to prevent respiratory complications.
D. Prevent pain by administering nerve block or Demerol as ordered.
E. Observe for signs of shock and hemorrhage. For patient on ventilator, use nasogastric tube to prevent abdominal distention and emesis, which can lead to aspiration.
F. Assist patient not on mechanical ventilator.
   1. Encourage turning, coughing, and hyperventilating every hour.
   2. Administer oxygen.
   3. Maintain IPPB therapy.
   4. Suction as needed.

Respiratory Tract Surgical Procedures

Submucus Resection (SMR)

Definition: Removal of part of deflected nasal septum.

Procedure

A. Lay back flap of mucous membrane.
B. Excise portion of septum.
C. Rationale.
   1. Restore normal breathing space.
   2. Permit more adequate sinus drainage.

Treatment and Nursing Care

A. Provide routine postoperative care.
B. Observe respiration.
C. Pack nasal cavity.
D. Apply mustache dressing.

Laryngectomy

Definition: Partial or total removal of larynx (epiglottis, thyroid cartilage, hyoid bone, cricoid cartilage, and part of trachea); may sometimes include removal of neck tissue.

Procedure

A. Bring out stump of trachea and suture to neck skin.
B. Close portion of pharynx.
   1. Procedure is permanent.
   2. Breathing through nose is eliminated.
C. If neck tissue and lymph nodes involved, radical neck resection performed.
D. Rationale: removal of benign or malignant tissue, tumors, or lymph nodes, if involved.

Treatment and Nursing Care

A. Suction frequently with sterile technique until area has healed; then use clean technique.
B. Observe for hemorrhage from surgical site.
C. Instruct patient regarding means for communication.
   1. Patient will not be able to speak immediately after surgery.
   2. Inform patient of available speech rehabilitation after healing has occurred.
D. Feed through nasogastric tube.

E. Encourage normal eating patterns after healing has occurred.

F. Instruct patient how to care for opening.

G. Possibly refer patient to the Lost Cord Club.

Tracheostomy

Definition: Creation of an external opening into the trachea for insertion of a breathing tube.

Procedure

A. Position patient so trachea is prominent.

B. Midline incision for tubal insertion.

C. Rationale.
1. Remove tracheobronchial secretions for patient unable to adequately cough.
2. Use with mechanical ventilators.
3. Use as emergency measure for unconscious patients.

Treatment and Nursing Care

☆A. Care for and maintain cuffed tracheostomy tube.
1. Release of cuff pressure five minutes out of every hour. Hyperventilation of patient before and after cuff is deflated with ambu bag.
2. Tracheal suction as ordered or prn.
   a. Always apply oral or nasal suction first so that, when cuff is deflated, secretions will not fall into lung from area above cuff.
   b. Catheter must be changed before tracheostomy suctioning.
3. Humidification with tracheostomy mist mask if patient not on ventilator.

B. Observe for hemorrhage from tracheostomy site.

C. Change dressings (nonraveling type) and cleanse surrounding area with hydrogen peroxide at least every four hours.

D. Care for and maintain silver tracheostomy tube.
1. Removal of inner cannula for soaking in hydrogen peroxide solution to loosen mucus accumulation.

2. Cleansing of inner and outer aspects of tube with brush.
3. Sterile saline or water rinse.
4. Suction of outer cannula before reinsertion.
5. Special orders for tube care.
   a. Disinfect tube by boiling for five minutes.
   b. Leave tube in disinfectant solution for varying lengths of time.
   c. Inner cannula is usually replaced by an interchangeable part every four hours.

Thoracic Cavity Surgical Procedures

Types of Procedures

A. Exploratory thoracotomy is an incision of the thoracic wall for locating bleeding, injuries and/or tumors.

B. Thoracoplasty is the removal of ribs or portions of ribs to reduce the size of the thoracic space.

C. Pneumonectomy is the removal of entire lung.

D. Lobectomy is the removal of a lobe of the lung.

E. Segmented resection is the removal of one or more segments of the lung.

F. Wedge resection is the removal of a small, localized area of disease near the surface of the lung.

Postoperative Nursing Care

A. Employ closed chest suction for all surgeries but pneumonectomy.
1. In pneumonectomy, it is desirable that the fluid accumulate in empty thoracic space.
2. Eventually the thoracic space fills with serous exudate which consolidates, preventing extensive mediastinal shifts.

B. Maintain patent chest tube; drain by chest tube stripping.

C. Maintain respiratory function.
   1. Patient to turn, cough, and deep breathe.
   2. Suction if necessary.
   3. Oxygen therapy.
   4. IPPB therapy.
   5. Mechanical ventilation if necessary.
D. Ambulate patient to enhance adequate ventilation and prevent postoperative complications.
E. Provide range-of-motion exercises to all extremities for promotion of adequate circulation.
F. Monitor for signs of increased central venous pressure which indicates impaired venous return to heart.
G. Positioning of patient.
   1. Semi-Fowler's position to facilitate lung expansion when vital signs are stable.
   2. Specific positions that require readjustment every one to two hours.
      a. Pneumonectomy.
         (1) Position on operated side for back care only.
         (2) Position on back or unoperated side only. (Some physicians will allow positioning on either side after twenty-four hours.)
      b. Segmental resection or wedge resection.
         (1) Position on back or unoperated side.
         (2) Position enhances expansion of remaining pulmonary tissue.
      c. Lobectomy.
         (1) Turn to either side.
         (2) Expands lung tissue on both sides.
H. Encourage postoperative arm and shoulder exercises.
   1. Affected arm should be put through both active and passive range of motion every four hours.
   2. Exercises should start within four hours after surgery when patient has returned to room.
   3. Exercising prevents formation of adhesions.

Postoperative Complications

Respiratory Complications

A. Causes.
   1. Inadequate ventilation.
   2. Airway obstructed by accumulation of secretion.
   3. Atelectasis (collapsed or airless lung) from underexpansion of lungs and anesthetic agents during surgery.
   4. Hypoventilation and carbon dioxide build-up from incisional splinting as a result of pain.
   5. Depression of CNS from overuse of medications.
B. Tension pneumothorax.
   1. Air leak through pleural incision lines.
   2. Mediastinal shift can occur.
C. Pulmonary embolism.
D. Bronchopulmonary fistula.
   1. Subcutaneous emphysema from escape of air into pleural space which is then forced into subcutaneous tissue around incision.
   2. Inadequate closure of bronchus during resection.
   3. Alveolar or bronchiolar tears in surface of lung (particularly following pneumonectomy).
E. Atelectasis and/or pneumonia from airway obstruction or as result of anesthesia.
F. Possible respiratory arrest.

Circulatory Complications

A. Hypovolemia from loss of fluid or blood; can result in cardiac arrest.
B. Arrhythmias from underlying myocardial disease; can result in cardiac arrest.
C. Pulmonary edema from fluid overload of circulatory system.

Management of Thoracic Surgical Equipment

Chest Tubes

General Principles

A. Purpose is the removal of air and serosanguineous fluid from pleural space following thoracic surgery.

B. Tubes are placed in pleural cavity and attached to water seal suction to maintain closed system.

C. Tubes are attached to water seal suction to maintain closed system.
1. All connectors are taped.
2. Bottle stoppers should fit tightly.
3. Bottles kept below level of bed.
4. Suction level maintained where ordered (be sure that bubbling is not excessive in the pressure-regulating bottle).
5. Water level maintained in bottle.

D. Mechanics of system.
1. Used after some intrathoracic procedures.
2. Chest tubes placed intrapleurally.
3. Breathing mechanism operates on principle of negative pressure.
   a. Pressure in chest cavity is lower than pressure of atmosphere.
   b. An injury that breaks into chest cavity (such as stab wound) will cause atmospheric air to then rush into the cavity.
   c. Vacuum must be applied to chest to reestablish negative pressure when chest has been open.
4. Closed water seal drainage is method of reestablishing negative pressure.
   a. Water acts as a seal and keeps the air from being drawn back into pleural space.
   b. Open drainage system would allow air to be sucked back into chest cavity and cause collapse of lung.
5. Closed drainage is established by placing catheter into pleural space and allowing it to drain under water.
   a. The end of the drainage tube is always kept under water.
   b. Air will not be drawn up through catheter into pleural space when tube is under water.
6. Drainage can be accomplished with one, two, or three bottles.
7. Some physicians do not allow clamping or milking of chest tubes. Follow physician's orders.

☆ Nursing Care

A. Assist physician in placement of tubes.
1. Tubes placed in pleural cavity following thoracic surgery.
2. Provides for removal of air and serosanguineous fluid from pleural space.

B. Attach to water-seal suction—maintains closed system.
1. Tape all connectors.
2. Ensure that all stoppers in bottles are tight fitting.

C. Apply suction.
1. Keep bottles below level of bed.
2. Keep suction level where ordered (be sure that bubbling is not excessive in the pressure-regulating bottle).
3. Maintain water level in bottle.

D. Maintain patency.
1. Milk chest tubes every 30 to 60 minutes if clots or debris present.
   a. Milk away from patient toward the drainage receptacle.
   b. Pinch tubing close to the chest with one hand as the other hand milks the tube. Continue going down tube in this method until coming to the drainage receptacle.
2. Use lotion or alcohol wipes to provide ease of stripping.

E. Maintain safety.
1. Keep rubber-tipped hemostats at bedside so that tube can be clamped off near to chest insertion site. Clamp to locate source of air leak.
2. Clamp if drainage system is interrupted or drainage bottle is to be replaced as ordered.
3. It is best to leave open to prevent tension pneumothorax.

180

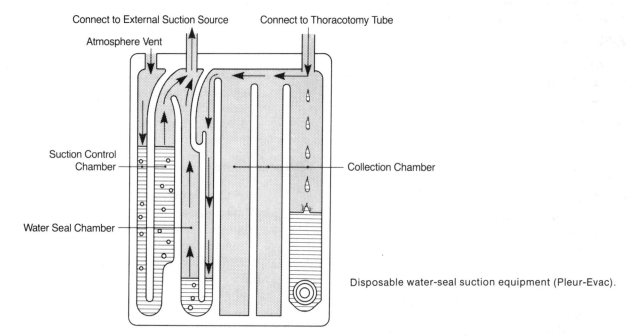

Connect to External Suction Source

Connect to Thoracotomy Tube

Atmosphere Vent

Suction Control Chamber

Water Seal Chamber

Collection Chamber

Disposable water-seal suction equipment (Pleur-Evac).

F. Monitor intake and output.
   1. With Pleur-evac suction equipment, visually measure chest drainage (holds up to 2800 to 3000 cc drainage). With two or three-bottle suction, tape or bottle markings may approximate the amount of drainage (similar to Pleur-evac).
   2. Change equipment only when the drainage chamber is full.

Water-Seal Chest Drainage

Assessment

A. Assess patient's respiratory rate, rhythm, and breath sounds for signs of respiratory distress.
B. Check that all connections on tubing are airtight and suction control is connected.
C. Examine system to see if it is set up and functioning properly.
D. Identify any malfunctions in system, i.e., air leaks, negative pressure, or obstructions.

Nursing Care

A. Maintain water-seal suction system.
B. Cessation of fluctuations indicates reexpansion of lung.
C. If chest tubes are used for lung reexpansion, bubbling will occur in the water-seal bottle.

One-Bottle Suction System

1. There is only one bottle; it functions as a collection bottle for drainage as well as to prevent air from leaking into pleural cavity.
2. As the drainage increases in amount, the water-seal tube (immersed in the drainage) is pulled up slightly to decrease the amount of force that is required to permit the fluid to be drained from the pleural space.
3. The depth to which the water-seal tube is immersed below the fluid in the bottle determines the pressure exerted by the water.
4. Vent is used to prevent pressure build-up and to allow continuous air removal.

Two-Bottle Suction System

1. Two-bottle suction.
   a. Drainage bottle (bottle number one) is connected from client and is between the patient and the water-seal bottle (or bottle number two).
      (1) Short tube goes from patient into drainage bottle (not to extend below drainage level).
      (2) Short tube with rubber tubing goes from the drainage bottle to water-seal bottle.
      (3) This tube extends below water level in the water-seal bottle.
   b. Mark drainage level on outside of bottle.
2. Bottle number two.
   a. The long tube extends below water level about 2 cm.
   b. A second short tube provides an air vent.
   c. Water in this bottle goes up the tube when patient inhales and down the tube when patient exhales. Fluctuates 5-10 cm.
   d. Water in this bottle should not bubble constantly.

Three-Bottle Suction System

1. One bottle is connected to suction motor—called a pressure regulator bottle.
2. Bottle number three regulates the amount of pressure in the system. (Bubbles constantly.)
3. Three tubes.
   a. Short tube, above water level, comes from water-seal bottle.
   b. Short tube connected to suction motor.
   c. Third tube, below water level in bottle, opens to the atmosphere outside of bottle.
   d. The depth to which third tube is submerged in the water determines the pressure within the drainage system.
4. When control bottle fluid becomes too low, outside air is sucked into the system. Depth

ONE BOTTLE SUCTION

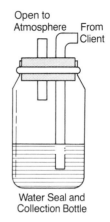

Open to Atmosphere   From Client

Water Seal and Collection Bottle

TWO BOTTLE SUCTION

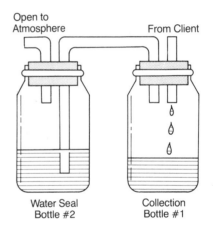

Open to Atmosphere   From Client

Water Seal Bottle #2   Collection Bottle #1

THREE BOTTLE SUCTION

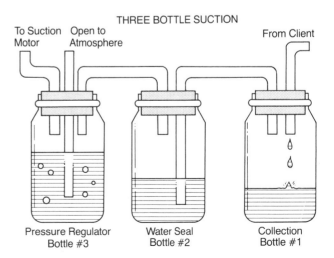

To Suction Motor   Open to Atmosphere   From Client

Pressure Regulator Bottle #3   Water Seal Bottle #2   Collection Bottle #1

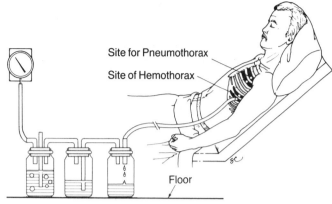

Site for Pneumothorax

Site of Hemothorax

Floor

Provide a straight line of tubing from chest tube to collection system. Keep collection system below level of chest tube insertion site (on the floor).

of control tube under water determines suction level of system.

5. Whenever the motor is off, drainage system must be open to the atmosphere.
    a. Intrapleural air can escape from the system.
    b. Vent prevents pressure build-up which interferes with drainage from patient.

Suctioning Equipment

A. Nasotracheal.
    1. Equipment needed.
        a. Sterile suction catheter, usually No. 14 or No. 16 French.
        b. Sterile saline.
        c. Suction machine.
        d. Sterile gloves.
    ☆2. Procedure.
        a. Lubricate catheter with normal saline.
        b. Insert catheter 6–8 inches into the nose.
        c. Do not apply suction while introducing catheter.
        d. When advanced as far as possible, begin suctioning by withdrawing catheter slowly, rotating it with pressure applied. (Usually a whistle tip catheter or Y connector tube is used to apply pressure.)
B. Tracheostomy.
    1. Equipment needed.
        a. Same equipment as for nasotracheal.
        b. Sterile syringe (5 cc) and sterile saline for instillation into tracheostomy tube.

☆2. Procedure.
    a. Be sure that suction catheter is not more than half the diameter of the tracheostomy tube.
    b. Lubricate with sterile saline.
    c. Insert catheter through tracheostomy tube for 8–12 inches with suction turned off.
    d. Do not suction for more than ten seconds.
    e. Rotate catheter while withdrawing it.
    f. Do not repeat procedure for at least three minutes, unless necessary to withdraw more secretions to permit adequate ventilation.
    g. If secretions are very tenacious, 3–5 cc of sterile saline may be inserted through tube and allowed to remain for a few seconds before suctioning (this increases viscosity of secretions and facilitates removal).
    h. To remove secretions from right bronchus, turn patient's head to left; vice-versa for left bronchus.

Common Respiratory Drugs

Bronchodilators Commonly Used

A. Aminophylline.
    1. Relaxes smooth muscle of the tracheobronchial tree.
    2. Intravenous, oral, elixir.
    3. Should be taken on an empty stomach since it is not absorbed well in an alkaline

medium.

    4. Side effects.

      a. Gastric irritation.

      b. Nausea.

      c. Cardiac arrhythmias (tachycardia, ventricular ectopy).

B. Tedral.

    1. Relaxes smooth muscle of the tracheobronchial tree, reduces congestion, and aids in preventing histamine-induced bronchospasm.

    2. Tablet, elixir—contain phenobarbital (habit forming).

    3. Caution necessary for patients with cardiovascular disease, hypertension, hyperthyroidism, prostatic hypertrophy, and glaucoma.

    4. Side effects.

      a. Drowsiness.

      b. Epigastric distress.

      c. Difficulty of urination.

      d. Palpitations.

      e. Insomnia, CNS stimulation.

C. Ephedrine.

    1. Relaxes smooth muscle of the tracheobronchial tree, reduces congestion, and acts as a vasoconstrictor.

    2. Tablet, parenteral.

    3. Side effects.

      a. Anxiety, tremulousness, palpitations.

      b. Insomnia.

      c. Difficulty of urination.

      d. CNS stimulation.

D. Isuprel.

    1. Relaxes smooth muscle of the tracheobronchial tree, relieves bronchospasm, and acts as a cardiac stimulant (increases cardiac output and venous return to the heart).

    2. Mistometer, solution for nebulization, IV (requires ICU).

    3. Caution necessary for patients with existing cardiac arrhythmias associated with tachycardias.

      a. It may result in aggravation of arrhythmias.

      b. Should not be used with epinephrine since both are cardiac stimulants and the combined effect may produce serious arrhythmias.

    4. Side effects.

      a. Tachycardia, nervousness, palpitations.

      b. Arrhythmias.

      c. Nausea.

      d. Headaches.

      e. Flushing, tremor, dizziness.

      f. Weakness.

      g. Diaphoresis.

      h. Chest pain.

E. Bronkosol.

    1. Relaxes smooth muscle of the tracheobronchial tree.

      a. Acts as bronchovasoconstrictor and reduces congestion.

      b. Less effective than Isuprel in its bronchodilating effect, but more potent than epinephrine.

    2. Hand nebulizer and solution for aerosolization.

    3. Precautions are the same as for Isuprel, but the side effects seem to appear less frequently.

F. Choledyl.

    1. Relaxes smooth muscle of the tracheobronchial tree.

      a. Relieves bronchospasm.

      b. Useful in long-term therapy of bronchospasm.

    2. Tablet, elixir.

    3. Concomitant use with other bronchodilators may increase side effects, especially CNS stimulation.

    4. Side effects.

      a. Gastric distress.

      b. Palpitations.

      c. CNS stimulation.

General Respiratory Drugs

A. Quibron.

    1. Relieves bronchiolar constriction and assists in removal of mucus.

    2. Capsule or elixir.

    3. Should not be given within 12 hours of rectal doses of theophylline.

    4. Side effects.

a. Gastrointestinal upset.

b. Nausea and vomiting.

B. Epinephrine.

1. Acts directly on beta cells of the bronchi, increases tidal volume, and relieves congestion in bronchial mucosa and constricting pulmonary vessels.

2. Used in anaphylaxis and asthma.

3. Subcutaneous injection.

4. Strong cardiotonic.

5. Vital signs should be monitored during use.

6. Side effects.

   a. Palpitations and tachycardia.
   b. Headache.
   c. Tremor, weakness, and vertigo.

Mucolytics

A. Mucomyst.

1. Reduces viscosity of purulent and nonpurulent secretions by breaking disulfide bond; assists in removal of secretions.

2. Inhalation medication.

3. Inactivates many antibiotics, including penicillin.

4. Side effects.

   a. Stomatitis.
   b. Hemoptysis.
   c. Nausea.

B. Potassium iodide.

1. Expectorant liquefies tenacious bronchial secretions.

2. Enseal (enteric-release) capsule.

3. Not used in acute bronchitis.

4. Thyroid abnormalities can occur with use.

Gastrointestinal System

The alimentary tract's primary function is to provide the body with a continual supply of nutrients, fluids, and electrolytes for tissue nourishment. This system has three components: a tract for ingestion and movement of food and fluids; secretion of digestive juices for breaking down the nutrients; and absorption mechanisms for the utilization of foods, water, and electrolytes for continuous growth and repair of body tissues.

Anatomy and Physiology

Alimentary Tract

A. Mouth.
1. Cheeks.
2. Hard and soft palates.
3. Muscles.
4. Maxillary bones (jaw).
5. Tongue—aids in chewing, swallowing, and speaking; contains taste buds.
6. Salivary glands.
   a. Constant secretions form saliva.
   b. Three pairs of glands located in the mucous membrane of the oral cavity.
      (1) Parotid—below the ear.
      (2) Submaxillary—floor of mouth.
      (3) Sublingual—floor of mouth.
7. Teeth—assist in mastication and in mixing saliva with food.
8. Digestive process starts in the mouth.
B. Pharynx.
1. Tubal structure that extends from the base of the skull to the esophagus.
2. Serves as a passageway for air from nasal cavity to larynx and for food from mouth to esophagus.
3. Parts.
   a. Nasopharynx.
   b. Oropharynx.
   c. Laryngopharynx.

C. Esophagus.
1. Muscular canal.
2. Extends from pharynx to stomach.

D. Stomach.
1. Distensible pouch located between the esophagus and the duodenum.
2. Divisions.
   a. Fundus which forms upper portion is located immediately below the cardiac sphincter.
   b. Body which forms the largest and central portion.
   c. Pylorus forms the lower portion.
3. Sphincters.
   a. Cardiac sphincter is muscle around the lower end of the esophagus where it opens into the stomach.
   b. Pyloric sphincter is muscle around the lower end of the stomach where it opens into the duodenum.
4. Curvatures.
   a. Lesser curvature.
   b. Greater curvature.
5. Layers.
   a. Serous coat is the outer layer which forms the visceral peritoneum; the peritoneum folds and forms the omentum, which hangs over the intestines like an apron.
   b. Muscular layer formed of three directional (circular, longitudinal, and oblique) muscle fibers.
   c. Submucous layer contains blood vessels and lymphatics.
   d. Mucous layer contains microscopic glands which assist in digestion.
6. Glands.
   a. Mucous gland secretes mucus.
   b. Gastric gland secretes gastric juice containing hydrochloric acid and digestive enzymes.
7. Function.
   a. Mechanical digestion.
      (1) Most digestion occurs near pyloric area where peristalsis is more forceful.

(2) Peristalsis is stimulated by the vagus nerve.

b. Chemical digestion—excretes gastric juice containing hydrochloric acid and enzymes.

E. Small intestine.

1. Convoluted tube approximately 23 feet in length.

2. General functions.

a. Digestion and absorption.

b. Receives bile and pancreatic juices.

3. Segments.

a. Duodenum begins at the pylorus and connects with the jejunum where it ends; it is approximately ten inches long.

b. Jejunum is the middle portion which is approximately eight feet long and lies coiled around the umbilical region.

c. Ileum is the terminal section which joins the colon at the ileocecal valve; it is approximately twelve feet long.

4. Folds.

a. Extend around the intestinal lumen; most numerous in the duodenum but disappear in the lower ileum.

b. Contain numerous villi through which products of digestion are absorbed. Each villus has an arteriole, venule and lymph vessel.

c. Folds provide a large surface area which assists digestion, secretion, and absorption.

F. Large intestine.

1. Extends from the ileocecal valve to the anus; it is five to six feet long and is wider than the small intestine.

2. Segments.

a. Cecum connects with the ileum at the ileocecal valve; appendix attaches to the distal end.

b. Ascending colon continues up the right side of the abdomen to lower borders of the liver where it turns.

c. Transverse colon continues from the ascending colon across the abdomen (front of stomach) to lower border of the spleen.

d. Descending colon continues from the transverse colon down the left side of the abdomen to the brim of the pelvis.

e. Sigmoid colon is the S-shaped portion which extends to the rectum.

f. Rectum is six to eight inches long and ends at anus.

3. General functions.

a. Reabsorption of fluids, electrolytes, glucose, and urea.

b. Mechanical digestion.

c. Peristalsis and defecation.

d. Elimination of wastes.

Accessory Organs

A. Liver.

1. Located in the right upper abdomen and protected by lower ribs.

2. Largest organ in the body.

3. General functions.

a. Metabolism of carbohydrates, fats, and proteins.

b. Detoxification of harmful substances in the blood.

c. Breakdown of old blood cells.

d. Constant secretion of bile, which drains from the liver through the hepatic duct into the common duct to the small intestine; bile is stored in the gallbladder.

e. Stores glycogen and vitamins A, B, B_{12}, and K.

f. Produces and stores heparin and fibrinogen.

B. Gallbladder.

1. Small sac of smooth muscle located in a depression at the edge of the visceral surface of the liver.

2. Functions as a reservoir for bile.

a. Bile from the hepatic duct enters the gallbladder through the cystic duct for storage.

b. Stored bile leaves the gallbladder through the cystic duct to flow through the common duct into the small intestine.

c. Bile activates the pancreas to release its digestive enzymes and an alkaline fluid.

C. Pancreas.
 1. Soft, pinkish-white organ that is six inches long and one inch wide; it adheres to the middle portion of the duodenum.
 2. Composed of exocrine and endocrine tissue.
    a. Exocrine cells secrete juices containing digestive enzymes.
    b. Endocrine cells secrete glucagon and insulin.

Diagnostic Procedures

Upper Gastrointestinal Roentgenography

A. Purpose.
 1. For visualizing GI tract.
    a. Structure and function of the esophagus.
    b. Size and shape of the right atrium.
    c. Size and shape of the stomach.
    d. Motility of the stomach.
    e. Ulcerations, tumor formations, and anatomic abnormalities of the stomach and small intestines.
    f. Emptying time of the stomach.
 2. For documenting in permanent records.
B. Procedure.
 1. Ingestion of barium or other contrast medium.
 2. Pass x-rays through the body so that GI tract will stand out in silhouette on film.
C. Preparation of the patient.
 1. NPO after midnight prior to the day of the test.
 2. Withhold medications.
 3. Explain procedure to the patient.

Barium Enema

A. Purpose.
 1. For visualizing the lower intestinal tract.
 2. For revealing abnormalities of structure and motility of the cecum and appendix.

B. Procedure.
 1. Barium enema given.
 2. X-ray film taken.
C. Preparation of the patient.
 1. Evacuate the intestinal tract by enema, laxatives, or suppositories until returning solution is clear.
 2. NPO after midnight (some methods allow clear liquids for breakfast).
 3. Explain procedure to patient.

Endoscopy

A. Purpose.
 1. For visualizing inside of body cavity to detect lesions.
 2. For taking biopsy.
 3. Secure washings for cytologic examination.
B. Preparation of the patient.
 1. NPO after midnight.
 2. Premedicate the patient.
 3. Give patient support during exam.
 4. Assist the physician.
 5. Topical anesthetic may be used to facilitate passage of the scope into the esophagus during exam. The anesthetic depresses the gag reflex.
C. Nursing care following an esophagogastroduodenoscopy (EGD).
 1. Withhold fluids or food by mouth until swallowing reflex returns.
 2. Observe carefully for swelling.
 3. Prevent aspiration if vomiting occurs.

Gastric Analysis

A. Purpose.
 1. For analyzing stomach contents for acid-fast bacilli, for volume, and for free acid.
 2. For detecting gastric bleeding.
B. Procedure.
 1. Insertion of nasogastric tube to aspirate stomach contents.
 2. Specimens obtained at varying times.

C. Preparation of the patient.
  1. NPO six to eight hours prior to exam.
  2. Collect specimens as ordered; label and send to lab.
  3. Remove nasogastric tube and provide oral hygiene.

Stool Analysis

A. Purpose.
  1. For examining amount, consistency, color, shape, blood, fecal urobilinogen, fat, nitrogen, parasites, food residue, and other substances.
  2. For culturing bacteria and viruses.
B. Procedure.
  1. Collect fresh, warm stool specimen for parasite analysis.
  2. Collect specimen in small amount for occult blood analysis (guaiac).
  3. Obtain a twenty-four hour collection for chemical analysis.
  4. Collect specimen in sterile container for C&S.
C. Stool characteristics.
  1. Color.
    a. Foods (spinach, cocoa) produce dark red.
    b. Medicines (senna) produce yellow.
    c. Iron produces black.
    d. Upper GI bleeding produces tarry black.
    e. Fresh, lower tract bleeding produces bright red.
  2. Stool abnormalities.
    a. Steatorrhea may be indicated by bulky, greasy, foamy, and foul-odored stools.
    b. Biliary obstruction may be indicated by light gray or clay-colored stools.
    c. Ulcerative colitis may be indicated by loose stools with copious amounts of mucus and/or pus.
    d. Constipation or obstruction may be indicated by small, hard-massed stools.

Gastrointestinal Disorders

Anorexia

Definition: Loss or lack of appetite for food.

Causes

A. Anxiety, depression.
B. Improper fit of dentures.
C. Illness, physical discomfort.
D. Constipation.
E. Intestinal obstruction.

Nursing Care

A. Become familiar with patient's eating habits, i.e., likes and dislikes in food, cultural and religious beliefs regarding food.
B. Permit, when possible, patient to choose own food.
C. Show interest, but don't force patient to eat.
D. Provide a pleasant and inviting environment.
E. Serve small portions of attractively prepared food.

Nausea and Vomiting

Definitions: Nausea is the distressing feeling that is felt when nerves ending in stomach and other body parts are irritated; may lead to vomiting. Vomiting is ejection of stomach contents through mouth.

Causes

A. Stress, fear, and depression.
B. Pain.
C. Acute febrile illness.
D. Medications.
E. Anesthesia.
F. Diseases of the stomach.
G. Intestinal obstruction.
H. Pregnancy.
I. Head injury.

Nursing Care

A. Administer relief-giving drugs.
B. Monitor fluid and electrolyte replacement.
C. Protect the patient from unpleasant sights, sounds, and smells.
D. Attempt to keep the stomach empty.
E. Promptly remove used equipment; change soiled linens and dressings.
F. Ventilate room and use unscented air fresheners.
G. Observe and record the character and quantity of emesis.

Constipation and Diarrhea

Definitions: Diarrhea is the rapid movement through intestines of loose, watery stools resulting from increased peristalsis. Constipation is the delay in the evacuation of feces, with passage of hard and dry fecal material.

Causes

A. Diarrhea—fecal impaction, ulcerative colitis, intestinal infections, drugs, or neurosis.
B. Constipation—lack of regularity, psychogenic causes, drugs, inadequate fluid intake, mechanical obstruction, lack of dietary bulk, or lack of exercise.

Nursing Care

A. Administer laxatives for constipation; antidiarrheals for diarrhea.
B. Observe stools for color, odor, shape, consistency, amount, presence of mucus, blood, or pus.
C. Provide perirectal skin care.

Oral Infections

Definitions: Stomatitis is an inflammation of the mouth. Glossitis is an inflammation of the tongue. Gingivitis is an inflammation of the gums.

Causes

A. Mechanical trauma.
B. Foods, drinks, allergies, or medications.
C. Poor oral hygiene.
D. Pathogens.

Signs and Symptoms

A. Anorexia.
B. Excessive salivation.
C. Foul breath (halitosis).

Treatment and Nursing Care

A. Remove causative factor.
B. Provide frequent, soothing oral hygiene.
C. Apply topical medications and administer systemic antibiotics.
D. Provide soft, bland diet.
E. Administer analgesic (may be topical application) thirty minutes before meals.

Malignant Tumors of the Mouth

Definition: Cancer of the mouth that usually affects the lips, tongue, or the mouth floor.

Predisposing Factors

A. Poor oral hygiene.
B. Chronic irritation.
C. Chemical and thermal trauma, i.e., tobacco, alcohol, and hot-spiced foods.

Treatment

A. Surgical removal of tumor.
B. Radiation therapy.

Esophageal Disorders

Definition: Local or systemic infection or chemical irritation from reflux of gastric juices into the lower esophagus.

Signs and Symptoms

A. Heartburn.
B. Intolerance of spices.
C. Alcohol and caffeine intolerance.
D. Dysphagia.

Treatment and Nursing Care

A. Give oral antacids.
B. Provide bland diet.
C. Elevate head of bed; do not recline after meals.

Esophageal Varices

Definition: Tortuous dilation of veins in the lower esophagus caused by portal hypertension and often associated with cirrhosis of liver.

Treatment and Nursing Care

A. Placement of Sengstaken-Blakemore tube to exert pressure against ruptured vessels.
   1. Maintain pressure in balloon.
   2. Do not deflate balloon.
B. Administer vitamin K.
C. Observe for hemorrhage and shock.
D. Provide frequent oral hygiene.

Cancer of Esophagus

Definition: Malignant tumors of the esophagus; carcinomas, constituting four per cent of all malignant tumors along the GI tract, are the most common form of tumor.

Signs and Symptoms

A. Dysphagia (most common).
B. Substernal pressure.

Treatment and Nursing Care

A. Radiation therapy.
B. Gastrostomy tube.
C. Watch for complications (rupture, hemorrhage).

Esophageal Hernia (Hiatus Hernia)

Definition: Protrusion of a portion of the stomach through the diaphragm and into the thorax.

Causes

A. Congenital weakness of the diaphragm.
B. Trauma.
C. Relaxation of the muscles.
D. Intra-abdominal pressure (obesity, ascites, pregnancy).

Signs and Symptoms

A. Heartburn and pain.
B. Dysphagia.
C. Vomiting.
D. Regurgitation (especially after large meals or ingestion of spicy foods).

Nursing Care

A. Provide small frequent meals (avoid highly seasoned foods).
B. Maintain patient in upright position during and after meals.
C. Administer antacids after meals and at bedtime.
D. Elevate head of bed to avoid regurgitation during sleep.
E. Advise patient against constrictive clothing about the waist.
F. Advise patient against sharp and forward bends.

Dyspepsia (Indigestion)

Definition: Imperfect digestion symptomatic of other GI diseases or disorders; characterized by heartburn and other abdominal discomforts.

Causes

A. Rapid ingestion.
B. Disease.
C. Altered gastric secretions.
D. Emotional problems.

Nursing Care

A. Provide bland diet.
B. Administer antispasmodics, tranquilizers, and antacids.
C. Advise patient to modify current eating habits.

Acute Gastritis

Definition: Inflammation of the stomach.

Causes

A. Ingestion of corrosive or erosive substances, (alcohol, aspirin, or contaminated food).
B. Acute systemic infections.
C. Radiotherapy or chemotherapy.
D. Infection.

Signs and Symptoms

A. Epigastric burning and pain.
B. Nausea and vomiting.
C. Malaise.
D. Hemorrhage.
E. Anorexia.
F. Headache.

Treatment and Nursing Care

A. Attempt to eliminate the cause; treat symptomatically.
B. Administer antacids and phenothiazines.

Principles of Nursing Care for Gastrointestinal Surgery

Preoperative Care

A. Psychological care.
   1. Allay fears regarding postoperative concerns.
   2. Familiarize the patient with hospital procedures.
      a. Show method for getting in and out of bed.
      b. Teach leg exercises.
      c. Teach deep breathing and coughing exercises.
      d. Explain pain medication schedule.
      e. Discuss recovery room routines.
   3. Encourage questions and feedback to determine what patient actually understands.
   4. Include family in preoperative explanations.
B. Physical care.
   1. Report any change in vital signs.
   2. Check and record each item on preoperative check list.
   3. Give enema to cleanse the lower colon.
   4. Remove all prostheses.
   5. Encourage patient to void.
   6. Administer preoperative medication (it will dry secretions and promote sense of well-being).
   7. Put side rails up.
   8. Remove valuables and place in safekeeping.

Postoperative Care

A. Check airway for obstruction.
B. Evaluate the need for pain medication.
C. Check for presence and patency of tubes.
D. Monitor IV.
   1. Check flow rate and contents of bottle.
   2. Check insertion site for pain and signs of inflammation.
E. Examine dressing for color and amount of drainage; record in nurse's notes.
F. Check vital signs frequently.
G. Observe for signs of hypovolemic shock.
   1. Drop in blood pressure.
   2. Increase in pulse or respirations.
   3. Change in color.
   4. Dyspnea.
H. Observe for first passage of flatus on all GI surgical patients. Bowel sounds or flatus indicate the return of peristalsis.
I. Record the time and amount of first voiding.

J. Turn patient every two hours.
   1. Encourage coughing and deep breathing.
   2. Support abdominal incision with pillow, hands, or blanket during patient coughing to reduce strain on incision and increase patient comfort.
K. Assist in ambulation as ordered.
L. Encourage taking of food as ordered and tolerated.
M. Follow general principles of nasogastric tube care.

Management of Postoperative Pain

A. Evaluate need for medication every three to four hours for the first twenty-four hours; give freely.
B. Do not give morphine to patients with biliary or pancreatic disorders as it results in spasms of the smooth muscle.

Management of Nasogastric Intubation and Decompression

A. Purpose of intubation.
   1. Prevent postoperative vomiting after GI surgery.
   2. Provide feedings.
   3. Relieve abdominal distention as a result of bowel obstruction or paralytic ileus.
   4. Provide rest for the GI tract.
B. Tubal types.
   1. Stomach tubes—flexible tubes introduced by way of nose to decompress stomach after surgery or for feedings.
      a. Salem sump—remove fluid accumulation.
      b. Levin tube—gastroduodenal catheter.
   2. Intestinal tubes—tubes placed in intestinal tract by way of nose to relieve gas pressure.
      a. Miller-Abbott—double-channel intestinal tube.
      b. Cantor tube—used for intestinal decompression.

C. Nursing care.
   1. Provide frequent oral and nasal care.
   2. Maintain patency of tubes with irrigation of normal saline as ordered.
   3. Check for placement of tubes before irrigation by listening with stethoscope for air bubble insertion via syringe.
   4. Observe color and amount of drainage.
   5. Record intake and output.
   6. Be alert to fact that vomiting or abdominal distention is an indication of obstruction.

Peptic Ulcer Disease (PUD)

Definition: Ulceration in the mucosal wall of the stomach, pylorus, or duodenum.

Predisposing Factors

A. Emotional and physical stress.
B. Irregular, hurriedly ingested meals.
C. Seasonal factor (spring and fall).
D. Excessive smoking.
E. Drugs, e.g., salicylates, phenylbutazone, and steroids.
F. Hereditary factors.

Signs and Symptoms

A. Boring, aching, gnawing or burning epigastric pain.
B. Pain usually occurring one half to three hours after eating.
C. Weight loss from reduced intake or weight gain from excessive intake in effort to relieve pain.
D. Vomiting which may result from pain or from pyloric obstruction due to ulcerations and to scarring that accompanies healing.
E. Occult blood in stool from bleeding.

Nursing Care

A. Promote healing process by preventing complications.
B. Provide symptomatic relief.

C. Eliminate irritating factors, e.g., alcohol, smoking, stress, and salicylates.

D. Administer antacids, anticholinergics, iron, ascorbic acid, or sedatives.

E. Observe emesis and/or stool closely (iron preparations may also result in dark stools).

F. Provide diet which eliminates gas-producing foods.

G. Observe and report significant physical and emotional responses to therapy.

H. Observe for indications of complications (i.e., hemorrhage, perforation).

I. Gastric surgery may be required if medical treatment is ineffective.

Gastric Surgical Procedures

A. Vagotomy—interruption of vagal innervation to reduce stimulation of hydrochloric acid production.

B. Gastrectomy or partial gastrectomy—removal of stomach portion that produces hydrochloric acid; anastamosis between remaining portion of stomach and small bowel (gastroenterostomy).

C. Gastrostomy, jejunostomy—creation of opening into the stomach or jejuneum for general purpose of maintaining nutritional status of patient when conditions make use of normal food route *not* feasible.

Postoperative Nursing Care

A. Provide routine care.
1. Observe and record vital signs.
2. Observe for signs of shock.
3. Check dressing for abnormal drainage or bleeding.
4. Provide bed rest.
5. Record intake and output.
6. Turn patient and encourage cough and deep breathing exercises every 2 hours.

B. Manage accessory equipment.
1. Foley and IV tubes.
2. Nasogastric tube.
   a. Ensure patency.
      (1) Irrigate with normal saline.
      (2) Maintain proper suction pressure.
      (3) Maintain correct position.
   b. Observe and record color, consistency, amount, and unusual odor of gastric contents.

C. Raise bed to semi-Fowler's position.

D. Following removal of NG tube provide diet of warm liquids; provide soft diet.

E. Control pain but avoid irritating medications such as salicylates.

F. Change incisional dressings as needed.

G. Prevent constipation.

H. Ambulate first postoperative day unless specified otherwise.

I. Discourage smoking.

J. Protect patient from stressful situations.

Postoperative Complications

A. Hemorrhage.
1. Indications.
   a. Emesis with coffee-grounds color.
   b. Tarry black stools (melena).
   c. Hematemesis (vomiting of bright-red blood).
2. Treatment—possible surgical procedure.

B. Perforation—erosion through stomach muscle into peritoneum.
1. Indications.
   a. Acute onset of severe, persistent pain that may be referred to shoulder or in between the scapulae.
   b. Tender, board-like rigidity of the abdomen.
   c. Thready, rapid pulse.
2. Treatment—surgical procedure.

C. Pyloric obstruction (scarring, edema, or inflammation at the pylorus from healing of chronic ulcerations).
1. Indications.
   a. Nausea and projectile vomiting.
   b. Pain.
   c. Weight loss.
   d. Constipation.

2. Treatment—gastric decompression or surgical repair to relieve the stenosis (narrowing).

D. "Dumping syndrome" (rapid emptying of large amounts of food into small bowel following gastrectomy).

1. Indications.
   a. Weakness, faintness.
   b. Diaphoresis.
   c. Palpitations.
2. Nursing care.
   a. Serve frequent meals of small proportions.
   b. Encourage drinking liquids between meals instead of with meals.
   c. Provide nutrients that are low in carbohydrates, high in proteins, and moderate in fats.
   d. Encourage thirty minute rest period after meals.
   e. Discourage use of table salt and sugars.

Gastric Cancer

Definition: Malignant tumor of the stomach.

Signs and Symptoms

A. *Early stage of carcinoma produces no symptoms.*
B. Weight loss.
C. Vague feeling of fullness and sensation of pressure.
D. Anemia as a result of blood loss.
E. Occult blood in stools.
F. Vomiting if pylorus becomes obstructed.
G. Late stage produces symptoms that include ascites, palpable mass, metastatic pain.

Treatment

A. Surgical resection.
B. Radiation therapy.
C. Chemotherapy.

Diverticulitis

Definition: Inflammation of diverticula (blind pouches) formed in the intestinal mucosa and walls of the sigmoid. Diverticulosis is the presence of multiple diverticula. Confirmed by upper-lower GI series and sigmoidoscopy.

Signs and Symptoms

A. Cramp-like pain.
B. Flatulence.
C. Nausea and fever.
D. Bowel irregularity.
E. Irritability, spasticity of intestine.

Treatment

A. Provide high residue diet that is high in protein, calories, vitamins, and iron. Low residue diet used in inflammatory phase of diverticulitis.
B. Administer antispasmodics.
C. Establish normal bowel habits for patient who has deviated from normal patterns.
D. Performance of surgery as necessary.

Ulcerative Colitis

Definition: Chronic ulcerous and inflammatory disease of the colon and rectum which commonly begins in the rectum and sigmoid colon and spreads upward; characterized by periods of exacerbation and remission.

Cause

A. Specific cause is unknown.
B. Autoimmune factors, allergic reactions and emotional instability are potential causative factors.
C. Bacterial infections may be causal factor.

Signs and Symptoms

A. Anemia and malnutrition.
B. Frequent stools that contain mucus, blood, and pus.

C. Anorexia, weight loss.

D. Cramp-like pain.

E. Abdominal tenderness.

Treatment and Nursing Care

A. Relieve anxiety, i.e., provide quiet environment, remove stress factor, and give medication.

B. Administer antibiotics for secondary bowel inflammation.

C. Administer steroid therapy for inflammation, toxicity, and emotional symptoms.

D. Administer anticholinergic drugs to relieve cramps and control diarrhea.

E. Provide high protein, high caloric diet with vitamin and iron supplements.

F. Allow patient to ventilate his or her feelings; extend acceptance to patient.

G. Administer no cathartics in acute stage; condition contraindicates cathartics.

H. Surgical treatment is indicated if medical management fails.

Complications

A. Dehydration.

B. Anemia and malnutrition (iron and vitamin K deficiency).

C. Magnesium and calcium imbalance.

D. Perforation, peritonitis, and hemorrhage.

E. Abscesses and strictures.

F. Hemorrhoids and anal fissures.

G. Tendency to bleed.

Intestinal Obstruction

Definition: Impairment of the forward flow of intestinal contents by partial or complete blockage.

Causes

A. Adhesions (fibrous bands of abdominal scar tissue which may become looped over a portion of the bowel).

B. Incarcerated or strangulated hernias.

C. Volvulus (twisting of the bowel).

D. Intussusception (telescoping of bowel upon itself).

E. Tumors.

F. Hematoma.

G. Fecal impaction.

H. Ileus (ineffective peristalsis due to toxic or traumatic disturbance of innervation to the bowel).

I. Loss of blood supply to the bowel with resulting necrosis.

Signs and Symptoms

A. Nausea and vomiting.

B. Reverse peristalsis with possible fecal vomiting.

C. Abdominal distention.

D. Absence of stools.

Treatment and Nursing Care

A. Intestinal decompression tube may be inserted to remove gas and fluid.

B. Monitor parenteral fluids and electrolytes.

C. Administer antibiotics.

D. Note and record in chart.
   1. Extent and nature of pain.
   2. Characteristics, amount, and frequency of stools, emesis, and flatus.
   3. Amount of intake and output.
   4. Vital signs.

E. Possible performance of surgery if medical therapy ineffective.

Colon Surgery

A. Ileostomy.
   1. Procedure—creation of opening into ileum brought through abdominal wall for purpose of eliminating bowel contents. Large intestine may or may not be removed.
   2. Conditions that may lead to ileostomy.
      a. Ulcerative colitis.
      b. Crohn's disease.
   3. Postoperative care.
      a. Observe and record vital signs.

b. Need not irrigate for evacuation as stool is always in liquid state.

c. Watch for excoriation of skin around stoma; condition may occur with ileostomy because of enzymatic action.

d. Increase fluid intake because reabsorption in large bowel is absent.

e. Provide low residue, high calorie diet; avoid foods that increase peristalsis or produce flatus.

☆ B. Colostomy.

1. Procedure—creation of abdominal stoma for bowel evacuation following removal of portion of lower (large) intestine.

2. Conditions indicating colostomy.

a. Cancer—usually requires permanent colostomy.

b. Traumatic injury—may require permanent or temporary colostomy.

c. Diverticulitis or obstruction—usually requires temporary colostomy.

3. Preoperative care.

a. Explain to patient the use of apparatus to be utilized in care of the colostomy.

b. Reassure patient that nurse will give assistance in learning to care for the colostomy.

c. Accept the patient's feelings about consequence of procedure; observe for depression, anxiety, and frustration.

d. Provide high calorie, low residue diet for several days.

e. Administer intestinal antiseptics with sulfa and neomycin (po) to decrease bacterial content of colon and to soften and decrease bulk of contents of colon.

f. Cleanse bowel by administering laxatives and enemas.

g. Provide adequate fluids and electrolytes.

4. Postoperative care.

a. Depends on which part of colon involved; contents are liquid to formed.

b. Patient has no voluntary control of bowel evacuation.

c. Ascending colostomy is hard to train for evacuation.

d. Evacuate bowel every twenty-four to forty-eight hours.

e. Control with diet and/or irrigation.

f. Maintain skin care around stoma.

g. Assure proper fit and placement of appliance.

h. Increase fluid intake.

i. Support and guide patient in learning to care for body function which henceforth will be accomplished differently.

Appendicitis

Definition: Inflammation of appendix as a result of bacterial infection.

Signs and Symptoms

A. Rebound tenderness (major symptom).

B. Generalized and severe abdominal pain.

C. Nausea and vomiting.

D. Elevated temperature.

E. Anorexia.

Surgical Procedure
Appendectomy.

A. Preoperative care.

1. Raise bed to semi-Fowler's position to relieve strain on abdomen.

2. Give nothing by mouth.

3. Insert nasogastric tube.

B. Postoperative care—routine for abdominal surgery.

C. Complications.

1. Rupture.

2. Peritonitis.

a. Indications.

(1) Severe abdominal pain localized in right lower quadrant.

(2) Elevated temperature.

(3) Elevated white cell count.

b. Treatment.

(1) Massive antibiotics.

(2) GI decompression.

(3) Bed rest.

(4) High Fowler's position to localize infection.

(5) Nothing by mouth.

Hernia

Definition: Protrusion of part of an organ through the structures normally containing it.

Types

A. Inguinal—occurring in the groin as result of increased abdominal pressure.
B. Femoral—occurring in the femoral canal.
C. Umbilical—occurring at the umbilicus.
D. Incisional—occurring at incisional site as a result of improper healing.

Classifications

A. Reducible hernia—can be replaced in normal cavity.
B. Irreducible hernia—cannot be replaced in the normal cavity.
C. Incarcerated—resulting edema of the affected structures.
D. Strangulated—gangrenous condition results due to trapped blood supply.

Treatment and Nursing Care

A. Surgical repair—hernioplasty; herniorrhaphy.
B. Advise patient not to cough following surgical repair.
C. Take measures to prevent urinary retention.
D. Encourage patient to ambulate soon after surgery to prevent postoperative complications.

Hemorrhoids

Definition: Dilated varicose veins of the anal canal that cause discomfort and bleeding.

Types

A. Internal—occurs above the internal sphincter, covered by mucous membrane.
B. External—occurs outside the external sphincter, covered by anal skin.
C. Thrombosed—infected, clotted, and painful.

Causes

A. By straining to evacuate when constipated.
B. Irritation and diarrhea.
C. Increased venous pressure from congestive heart failure.
D. Increased abdominal pressure as occurs in pregnancy.
E. Habitual toilet sitting (reading of magazines in the bathroom).

Signs and Symptoms

A. Anal itching.
B. Painful bowel evacuation.
C. Bleeding with bowel evacuation.

Treatment and Nursing Care

A. Treat constipation and other causes of increased pressure.
B. Relieve pain with heat, astringents, and topical and systemic analgesics.
C. Give frequent hot sitz baths.
D. Surgical removal by hemorrhoidectomy.
E. Postoperative care.
   1. Make routine observations including vital signs.
   2. Maintain meticulous perineal and rectal cleanliness.
   3. Apply topical anesthetics; give sitz baths for comfort.
   4. Maintain prone or on-side positions to prevent pressure and provide comfort.
   5. Administer medications before first postoperative bowel movement.
   6. Increase liquids and bulk with administration of stool softeners to decrease discomfort of first bowel movement.
   7. Give ordered enema with caution.
      a. Administer medications to relieve pain before giving enema.
      b. Use well-lubricated tip.
      c. Introduce tip with gentleness.

Diagnostic Procedures for Liver, Gallbladder, and Pancreas Disorders

Radiologic Techniques

A. Cholecystogram.
1. Purpose—visualize gallbladder by means of radiopaque dye given intravenously few minutes prior to exam or by means of Telepaque given orally the evening prior to exam.
2. Preprocedural nursing care (using Telepaque).
   a. Give patient low-fat meal evening prior to exam.
   b. Give Telepaque according to body weight at three to five minute intervals with 240 cc of water (minimum).
   c. Give nothing by mouth after midnight.
B. Cholangiography.
1. Purpose—visualize bile ducts by means of contrast radiopaque injected directly into biliary tree.
2. Preprocedural nursing care.
   a. Restrict fluids to concentrate dye.
   b. Cleanse intestinal tract.
C. Liver scan—visualize liver tissue by means of administered radioiodine (131) or similar substances and scintiscan to reveal its concentration in the liver.

Liver Biopsy

A. Purpose—facilitate diagnosis by sampling liver tissues with needle aspiration to determine tissue changes.
B. Preprocedural nursing care.
1. Obtain baseline vital signs.
2. Maintain NPO regime.
3. Assemble equipment, position patient, and assist the physician.
C. Postprocedural nursing care.
1. Position patient on right side over biopsy site to prevent hemorrhage.

2. Observe for complications (hemorrhage, shock).
3. Measure and record vital signs.

Laboratory Examination

A. Serum bilirubin level—abnormal amounts indicate biliary and liver disease leading to jaundice.
B. Carbohydrate metabolism—glucose tolerance levels should return to normal within one to two hours.
C. Blood ammonia—level rises in liver failure because liver converts ammonia to urea.
D. Enzyme production—elevation of enzymes reflects organ damage (SGPT, SGOT, LDH).
E. Prothrombin time—clotting ability reduced in liver cell damage.

Disorders of the Liver, Gallbladder, and Pancreas

Jaundice

Definition: Symptom of liver disorder characterized by yellow pigmentation of the skin and due to accumulation of bilirubin pigment in the blood. The degree of jaundice is best detected in the sclera of the eyes.

Indications

A. Rapid rate of red blood cell destruction (hemolytic jaundice).
B. Diseased liver cells.
C. Viral liver cell necrosis or cirrhosis of the liver.
D. Obstruction due to inflammation, tumors, or cholestatic agents.

Nursing Care

A. Relieve pruritus with starch baths, lotions, antihistamines, and mild sedatives.
B. Provide emotional support.

C. Prepare family for patient's altered skin and eye color.

D. Remove mirrors from patient's line of sight.

E. Encourage bed rest.

Viral Hepatitis

Definition: Inflammation of the liver caused by a virus.

A. Type A hepatitis (infectious hepatitis).
  1. Transmitted by excreta, infected blood transfusion, contaminated syringes and needles, contaminated food products, and possibly by way of respiratory tract.
  2. Signs and symptoms.
     a. Headache and fever.
     b. Nausea, anorexia, and vomiting.
     c. Abdominal pain with tenderness.
     d. If jaundiced, patient produces dark urine and clay-colored stools.
     e. Maculopapular rash.
  3. Nursing care.
     a. Isolate to prevent transmission of disease.
     b. Use disposable equipment.
     c. Provide high caloric, well-balanced diet.
     d. Encourage adequate rest.
     e. Stress the importance of continuing medical supervision after hospitalization.
     f. Advise patient never to be blood donor.
     g. Advise against use of alcoholic beverages.
     h. Encourage gamma globulin as preventive measure when in close contact with others.
B. Type B hepatitis (serum hepatitis, viral).
  1. Transmitted by oral or parenteral route by means of infusion, ingestion, or inhalation of the blood of an infected person; and by contaminated equipment, such as needles, syringes, and dental instruments.
  2. Signs and symptoms are similar to but more severe than infectious hepatitis.
  3. Treatment and nursing care.

     a. Encourage bed rest until symptoms have decreased in severity.
     b. Provide well-balanced diet supplemented with vitamins.
     c. Administer antacids for gastric acidity.

Hepatic Coma

Definition: Hepatic coma results from brain cell alterations due to build-up of ammonia levels.

Signs and Symptoms

A. Impaired memory, attention, concentration, and rate of mental response.

B. Confusion, inappropriate behavior, and depressed level of consciousness.

C. Untidy appearance.

D. Flapping tremor upon dorsiflexion of the hand.

E. Disorientation leading to eventual coma.

Nursing Care

A. Observe, measure, and record neurologic status daily (ability to perform simple task such as writing one's signature diminishes as the blood ammonia level increases).

B. Weigh patient daily because liver function decreases and ascites and edema increase.

C. Measure and record intake and output.

D. Administer sedatives and analgesics sparingly because failing liver unable to detoxify them.

E. Eliminate protein from the diet temporarily because the ammonia formed from the breakdown of proteins cannot be converted into urea for excretion.

Cirrhosis

Definition: Progressive disease of the liver characterized by diffuse damage (degeneration) to the cells which cannot be recovered or reversed.

Types

A. Alcoholic (nutritional).

B. Postnecrotic (e.g., precipitated by viral hepatitis).

Signs and Symptoms

A. Gastrointestinal distress, fatigue, low resistance to infection, gradual failing health.
B. Emaciation and ascites due to malnutrition.
C. Edema of lower extremities.

Nursing Care

A. Provide diet adequate in proteins and carbohydrates, low in salt, and with multivitamins.
B. Avoid administering sedatives and opiates.
C. Prevent infection by providing adequate rest and environmental control.
D. Provide good skin care and control pruritus resulting from elevated BUN.
E. Measure and record and compare vital signs to previous measurement.
F. Evaluate level of consciousness and be alert to personality changes and signs of increasing stupor.

Cholecystitis with Cholelithiasis

Definition: Inflammation of the gallbladder caused by cholelithiasis (presence of gallstones).

Signs and Symptoms

A. Pain in upper right quadrant of abdomen that is moderate to severe with passage of stones.
B. Nausea and vomiting.
C. Intolerance to fat.
D. Fever.
E. Jaundice will occur if common bile duct obstructed with stones.
F. Edema from inflammation.

Treatment and Nursing Care

A. Administer drugs for control of pain.
B. Insert nasogastric tube for suction.
C. Give nothing by mouth (low fat diet may be possible).
D. Measure and record intake and output.

E. Provide skin care.
F. Cholecystectomy is indicated if medical treatment ineffective.
G. Postoperative nursing care.
   1. Make and record routine postoperative observations.
   2. Prevent respiratory complication (diaphragmatic discomfort increased because of proximity of incision).
   3. Maintain nasogastric tube.
   ☆ 4. Maintain T-tube which provides for bile drainage from liver, allowing some of the bile to enter into the common duct. T-tube provides independent drainage.
      a. Ensure patency and avoid stress on the tube; carefully position after dressings are changed.
      b. Use measures to control infection.
      c. Note character and amount of drainage.
      d. Clamp and release regimen as initial step in preparation for T-tube removal.
   5. Prevent infection (patients are often obese and may have delayed healing).
   6. Observe for indications of biliary obstruction, such as clay-colored stool, jaundiced sclera and/or skin.
   7. Advise patient to remain on low-fat diet for at least two to three months.

Acute Pancreatitis

Definition: Inflammation of the pancreas. Cause is unknown, although alcoholic indulgence or biliary tract disease are thought to be predisposing factors.

Signs and Symptoms

A. Constant abdominal pain radiating to the back and flank.
B. Nausea and vomiting.
C. Fever.
D. Jaundice (observe stool for fat or clay color).
E. Abnormal glucose levels.

Treatment and Nursing Care

A. Give nothing by mouth.

B. Insert nasogastric tube for nausea and vomiting.

C. Provide skin care.

D. Administer analgesics, anticholinergics, antacids.

E. Monitor glucose levels with Clinitest and blood tests.

F. Maintain quiet, nonstressful environment.

G. Observe and record vital signs.

H. Weigh and record patient's weight.

I. Measure and record intake and output.

Genitourinary System

This system—the kidneys and their drainage channels—is essential for the maintenance of life. The organs of the GU system are responsible for excreting the end products of metabolism as well as regulating water and electrolyte concentrations of body fluids.

Anatomy and Physiology

Kidneys

A. Paired glandular organs located to the right and left of the midline, lateral to lower thoracic vertebrae, that have the ability to adapt to the body's changing needs for elimination of various substances.

B. Major functions.
1. Excrete most of the end products of body metabolism.
2. Maintain body acid-base and plasma electrolyte equilibrium.
3. Produce enzymes that act on plasma substance which is capable of raising blood pressure.

C. Composition.
1. Nephrons—microscopic filtering units.
2. Glomerulus—capillary clusters within nephron capsule; filtering unit of the nephron.
3. Tubule—collecting channel in nephron that converts the fluid to urine as it goes to the pelvis of the kidneys.
4. Pelvis—collecting funnel; leads into ureter.

D. Urine.
1. Composed of excess water and other soluable waste materials that are not reabsorbed into the tubules.
2. Characteristics of normal urine.
   a. Can be diluted or concentrated.
   b. Clear.
   c. Yellow-amber in color.
   d. Slightly acid.
   e. Specific gravity 1.015 to 1.025.
   f. Negative for bacteria, albumin, sugar, blood, ketones, or bilirubin.

Ureter

A. Paired tubes lined with mucosa connecting the kidneys with the bladder.

B. Conducts urine by rhythmic contractions.

Bladder

A. Round, hollow, membranous sac with muscular walls, located in the pelvis.

B. Extraperitoneal; however, peritoneum adheres to dome of bladder.

C. May hold 1000 cc in volume if outflow obstructed.

Urethra

A. Single tube which allows passage of urine from bladder to outside of body.

B. Female urethra approximately 3 to 5 cm in length.

C. Male urethra approximately 20 cm in length.

Diagnostic Procedures

A. Blood chemistry—blood urea nitrogen (BUN) analysis will indicate the ability of the kidney to excrete waste products.

B. Intravenous pyelogram (IVP)—injection of contrast dye for visualization on x-ray film of absence, presence, location, size, and configuration of each kidney, the filling of the renal pelvis, and outlines of the ureters.

C. Phenolsulfonphthalein (PSP)—a dye that tests the excretory function of the kidney.

D. Renal biopsy—needle inserted through renal tissue to extract tissue cells that are examined for evidence of malfunction; test can indicate the presence of disease, confirm a diagnosis, indicate prognosis, or give evidence of response to treatment.

E. Cystoscopy—direct visualization by cystoscope for purposes of inspection, biopsy, treatment, or removal of stones.

F. Retrograde pyelogram—insertion of cystoscope and placement of ureteral catheters followed by injection of contrast dye into the catheters for visualization on x-ray film of ureters and kidneys.

Disorders of the Kidney

Nonspecific Signs and Symptoms

A. Retention—inability to expel urine from the bladder due to obstruction or loss of innervation.

B. Incontinence—loss of voluntary control in discharge of urine.

C. Residual urine—urine remaining in bladder after voiding.

D. Anuria—suppression or failure of kidney to produce sufficient urine.

E. Oliguria—amount and frequency of urination are diminished.

F. Hematuria—blood in the urine, usually caused by infection or trauma.

Principles of Nursing Care

A. Maintain accurate measurement of intake and output.

B. Force or restrict fluids as ordered.

C. Observe and record characteristics of urine and times of voiding.

D. Record specific urinary complaints, e.g., urgency, burning, pain, frequency, bladder spasms, and inability to void (retention).

E. Strain all urine and take specimen to lab (if ordered) if renal lithiasis (stones) are suspected.

F. Maintain comfort of patient; position and provide analgesics and external heat for renal colic.

☆ Specialized Catheter Care

A. Maintain patency of catheters.

B. Types of urinary tract catheters.
   1. Foley catheter—designed with inflatable balloon which, upon inflation, anchors catheter within bladder.
   2. Three-way Foley catheter—provides for drainage of urine, balloon for anchoring, and a third channel to allow for irrigation of the bladder.
   3. Straight catheter—a simple rubber catheter that is inserted into bladder for drainage and then removed.
   4. Ureteral catheters—very small-gauge catheters inserted directly into ureters during cystoscopy for drainage of urine from the pelvis of the kidney or for injection of dye for diagnostic purposes; if left inserted, they are usually anchored with a Foley.

Acute Renal Failure

Definition: Sudden loss of kidney function caused by failure of renal circulation or tubular or glomerular damage.

Causes

A. Dehydration.

B. Shock.

C. Traumatic injury.

D. Toxic agents, e.g., sulfonamides, arsenic.

E. Infection.

Signs and Symptoms

A. Decreased urine output (volume of less than 400 to 500 ml/24 hours).

B. Hypertension may develop.

C. Nausea, vomiting, diarrhea, and convulsions leading to coma.

Treatment and Nursing Care

A. Treat cause of failure immediately.

B. Monitor body fluid volume and electrolytes.

C. Monitor urinary output (hourly basis may be indicated).

D. Weigh patient daily.

E. Follow diet restrictions: limited protein and sodium, with vitamin supplements.

F. Observe for complications of fluid overload, electrolyte disturbances, and CHF.

Chronic Renal Failure

Definition: Progressive impairment of kidney function which, without intervention, ends fatally in uremia.

Signs and Symptoms

A. Weakness, fatigue, and headaches.

B. Anorexia, nausea, and vomiting.

C. Hypertension with renal and heart failure.

D. Anemia.

E. Central nervous system signs (i.e., irritability, convulsions).

Treatment and Nursing Care

A. Monitor intake and output.

B. Weigh patient daily.

C. Provide diet low in salt and altered amounts of protein; prepare as attractively as possible.

D. Monitor blood pressure closely.

E. Provide emotional support because chronicity of disease may precipitate depression.

F. Assist with hemodialysis.

1. Procedure permits passage through a semipermeable membrane of substances, such as urea, creatinine, and uric acid, which diffuse through the pores of the membrane in the machine.

   a. The blood, which contains the waste products, flows from the patient into the dialysis machine where it comes into contact with the dialysate.

   b. The waste products are removed through contact of the blood as it flows into the machine and comes in contact with the dialysate.

2. In essence, the dialysis machine becomes the patient's "kidney."

G. Peritoneal dialysis.

1. A method of separating substances by interposing a semipermeable membrane. The peritoneum is used as the dialyzing membrane and substitutes for kidney function during failure.

2. Procedure allows for infusion of dialysate through a peritoneal catheter for "dwell time" in order that waste products in the blood may diffuse into the solution.

3. The dialysate is in direct contact with blood supply of mesentery.

4. After "dwell time" fluid is drained by gravity into receptacles, and sample is sent to laboratory for testing. The volume returned by gravity should equal or be in excess of the volume of the infusion.

Pyelonephritis

Definition: An acute or chronic infection and inflammation of one or both kidneys that usually begins in the renal pelvis.

Signs and Symptoms

A. Attacks of chills and fever, with malaise.

B. Tenderness and dull, aching pain in the back.

C. Frequency and burning with urination.

Treatment and Nursing Care

A. Record characteristics, frequency, and amount of voiding.

B. Provide diet high in calories and vitamin supplements and low in protein.

C. Give sufficient liquids to maintain urine volume of 1500 cc/24 hrs.

D. Observe for edema and signs of renal failure.

E. Teach principles of optimum personal hygiene to prevent further infections.

Acute Glomerulonephritis

Definition: Inflammatory disease of both kidneys that interferes with glomerular filtration; most commonly caused by repeated streptococcal infections in childhood.

Signs and Symptoms

A. Headache, malaise, and weakness.
B. Oliguria and puffiness around the eyes.
C. Hematuria.
D. Moderate to marked hypertension.
E. Tenderness at costovertebral angle is common.
F. Diagnostic urinalysis indicates erythrocyte casts.

Treatment and Nursing Care

A. Administer antibiotics and antihypertensives.
B. Encourage bed rest.
C. Provide diet low in protein, low in sodium, high in carbohydrates, and high in vitamins.
D. Restrict fluids based on previous day's output.
E. Do not permit increase of activity until blood pressure and BUN are normal for one to two weeks.
F. Record intake and output.
G. Weigh patient daily.
H. Observe for signs of overhydration, hypertension, and renal failure.

Kidney Surgery

Nephrectomy

Definition: Surgical removal of a kidney.

Indications

A. Severe injury producing irreparable damage to cells.
B. Chronic disease.
C. Permanent loss of kidney function.
D. Renal donor.

Nursing Care

A. Measure and record intake and output.
B. Encourage patient to take fluids.
C. Observe for signs of hemorrhage and shock.
D. Provide care for incision and Penrose drain.

E. Encourage postoperative exercises and early ambulation.
F. Control environment against infection from visitors and personnel.

Nephrostomy

Definition: Creation of surgical opening into kidney and placement of a catheter in the renal pelvis for urinary drainage.

Nursing Care

A. Record characteristics of drainage and urine.
B. Check for bleeding at surgical site as this is major complication.
C. Unless ordered, do not clamp catheter.
D. Unless ordered, do not irrigate (never irrigate with force; use only 5 to 10 cc of sterile solution; be especially careful not to contaminate).
E. In bilateral nephrostomy, maintain separate outputs.
F. Maintain patency of tubes when positioning patient and when changing dressings.

Urolithotomy

Definition: Removal of stones (calculi) formed in the urinary system (urolithiasis).

Types

A. Ureterolithotomy—removal of calculi from ureter which may be accomplished with use of cystoscope and stone crusher.
B. Pyelolithotomy—removal of stone from kidney pelvis.

Nursing Care

A. Force fluids.
B. Strain all urine.
C. Measure and record intake and output.
D. Observe and record characteristics of urine and time of voiding.
E. Prevent infection.
F. Observe for perforation of bladder, abdominal rigidity, anuria, chills, fever, and urine retention.

Bladder Disorders and Surgery

Cystitis

Definition: Inflammation of the bladder from infection or from obstruction of the urethra.

Signs and Symptoms

A. Frequency and urgency of urination.
B. Burning sensation in urethra during urination.
C. Suprapubic discomfort.
D. Dark and odorous urine.
E. Urinalysis reveals presence of bacteria and blood cells.

Treatment and Nursing Care

A. Attempt to remove cause of the infection.
B. Administer antibiotic therapy.
C. Collect uncontaminated urine specimen (catheterized or mid-stream).
D. Maintain adequate fluid intake.
E. Decrease patient's activity during the acute stage.
F. Teach principles of optimum personal hygiene to prevent recurrent infection.

Suprapubic Cystostomy

Definition: Creation of surgical opening and placement of catheter into bladder for urinary drainage.

Nursing Care

A. Change dressings frequently, and give skin care (avoid reinforcing and creating bulky, wet, odorous dressings that cause excoriation to the skin).
B. Maintain patency of catheter when applying dressing or positioning patient.
C. Provide clamp and release regimen until patient can void voluntarily.

Cystectomy

Definition: Removal of bladder (due to presence of tumors) with diversion of ureters into "bladder" constructed from loop of ileum which is brought through abdominal wall as an ileostomy opening.

Nursing Care

A. Provide routine postoperative care.
B. Maintain nasogastric tube.
C. Care for stoma with ileostomy procedure.
D. Measure and record intake and output.
E. Observe for development of fistula or dehiscence.
F. Refer patient to enterostomy therapist and a visiting nurse association.

Prostatectomy

Definition: Removal of prostate gland.

Indications

A. Enlargement of prostate (benign prostatic hypertrophy) which interferes with free urinary bladder flow.
B. Malignancy of prostate gland.

Symptoms of Enlargement

A. Recurring infection.
B. Urine stasis.
C. Nocturia.
D. Frequency.
E. Dysuria.
F. Straining to void.

Types of Prostatectomy

A. Transurethral resection (TUR).
  1. Insertion of a resectoscope into bladder through the urethra.
  2. The prostate is "shelled out in pieces," which are then irrigated from the bladder.
B. Suprapubic prostatectomy.
  1. Abdominal surgical incision for entering urinary bladder.
  2. The prostate gland is enucleated.

Postoperative Nursing Care

A. Maintain adequate bladder drainage via catheter.
   1. Suprapubic catheter used following suprapubic prostatectomy.
   ☆ 2. Continuous bladder irrigation (or triple lumen catheter) is used following transurethral resection.
      a. One lumen is used for inflating bag (usually 30 cc. bag), one for outflow of urine, and one for irrigating solution instillation.
      b. Run solution in rapidly if bright red drainage or clots are present; when drainage clears, decrease to about 40 drops/minute.
      c. If clots cannot be rinsed out with irrigating solution, irrigate with syringe as ordered.
B. Provide fluids to prevent dehydration (2 to 3 liters every twenty-four hours).
C. Provide high protein, high vitamin diet.
D. Observe for signs of hemorrhage and shock.

E. Traction is applied to Foley catheter (if not connected to three-way drainage) to help in hemostasis.
   1. Catheter is pulled on and taped to leg.
   2. Do not release traction without order (traction released after bright red drainage has diminished).
F. Instruct patient in perineal exercises to regain urinary control.
   1. Tense perineal muscles by pressing buttocks together; hold for as long as possible.
   2. Repeat this process ten times every hour.
G. Ambulate early (after urine has returned to nearly normal color).
H. Observe for complications.
   1. Epididymitis (most frequent).
   2. Gram negative sepsis.
I. Administer urinary antiseptics or antibiotics as ordered to prevent infection.
J. Provide wound care for suprapubic and retropubic prostatectomies (similar to that for abdominal surgery).
K. Provide sitz bath and heat lamp treatments to promote healing.

Endocrine System

The endocrine system is one of the integrative body systems that regulates body functions. It is made up of a series of glands which function individually or conjointly to integrate and control innumerable metabolic activities of the body. These glands automatically regulate various body processes by releasing chemical signals called hormones.

Anatomy and Physiology

Endocrine Glands

A. Secrete hormones directly into the bloodstream.

B. Located in various parts of the body.

C. Each gland has a specific function; actions of glands are also interrelated, influencing one another.

    1. Tropic hormones.

        a. Secreted by anterior lobe of pituitary gland.

        b. Influence several other glands' secretion of hormones.

    2. Target glands—those glands affected by tropic hormones.

        a. Thyroid.

        b. Adrenal cortex.

        c. Gonads.

D. Also called *ductless glands* since they secrete directly into the bloodstream.

E. See Appendix 1 for a tabulation of gland function, hormones, and glandular disorders.

Hormones

A. Secreted in minute amounts but exert powerful influence on the body.

    1. Growth and development.

    2. Metabolism.

    3. Reproduction.

    4. Development of personality.

B. Influence is integrative and regulating; they control rate, but do not initiate cellular processes.

C. Effect of hormone on the body may occur in area far removed from secreting gland.

Endocrine System Assessment

A. Assess for growth imbalance.

    1. Excessive growth.

        a. Pituitary or hypothalamic disorders.

        b. Excess adrenal, ovarian, or testicular hormone.

    2. Retarded growth.

        a. Endocrine and metabolic disorders; difficult to distinguish from dwarfism.

        b. Hypothyroidism.

B. Evaluate obesity.

    1. Sudden onset suggests hypothalamic lesion (rare).

    2. Cushing's syndrome (with characteristic buffalo hump).

C. Assess abnormal skin pigmentation.

    1. Hyperpigmentation may coexist with depigmentation in Addison's disease.

    2. Thyrotoxicosis may be associated with spotty brown pigmentation.

    3. Pruritus is a common symptom in diabetes.

D. Check for hirsutism.

    1. Normal variations in body occur on nonendocrine basis.

    2. First sign of neoplastic disease.

    3. Indicates changes in adrenal status.

E. Evaluate appetite changes.

    1. Polyphagia is a common sign of uncontrolled diabetes.

    2. Indicates thyrotoxicosis.

    3. Nausea and weight loss may indicate addisonian crisis or diabetic acidosis.

F. Check for polyuria and polydipsia.

    1. Symptoms usually of nonendocrine etiology.

    2. If sudden onset, suggest diabetes mellitus or insipidus.

    3. May be present with hyperparathyroidism or hyperaldosteronism.

G. Assess mental changes.

    1. Though often subtle, may be indicative of underlying endocrine disorder.

        a. Nervousness and excitability may in-

dicate hyperthyroidism.
  b. Mental confusion may indicate hypopituitarism, Addison's disease, or myxedema.
  2. Mental deterioration is observed in untreated hypoparathyroidism and hypothyroidism.
H. Assess for coma state.
  1. Drowsiness.
  2. Hypernea.
  3. Tachycardia.
  4. Subnormal temperature.
  5. Fruity odor to breath.
  6. Acetone in urine (test done if over 2+ sugar in urine).
  7. Stupor leading to coma.

Diagnostic Procedures

Radioactive Iodine (RAI) Uptake (Radioiodine ^{131}I)

A. Purpose: measures the absorption of the iodine isotope to determine how the thyroid gland is functioning.
B. Drug given by mouth or IV.
C. Results.
  1. Normal values: 5 to 35 percent in 24 hours (recently lowered values in United States due to increased ingestion of iodine).
  2. Elevated values indicate: hyperthyroidism, thyrotoxicosis, hypofunctioning goiter, iodine lack, excessive hormonal losses.
  3. Depressed values indicate: low T_4, antithyroid drugs, thyroiditis, myxedema, or hypothyroidism.

T_3 and T_4 Resin Uptake Tests

A. Purpose: both of these are used as screening tests for diagnosis in thyroid disorders. T_4 is 90 percent accurate in diagnosing hyperthyroidism and hypothyroidism.
B. Results.
  1. Normal values.
    a. T_4: 3.8 to 11.4%.
    b. T_3: 25 to 35%.
  2. T_4.
    a. Elevated: hyperthyroidism, early hep-

atitis, exogenous T_4.
    b. Decreased: hypothyroidism, abnormal binding, exogenous T_3.
  3. T_3.
    a. Elevated: hyperthyroidism, T_3 toxicosis.
    b. Decreased: advancing age.

Disorders of the Pituitary Gland

Acromegaly

Definition: Overproduction of growth-stimulating hormone by the anterior lobe, occurring in adulthood after closure of the epiphyses of the long bones.

Signs and Symptoms

A. Excessive growth of short, flat bones.
  1. Large hands and feet.
  2. Thickening and protrusion of the jaw and orbital ridges.
  3. Coarse facial features.
  4. Pain in joints.
B. Increased diaphoresis.
C. Oily, rough skin.
D. Increased hair growth over the body.
E. Menstrual disturbances; impotence.
F. Symptoms associated with local compression of brain by tumor.
  1. Headache.
  2. Visual disturbances; blindness.
G. Related hormonal imbalances may develop.
  1. Diabetes mellitus.
  2. Cushing's syndrome.
H. Increased growth-stimulating hormone level as indicated by laboratory tests.

Treatment and Nursing Care

A. Provide emotional support.
  1. Encourage expression of patient's feelings.
  2. Avoid situations which may be embarrassing to the patient.
  3. Encourage family to give support to and and to communicate with the patient.

B. Give frequent skin care.

C. Provide proper positioning and support for painful joints.

D. Test urine for sugar and acetone.

E. Be aware of possible needed treatment.

1. Irradiation of the tumor.

2. Hypophysectomy.

3. Lifelong replacement of hormones as a result of above treatments.

Hypophysectomy

Definition: Excision of the pituitary gland.

A. General preoperative care.

1. Emotional support.

2. Explanation of procedure to be performed.

B. General postoperative care.

1. Signs of related hormonal disturbances and deficiencies.

   a. Adrenal insufficiency.

   b. Hypothyroidism and acute thyroid crisis.

   c. Diabetes insipidus.

   d. Severe hypoglycemia.

2. Education.

   a. Importance of continual medical supervision.

   b. Safe self-administration of replacement hormones.

      (1) Cortisone.

      (2) Thyroid.

      (3) Sex hormones.

      (4) Vasopressin tannate.

   c. Avoidance of over-the-counter drugs.

   d. Measures to prevent infections; prompt reporting to physician if infections appear.

   e. Recognition of stress and avoidance of stress-producing situations.

   f. Importance of medic-alert band and carrying emergency medications.

   g. Avoidance of forceful blowing of nose and of coughing.

3. Need for emotional support and involvement of family in ongoing care.

Gigantism

Definition: Overproduction of growth-stimulating hormone by the anterior lobe, occurring in childhood prior to closure of the epiphyses of the long bones.

Signs and Symptoms

A. Symmetrical overgrowth of the long bones.

B. Increased height in early adulthood of eight to nine feet.

C. Deterioration of mental and physical processes, which may occur in early adulthood.

Treatment

A. Irradiation of pituitary.

B. Hypophysectomy.

Dwarfism

Definition: Underproduction of growth-stimulating hormone by the anterior lobe.

Signs and Symptoms

A. Severe retardation of physical growth.

B. Premature body-aging processes.

Treatment

A. Human growth-stimulating hormone injections (HGH).

B. Given if the imbalance is diagnosed and treated in early stage.

Diabetes Insipidus

Definition: Antidiuretic hormone (ADH) deficiency resulting from damage or tumors occurring in the posterior lobe of the pituitary gland.

Signs and Symptoms

A. Severe polyuria.

B. Severe polydipsia.

C. Dehydration.

D. Weight loss; muscle weakness.

E. Laboratory values—low urinary specific gravity (1.001 to 1.005).

Treatment and Nursing Care

A. Administer vasopressin tannate (Pitressin Tannate) IM or nasal spray.

B. Administer benzothiadiazide diuretics for mild cases.

C. Be aware that hypophysectomy may be required if tumor is present.

D. Provide adequate fluids; avoid fluids with diuretic-type actions.

E. Measure intake, output, and weight.

F. Advise patient of importance of wearing medic-alert band.

Disorders of the Adrenal Gland

Addison's Disease

Definition: Hypofunction of adrenal cortex of adrenal gland, resulting in deficiency of steroid hormones (glucocorticoids, mineralocorticoids, and androgens).

Signs and Symptoms

A. Slow and insidious onset: eventually fatal if untreated.

B. Lassitude, lethargy, and generalized weakness.

C. Gastrointestinal disturbances, e.g., nausea, diarrhea, and anorexia.

D. Hypotension.

E. Increased pigmentation of the skin.

F. Emotional disturbances.

G. Weight loss.

H. Elevated serum potassium, decreased serum sodium, elevated BUN levels, and low blood sugar.

Treatment and Nursing Care

A. Be aware that lifelong replacement therapy with synthetic corticosteroid drugs will be required.

B. Provide emotional support.

C. Weigh patient daily; monitor vital signs qid.

D. Observe for side effects of replacement hormones.

   1. Cortisone and hydrocortisone side effects.

      a. Sodium and water retention.

      b. Potassium depletion.

      c. Drug-induced Cushing's syndrome.

      d. Gastric irritation (give medication with meal or antacid).

      e. Mood swings.

      f. Local abscess at injection site when given IM (inject deeply into gluteal muscle).

      g. Addison's crisis, which might be produced by sudden withdrawal of medication.

   2. Fludrocortisone acetate side effects—the same as for cortisone and hydrocortisone, particularly sodium retention and potassium depletion.

   3. Deoxycorticosterone acetate side effects—sodium retention and potassium depletion.

E. Protect patient from exposure to infection and from stress.

F. Provide high carbohydrate, high protein diet in frequent small feedings.

G. Maintain strict intake and output records.

Addisonian Crisis

Definition: Condition caused by adrenal insufficiency, which may be precipitated by infection, trauma, stress, surgery, or diaphoresis with excessive salt loss.

Signs and Symptoms

A. Severe headache; abdominal, leg, and lower back pain.

B. Extreme, generalized muscular weakness.

C. Severe hypotension and shock.

D. Irritability and confusion.

E. Death from shock, vascular collapse, or hyperkalemia.

Treatment and Nursing Care

A. Monitor IV fluid replacement to restore fluid and electrolyte balance.

B. Steroid replacement.

C. Monitor vital signs and intake and output continually and closely until crisis passes.

D. Take measures to protect patient from infection.

E. Do not allow patient to do anything for self and encourage remaining as quiet as possible; perform no unnecessary nursing procedures.

Cushing's Syndrome

Definition: Disease produced by hyperfunction of the adrenal cortices of the adrenal glands, resulting in hypersecretion of the glucocorticoid steroid hormones.

Signs and Symptoms

A. Abnormal adipose tissue distribution.
1. Moon-like fullness of face.
2. Buffalo hump (fatty swellings on body).
3. Obese trunk with thin extremities.

B. Reddish purple striae of skin stretched with fat tissue.

C. Fragile skin; easily bruised.

D. Osteoporosis; susceptible to fractures.

E. Hyperglycemia; may eventually develop diabetes mellitus.

F. Mood swings from euphoria to depression.

G. High susceptibility to infections; diminished immuno-response to infections once they occur.

H. Lassitude and muscular weakness.

I. Masculine characteristics in females.

J. Potassium depletion.

K. Sodium and water retention.

L. Elevated blood sugar and glycosuria.

M. Elevated white blood count with depressed eosinophils and lymphocytes.

N. Elevated plasma cortisone levels.

O. Elevated 17-hydroxycorticosteroids in urine.

Treatment and Nursing Care

A. Take measures to protect from infections.

B. Protect patient from accidents or falls.

C. Give meticulous skin care, avoiding harsh soaps.

D. Provide low caloric, high protein, high potassium diet.

E. Provide emotional support.
1. Encourage ventilation of patient's feelings.
2. Avoid reacting to patient's appearance.
3. Anticipate the needs of the patient.
4. Explain to patient that changes in body appearance and emotional lability should improve with treatment.

F. Measure intake and output; test for urinary sugar; weigh daily.

G. Provide specialized care if adrenalectomy is necessary.
1. General preoperative care.
2. Postoperative care.
   a. Frequent monitoring of vital signs and intake and output.
   b. Careful administration of parenteral fluids and medications as ordered.
   c. Strict adherence to sterile techniques when changing dressings.
   d. Observation for shock, hypoglycemia.

H. Be aware that chemotherapy may be administered for inoperable, cancerous tumors.

Disorders of the Thyroid Gland

Myxedema

Definition: Adult form of decreased synthesis of thyroid hormone resulting in a hypothyroid state.

Signs and Symptoms

A. Occurs primarily in older age group, five times more frequent in women than in men.

B. Slowed rate of body metabolism.
1. Lethargy, apathy, and fatigue.
2. Intolerance to cold.
3. Hypersensitivity to sedatives and barbiturates.
4. Weight gain.
5. Cool, dry, rough skin.
6. Coarse, dry hair.

C. Personality changes.
1. Forgetfulness and loss of memory.
2. Complacency.

D. Anorexia, constipation, and fecal impactions.

E. Interstitial edema.
1. Nonpitting edema in the lower extremity.
2. Generalized puffiness.

F. Decreased diaphoresis.

G. Menstrual disturbances.

H. Cardiac complications.
1. Coronary heart disease.
2. Angina pectoris.
3. Myocardial infarction and congestive heart failure.

I. Anemia.

J. Below normal test results.
1. PBI.
2. ^{131}I.
3. T_3 and T_4.

K. Elevated serum cholesterol level.

Treatment and Nursing Care

A. Administer thyroid replacement (initial small dosage, increased gradually).

B. Individualize maintenance dosage.
1. Desiccative thyroid.
2. Sodium levothyroxine (Synthroid Sodium).
3. Triiodothyronine (Cytomel).

C. Observe for symptoms of overdosage in thyroid preparations.

1. Myocardial infarction, angina, and cardiac failure, particularly in patients with cardiac problems.
2. Restlessness and insomnia.
3. Headache and confusion.

D. Provide time for patient to complete activities.

E. Provide warm environment with extra blankets and other modes of warming.

F. Give meticulous skin care.

G. Orient patient as to date, time, and place.

H. Take measures to prevent constipation.

I. Administer sedatives or narcotics as ordered by physician. (Usually one-half to one-third normal dosage is ordered.)

Hyperthyroidism (Thyrotoxicosis)

Definition: A result of increased synthesis of thyroid hormone often accompanied by exophthalmic goiter (Grave's disease).

Signs and Symptoms

A. Occurs four times more frequently in women than in men; usually occurs between twenty to forty years of age.

B. Increased rate of body metabolism.
1. Weight loss despite ravenous appetite and ingestion of large quantities of food.
2. Intolerance to heat.
3. Nervousness, jitters, and fine tremor of hands.
4. Smooth, soft skin and hair.
5. Tachycardia and palpitation.
6. Diarrhea.

C. Personality changes.
1. Irritability and agitation.
2. Exaggerated emotional reactions.
3. Mood swings from euphoria to depression.

D. Enlargement of the thyroid gland (goiter).

E. Exophthalmos.
1. Fluid collects around eye sockets, causing eyeballs to protrude.
2. Condition not always in evidence.
3. Usually does not improve with treatment.

F. Cardiac complications common.

G. Above normal test results.

   1. PBI.

   2. ^{131}I.

   3. T_3 and T_4.

H. Relatively low serum cholesterol.

Treatment and Nursing Care

A. Administer drugs if ordered by physician.

   1. Antithyroid drugs.

      a. Most common are propylthiouracil and methimazole (Tapazole).

      b. Possible side effect of agranulocytosis.

   2. Iodine preparations.

      a. Saturated solution of potassium iodide (SSKI).

      b. Lugol's Solution.

   3. Radioiodine therapy.

      a. Useful for patients who are poor surgical risks.

      b. Uptake of ^{131}I by thyroid gland results in destruction of thyroid cells.

      c. Mxyedema may occur as complication.

B. Provide for adequate rest.

   1. Bed rest.

   2. Calming diversionary activities.

C. Provide cool, quiet, stable environment.

D. Maintain diet high in calories, protein, and vitamins; no stimulants.

E. Weigh daily.

F. Provide emotional support to patient.

   1. Be aware that exaggerated emotional responses are a manifestation of hormone imbalance.

   2. Be sensitive to patient's needs.

   3. Avoid stress-producing situations.

G. Adhere to regular schedule of activities.

H. Provide specialized care if thyroidectomy (subtotal or total removal of thyroid gland) is required.

   1. Ensure that patient is in required preoperative state.

      a. Return of thyroid function tests to normal.

      b. Adequate nutritional status.

      c. Marked decrease in signs of thyrotoxicosis.

      d. Absence of cardiac problems.

   2. Provide postoperative care.

      a. Monitor vital signs carefully.

      b. Observe closely for signs of complications.

         (1) Hemorrhage.

         (2) Respiratory distress.

         (3) Laryngeal nerve injury.

         (4) Tetany and hypocalcemia.

         (5) Thyroid "storm."

      c. Have tracheostomy tray suction equipment, and oxygen equipment at bedside.

      d. Raise bed to semi-Fowler's position; avoid strain to suture line.

      e. Encourage head and neck range-of-motion exercises when ordered.

Thyroid "Storm"/Thyroid Crisis

Definition: Acute, potentially fatal hyperthyroid condition which may occur as a result of surgery, inadequate preparation for surgery, severe infection, or from stress.

Signs and Symptoms

A. High fever (may rise to 106°F) and dehydration.

B. Tachycardia.

C. Irritability and restlessness leading to delirium and coma.

Treatment and Nursing Care

A. Administer drugs and take special measures as ordered.

   1. Hypothermic measures.

   2. Hydration.

   3. Antithyroid drugs and iodine preparations.

   4. Adrenergic and catecholamine blocking agents.

   5. Corticosteroids.

B. Monitor vital signs, intake and output.

C. Take safety measures if agitated or comatose.

D. Provide calm, quiet environment.

E. Protect from infection.

Disorders of the Parathyroid Glands

Hypoparathyroidism

Definition: Condition caused by acute or chronic and deficient hormone production by the parathyroid gland.

Signs and Symptoms

A. Acute hypocalcemia.
1. Numbness, tingling, and cramping of extremities.
2. Acute, potentially fatal tetany.
   a. Painful muscular spasms.
   b. Seizures.
   c. Irritability.
   d. Positive Chvostek's sign.
   e. Positive Trousseau's sign.
   f. Laryngospasm.
   g. Cardiac arrhythmias.
B. Chronic hypocalcemia.
1. Poor development of tooth enamel.
2. Mental retardation.
3. Muscular weakness with numbness and tingling of extremities.
4. Loss of hair and coarse, dry skin.
5. Personality changes.
6. Cataracts.
7. Cardiac arrhythmias.
8. Renal stones.
C. Laboratory values.
1. Low serum calcium levels.
2. Increased serum phosphorus level.
3. Low urinary calcium and phosphorus output.
4. Increased bone density on x-ray examination.

Treatment and Nursing Care

A. General care.
1. Frequently check for increasing hoarseness.
2. Observe for irregularities in urine.
3. Force fluids as ordered.
B. Acute care.
1. Prepare for administration of IV calcium gluconate solution.
2. Administer anticonvulsants and sedatives.
3. Prepare for tracheostomy if laryngospasm has caused obstruction.
C. Chronic care.
1. Administer oral calcium salts and vitamin D preparations.
2. Provide high calcium, low phosphorus diet.

Hyperparathyroidism

Definition: Abnormal, excessive hormone production by the parathyroid gland.

Signs and Symptoms

A. Bone demineralization with deformities, pain, high susceptibility to fractures.
B. Hypercalcemia.
1. Calcium deposits in various body organs such as eyes, heart, lungs, and kidneys (stones).
2. Gastric ulcers.
3. Personality changes, depression, and paranoia.
4. Nausea, vomiting, anorexia, and constipation.
5. Polydipsia and polyuria.

Treatment and Nursing Care

A. Be aware that subtotal surgical resection of parathyroid glands may be necessary.
B. Administer additional oral calcium as ordered, for bone rebuilding processes may be required for several months.
C. Force fluids (include juices to make urine more acidic).

D. Take safety measures to prevent accidents and injury.
E. Provide a diet high in phosphorus.
F. Measure intake and output.
G. Observe urine closely for stones.
H. Observe for digitalis toxicity if patient is taking digitalis.

Disorders of the Pancreas

Diabetes Mellitus (Type I, Type II)

Definition: A group of disorders that have a variety of genetic causes, but have glucose intolerance as a common thread. Condition is caused by absence or lack of insulin or inability of cells to use insulin effectively.

Characteristics

A. Classifications.
   1. Type I—insulin dependent diabetes mellitus (IDDM).
   2. Type II—noninsulin dependent diabetes mellitus (NIDDM).
   3. Gestational (GDM)—increased blood glucose levels during pregnancy.
   4. Impaired glucose tolerance (IGT). Plasma glucose levels vacillate between normal or increased (formerly latent, borderline, and subclinical diabetes).
B. Distinguishing features of Type I and Type II diabetes.
C. Risk factors.
   1. Patient history—hereditary predisposition.
   2. Weight—presence of obesity.
   3. High stress levels.
D. Results of laboratory values.
   1. Elevated fasting blood sugar; postprandial blood sugar; glucose tolerance test or tolbutamide (Orinase) tests.
   2. Clinitest and Testape.
      a. Indicate presence of sugar in urine, i.e., 1+ to 4+.
      b. Clinitest: 2-drop and 5-drop method: from no sugar (blue) to 4+ or 2 percent (orange-rust).
      c. Values of the two tests are not interchangeable.
   3. Acetest and Ketostix—may be positive for presence of acetone in urine.
   4. Elevated cholesterol and triglyceride levels.
   5. Capillary blood glucose (finger stick).
   6. Glycosylated hemoglobin test.
      a. Abnormally high in diabetics with chronic hyperglycemia.
      b. Values.
         (1) Normal 3.5-6.2%.
         (2) Good control less than 7.5%.
         (3) Fair control 7.6-8.9%.
         (4) Poor control more than 9.0%.

Signs and Symptoms

A. Early symptoms.
   1. Common to both Type I and Type II.
      a. Polyuria.
      b. Polydipsia.
      c. Polyphagia.
      d. Blurred vision.
      e. Fatigue.
      f. Abnormal sensations (prickling, burning).
      g. Infections (vaginitis).
   2. Type I.
      a. Anorexia.
      b. Nausea, vomiting.
      c. Weight loss.
   3. Type II.
      a. Obese.
      b. Slow wound healing.

Complications

A. Ketoacidosis.
   1. Onset.
      a. Acute or over several days.
      b. Result of stress, infection, surgery, or lack of effective insulin.
      c. Overeating may contribute to but does

not cause onset.

d. Life-threatening situation.

2. Hyperglycemia, glucosuria, ketosis, ketonuria, and low CO_2 combining power.

3. Polyuria, polydipsia, and dehydration.

4. Nausea, vomiting, and anorexia.

5. Flushed, warm skin.

6. Blurred vision.

7. Acetone odor (sweet) on breath.

8. Kussmaul respirations (rapid, deep).

9. Cardiac failure and coma.

B. Infections.

C. Vascular disease.

1. Microangiopathy—affects basement membrane of almost all small blood vessels throughout body.

a. Retinopathy.

b. Nephropathy.

2. Large vessel.

a. Coronary heart disease.

b. Atherosclerosis, arteriosclerosis.

D. Neuropathy.

E. Cataracts.

Treatment

A. Diet.

1. The cornerstone of management, interdependent with medication and exercise.

2. Attainment of normal weight may clear symptoms.

3. Total calories are individualized.

4. ADA exchange diet.

a. Seven exchange lists.

b. Prescribed as to total calories and number of exchanges from each group.

c. Calories divided into:

(1) 50% CHO.

(2) 30% Fat.

(3) 20% Protein.

B. Medications.

1. Insulin.

a. Types.

(1) Short acting.

(a) Regular.

(b) Semilente.

(c) Humulin.

(2) Intermediate acting.

(a) NPH.

(b) Lente.

(c) Humulin.

(3) Long acting.

(a) PZI.

(b) Ultralente.

(4) Available in U-100.

b. Insulin pumps deliver low-dose insulin at a continuous rate.

2. Oral hypoglycemic drugs.

a. Sulfonylureas.

(1) Thought to stimulate beta cells to increase insulin release.

(2) Tolbutamide (Orinase), short acting.

(3) Chlorpropamide (Diabinese), long acting.

(4) Acetohexamide (Dymelor), intermediate acting.

(5) Tolazamide (Tolinase), intermediate acting.

b. Second generation sulfonylureas.

(1) Glyburide, intermediate acting.

(2) Glipizide, short acting.

C. Exercise.

1. Decreases body's need for insulin.

2. Regular, ongoing activities important.

3. Administer 10 gm CHO before exercise.

Nursing Care

A. Give meticulous skin care, particularly of lower extremities.

B. Take measures to protect patient from infection, injury, stress.

C. Observe for signs of insulin reaction and ketoacidosis.

D. Take second voided specimen for accurate sugar and acetone urine test.

E. Measure intake and output.

F. Provide emotional support.
   1. Encourage patient to verbalize feelings.
      a. Necessity for changes in life style, diet, and activities.
      b. Possible change in self-image and self-esteem.
      c. Fear of future and complications.
   2. Encourage involvement of family.

G. Educate patient in effective self-management.
   1. Determine patient's current status.
      a. Level of knowledge.
      b. Cultural, socioeconomic, and family influences.
      c. Daily dietary and activity patterns.
      d. Emotional and physical status and effect on current ability to learn.
   2. Inform patient about insulin and insulin injections.
      a. Keep insulin at room temperature; refrigerate extra supply of insulin.
      b. Rotate insulin bottle gently prior to drawing up insulin.
      c. Use sterile injection techniques.
      d. Rotate injection sites.
      e. Watch for signs of under- and over-dosage.
   3. Advise patient about oral medications.
      a. Take medications regularly.
      b. Watch for hypoglycemic reactions occurring with sulfonylureas.
      c. Be aware that alcohol ingestion in conjunction with sulfonylureas produces Antabuse effects.
   4. Advise patient to take all possible measures to prevent infection and injury.
      a. Report infection or injury promptly to physician.
      b. Maintain meticulous skin care.
      c. Maintain proper foot care.
      d. Be aware that insulin requirements may need to be increased when suffering from infections.
      e. Be prepared for impairment of healing process.
      f. Avoid tight-fitting garments and shoes.
      g. Avoid "bathroom surgery" for corns and callouses.
   5. Stress the importance of diet.
      a. No variation in meal times.
      b. Importance of patient's individual dietary goals.
      c. Incorporation of diet into life style, cultural and socioeconomic food patterns, and daily activities.
      d. Need for increase of intake when vigorously exercising.
   6. Stress the importance of exercise.
      a. Regularity and amount of exercise important.
      b. Sporadic, vigorous activities should be avoided.
      c. With careful planning, participation in most activities and sports is possible.
      d. Increased or decreased food intake might be required according to anticipated level of activity.
   7. Advise patient to wear medic-alert band or carry other identification regarding diabetic status.
   8. Advise patient to carry a form of concentrated sugar at all times.

Functional Hyperinsulinism (Hypoglycemia)

Definition: Condition that is the result of excess secretion of insulin by the beta cells of the pancreas gland.

Signs and Symptoms

A. Personality changes.
   1. Tenseness.
   2. Nervousness.
   3. Irritability.
   4. Anxiousness.
   5. Depression.
B. Excessive diaphoresis.
C. Excessive hunger.
D. Muscle weakness and tachycardia.
E. May be associated with "dumping syndrome" following gastrectomy.

F. May occur prior to development of diabetes mellitus.

G. Laboratory values—low blood sugar during hypoglycemic episodes.

Treatment and Nursing Care

A. Provide high protein, low carbohydrate diet.

B. Take measures to reduce anxiety and tenseness; may be attained through counseling.

Ketoacidosis

Definition: The two major metabolic problems that are the source of this condition are hyperglycemia and ketoacidemia, both due to insulin lack associated with hyperglucagonemia.

Signs and Symptoms

A. Ketoacidotic coma is usually preceded by a few days of polyuria and polydipsia with associated symptoms.
  1. Fatigue.
  2. Nausea and vomiting.
  3. Mental stupor.

B. Physical assessment indicates dehydration, rapid breathing, and fruity odor of acetone to breath.

Nursing Care

A. Maintain fluid and electrolyte balance.
  1. Normal saline IV until blood sugar reaches 250–300 mg; then a dextrose solution is started.
  2. Potassium added to IV after renal function is evaluated and hydration is adequate.

B. Provide insulin management.
  1. Give ½ dose IV and ½ dose sub q.
  2. Give with small amounts of albumin as insulin adheres to IV tubing.
  3. Hourly dosage depends on S & A and blood sugar levels.

C. Provide patent airway and adequate circulation to brain.

D. Obtain hourly sugar and acetone urine tests.

E. Test blood sugar level q 1–2 hours. Keep sugar and acetone at 1+.

F. Maintain personal hygiene.

G. Protect from injury if comatose.

Table 1. Insulin Treatment

Category	Types	Onset	Peak	Duration	Time and Symptoms of Untoward Reaction
Rapid acting	Regular	30-60 min.	2-3 hours	5-10 hours	15 minutes to 4-5 hours: hunger, trembling, visual disturbance, cold perspiration, weakness, coma
	Semilente	30-60 min.	5-7 hours	12-16 hours	
	Humulin R	30-60 min.	2-3 hours	5-7 hours	
Intermediate acting	NPH	1-1½ hours	8-12 hours	24 hours	4-6 hours: majority of attacks occur in early morning or evening—extreme fatigue may be only symptom
	Lente	1-2 hours	7-15 hours	24 hours	
	Humulin N	1½-3½ hours	8-12 hours	18-24 hours	
Slow acting	Protamine Zinc (PZI)	4-8 hours	10-20 hours	36 hours	12-24 hours: usually early morning, gradual onset, sleeplessness, nausea, headache, mental confusion
	Ultralente	4-8 hours	10-20 hours	36 hours	

*Times of onset, peak, and duration vary depending on manufacturer of insulin and client response. Check package inserts.

Table 2. Complications Associated With Diabetes

Clinical Manifestations	Hypoglycemia	Diabetic Ketoacidosis (DKA)	Hyperglycemic Hypersmolar Nonketotic Coma (HHNK)
	Type I	**Type I**	**Type II**
Cause	Too much insulin or too little food	Absence or inadequate insulin	Uncontrolled diabetes or oral hypoglycemic drugs
Onset	Rapid (within minutes)	Slow (about eight hours)	Slow (hours to days)
Appearance	Exhibits symptoms of fainting	Appears ill	Appears ill
Respirations	Normal	Rapid and deep, shortness of breath	Rapid and deep; absence of Kussmaul's
Breath odor	Normal	Sweetish due to acetone	Normal
Pulse	Tachycardia	Tachycardia	Tachycardia
Blood pressure		Lowered blood pressure	Decreased blood pressure
Hunger	Hunger pangs in epigastrium	Loss of appetite	Hunger
Thirst	None	Increased	Increased, dehydration
Vomiting	Nausea; vomiting rare	Common	Common
Eyes	Staring, double vision	Appear sunken	Visual loss
Headache	Common	Occasionally	Occasionally
Skin	Pallor, perspiration, chilling sensation	Hot, dry skin	Hot, dry skin
Muscle action	Twitching common, unsteady gait	Twitching absent	Twitching absent
Pain in abdomen	None	Common	Common
Mental status	Confusion, erratic, change in mood, unable to concentrate	Malaise, drowsy, confusion coma	Confused, dull, coma
Lab findings			
Sugar in urine	None after residual is discarded	Present	Present
Blood sugar	Below 50–70 mg/dl blood	High, 350–900 mg/dl	Very high, 800 mg/dl up to 2400 mg/dl
Ketones	Absent	High	Absent
Ketones in blood plasma	Absent	4+ present	Absent

Appendix 1. Endocrine Gland Function, Hormones, and Disorders

Gland	Hormones Produced	Function	Endocrine Disorder

Pituitary
 	
Location: Base of the brain
	Anterior Lobe
	  Adrenocorticotropic
	    hormone (ACTH)
	  Thyrotropic hormone
	    (TSH)
	  Somatotropic hormone
	    (STH)
	  Gonadotropic hormones
	    (FSH, LH, LTH)
	Posterior Lobe
	  Vasopressin
	  Oxytocin
	  Melanocyte stimulating
	    hormone (MSH)
		Directly affects the function of other endocrine glands; termed "master gland."
		Controls sexual development and function.
		Promotes growth of body tissues.
		Influences water absorption by kidney.
		Influenced by hypothalamus.
			Anterior pituitary
			  Gigantism
			  Acromegaly
			  Cushing's disease
			  Dwarfism
			Posterior pituitary
			  Diabetes insipidus

Adrenal
 	
Location: Above each kidney
	Cortex
	  Glucocorticoids
	    Cortisol
	    Cortisone
	    Cortisterone
	  Mineralocorticoids
	    Aldosterone
	    Desoxycorticosterone
	    Corticosterone
	  Sex hormones
	    Androgens
	    Estrogens
	Medulla
	  Epinephrine
	  Norepinephrine
		Regulates sodium and electrolyte balance.
		Affects carbohydrate, fat, and protein metabolism.
		Influences the development of sexual characteristics.
		Stimulates "fight or flight" response to danger.
			Addison's disease
			Cushing's syndrome
			Pheochromocytoma
			Primary aldosteronism

Thyroid Location: Anterior part of the neck	Thyroxine Triiodothyronine Thyrocalcitonin	Controls rate of body metabolism, growth, and nutrition.	Goiter Cretinism Myxedema Hyperthyroidism (Grave's disease)
Parathyroid Location: Near thyroid	Parathormone (PTH)	Controls calcium and phosphorus metabolism.	Hypoparathyroidism Hyperparathyroidism
Islets of Langerhans of Pancreas Location: Posterior to stomach and liver	Insulin Glucagon	Influences carbohydrate metabolism. Indirectly influences fat and protein metabolism.	Diabetes mellitus Hyperinsulinism
Ovaries Location: Pelvic cavity	Estrogen and progesterone Testosterone	Controls development of secondary sex characteristics.	Lack of acceleration or regression of sexual development

Integumentary System

The integumentary system comprises the enveloping membrane or skin of the body. It consists of the outer epidermis and inner layer of dermis. The hair, nails, and various glands are outgrowths of the skin. The skin performs many vital body functions that include protection against negative elements in the environment and reception of temperature, touch, and pressure.

Anatomy and Physiology

Skin

A. Skin comprises about 15 percent of the body weight and forms a barrier between the internal organs and the external environment.
B. The epidermis, dermis, and subcutaneous tissue compose the skin's three layers.
C. Skin is the largest sensory organ of the body. It contains nerves and specialized sensory organs sensitive to pain, touch, pressure, heat, and cold.
D. Chief pigment is melanin, produced by basal cells.
E. Skin harbors bacterial flora.
   1. Bacteria normally present in varying amounts.
   2. Organisms are shed with normal exfoliation of skin; bathing and rubbing may also remove bacteria.
   3. Normal pH of skin (4.2 to 5.6) retards growth of bacteria.
   4. Damaged areas of skin are potential points of entry for infection.
F. Functions of skin.
   1. Protection.
   2. Temperature regulation.
   3. Sensation.
   4. Storage.

Hair

A. Keratinous structures growing out of tubular invaginations of the epidermis called hair follicles.
B. Hair goes through cyclic changes of growth, atrophy, and rest.
C. Melanocytes present in the bulb of each hair account for color.
D. All parts of the body except the palms, soles of the feet, distal phalanges of fingers and toes, and the penis are covered with some form of hair.

Sweat Gland

A. Aggregate of cells that produce a liquid (perspiration) salty to the taste and with a pH ranging from 4.5 to 7.5.
B. Contains duct that opens out at the surface of the skin.
C. Chief components of sweat are water, sodium, potassium, chloride, glucose, urea, and lactate.

System Assessment

A. Assess color.
   1. Assess color of skin, including deviations from the normal range within the individual's race.
      a. Use a nonglare daylight or 60-watt bulb.
      b. Note especially the bony prominences.
      c. Observe for pallor (white), flushing (red), jaundice (yellow), ashen (gray), or cyanosis (blue) coloration.
      d. Check mucous membranes to be accurate.
   2. Observe for increased or decreased areas of pigmentation.
   3. Observe for various skin discolorations: ecchymosis, petechiae, purpura, or erythema.
B. Evaluate skin temperature.
   1. Palpate skin (especially areas of concern) for temperature.
   2. Note changes in different extremities.

C. Assess turgor.
  1. Observe skin for its ease of movement and speed of return to original position.
  2. Observe for excessive dryness, moisture, wrinkling, flaking and general texture.
  3. Observe for a lasting impression or dent after pressing against and removing finger from skin—indicates edema or fluid in the tissue.
D. Assess skin sensation.
  1. Ability to detect heat, cold, gentle touch, and pressure.
  2. Note complaints of itching, tingling, cramps, or numbness.
E. Observe cleanliness.
  1. Observe general state of hygiene. Note amount of oil, moisture, and dirt on the skin surface.
  2. Note presence of strong body odors.
  3. Investigate hair and scalp for presence of body lice.
F. Assess integrity (intactness of skin).
  1. Note intactness of skin. Observe for areas of broken skin (lesions) or ulcers.
  2. Assess any lesion for its location, size, shape, color(s), consistency, discomfort, odor, and sensation associated with it.
G. Assess skin conditions (see Appendix 1 for types of skin lesions).

Skin Disorders and Burns

General Nursing Care for the Skin

A. Determine type of lesion or area of altered tissue (see Appendix 1 for types of skin lesions).
  1. Primary lesion is initial, or first, lesion.
  2. Secondary lesion is a result of a change or complication that involves a primary lesion.
B. Provide psychological support.
  1. Encourage patient to express feelings.
    a. May be embarrassed about appearance.
    b. May be fearful of scarring.
    c. May be depressed about long duration and chronicity of disorder.
  2. Accept patient as he or she is; nonverbal communication is therapeutic (touch).
C. Take measures to prevent damage to healthy skin.
  1. Prevent scratching.
    a. Keep fingernails smooth and short.
    b. Encourage patient to wear cotton gloves as reminder not to scratch.
    c. Restrain if ordered.
  2. Use hot and cold applications with caution.
D. Take measures to prevent secondary infections.
  1. Use medical aseptic technique.
  2. Maintain isolation if lesions are infectious.
  3. Careful handwashing.
E. Take measures to reverse inflammatory process.
  1. Relieve symptoms.
    a. Control room temperature and humidity.
    b. Decrease local irritation.
  2. Give medication and treatment as needed.

Allergic Reactions

Contact Dermatitis

Definition: Skin reaction caused by contact with a substance to which the skin is sensitive. Reaction is characterized by inflammation as evidenced by itching, redness, and skin lesions.

Causes

A. Contact with chemicals.
  1. Clothing (especially woolens).
  2. Cosmetics.
  3. Household products (especially detergents).
  4. Industrial substances (paints, dyes, cements).
B. Contact with toxic irritants: poison oak, poison ivy, or poison sumac.

Signs and Symptoms

A. Papules.
B. Vesicles.
C. Severe itching (pruritus).

Preventive Measures

A. Avoid irritant or remove irritating clothing.
B. Do not use detergent.
C. Wear rubber gloves for household chores.
D. Make request of industry to provide protective clothing; or allow change of job site for highly sensitive individuals.

Treatment and Nursing Care

A. Cleanse skin of plant oils.
B. Apply lotion.
C. Administer steroids for severe reactions.
D. Apply cold wet dressings of Burrow's Solution to relieve itching.

Eczema

Definition: Superficial inflammatory process involving primarily the epidermis.

Signs and Symptoms

A. Local eruptions.
   1. Erythema, papules, vesicles may be present.
   2. Area may be edematous, weeping, eroded, and/or crusted.
B. Swelling of regional lymph nodes.
C. May occur at any age, but particularly common in infancy.
D. Runs a chronic course with remission and exacerbation.
   1. Patient usually becomes irritable.
   2. Skin may be thickened, scaled, and fissured.

Treatment and Nursing Care

A. Seek the cause which may be foods, emotional problems, or familial tendencies.
B. Do not allow the patient to be vaccinated for smallpox; isolate from individuals recently vaccinated.
C. Control skin eruptions.
   1. Encourage patient to withhold scratching.
   2. Apply wet dressings or give therapeutic baths (no soaps during acute stages).
   3. Apply mild lotion (calamine) when no oozing or vesiculation is present.
   4. Apply cornstarch paste to remove crusts.
   5. Rub cornstarch into bed linen, and do not use woolen blankets.

Bacterial Infections

Impetigo

Definition: Bacterial disease caused by streptococcal, staphylococcal, or combined infection.

Signs and Symptoms

A. Local vesicles.
B. Pustules evolving from vesicles that become crusted.

Treatment and Nursing Care

A. Prevent the spread of disease.
B. Dry the lesions by exposure to air (use compresses of Burrow's Solution to remove the crusts so as to allow better exposure to air).
C. Apply local antibiotic ointments or bland emollients to prevent cracking and fissures as directed by physician.
D. Caution family to use only hexachlorophene soap, to use other hygienic care materials, and to use separate towels to prevent the spread of the disease.

Furuncle (Boil)

Definition: Bacterial inflammation of skin caused by staphylococcal infection of a hair follicle.

Signs and Symptoms

A. Onset is sudden; the skin becomes red, tender, and hot around the hair follicle.
B. The center forms pus, and the core may be extruded spontaneously or by excision and manipulation.

Treatment and Nursing Care

A. Isolate towels, soap, and clothing; necessary to maintain scrupulous cleanliness.
B. Administer systemic antibiotics if a series of furuncles occur and if ordered.
C. Check for presence of diabetes mellitus. Should be ruled out only after tests prove negative.

Viral Infections

Herpes Simplex

Definition: Infectious condition (cold sore) caused by a virus that may occur on lips, face, or genitalia.

Signs and Symptoms

A. Local burning, tingling, itching.
B. Local erythema.
C. Vesicles appear later.

Nursing Care

A. Keep lesion dry and clean.
B. Advise patient to avoid sexual or direct contacts.
C. Encourage patient to request physician to periodically reexamine lesion.

Herpes Zoster

Definition: Acute infectious process caused by viral invasion of central nervous system.

Signs and Symptoms

A. Pain and discomfort.
B. Cutaneous lesions usually located along major nerve root.

Burns

Definition: Destruction of skin layers by thermal, chemical, or electrical agents.

Classification of Burns

A. Degree of burn—determined by layers involved.
  1. First degree.
    a. Involves epidermis.
    b. Area is red or pink.
    c. Moderate pain.
    d. Spontaneous healing.
  2. Second degree.
    a. Involves epidermis and dermis to the basal cells.
    b. Blistering.
    c. Severe pain.
    d. Regeneration in one month.
    e. Scarring may occur.
  3. Third degree.
    a. Involves epidermis, dermis, and subcutaneous tissue and may extend to the muscle in severe burns.
    b. White, gray, or black in appearance.
    c. Absence of pain.
    d. Edema of surrounding tissues.
    e. Eschar formation.
    f. Grafting needed due to total destruction of dermal elements.
  4. Fourth degree.
    a. Involves muscle and bone.
    b. Increased destruction of RBCs.

B. Classification according to the percentage of body area destroyed.
1. Critical burns—30 percent or more of the body has sustained second degree burn and 10 percent has sustained third degree burn; further complicated by respiratory involvement, smoke inhalation, fractures, and other tissue injury.
2. Moderate burns—less than 10 percent of the body has sustained third degree burn and 15 to 30 percent has sustained second degree burn.
3. Minor burns—less than 15 percent of the body has sustained second degree burn and less than 2 percent has sustained third degree burn.
4. Estimation of percentage of total body surface involved with "Rule of Nine" (see Appendix 2).

C. Classification according to cause.
1. Thermal burns: flame burns, scalding with hot liquids, or radiation.
2. Chemical burns: strong acids or strong alkali solutions.
3. Electrical burns.
   a. Most serious type of burn.
   b. Body fluids may conduct an electrical charge through body (look for entrance and exit area).
   c. Cardiac arrhythmias may occur.
   d. Toxins are created postburn that injure kidneys.
   e. Voltage and ampere information important in history taking.

Problems Associated with Burns

A. Fluid and electrolyte imbalance.
1. Edema appears around the wound as a result of damage to capillaries.
2. There is a loss of fluid at the burn area.

B. Pulmonary changes from inhalation injury.
1. Pulmonary edema.
2. Obstruction of the air passages from edema of the face, neck, trachea, and larynx.
3. Restriction of lung mobility from eschar on chest wall.

C. Renal changes.

1. In burns of 15 to 20 percent of the body surface, there is a decreased urinary output, which must be avoided or reversed.
2. Urinary tract infections are frequent.

D. Gastrointestinal changes.
1. Acute gastric dilation.
2. Paralytic ileus.
3. Curling's ulcer that produces "coffee ground" aspirant.

E. Factors which determine seriousness of burn.
1. Age.
   a. Below eighteen months.
   b. Above sixty-five years.
2. General health.
3. Site of burn.
4. Associated injuries (fractures).
5. Causative agents.

Nursing Care

A. Maintain patent airway.
B. Maintain aseptic area.
C. Provide fluid replacement therapy.
1. Shock phase.
   a. First 24 to 48 hours postburn, fluid shifts from plasma to interstitial space.
   b. Potassium levels rise in plasma.
   c. Blood hemoconcentration and metabolic acidosis occur.
   d. Fluid loss is mostly plasma.
   e. Nursing responsibilities.
      (1) Monitor vital signs frequently.
      (2) Monitor urinary output (50 to 100 cc/hour).
      (3) Give one half of total fluids in first eight hours.
2. Postshock phase (diuretic phase).
   a. Capillary permeability stabilizes and fluid begins to shift from interstitial spaces to plasma.
   b. Hypokalemia, hypernatremia, hemodilution, and pulmonary edema are potential dangers.
   c. Nursing responsibilities.
      (1) Monitor CVP.
      (2) Observe lab values.
      (3) Maintain adequate urine output.

D. Relieve pain with morphine sulfate as ordered. Give small doses frequently. Given IV.

E. Assess peripheral circulation.

F. Provide adequate heat to maintain patient's temperature.

G. Promote good body alignment: begin range of motion early.

H. Administer antacids to prevent stress ulcer.

I. Maintain reverse isolation.

J. Maintain wound care.
1. Initial excision: mainly for electrical burns.
2. Occlusive dressings.
   a. Painful and costly.
   b. Decreases water loss.
   c. Limits range-of-motion exercises.
   d. Helps to maintain functional position.
   e. Advent of topical antibiotics has led to decreased use.
3. Exposure method.
   a. Allows for drainage of burn exudate.
   b. Eschar forms protective covering.
   c. Use of topical therapy.
   d. Skin easily inspected.
   e. Range-of-motion exercises easier to perform.

☆K. Apply topical preparations to wound area.
1. Mafenide (Sulfamylon).
   a. Exerts bacteriostatic action against many organisms.
   b. Penetrates tissue wall.
   c. Dressings not needed when used.
   d. Breakdown of drug provides heavy acid load. Inhibition of carbonic anhydrase compounds situation. Individual compensates by hyperventilating.
   e. Alternate use with Silvadene.
2. Silvadene.
   a. Broad antimicrobial activity.
   b. Effective against yeast.
   c. Inhibits bacteria resistant to other antimicrobials.
      (1) Not usually used prophylactically.
      (2) Given for specific organism.
      (3) Not helpful first 48 hours due to vessel thrombosis.
   d. Can be washed off with water.

L. Administer systemic antibiotics.

M. Debridement and eschar removal daily.

N. Provide long-term care.
1. Maintain good positioning to prevent contractures.
2. Provide adequate rest.
3. Prevent infection.
4. Maintain adequate protein and caloric intake to promote healing.
5. Monitor hydration status.
6. Protect skin grafts.
7. Provide psychological support (as important as physical care).
   a. Deal with the patient's fear of disfigurement and immobility from scarring.
   b. Provide constant support, as plastic repair is lengthy and painful.
   c. Involve the family in long-term planning and day-to-day care.

☆**Isolation Protocol**

A. Protocol for entering isolation room
1. Put on cap.
2. Put on and tie mask.
3. Put on gown and tie.
4. Wash hands and put on gloves.

B. Protocol for leaving isolation room
1. Untie gown at waist.
2. Take off gloves.
3. Wash hands.
4. Take off cap.
5. Untie gown at neck.
6. Pull gown off and place in laundry hamper.
7. Take off mask.
8. Leave room and wash hands.

Skin Disorders as Manifestation of Internal Disease

Lupus Erythematosus

Definition: Collagen disease of the connective tissue that leads to a skin rash. The disease may involve any organ of the body.

Signs and Symptoms

A. Discoid eruption—a chronic, localized scaling erythematous skin eruption over nose, cheeks, and forehead producing characteristic "butterfly" appearance.
B. Fever, malaise and weight loss.
C. Exacerbation and remission of symptoms.
D. Sensitivity to sunlight (photophobia).
E. Systemic (disseminated) lupus erythematosus may involve multiple organs and lead to death.

Treatment and Nursing Care

A. Protect patient from sunlight and avoid antibiotic ointments that may spread the lesions.
B. Administer steroid treatment to prevent progression of the disease.
C. Advise patient that strict personal hygiene is an absolute requirement.
D. Be aware that there is no development of immunity and recurrence is common.

Syphilis

Definition: Contagious venereal disease that leads to many structural and cutaneous lesions caused by the spirochete *Treponema pallidum.* The disease is transmitted by direct, intimate contact or in utero.

Stages

A. Primary stage.
1. Incubation period is ten days to three weeks.
2. Characteristic lesion is red, eroded, indurated papule; the sore or ulcer at the site of the invasion by the spirochete is called a *chancre.*
3. Accompanied by enlarged lymph node in drainage area of chancre.
4. May be painless or painful.
5. This stage is highly infectious.
B. Secondary stage.
1. Develops if the individual is not treated in the primary stage.
2. May be mild enough to pass unnoticed or it may be severe, with a generalized rash on skin and mucous membrane.

Characteristics

A. Fever and sore throat.
B. Malaise may be present.
C. Transmitted most commonly by sexual intercourse, but infants may become infected during the birth process.
D. No age or race is immune to the disease.
E. Diagnosed by serum studies and/or dark field examination of secretions of the chancre.

Treatment and Nursing Care

A. Administer, if ordered, long-acting Bicillin as primary treatment.
B. Advise patient to avoid sexual contact until clearance is given by physician.

Malignant Tumors of Skin

Basal Cell Epithelioma

Definition: Tumor arising from the basal layer of the epidermis. Lesion is a small, smooth papule with telangiectasis and atropic center.

Signs and Symptoms

A. Starts as a papule and grows slowly.
B. Central area may become depressed and ulcerated, forming a classic rodent ulcer.
C. Locally invasive and seldom metastasizes.

Treatment and Nursing Care

A. Surgical excision is preferred.
B. Radiation therapy is administered for lesions of the eyelid and nose.
C. Watch for potential malignancy in other locations.

Squamous Cell Carcinoma

Definition: Tumor of the epidermis that frequently arises out of keratosis and is considered an invasive cancer. The lesion begins as erythematous macules or plaques with indistinct margins; surface often becomes crusted.

Signs and Symptoms

A. Lesions enlarge more rapidly than in basal-cell epithelioma and may metastasize.
B. A nodular tumor usually appears on the lower lip, tongue, head, or neck.

Treatment

A. Excision is preferred.
B. Irradiation.

Melanoma

Definition: Malignant pigmented tumor that arises out of melanocytes and is often fatal. May arise from so-called blue-black mole.

Treatment

A. Surgical excision preferred.
B. Cancer-destroying drugs may be used.

Appendix 1. Types of Skin Lesions

Primary lesions

Bulla	Large vesicle; elevation of skin filled with serous fluid.
Erythema	Form of macula showing redness over skin.
Lichenification	Thickening of affected tissue.
Macule	Flat, discolored patch on skin of various colors and shapes.
Papule	Raised, solid elevation of skin usually smaller than one cm.
Pustule	Small elevation of skin filled with purulent fluid.
Telangiectasis	Dilation of capillary, producing visible, red, irregular line.
Vesicle	Elevation of skin filled with clear, serous fluid; "blister."
Wheal	Irregularly shaped elevation that is caused by edema.

Secondary lesions

Crust	Dried serum from open lesion mixed with surface dirt and dead cells; "scab."
Scale	Flake of shed dry epidermis.

Appendix 2. "Rule of Nine"

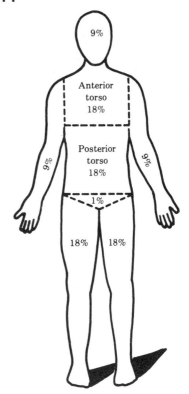

Musculoskeletal System

Skeleton provides body with support and protection. The skeleton is used in locomotion but requires muscles to supply source of power and added support. Musculoskeletal system assists in unifying actions of whole body and helps it adjust to environmental changes.

Anatomy and Physiology

Skeletal System

A. System of separate bones (206) bound together by ligaments.
B. System responsible for supporting, moving, and giving shape to the body.
   1. Supports surrounding tissues and provides body with framework.
   2. Protects vital organs and soft tissues.
   3. Provides leverage and source of attachment for skeletal muscles.
   4. Forms erythrocytes, granular leukocytes, and thrombocytes in red marrow of bone.
   5. Stores calcium and other minerals.

Classification

A. According to body region.
   1. Axial skeleton—includes head and trunk which form central axis to which appendicular skeleton is attached.
      a. Composed of 80 bones.
      b. Includes skull, spine, ribs, sternum, and hyoid bone.
   2. Appendicular skeleton—includes shoulder girdle, arm bones, pelvic girdle, and leg bones.
      a. Composed of 126 bones.
      b. Shoulder (pectoral girdle from which arms hang).
         (1) Consists of two clavicles (collarbones).
         (2) Consists of two scapulae (shoulder blades), which are attached to clavicle.
      c. Arm bones.
         (1) Humerus (upper arm bone) is connected at elbow to ulna and radius (lower arm bones).
         (2) Carpals make up wrist.
         (3) Metacarpals form hand palm.
         (4) Phalanges form finger bones.
      d. Pelvic girdle (hip).
         (1) Pelvis formed from pelvic girdle, plus bones of sacrum and coccyx.
         (2) Encircles and protects genitourinary organs.
         (3) Sockets in girdle fit femur leg bone.
      e. Leg bones.
         (1) Constructed similarly to arm bones but heavier and stronger.
         (2) Femur (thigh bone) extends from pelvis to knee.
         (3) Tibia and fibula extend from knee to ankle.
         (4) Knee is separate bone (patella).
         (5) Ankle bones (tarsals); foot bones (metatarsals); toe bones (phalanges).
B. According to shape.
   1. Long bones—made up of a shaft (diaphysis) and two flared ends (epiphyses); include radius and femur.
   2. Short bones; include carpals and tarsals.
   3. Flat bones; include ribs and skull.
   4. Irregular bones; include vertebrae.

Development

A. The bone-like tissue of very young is mostly cartilage.
B. Cartilage is replaced by bone tissue through process of ossification.
   1. Calcium collects in cartilage and becomes hardened.
   2. Some cartilage cells break loose so that channels develop in bone shaft.

3. Blood vessels enter channels carrying small cells of connective tissue; some tissue cells (osteoblasts) form true bone.
   a. Osteoblasts enter hardened cartilage, forming layers of hard bone.
   b. Other cells work to tear down old bone structure (osteoclasts) so osteoblasts can rebuild with new bone.
C. Bone-growth process occurs by mechanism of cartilage formation followed by replacement of cartilage with hard material.
   1. Cartilage grows over hardened bone.
   2. Cartilage hardens with addition of calcium.
   3. Process continues until full growth of body is reached.
D. Amount of calcium deposited and reabsorbed into blood is regulated by the parathyroid and thyroid glands.

Structure

A. Bone is formed of dense connective tissue.
   1. Tissue consists of bone cells (osteocytes).
   2. Cells embedded in matrix made up of calcified intercellular substance.
   3. Bone consists of 50 percent water and 50 percent solid matter.
   4. Calcium phosphate is the basic bone chemical that gives hardness and strength.
B. Bone is comprised of concentric cylindrical layers.
   1. Periosteum (the exterior covering, outer layer)—thin, tough membrane of fibrous tissue.
      a. Supports tendons connecting muscle to bone.
      b. Serves as protective sheath.
      c. Serves to extend blood supply to bone.
   2. Compact bone layer—dense hard layer of bone tissue.
      a. Fibrous composition to give resiliency to bone.
      b. Compact tissue tunneled by central canal or hollow cavity.
         (1) Marrow (soft tissue, medulla) contained in compact bone hollow.

(2) Contains fine branching canals (haversian system) through which small blood vessels and lymphatics run.
(3) Porous bone layer—spongy (cancellous) tissue that contains sponge-like hollows.

Joints

A. Articulation is a union or junction of two or more bones.
B. Function of joint is skeletal flexibility and motion.
C. Classification—according to structural variations that allow for different kinds of movement.
   1. Diarthrotic joints are freely movable.
      a. This type of joint is a cavity enclosed by a capsule lined with synovial membrane that secretes a lubricant.
      b. Capsule is reinforced by ligaments.
      c. Articular cartilage covers ends of bones.
      d. Types of joint movement make for structural variations.
         (1) Hinge type allows single directional movement (elbow).
         (2) Ball-and-socket type allows bending (hip).
         (3) Saddle type allows multidirectional shifting (thumb).
         (4) Pivot type allows rotary movement.
         (5) Gliding type allows limited sliding of bones against each other (wrist, ankle, invertebral joints).
         (6) Ellipsoidal type.
   2. Synarthrotic joints are immovable.
      a. Tissue grows between articulating surfaces.
      b. Includes suture lines of skull.
   3. Amphiarthrosis is a joint with limited movement.

Muscular System

A. System of fibers (more than 600) attached to bones and marked by striation.

B. System allows body movement under control of voluntary nervous system.
 1. Provides for body movement, locomotion.
 2. Provides support for the body.
 3. Performs body functions such as partial production of heat.

Classification

A. According to location—posterior tibial allows inversion of foot.
B. According to direction of fibers—muscle of tongue allows for change in shape for eating.
C. According to action—flexor muscle of toe allows toe to bend on itself; extensor muscle of toe allows extension of toe.
D. According to size and shape—trapezius of neck and shoulder allows for elevation and rotation of shoulder.
E. According to number of origin heads—biceps of arm allow for flexing and turning arm upward.
F. According to points of attachment—sterno-cleidomastoid allows for flexion and rotation of head.

Cell Structure

A. Fibers of voluntary muscles grouped together in sheath of connective tissue.
B. Each bundled group of muscle fibers surrounded by connective tissue sheath.
C. Sheath tissue may be continuous with fibrous tissue that extends from the muscle as a tendon.

Properties

A. Excitability—capacity of muscle to respond to stimulus without intervention of motor nerves.
B. Contractility—ability of muscle to shorten, tighten, and contract.
C. Tonicity—ability of muscle to maintain steady contraction which determines its firmness.
D. Extensibility—ability of muscle to stretch in response to applied force.
E. Elasticity—ability of strained muscle to regain original size and shape when applied force is removed.

Contraction

A. For muscle contraction and other fine movements to occur, muscle tissue must be stimulated.
 1. Each fiber receives own neural impulse from somatic motor neuron.
 2. Signal of impulse along nerve muscle fiber changes chemical to mechanical energy.
 3. Each fiber has stored supply of fuel for contraction energy source.
  a. Stimulus releases calcium to cause fiber filament movement.
  b. Nerve stimulates breakdown of ATP.
B. Area where motor neuron ends in muscle fiber is called myoneural junction.

Movement

A. Skeletal muscles produce body movement by pulling on bones.
B. Bones serve as levers, and joints serve as fulcrums of these levers.
 1. Each muscle has a point of origin and a point of insertion that are usually attached to bone.
 2. The point of origin is the more fixed point of attachment.
 3. The point of insertion is the more movable end.
C. Muscles that move a body part usually do not extend over that part.
D. Skeletal muscles usually perform with group action; some contract while others relax.
 1. Prime movers are muscles responsible for the primary movement of contraction.
 2. Antagonists are muscles that exert an action opposing that of prime mover.
 3. Synergists are muscles that enhance action of prime mover.

E. Accessory parts.
   1. Ligaments—cord-like connective tissue that holds bones together.
   2. Tendons—attach muscles to bones.

Musculoskeletal Disorders

Fractures

Definition: A break in the continuity of bone.

Causes

A. Direct application of force at site.
B. Distant application of force but transmitted to fracture site.
C. Sudden muscle contraction.
D. Spontaneous break as result of disease.

Classification

A. According to severity.
   1. Simple (closed)—a break is present but no external wound in skin.
   2. Compound (open)—a break is present and there is external wound in skin over or leading to fracture site.
   3. Comminuted—bone has splintered into fragments.
   4. Greenstick—one side of the bone broken but the opposite side is bent.
B. According to direction and location.
   1. Oblique—break runs in slanting direction.
   2. Spiral—break coils around bone.
   3. Extracapsular—break occurs outside the joint.
   4. Intracapsular—break occurs inside the joint.

Signs and Symptoms

A. Deformity.
B. Loss of power or movement.
C. Pain, tenderness, and muscle spasm over fracture site.
D. Edema.
E. Discoloration from bruising.
F. Possible shock.

Emergency Nursing Care

A. Keep limb or part stable until immobilized.
B. Take measures to prevent shock.
C. Cover open wound with dry and clean or sterile dressing.

Treatment

A. Objectives.
   1. Regain correct alignment through reduction.
   2. Maintain alignment.
   3. Regain function of affected part.
B. Fractures treated by reduction; broken ends pulled into alignment and continuity of bone established so healing can occur.
   1. Methods of reduction.
      a. Closed—fractured bone brought into alignment by manual manipulation; no incision made.
      b. Open—surgical incision made and bone aligned under direct visualization; also performed to cleanse open fracture or to stabilize alignment with inserted fixators.
   2. Forms of alignment.
      a. Closed—application of cast, splint, and/or traction.
      b. Open—fixation with metallic pins, wires, screws, plates, nails, or rods.

☆Principles of Cast Care

A. After application of cast, allow twenty-four to forty-eight hours for drying.
   1. Cast will change from dull to shiny substance when dry.
   2. Heat can be applied to assist in drying process.

B. Do not handle cast during drying process as indentations from fingermarks can cause skin breakdown under cast.

C. Keep extremity elevated to prevent edema.

D. Provide for smooth edges surrounding cast.
   1. Prevents crumbling and breaking down of edges.
   2. Stockinet can be pulled over edge and fastened down with adhesive tape to outside of cast.

E. Observe casted extremity for signs of circulatory impairment. Cast may have to be cut if edematous condition continues.

F. If there is an open, draining area on affected extremity, a window (cut out portion of cast) can be utilized for observation and/or irrigation of wound.

G. Keep cast dry; it can break down when water comes in contact with plaster. Plastic bags or plastic coated bed chux can be utilized during the bath or when using bedpan, to protect cast material.

H. Utilize isometric exercises to prevent muscle atrophy and to strengthen the muscle. Isometrics prevent joint from being mobilized.

I. Position patient with pillows to prevent strain on unaffected areas.

J. Turn every two hours to prevent complications. Encourage to lie on abdomen four hours a day.

The Immobilized Patient

A. Prevent respiratory complications.
   1. Have patient cough and deep breathe every two hours.
   2. Turn every two hours if not contraindicated.
   3. Provide suction if needed.

B. Prevent thrombus and emboli formation.
   1. Apply antiembolic stockings.
   2. Initiate isometric and isotonic exercises.
   3. Start anticoagulation therapy, if indicated.
   4. Turn every two hours.
   5. Observe for signs and symptoms of pulmonary and/or fat emboli.

C. Prevent contractures.
   1. Start range-of-motion exercises to affected joints qid, all joints bid.
   2. Provide foot board and/or foot cradle.
   3. Position and turn every two hours.

D. Prevent skin breakdown.
   1. Massage with lotion once a day to prevent drying.
   2. Use alcohol for back care to toughen skin.
   3. Massage elbows, coccyx, heels bid.
   4. Turn every two hours.
   5. Alternate pressure mattress, sheepskin.
   6. Use stryker boats or heel protectors.
   7. Use elbow guards.

E. Prevent urinary retention and calculi.
   1. Force fluids.
   2. Monitor intake and output.
   3. Administer urinary antiseptic (Mandelamine, etc.).
   4. Offer bedpan every four hours.

F. Prevent constipation.
   1. Force fluids.
   2. Provide high fiber diet.
   3. Administer laxative or enema.
   4. Offer bedpan at same time each day—encourage to establish good bowel habits.

G. Provide psychological support.

Traction

A. Traction is force applied in two directions.

B. Purpose is to reduce and/or immobilize a fracture, to provide proper bone alignment and regain normal length, or to reduce muscle spasm.

Skeletal Traction

A. Mechanical—applied to bone, using pins (Steinmann), wires (Kirschner), tongs (Crutchfield).

B. Most often used in fractures of femur, tibia, humerus.

C. Nursing care.
   1. Observe pin or tong insertion site for drainage, odors, erythema, edema (usually

indication of inflammatory process or infection).
2. Watch for skin breakdown if bandage is used to apply traction.
3. Cover end of pins or wires with rubber stoppers or cork to prevent puncture of nursing personnel or patient.
4. Cleanse area surrounding insertion site of pin or tongs with hydrogen peroxide or Betadine. Some physicians order antibiotic ointments to be applied to area.

Balanced Suspension Traction

A. Thomas's splint with Pearson attachment is used in conjunction with skin or skeletal traction (used particularly with skeletal traction for fractured femur).
B. Balanced suspension traction is produced by a counterforce other than the patient.
☆C. Nursing care.
1. Maintain proper alignment.
2. Protect skin from excoriation, particularly around the top of Thomas's splint. Pad with cotton wadding or ABD's.
3. Prevent pressure points around the top of Thomas's splint by keeping patient pulled up in bed.
4. Maintain at least 20-degree angle from thigh to the bed.
5. Provide foot plate to prevent foot drop.
6. Keep heels clear of Pearson attachment to prevent skin breakdown and decubitus.
7. Position patient frequently from side to side (as ordered).
8. Unless contraindicated, head of bed can be elevated for comfort and facilitating adequate respiratory functions.
9. Place overbed table on unaffected side.

Skin Traction

A. Traction applied by use of elastic bandages, moleskin strips, or adhesive.
B. Used most often in alignment or lengthening (for congenital hip displacement, etc.).

C. Most common types.
1. Russell traction.
☆2. Buck's extension (most common).
   a. Pull is exerted in one plane.
   b. Used for temporary immobilization.
   c. Apply moleskin or adhesive material to leg. Follow with application of ace wrap.
   d. Attach a foot block with a spreader and rope which goes into a pulley.
   e. Attach weight to pulley and hang freely over edge of bed. (Not more than eight to ten pounds of weight can be applied.)
   f. Observe and readjust bandages for tightness and smoothness (can cause constriction which leads to edema or even nerve damage).
☆3. Cervical traction (used for whiplashes and cervical spasm).
   a. Use head harness (or halter).
      (1) Pad chin.
      (2) Protect ears from friction rub.
   b. Elevate head of bed and attach weights to pulley system over head of bed.
   c. Observe for skin breakdown.
      (1) Powder areas encased in the halter.
      (2) Place back of head on padding.
☆4. Pelvic traction (used for low back pain).
   a. Apply girdle snugly over patient's pelvis and iliac crest; attach to weights.
   b. Observe for pressure points over iliac crest.
   c. Keep patient in good alignment.
   d. May raise foot of bed slightly (12 inches) to prevent patient from slipping down in bed.
☆D. Care of traction apparatus.
1. Weights should hang freely and not touch the floor.
2. Pulleys should not be obstructed.
3. Ropes in the pulley should move freely.
4. Knot should be secured in rope to prevent slipping.
5. Proper body alignment (up in bed, in direct line with traction) and proper countertraction should be maintained.

6. Weights should not be removed or lifted without specific order. (Exceptions are pelvic and cervical traction that patients can remove at intervals.)
7. Sharp edges from traction apparatus should be covered with hollowed out rubber balls to prevent injury to nursing personnel if they bump into equipment.

☆E. Care of patient in traction.
1. Maintain correct alignment.
2. Maintain counterbalance or correct pull.
   a. Pull is exerted against traction in opposite direction (balanced suspension).
   b. Pull is exerted against a fixed point.
   c. Bed is elevated under area involved to provide the countertraction.
3. Provide firm mattress or bedboards.
4. Observe for complications.
   a. Osteomyelitis (infections of bone).
   b. Bone deformities.
   c. Skin breakdown.
5. Provide range-of-motion exercises for unaffected extremities.
6. Observe for circulatory impairment.
   a. Blanching of nailbeds (color should return quickly when nailbeds are depressed).
   b. Extremity should be pink and warm.
   c. Check for edema in affected extremity.
   d. Patient should be able to wiggle finger or toes.
   e. Patient should not have tingling or loss of sensation in affected extremity.
7. Prevent foot drop.
   a. Provide footplate.
   b. Encourage dorsiflexion exercises.
8. Provide overhead trapeze to allow patient to assist in activities (turning, moving up in bed, using bedpan, etc.).
9. Prevent postoperative complications.

Hip (Proximal) Fracture

Definition: Bone discontinuity of proximal end of femur, intracapsular or extracapsular, which occurs most frequently in elderly women.

Preoperative Nursing Care

A. Provide care as given to patients in skin traction.
B. Give special care if patient's increased age is a factor.
C. Observe for elimination regularity.
D. Encourage proper exercises.
E. Maintain proper positioning.
F. Assist patient with eating; nourishing diet essential for healing process.

Operative Procedure

A. Surgical fixation with nails, plates, or screws.
B. Possible prosthesis.

Postoperative Nursing Care

A. Turn patient from unaffected side to back as routine; a physician's order is required to turn from side to side.
B. Turn patient with hip prosthesis by always placing pillows between legs to avoid adduction.
C. Elevate head (may be limited to 30 to 40 degrees) to avoid acute hip flexion.
D. Introduce quadricep and gluteal setting muscle exercises; encourage use of overhead trapeze for assistance in moving.
E. Take measures to protect patient when moving from bed to chair (patient not to bear weight on affected leg).
F. Provide routine postoperative measures to ensure patient's comfort.
G. Take measures as necessary to prevent complications.

Hip Arthroplasty (Total Hip Replacement)

Definition: Amputation of femoral head with implantation of a steel ball and stem and placement of polyethylene or metal cupin for the acetabulum; its purpose is the alleviation of pain and the restoration of movement for those with osteoarthritis or rheumatoid arthritis.

Postoperative Nursing Care

A. Early nursing care.
  1. Inform patients that they may remain on back for several days or that they may be up and out of bed after one day.
  2. Leg is initially suspended in a Marmar sling with 5 pounds Buck's extension.
  3. Do not make these interventions.
     a. Hyperadduct leg.
     b. Internally rotate leg.
     c. Flex hip more than 60 degrees.
B. Place abduction pillow at site to keep hip in stable position.
C. Elevate head of bed gradually several days after surgery, allowing only minimal flexion of the hip.
D. Monitor dressing and drainage apparatus.
E. Perform routine postoperative nursing actions.
F. Encourage patient to carry out prescribed isometric exercise program (quadricep and gluteal muscle setting), progressing to flexion and extension of hip, knee, and foot by use of a sling with traction apparatus.
G. Inform patient that physical therapist will supervise exercise regimen.

Arthrotomy (Knee Surgery)

Definition: Incision of joint for removal of cartilage.

Nursing Care

A. Encourage and assist with bed exercises.
B. Begin quad setting, straight-leg raising exercises (should be done for five minutes every half hour).
  1. Quad-setting exercises—tightening or contracting the muscles of anterior thigh (knee cap is drawn up toward thigh).
  2. Straight-leg raising—lifting leg straight off the bed, keeping knee extended and foot in neutral position.
C. Encourage and assist with dorsiflexion and plantar flexion of feet and ankles.

D. Apply ice bags to knee to reduce edema as necessary.
E. Help patient out of bed first postoperative day (use three point crutch walking gait without weight-bearing).
F. Give routine postoperative care as necessary.

Total Knee Replacement

Definition: Implantation of a metallic upper portion which substitutes for the femoral condyle and a lower, high polymer plastic, portion which substitutes for the tibial joint surfaces.

Nursing Care

A. Provide quad setting and straight-leg raising exercises every hour.
B. Provide and encourage general bed exercises.
C. Provide cast care as patient usually has a cast or splint.
D. Do not dangle leg; may result in dislocation.
E. Insert hemovac to drain excessive blood and drainage.
  1. Record and measure intake and output accurately.
  2. Observe for hemorrhage and infection.
F. Instruct patient how to walk with crutch.
G. Provide general postoperative care.

Amputation

Definition: Surgical removal of part or all of an extremity; connecting bones may be separated at joint (disarticulation).

Types

A. Closed, or flapped—skin closed over bone end of stump.
B. Open, or guillotine—skin not closed over stump end in order that drainage can occur.

Preoperative Nursing Care

A. Support patient emotionally and listen to patient's expressed concerns regarding limb loss.

B. Help patient strengthen muscles of upper extremity (if lower extremity affected) as preparation for crutch walking.
   1. Extend and flex arms while holding weights.
   2. Do push-ups if condition permits.
C. Inform patient of possible occurrence of phantom pain following surgery. The sensation may last from a few hours to a longer period of time.

Postoperative Nursing Care

⭐A. Delayed fitting of prosthesis.
   1. Observe stump for excessive bleeding (keep tourniquet ready in event of hemorrhage).
      a. Reinforce or change dressing only if ordered.
      b. Observe drainage especially if Penrose drain inserted.
   2. Elevate extremity.
      a. Elevation of bed is preferred.
      b. If pillow used, remove within 48 hours to avoid flexion contracture.
   3. Turn patient to prone position first postoperative day for brief period and gradually increase time.
   4. Exercise all extremities.
   5. Assist with transfer of patient to wheelchair.
   6. Assist with and encourage crutch walking several days postoperatively.
   7. Apply ace bandage properly (avoid tightness while maintaining tension); helps to condition stump.
   8. Observe for signs of depression; listen to patient's expression of feelings.
   9. Encourage physical and psychological progress.
B. Immediate fitting of prosthesis.
   1. Immediate fitting causes less pain and hastens healing.
   2. Immediately following surgery, sterile dressing is applied to stump followed by rigid plastic dressing.
   3. Prosthetic device is attached.

4. If cast falls off, wrap stump immediately with ace bandage and call physician; normally, cast will be changed and reapplied 10 to 14 days postoperatively.
5. Observe for drainage and mark site with pen.
6. Elevate extremity stump for only 24 hours.
7. Assist patient in dangling and walking first day postoperatively (first use parallel bars, then crutches).
8. Be aware that exercises are usually not required because of early ambulation.

Laminectomy

Definition: Removal of posterior arch of vertebrae (lamina) to expose the spinal cord; performed on the cervical or lumbar area of vertebra for removal of spinal cord tumors or herniated disc.

Postoperative Nursing Care

A. Observe neurovascular signs.
B. Monitor dressing for clear or bloody drainage.
C. Place pillow between patient's legs and turn patient from side to side as a unit (log roll) every two hours.
D. Head of bed is usually kept flat for lumbar laminectomy but elevated for cervical laminectomy.
E. Roll patient onto bedpan (as used with fractures), supporting back with pillow.
⭐F. Give assistance in preparation for ambulation.
   1. Turn patient on side.
   2. Reach under shoulder that is resting on bed.
   3. Help raise patient as he or she uses arms to push up from bed.
   4. Help patient swing over edge of bed.
G. Instruct patient in proper movement and position.
   1. Turn as a unit.
   2. Sit with back straight.
   3. When necessary to reach floor with hands, squat and maintain straight back.
H. Give routine postoperative care.

Spinal Fusion

Definition: Removal of bone from iliac crest for fusing with spinal vertebrae.

Postoperative Nursing Care

A. Keep patient supine for first eight hours to reduce possibility of compression if ordered by physician (most physicians order patient to be off back first 48 hours).
B. Monitor both surgical sites.
C. Brace is applied when patient is ambulated; beginning of ambulation varies from three to four days to eight weeks, depending on extent of fusion.
D. Patient is not to lift, bend, stoop, or sit for prolonged periods for at least three months.
   1. Grafts are stable by one year.
   2. Some limitation to flexion of spine, depending on extent of fusion.
E. Provide routine care as for postlaminectomy.

Osteoarthritis

Definition: Degeneration of articular cartilage in the joints resulting from prolonged wear and tear on joint surfaces.

Predisposing Factors

A. Aging.
B. Faulty body posture, joint trauma.
C. Familial tendency.
D. Being female (females more frequently affected than males).
E. Obesity.

Signs and Symptoms

A. Onset usually insidious and gradual.
B. Stiffness of joints.
C. Aching of joints (more noticeable after exercise).
D. Limited joint movement.
E. Nodular bony enlargements on the distal joints of fingers (Heberden's nodes).
F. Occurs usually in hip, knee, vertebra, and finger joints.

Treatment and Nursing Care

A. Arrange for weight reduction if indicated.
B. Provide rest periods; avoid excessive exercise of joints.
C. Apply warm moist packs; give tub baths and paraffin dips.
D. Assist with exercise program to improve posture.
E. Provide range of motion exercises.
F. Administer medications as ordered.
   1. Antiinflammatory drugs, e.g., phenylbutazone, acetylsalicylic acid.
   2. Analgesics, e.g. acetylsalicylic acid.
   3. Corticosteroid intraarticular injections.
G. Be aware of possible need for surgical procedure (synovectomy, arthrodesis, or arthroplasty).
H. Instruct patient in use of proper body mechanics.
I. Advise patient to avoid emotional stress to lessen strain on muscles and joints.
J. Encourage patient to engage in prescribed exercises, to take prescribed medications, and to avoid being overweight.

Rheumatoid Arthritis

Definition: Chronic systemic disease affecting any or all of the body systems and characterized by recurrent inflammation involving the linings of the joints; joint capsule progressively changes and ankylosis occurs. Actual cause is unknown; suspected causes may be an autoimmune disorder or hereditary factors.

Signs and Symptoms

A. Easily fatigued.
B. Loss of weight.
C. Joint pain and stiffness, especially in the morning.

D. Painful and stiff joints that become swollen, reddened, and tender.

E. Subcutaneous nodules over bony prominences.

F. Anemia.

G. Periods of remission and exacerbation.

Treatment and Nursing Care

A. Encourage adequate rest periods; extent of rest depends on current status of disease.

1. During day as necessary.

2. Use of firm mattress and no pillows; improper positioning of joints can result in contracture.

3. Use of splints for supporting joints.

4. Relief from emotional stress.

B. Administer medications as ordered.

1. Antiinflammatory analgesics (see osteoarthritis medications).

2. Corticosteroids, e.g., prednisone.

3. Intraarticular corticosteroid injections into joint.

4. Gold salts.

C. Apply moist heat, i.e., baths, packs, paraffin dips.

D. Encourage exercise of joints within limits of tolerance.

E. Be aware of possible need for surgery (see osteroarthritis).

F. Discuss aspects of the disease with the patient in a realistic and optimistic manner.

G. Assist patient in maintaining independence.

H. Advise patient to call on physician for any problems; caution against promises for quick cures, whatever the source.

Osteoporosis

Definition: Decrease in the amount of bone capable of maintaining structural integrity of the skeleton. Etiology is unknown.

Signs and Symptoms

A. Backache with pain radiating around trunk.

B. Skeletal deformities.

C. Pathologic fractures.

D. Lab findings.

1. Serum calcium, phosphorus and alkaline phosphatase are usually normal.

2. Parathyroid hormone may be elevated.

Treatment and Nursing Care

A. Provide pain control.

B. Prevent fractures.

1. Instruct in safety factors—watch steps, avoid use of scatter rugs.

2. Keep side rails up to prevent falls.

3. Move gently when turning and positioning.

4. Assist with ambulation if unsteady on feet.

C. Administer medications as ordered.

1. Estrogen—decreases rate of bone resorption.

2. Calcium and vitamin D—support bone metabolism.

D. Instruct in regular exercise program.

1. Range-of-motion exercises.

2. Ambulation several times per day.

E. Instruct in good use of body mechanics.

F. Provide diet high in protein, calcium, vitamin D.

Oncology Nursing

Oncology is the area of nursing that focuses on the patient with cancer. Cancer is the second leading cause of death in the United States. As such, it is an area that will demand more nursing care and involvement in the future. This section focuses on the concepts of oncology nursing.

Neoplastic Diseases

Definition: Cancer is a group of neoplastic diseases in which there is a new growth of abnormal cells.

Characteristics

A. Etiology.
  1. Unknown.
  2. Environmental factors (50 to 80 percent of cases).
  3. Biological factors.
  4. Heredity.
  5. Theory—caused by a virus.
B. Pathophysiology.
  1. Cell growth is unregulated, and cell division is uncontrolled.
  2. Cells reproduce and divide more quickly than normal cells until a tumor mass is formed.
  3. Tumors grow in a disorganized fashion, interrupting bodily function.
  4. Malignant cells spread by:
    a. Direct extension.
    b. Metastasis through blood and lymph circulation and body fluid diffusion.
C. Classification of cancers.
  1. Classed according to type of tissue from which they evolve.
    a. Carcinomas.
      (1) Begin in epithelial tissue.
      (2) Example: skin, mucous membrane.
    b. Sarcomas.
      (1) Begin in nonepithelial tissue.
      (2) Example: bone, muscle, fat, lymph system.
  2. Type of cell in which they arise.
    a. Cell type affects appearance, rate of growth and degree of malignancy.
    b. Examples.
      (1) Basal cell carcinomas.
      (2) Melanoma.
      (3) Lymphoma.
D. Staging.
  1. Describes extent of tumor.
  2. Basic components.
    a. T: primary tumor.
    b. N: regional nodes.
    c. M: metastasis.
  3. Describe extent to which malignancy has increased in size.
  4. Involvement of regional nodes.
  5. Metastatic development.

Comparison of Benign and Malignant Tumors

	Malignant	Benign
Cell type	Abnormal from those of original tissues	Close to those of original tissues
Growth	Rapid; infiltrates surrounding tissue in all directions	Slow and noninfiltrating
Encapsulated	Infrequent	Frequent
Metastasis	Through blood, lymph, to new tumor sites	None
Effect	Terminal without treatment	Can become malignant or obstruct vital organs

Assessment

A. Diagnostic tests.
  1. Annual pap smear.
  2. Annual colon-rectum exam for patients over 40 years.
  3. Annual chest x-ray.
  4. Annual examination of mouth and teeth.
  5. Annual physical exam, including urine and blood work.
  6. Monthly breast self-exam.

B. Risk factors.
  1. Smoking.
  2. Excessive exposure to sunlight.
  3. Excessive exposure to certain chemicals.
C. Warning signs.
  1. Open sore or wound that does not heal.
  2. Indigestion or difficulty swallowing.
  3. Change in normal bowel or bladder habits.
  4. Changes in moles or warts.
  5. Unusual bleeding or discharge.
  6. Thickening or lump in breast or other tissue.
  7. Nagging cough or hoarseness.

Radiation Therapy

Characteristics

A. Categories
  1. Curative (primary treatment for Hodgkin's disease).
  2. Palliative (reduces pain from breast tumor).
  3. Adjunctive therapy (used with surgery and/or chemotherapy).
B. Types.
  1. External: gamma rays, cobalt, linear accelerater, delivered via machine to lesion on body.
  2. Internal: isotope placed into a body cavity or interstitially; cellular DNA is the target.
C. Side effects.
  1. Severe nausea and vomiting.
  2. Diarrhea.
  3. Hematuria.
  4. Anemia.
  5. Skin: scaling and dryness; "wet" reaction.
  6. Hair loss (alopecia).
D. Precautions to excessive exposure of internal radiation.
  1. Distance.
    a. Work as far away from source as possible.
    b. Intensity of radiation decreases rapidly the further away from source.
  2. Shielding.
    a. Lead shield—keep between source and staff.
    b. Radioactivity material stored in lead-shielded container when not in use.
    c. Do not touch radioactive material with hand.
  3. Time.
    a. Work efficiently.
    b. Review procedures before beginning them.
    c. Trade-off between distance and time (the further away from source, the more time that can be spent around source).

Nursing Care

A. External radiation.
  1. Offer psychological support.
  2. Educate patient.
    a. What to expect from treatment.
    b. Explanation of radiotherapy room.
    c. Possible side effects and ways to minimize them.
  3. Encourage diet: high protein, high carbohydrate, fat free, and low residue.
    a. Foods to avoid: tough, fibrous meat; poultry; shrimp; all cheeses (except soft); coarse bread; raw vegetables; irritating spices.
    b. Foods allowed: soft-cooked eggs, ground meat, pureed vegetables, milk, cooked cereal.
    c. Increase fluids.
    d. Diet supplement to increase calorie and fluid intake.
    e. Do not eat several hours before treatment.
  4. Administer medications.
    a. Compazine—nausea.
    b. Lomotil—diarrhea.
  5. Provide skin care—radiodermatitis may occur three to six weeks after start of treatment.
    a. Avoid creams, lotions, perfume to irradiated areas.
    b. Wash and lukewarm water, pat dry (some physicians allow mild soap).
    c. Avoid exposure to sunlight or artificial

heat such as heating pad.

   d. Baby oil may be ordered t.i.d.

⭐B. Internal radiation.

1. Maintain bedrest when radiation source in place.

2. Restrict movement to prevent dislodging radiation source.

3. Position patient except on back (when cesium needle in tongue or cervix).

4. Administer range-of-motion exercise q.i.d.

5. Avoid direct contact around implant site; avoid washing areas, etc.

6. Take vital signs every four hours (report temperature over 100°F).

7. Observe for dehydration or G.I. tract changes.

8. Observe and report skin eruption, discharge, abnormal bleeding.

9. Provide clear liquid diet (low residue is sometimes ordered) and urge fluids.

10. Insert Teflon Foley catheter (radiation decomposes rubber) to avoid necessity of bedpan.

11. Observe frequently for dislodging of radiation source (especially linen and dressings).

12. If radiation source falls out:

   a. Do not touch with hands.

   b. Pick up source with foot-long applicator.

   c. Put source in lead container and call physician.

   d. If unable to locate source, call physician immediately and bar visitors from room.

13. After source removed:

   a. Administer Betadine douche if ordered following cervical implant.

   b. Give Fleet Enema, if ordered.

   c. Patient may be out of bed.

   d. Avoid direct sunlight to radiation areas.

   e. Apply cream to relieve dryness or itching.

   f. Patient may resume sexual intercourse within seven to ten days.

   g. Notify physician if nausea, vomiting, diarrhea, frequent urination or bowel movements, or temperature above 100°F is present.

Chemotherapy

Characteristics

A. Purpose.

1. Interferes with cell doublings.

2. Destroys all cancer cells.

B. Action.

1. Damages cells only during process of dividing.

2. To eradicate malignant tumor, large doses are administered or treatment started when the number of cells is small enough to allow tumor destruction.

3. Used in conjunction with surgery and/or radiotherapy early in disease process.

4. Combination of antineoplastic drugs frequently used for synergistic effect.

5. Sequential antineoplastic therapy may be used, particularly with remissions.

C. Factors for deciding dosage and timing of drugs.

1. Dosage calculated on body surface area and kilograms of body weight.

2. Time lapse between doses to allow recovery of normal cells.

3. Side effects of each drug and when they are likely to occur.

4. Liver and kidney function, as most antineoplastics are metabolized in one of these organs.

D. Common side effects.

1. Damage to rapidly growing normal cells.

   a. Bone marrow (most serious damage).

     (1) Infection.

     (2) Abnormal bleeding.

   b. Hair follicles—alopecia.

   c. Mucus lining of gastrointestinal tract.

     (1) Nausea, vomiting, anorexia.

     (2) Fluid and electrolyte imbalances.

     (3) Dietary deficiency.

     (4) Stomatitis.

2. Elevated uric acid and crystal and urate stone formation.
3. Time of most severe depression of cells (termed nadir); different for each type of cell.
4. Chemotherapeutics—have specific side effects in addition to these.

E. Classification of chemotherapeutic agents.
1. Alkylating agents: nitrogen mustard, cyclophosphamide.
2. Antimetabolites: 5-FU, methotrexate.
3. Antibiotics: Adriamycin, Bleomycin, Dactinomycin.
4. Plant alkaloids (antimitotics): vincristine, vinblastine.
5. Hormones: estrogens, progesterones.
6. Miscellaneous: procarbazine, cis-Platinum.

Nursing Care

A. Minimize scalp hair loss by tourniquet application around scalp during IV administration and for 15 minutes after dose.

B. Observe frequently for signs of bleeding or infection.
C. Provide emotional support for alteration in body image or grieving process.
D. Administer IV dose slowly to prevent toxic effects.
E. Discontinue IV administration of drug to prevent tissue damage if extravasation occurs.
F. Maintain intake and output to observe kidney function.
G. Urge fluids to increase uric acid excretion and decrease crystal and urate stone formation.
H. Administer allopurinol to lower uric acid.
I. Provide small, frequent meals with nutritious snacks with main meal early in morning.
J. Provide high calorie dietary supplements.
K. Provide frequent oral hygiene to decrease severity of stomatitis.
L. Diet for diarrhea: bland, low residue, high in constipating food.
M. Avoid exposure to infected persons. (Patient is more susceptible to infection.)

Review Questions

1. Angina pectoris is caused by which one of the following?

    A. Inadequate cardiac output.
    B. Too much physical activity.
    C. Increased cardiac output.
    D. Inadequate supply of oxygen to myocardium.

2. Nitroglycerin is given sublingually because

    A. Superficial blood vessels promote rapid absorption.
    B. They are excreted in the gastrointestinal tract.
    C. In all cases dyspnea is present.
    D. They are too rapidly absorbed in the gastric area.

3. Severe pruritus is a common symptom of Hodgkin's disease. Pruritus means

    A. Enlarged liver.
    B. Enlarged spleen.
    C. Inflamed gums.
    D. Itching.

4. Which of the following drugs is a steroid and used in the treatment of a patient with acute leukemia?

    A. Prednisone.
    B. Cytoxan.
    C. Nitrogen mustard.
    D. Leukeran.

5. Jill Adams, a twenty-one-year-old patient, is admitted to the hospital with the diagnosis of possible brain tumor. Soon after admission, Jill has a grand mal seizure. Which one of the following interventions would you carry out?

    A. Call the doctor immediately.
    B. Restrain the patient to prevent injury.
    C. Record the type of muscular activity involved in the seizure.
    D. Place tongue blade between teeth, by force if necessary.

6. The presence of which of the following reflexes is the most important indicator of neurological pathology?

    A. Homan's.
    B. Babinski.
    C. Gag.
    D. Moro.

7. The doctor schedules Jill for a craniotomy and orders a neurological exam. Which of the following is *not* a common preoperative procedure for a patient scheduled for a craniotomy?

    A. Good mouth care.
    B. Cleansing enema.
    C. Complete bath including shampoo.
    D. Quiet, nonstimulating environment.

8. A neurological exam or craniocerebral test does *not* include which of the following?

    A. Hand grip or strength of extremities.
    B. Movement of legs.
    C. Level of consciousness.
    D. Pulse deficit.

9. Postoperative nursing care for Jill will include

    A. Placing her in Trendelenburg's position.
    B. Administering morphine sulfate for pain.
    C. Restraining her with posey belt and soft wrist restraints.
    D. Recording rectal temperatures frequently.

10. Jill develops increased intracranial pressure. Which of the following is *not* indicative of intracranial pressure?

    A. Vomiting.
    B. Increased blood pressure.
    C. Decreased pulse rate.
    D. Agitation.

11. Which one of the following measures would *not* be effective for preventing increased intracranial pressure?

    A. Administration of hypotonic IV solutions.
    B. Restricting intake to 1200 cc per day.
    C. Administering osmotic diuretics, such as mannitol.
    D. Administering corticosteroids, such as Decadron.

12. Which one of the following instructions in the use of tissues is correct?

    A. Wash hands after use.
    B. Cover nose and mouth.
    C. Dispose of tissue after use.
    D. All of these.

13. Which one of the following would help to ease dyspnea?

    A. Elevate the head of the bed.
    B. Keep patient warm.
    C. Keep mouth moist.
    D. Turn on side.

R 14. Care for a patient following a bronchoscopy will include

   A. Withholding food and liquids until the gag reflex returns.
   B. Providing throat irrigations every four hours.
   C. Having patient refrain from talking for several days.
   D. All of these.

R 15. The examination in which a special instrument is inserted into the trachea and major bronchi for direct visualization is called a

   A. Chest x-ray.
   B. Bronchography.
   C. Bronchoscopy.
   D. Thoracentesis.

G 16. Mrs. Thompson, a housewife, consulted her doctor because of fatigue, weight loss, anorexia with nausea, constipation, and occasionally a small amount of blood in her stools. The doctor orders an upper GI series and a barium enema. Mrs. Thompson is very anxious. The nurse reassures her and tries to relieve her anxiety by

   A. Asking the dietician to explain the diet.
   B. Diverting Mrs. Thompson's attention by discussing television.
   C. Asking Mrs. Thompson why she dreads the examinations.
   D. Telling Mrs. Thompson not to worry because the x-ray department does these every day.

G 17. The primary purpose of an upper GI series is to

   A. Visualize the gallbladder.
   B. Determine the necessity of surgery.
   C. Study the structure and function of the upper digestive tract.
   D. Diagnose cancer of the transverse colon.

G 18. That evening you collect a stool specimen for occult blood. The specimen

   A. Is collected in a sterile container.
   B. Must fill the container.
   C. Requires only a small amount and a clean container.
   D. Cannot be collected until the patient has had an enema.

G 19. After barium studies, constipation must be avoided. The common complaints of a patient suffering from constipation include all of the following *except*

   A. Anal irritation.
   B. Anorexia.
   C. Abdominal distention.
   D. Nausea.

G 20. Because these studies might be inconclusive, the physician scheduled a sigmoidoscopy before the barium studies. The purpose of this exam is to

   A. Visualize the lower portion of the colon.
   B. Administer steroids.
   C. Examine external hemorrhoids.
   D. Visualize the ascending colon.

G 21. It was decided that Mrs. Thompson might have a malignancy, and surgery was indicated. Neomycin is administered preoperatively to

   A. Prevent infection postoperatively.
   B. Eliminate the need for preoperative enemas.
   C. Decrease and retard the growth of normal bacteria in the intestines.
   D. Treat cancer of the colon.

22. The surgical procedure confirmed carcinoma of the colon. Mrs. Thompson returned from surgery with which one of the following procedures?

   A. Permanent colostomy.
   B. Ileostomy.
   C. Temporary colostomy.
   D. Gastrostomy.

23. After she recovers, but before dismissal, Mrs. Thompson will be taught all of the following *except*

   A. Care of her colostomy.
   B. How to give her own narcotics daily.
   C. To avoid foods that have previously caused diarrhea or gas.
   D. The necessity of continuing medical supervision.

24. When Mrs. Thompson developed dyspepsia, the nurse selected an antacid from prn meds because antacids

   A. Relieve epigastric pain.
   B. Neutralize stomach acid, thereby relieving the discomfort.
   C. Will prevent vomiting that often follows indigestion.
   D. Relieve anxiety.

H 25. A myocardial infarction results from

   A. Critical reduction in blood supply to myocardium.
   B. Marked increase in cardiac output.
   C. Sudden irregularity of cardiac contraction.
   D. Marked decrease in cardiac output.

H 26. Oxygen therapy may be ordered for a patient with myocardial infarction to

   A. Minimize the extent of myocardial necrosis.
   B. Increase cardiac output.
   C. Decrease cardiac output.
   D. Dilate coronary blood vessels.

27. A soft diet is often ordered for a patient with myocardial infarction. The purpose of this soft diet is to

    A. Minimize the effort of mastication and digestion.
    B. Enhance elimination.
    C. Add to the palatability of the diet.
    D. Reduce the caloric intake.

28. Anticoagulants are ordered for patients with myocardial infarction to

    A. Relieve pain from myocardial damage.
    B. Prevent extension of a coronary thrombus.
    C. Improve coronary circulation.
    D. Improve cardiac output.

29. Phlebotomy is used to treat which one of these disorders?

    A. Ruptured spleen.
    B. Acute leukemia.
    C. Polycythemia vera.
    D. Hodgkin's disease.

30. Gamma globulin in blood plasma is an example of which of the following?

    A. An organic salt.
    B. A protein.
    C. A hormone.
    D. An enzyme.

31. The use of reverse isolation to prevent infections is often used as a nursing measure for a patient with

    A. Pernicious anemia.
    B. Ruptured spleen.
    C. Hepatomegaly.
    D. Acute leukemia.

32. Mr. Schmidt, a thirty-five-year-old patient, has routine testing daily for urine sugar and acetone. The practical nurse will realize that the patient probably has

    A. Urinary tract infection.
    B. Diabetes mellitus.
    C. Pyelonephritis.
    D. Prostatic hypertrophy.

33. When the charge nurse asked if the specimen was fresh, the practical nurse would have replied,

    A. "Yes, he voided as soon as he awakened this morning."
    B. "No, but he hadn't eaten since he voided."
    C. "I followed the double voiding collection procedure."
    D. "Yes, because I collected a midstream specimen."

34. When it was discovered that Mr. Schmidt did indeed have a urinary tract infection, the vocational nurse

realized adequate fluid intake would be essential, especially if which of the following drugs was ordered?

    A. Analgesics to relieve the pain.
    B. Sulfonamides to combat the infection.
    C. Opiate derivatives to relieve the bladder spasm.
    D. Tranquilizers to relieve the anxiety.

35. During any infectious process within the body, the increase of the white blood cells is identified as

    A. Leucocytosis.
    B. Histoplasmosis.
    C. Phagocytosis.
    D. Erythropoiesis.

36. Prolonged bed rest, as is sometimes required, increases the incidence of which of the following complications due to urinary stasis?

    A. Urolithiasis and cystitis.
    B. Pyelitis.
    C. Addison's disease.
    D. Renal failure.

37. If renal failure occurs, the vocational nurse will realize that one form of treatment now available is

    A. Paracentesis.
    B. Nephrostomy.
    C. Hemodialysis.
    D. Cystostomy.

38. The outermost layer of the integumentary system is

    A. Melanin.
    B. Dermis.
    C. Epidermis.
    D. Subcutaneous.

39. It is important to maintain the normal pH of the skin in order to

    A. Retard bacterial growth.
    B. Maintain the body's acid-base balance.
    C. Facilitate repair of tissue cells.
    D. Accomplish all of these.

40. Acromegaly is due to an

    A. Oversecretion of growth hormone in a child.
    B. Oversecretion of growth hormone in an adult.
    C. Undersecretion of growth hormone in an adult.
    D. Undersecretion of growth hormone in a child.

41. Mr. Adams has severe diabetes insipidus. You would expect Mr. Adams's urine to have a specific gravity of

    A. -1.000.
    B. 1.001-1.005.
    C. 1.010-1.015
    D. 1.020 and over.

42. The drug of choice in diabetes insipidus is

   A. ACTH.
   B. Diabinese.
   C. Vasopressin.
   D. Dessicated thyroid.

43. Your neighbor's husband, Mr. Thomas, has fallen down the basement steps and suspects a fracture of the lower leg. Fracture is best defined as

   A. The manipulation of a bone.
   B. A break in the continuity of the bone.
   C. A break in the skin over a bone.
   D. A bending of the bone.

44. Which of the following symptoms would *not* indicate the possibility of a fracture of Mr. Thomas's leg?

   A. Deformity of the part.
   B. Pain and muscle spasm.
   C. Loss of function.
   D. Foul odor.

45. Mr. Thomas sees a doctor who confirms that his leg is fractured. The doctor hospitalizes Mr. Thomas and applies a leg cast. The nurse should check Mr. Thomas's toes for

   A. Change in temperature.
   B. Change in color.
   C. Edema.
   D. All of the above.

46. Mr. Thomas is unable to feel you apply pressure on his toes and complains of tingling. These signs would indicate

   A. Pressure on a nerve.
   B. Phantom pain syndrome.
   C. Overmedication of an analgesic.
   D. Improper alignment of the fracture.

47. A wet cast should be

   A. Placed on a firm surface.
   B. Handled only with the palms of the hands.
   C. Dry in 3 to 4 hours.
   D. Petaled to lessen chance of irritation to the patient.

48. Isophageal varices are frequently a complication associated with cirrhosis of the liver. Which one of the following statements is *not* true about this condition?

   A. The veins of the esophagus and stomach are distended, and this results in large amounts of blood being vomited when varices rupture.
   B. Associated dilated veins can also be found in the anal area in the form of hemorrhoids.

   C. Hemorrhage can be controlled by administering large amounts of vitamin K.
   D. The condition is often associated with alcoholism.

49. The usual treatment of choice for patients with esophageal varices is

   A. Placement of a Miller-Abbott tube.
   B. Placement of a Levin tube.
   C. Placement of a Sengstaken-Blakemore tube.
   D. Placement of a Johnston tube.

50. John Petry was admitted to the hospital with a head injury incurred when he fell off a ladder. John's restlessness is probably caused by

   A. Decreased ocular pressure.
   B. Cerebral anoxia.
   C. Dehydration.
   D. Decreased pain sensation.

51. John developed increased intracranial pressure due to a blood clot at the injury site. Which one of the following clinical manifestations is *not* indicative of increased intracranial pressure?

   A. Pulse rate of 56.
   B. Respiratory rate of 10 and irregular.
   C. Blood pressure 100/80.
   D. Temperature 100°F orally.

52. John is placed on several intravenous medications postoperatively. Which one of the following would least likely be ordered?

   A. Mannitol.
   B. Solu-Cortef.
   C. Dilantin.
   D. Glucagon.

53. Which one of these is a major objective of dermatological nursing?

   A. Reverse the inflammatory process if present.
   B. Prevent secondary infections.
   C. Prevent damage to healthy skin.
   D. All of the above.

54. Which of the following statements best describes a guiding principle in treating dermatoses?

   A. It is better to leave the skin alone than to experiment with several interventions.
   B. Use heat for the first twenty-four hours; then apply tepid compresses.
   C. Debridement of pustules is essential before applying a topical substance.
   D. Irritants frequently are valuable to produce erythema and an increased blood supply.

55. Judy Moore is a twenty-seven-year-old housewife and mother of two with a diagnosis of pneumococcal pneumonia. She has been ill for four days. Pneumonia is defined as

    A. Distention of the alveoli.
    B. Inflammation of the pleura.
    C. Constriction of the bronchi.
    D. Inflammation of the tissues of the lungs.

56. When giving the nursing care for Mrs. Moore, the nurse should remember that one of the most important aims in the treatment of pneumonia is

    A. Keeping the patient clean.
    B. Administering laxatives.
    C. Conserving the patient's energy.
    D. Explaining the nursing procedures.

57. Care must be taken when handling nasal and bronchial secretions from Mrs. Moore because

    A. Bloody sputum will be present.
    B. These secretions are contagious.
    C. The sight may be upsetting to the patient.
    D. The patient may be running an elevated temperature.

58. When instructing Mrs. Moore in the proper method of disposing of used tissues, the nurse would explain to place the tissues in

    A. A waste basket conveniently located.
    B. The bed pan.
    C. An emesis basin near the bed.
    D. A cuffed paper bag.

59. Mrs. Santell, eighty-two years old, was admitted to the hospital with a fractured hip. The doctor places her in Buck's traction to help reduce the fracture. This type of traction is known as

    A. Skeletal.
    B. Skin.
    C. Balanced suspension.
    D. Overhead.

60. When checking the traction apparatus, the nurse should make which of the following observations?

    A. Check that the weights are hanging free.
    B. Check that the rope is on the pulley.
    C. Check that the foot plate is not resting against the pulley.
    D. All of the above.

61. Mrs. Santell has an open reduction with fixation by the use of a nail. Postoperatively, the nursing interventions include all of the following except

    A. Avoid acute hip flexion.
    B. Elevate affected leg to avoid edema.

    C. Encourage patient to use overhead trapeze when moving.
    D. Encourage patient to perform quadriceps exercises.

62. Nursing interventions for the patient in skeletal traction would include all of the following except

    A. Observing the pin site for inflammation.
    B. Providing isotonic exercises of unaffected extremities.
    C. Performing a neurovascular check.
    D. Giving the patient a bath each day.

63. Jack Johnson was admitted to the hospital with ulcerative colitis. He has had the disease for eight years. He had been poorly controlled on a medical regime and is now scheduled for surgical correction. The usual surgical intervention of ulcerative colitis is

    A. Ureterostomy.
    B. Ileostomy.
    C. Abdominal perineal resection.
    D. Ureteroileostomy.

64. Mr. Johnson's symptoms include all of the following except

    A. Abdominal cramping.
    B. Constipation.
    C. Fever.
    D. Bloody diarrhea.

65. Preoperatively, his diet will consist of which one of the following diet regimes?

    A. Bland, high residue, high protein diet.
    B. Bland, low residue, high protein diet.
    C. Bland, low residue, low protein diet.
    D. Bland, high residue, low fat diet.

66. Postoperatively, Mr. Johnson's nursing care will include all of the following interventions except

    A. Daily stoma irrigations.
    B. Appliance secured closely around stoma.
    C. Good skin care around stoma.
    D. Force fluids.

67. Ms. Jones is being admitted to your medical-surgical unit. She has Addison's disease, has been taking her medications as ordered, and is scheduled for a bilateral adrenalectomy. To which of the following patients' rooms would it be inappropriate to assign Ms. Jones?

    A. Ms. R., a forty-five-year-old female, five days postoperative gastrectomy.
    B. Ms. S., a thirty-four-year-old female, ten days postoperative craniotomy.

C. Ms. T., a fifty-eight-year-old female, diabetic, admitted yesterday, leg ulcer with drainage (culture and sensitivity not reported yet).

D. Ms. U., a thirty-year-old female, with breast cancer.

68. Common symptoms associated with Addison's disease include

A. Generalized weakness, increased pigmentation of the skin, hypotension, and emotional disturbances.

B. Buffalo hump, weight gain, and striae of the skin.

C. Hyperglycemia, increased frequency of infections, and polyuria.

D. Grotesque appearance, increased oiliness of skin and hair, headaches, and impotence.

69. Mr. Brown is a thirty-five-year-old patient with an admitting diagnosis of head injury following an auto accident. What is the most sensitive indication of a patient's clinical condition following a head injury?

A. Pupillary changes.

B. Level of consciousness.

C. Blood pressure and pulse.

D. Motor function.

70. Which vital sign is the most sensitive index of increasing intracranial pressure?

A. Pulse.

B. Blood pressure.

C. Respiration.

D. Temperature.

71. Mr. Brown has all of the following needs, but which one should receive first priority?

A. Control of pain and restlessness.

B. Maintenance of open airway.

C. Maintenance of fluid-electrolyte balance.

D. Monitoring of neurological status, including vital signs.

72. Mr. Brown is complaining of a severe headache and demonstrates nuchal rigidity and Kernig's sign. Which complication is most likely?

A. Subdural hemorrhage.

B. Increased intracranial pressure.

C. Shock.

D. Subarachnoid hemorrhage.

73. The follicle-stimulating hormone (FSH) and the luteinizing hormone (LH) are

A. Corticotropic.

B. Gonadotropic.

C. Somatotropic.

D. Adrenotropic.

74. Which one of these hormones is *not* produced by the posterior lobe of the pituitary?

A. Oxytocin.

B. Vasopressin.

C. Adrenocorticotropic (ACTH).

D. All are produced by the pituitary.

75. The so-called master gland is the

A. Parathyroid.

B. Thyroid.

C. Adrenal.

D. Pituitary.

76. A primary objective of treatment for patients with congestive heart failure is to

A. Reduce the workload of the heart.

B. Promote rest for the heart.

C. Reduce fluid retention.

D. Reduce circulating blood volume.

77. The dyspnea associated with left-sided heart failure is due to

A. Accumulation of fluid in the alveoli.

B. Obstruction in the lungs by mucus.

C. Compression of the lungs by an enlarged heart.

D. Accumulation of blood in the left atrium.

78. A nursing measure utilized to relieve dyspnea associated with congestive heart failure is to place the patient in which one of the following positions?

A. Supine.

B. Trendelenburg's.

C. Reverse Trendelenburg's.

D. Fowler's.

79. Pulmonary edema is due to failure of the

A. Right atrium.

B. Left atrium.

C. Right ventricle.

D. Left ventricle.

80. The purpose of applying rotating tourniquets in the presence of pulmonary edema is to

A. Reduce the workload of the lungs.

B. Contain blood volume within the vital organs.

C. Reduce the workload of the heart.

D. Reduce peripheral arterial stasis.

81. Nursing measures for the patient with rotating tourniquets include

A. Rotate tourniquets every 30 minutes.

B. Remove all tourniquets once every hour.

C. Diagram tourniquet rotation.

D. All of the above.

82. Which of these is the technical term for "red blood cell"?

A. Leukocyte.
B. Thrombocyte.
C. Erythrocyte.
D. Lymphocyte.

83. Mr. Raggers was admitted to the hospital with a diagnosis of acute glomerulonephritis. His symptoms were mild and consisted of fatigue, anorexia, mild hypertension, and a slight edema of the extremities. Mr. Raggers had had a routine physical examination as part of a company program to keep their executives in good health. Acute glomerulonephritis was suspected after the results came back from which of the following tests?

A. Blood workup.
B. Routine urinalysis.
C. Blood pressure and vital signs.
D. Renal biopsy.

84. One of the primary objectives of treatment for Mr. Raggers's illness would be to

A. Restore fluid and electrolyte balance.
B. Encourage bed rest during the acute phase.
C. Give high protein diet to restore nutritional status.
D. Treat hypertension.

85. Mr. Raggers's condition suddenly worsens, and renal failure is suspected. All of the following symptoms would be present *except*

A. Hypertension.
B. Proteinuria.
C. Hypotension.
D. Oliguria.

86. Mr. Raggers is put on Lasix. The main action of this drug is to

A. Decrease blood flow to the renal cortex.
B. Increase intrarenal vascular resistance.
C. Prevent infection.
D. Increase the production of urine.

87. Mr. Raggers is put on a special diet. The main objective of diet control during the acute stage of renal failure is to

A. Increase the sodium intake to retain body fluids.
B. Reduce calories since the patient is on bed rest.
C. Reduce protein due to decreased ability of the kidney to filter.
D. Increase protein to encourage healing.

88. In addition to intake and output, which one of the following procedures is routine for patients with acute glomerulonephritis?

A. Fasting blood sugars.
B. Daily urinalysis.
C. Daily weight.
D. Warm, soapy baths twice daily.

89. Mrs. Stansell, a mother of four and thirty-eight years old, is admitted to the hospital. She is obese with complaints of fever, malaise, nausea, vomiting, and right upper quadrant tenderness. Realizing the patient is jaundiced, the practical nurse recognizes the need for

A. Taking enteric precautions until diagnosis is confirmed.
B. Keeping the patient sedated.
C. Restricting oral fluids containing milk.
D. Postponing application for insurance until diagnosis is confirmed.

90. The practical nurse knows that jaundice can be related to biliary obstruction and expects that

A. Carbohydrates will be limited.
B. Fatty foods will be restricted.
C. Juices will be avoided.
D. Patient will be managed with parenteral fluids for one week.

91. When the patient remarks that there has never been any gallbladder disease in her family, the nurse's best reply would be to tell the patient that

A. This condition is usually inherited.
B. This condition has a higher incidence in overweight, early middle-aged females who have had children.
C. This disease occurs only once.
D. It is extremely important to tell the physician the family history.

92. Mr. Moran is thrown from a car during a traffic accident. He appears to be paralyzed from the waist down. The *first* emergency measure to be taken at the scene of the accident is to

A. Check for hemorrhage and stop it.
B. Open airway and maintain it.
C. Check for paralysis and attempt to prevent it.
D. None of these.

93. On admission he is moved from the ambulance stretcher to a bed. Moving the patient is done carefully to

A. Avoid hemorrhage of internal organs.
B. Maintain an adequate airway.
C. Prevent possible further injury to spinal cord.
D. Provide reduction of any fractures.

94. A patient has been admitted with a diagnosis of severe hyperthyroidism. Which aspect of nursing care do you anticipate will be the most difficult?

A. Adequate rest.
B. Eye care.
C. Diet.
D. Skin care.

95. Exophthalmos, a symptom of hyperthyroidism, is

A. Perspiration.
B. Belching.
C. Bulging eyes.
D. None of these.

96. A common postoperative complication of thyroidectomy is

A. Pineal damage.
B. Facial nerve damage.
C. Hypercalcemia.
D. Respiratory distress.

97. Mr. Robert Jarvis is a thirty-five-year-old insurance salesman. He was admitted to the nursing unit four hours ago with a diagnosis of asthma. The primary cause of asthma is thought to be

A. Viral infection.
B. Bacterial infection.
C. Allergy to a certain substance.
D. Lack of proper nutrition.

98. The characteristic symptom of asthma is

A. Flushed skin.
B. Wheezing type of respiration.
C. Hemoptysis.
D. Chest pain.

99. Which of the following types of medication would probably be ordered for Mr. Jarvis?

A. Bronchodilators.
B. Analgesics.
C. Antipyretics.
D. Antibiotics.

100. When caring for Mr. Jarvis, the nurse should remember to

A. Check temperature frequently.
B. Limit fluid intake.
C. Increase fluid intake.
D. Remain calm and supportive.

101. The following are all characteristics of osteoarthritis *except*

A. It is found mostly in the aging obese person.
B. It is thought to be an autoimmune disease.
C. Joints are stiff.
D. Onset is slow and gradual.

102. Some comfort measures for persons with osteoarthritis include

A. Applying warm, moist packs to joints.
B. Undertaking exercises that provide stress to muscles.
C. Wearing a copper bracelet to lessen pain.
D. Using a soft mattress to ease pain.

103. Arthroplasty of the hip can be used as a treatment for osteoarthritis. This procedure is

A. Fixation of the joint.
B. Replacement of the femoral head and acetabulum with metal and plastic.
C. Replacement of the femoral head with a metal prosthesis.
D. Amputation of the head and neck of the femur.

104. Postoperative nursing interventions for the patient with a hip arthroplasty include

A. Observe the dressing and hemovac for amount of drainage.
B. See that abduction of the affected hip is maintained.
C. Avoid acute flexion of the hip.
D. All of the above.

105. Acetylsalicylic acid is helpful to people with osteoarthritis because of what type of action?

A. Analgesic.
B. Antipyretic.
C. Adrenergic blocking.
D. Antispasmodic.

106. Eczema is caused by

A. A cancer cell.
B. An allergy.
C. A pathogen.
D. None of the above.

107. Which one of the following activities is contraindicated in infantile eczema?

A. Have child vaccinated to prevent childhood diseases.
B. Cover hands and feet with cotton materials.
C. Apply open wet dressings or corn starch paste.
D. Adhere strictly to elimination diet.

108. Miss Carson has been unconscious for several days. The doctor states that her brain is bruised. This condition would be called

A. Concussion.
B. Contusion.
C. Skull fracture.
D. Convulsion.

109. Miss Carson develops an elevated temperature. The doctor orders alcohol and water sponge and the drug chlorpromazine. The best rationale for administering this medication is to

    A. Reduce restlessness and pain.
    B. Control shivering.
    C. Lower temperature.
    D. Prevent vomiting.

110. Mrs. Olsen was admitted for a gastric resection as treatment for duodenal ulcer. Which of the following observations of her pain pattern will be included in your nursing assessment?

    A. Pain is constant over epigastric area when eating.
    B. Pain is experienced about two to three hours after eating.
    C. Pain occurs about one-half hour after eating.
    D. There is no correlation between food intake and pain.

111. Your nursing assessment should include observations for possible complications associated with duodenal ulcer disease. Which one of the following manifestations would *not* be indicative of this type of complication?

    A. Pain radiating to scapular area.
    B. Hematemesis.
    C. Bright-red bloody stools.
    D. Tarry stools.

112. Instructions to a patient receiving preoperative atropine would include the fact that

    A. He might experience ringing in his ears.
    B. He will become drowsy.
    C. His mouth will feel dry.
    D. His pain will be decreased.

113. Anticholinergic drugs are used to treat patients with gastric ulcer disease. Which one of the following pharmacological actions is *not* true in relation to anticholinergic drugs?

    A. They decrease gastric emptying.
    B. They suppress gastric secretions.
    C. They block the effects of vagus nerve impulses on smooth muscle.
    D. They decrease the responsiveness of the patient.

114. Nursing interventions carried out within an hour prior to any major surgery would most likely include which one of the following?

    A. Putting the side rails up following preoperative medication.
    B. Giving an enema.
    C. Performing preoperative shave and scrub.
    D. Checking for history and physical on chart.

115. Nursing responsibilities for the preoperative period would include notifying the physician if

    A. The erythrocyte count is 6 mil/cc mm.
    B. The temperature is 99.6°F orally.
    C. The hemoglobin is 14 gm/100 ml.
    D. The urine report indicated ketonuria.

116. Mrs. Olsen returns with a nasogastric tube. Which one of the following complications may occur?

    A. Electrolyte imbalance.
    B. Gastric distention.
    C. Ulcerative colitis.
    D. Infection.

117. An early complication following gastric resection is

    A. Constipation.
    B. Clay-colored stools.
    C. Infection.
    D. Hemorrhage.

118. The most common late-occurring complication following a subtotal gastric resection is

    A. Adhesions.
    B. Hemorrhage.
    C. Dumping syndrome.
    D. Intractable pain.

119. The absence of the blink reflex predisposes the patient to

    A. Loss of vision.
    B. Blurring of vision.
    C. Corneal drying and ulceration.
    D. None of these.

120. Mr. Samuels has grand mal epilepsy. Which of the following is the first sign or symptom of this type of seizure?

    A. Fall.
    B. Cry.
    C. Incontinence.
    D. Aura.

121. During a seizure, what should the nurse do first?

    A. Yell for help.
    B. Protect the patient's head and body from damage.
    C. Hold him down firmly.
    D. Monitor pupil reactions.

122. Mr. Samuels should be advised by the nurse to avoid all of the following *except*

    A. Emotional stress.
    B. Physical activity.
    C. Physical exhaustion.
    D. Alcoholic beverages.

254

123. Nursing care for a patient who has pleurisy with effusion would include

   A. Medication to prevent coughing.
   B. Moderate activity.
   C. Position on side of effusion.
   D. Antibiotics.

124. Mr. Levin is going to have an above-the-knee amputation with a delayed prosthesis fitting. Preoperatively, the nurse can assist the patient by all the following *except*

   A. Have him do sit-up exercises.
   B. Advise him of the possibility of phantom limb sensation.
   C. Have him lift weights.
   D. Listen to his concerns about his loss.

125. Immediate postoperative nursing interventions for Mr. Levin would include

   A. Change the dressing as necessary.
   B. Keep a tourniquet at his bedside.
   C. Turn on abdomen immediately to prevent contracture.
   D. Maintain his position on affected side to lessen chances of hemorrhage.

126. The advantages to the patient for an immediate prosthesis fitting following an amputation are

   A. Ability to ambulate sooner.
   B. Less chance of phantom limb sensation.
   C. Dressing changes not necessary.
   D. All of the above.

127. Ms. White is admitted with a diagnosis of Cushing's syndrome. Which of the following comprise the most important components of her nursing care?

   A. Acceptance of her appearance, careful administration of steroids as ordered, and diversionary activities.
   B. Acceptance of her appearance, meticulous skin care, close observation for potassium retention and sodium and water depletion, and provision of a quiet environment.
   C. Acceptance of her appearance, meticulous skin care, protection from infection and injuries, and observation for potassium depletion.
   D. Acceptance of her appearance, meticulous skin care, preparation for hypophysectomy, and observation for sodium and water retention.

128. Mrs. Allen is admitted with severe contact dermatitis of the lower legs. Her skin is erythematous and has many vesicles. Vesicles are

   A. Skin elevations filled with clear fluid.
   B. Skin elevations filled with purulent material.
   C. Firm skin areas.
   D. Flat, discolored areas.

129. Since Mrs. Allen's skin is erythematous, you would expect it to be

   A. Bumpy but intact.
   B. Bluish gray.
   C. Red.
   D. Smooth and intact.

130. Mrs. Allen has had contact dermatitis for many years and has developed lichenification. *Lichenification* means

   A. Constant oozing from the affected area.
   B. Lack of pigmentation.
   C. Thickening of the affected skin.
   D. Stable condition.

131. A patient with emphysema was ordered postural drainage. The purpose of this procedure is to

   A. Increase oxygen intake.
   B. Remove mucus that collects in the lower bronchial tree.
   C. Force air out of the pleural cavity.
   D. Strengthen the muscles of respiration.

132. Mr. Banning is admitted with a diagnosis of myxedema. This disorder is due to a dysfunction of the

   A. Pituitary.
   B. Parathyroid.
   C. Thyroid.
   D. Ovary.

133. Mrs. Benson is admitted with multiple sclerosis. The actual cause of multiple sclerosis is unknown. Which of the following is thought to be a possible cause?

   A. Continuous metal poisoning.
   B. Autoimmune process.
   C. Decreased blood supply to the brain.
   D. Absence of oxidizing enzyme.

134. The pathophysiology of multiple sclerosis consists of

   A. Formation of fluid-filled cavities in the central part of the spinal cord.
   B. Formation of fibrous tissue causing pressure on nerve roots.
   C. Chronic inflammation of the coverings of the central nervous system.
   D. Patchy destruction of the myelin sheath.

135. Which of the following symptoms is not common to multiple sclerosis?

   A. Spastic weakness of lower extremities.
   B. Nystagmus.
   C. Visual disturbances.
   D. Generalized pain.

136. Prednisone, a corticosteroid, is ordered for Mrs. Brown. The chief purpose of administering the drug in her case is to

    A. Prevent complications.
    B. Cure her disease.
    C. Reduce her symptoms.
    D. Maintain and rebuild tissues.

137. A diagnostic test to determine brain death is

    A. A pneumoencephalogram.
    B. A ventriculogram.
    C. An electroencephalogram.
    D. A myelogram.

138. A patient with influenza may be encouraged to take aspirin to

    A. Relieve headache.
    B. Reduce fever.
    C. Relieve muscular aching.
    D. All of these.

139. The most important aspect of nursing care for the patient with impetigo is

    A. Prevention of scarring.
    B. Psychological support.
    C. Prevention of spread of the disease.
    D. None of these.

140. Mr. Wood has Parkinson's disease with progressive disability. The primary goal of nursing interventions should be that Mr. Wood

    A. Maintain a cheerful, positive outlook.
    B. Be physically active and independent.
    C. Be in a quiet environment without excessive external stimuli.
    D. Maintain good personal hygiene.

141. The nurse is particularly observant of Mr. Wood's tremor of his fingers at rest. This action is called

    A. Pill-rolling.
    B. Cog-wheeling.
    C. Euphoric birding.
    D. Tonic-clonic.

142. Mr. Wood's tremors seem to be worse in which of the following situations?

    A. When he tries to do a manipulative task.
    B. When he is excited, tense, or fatigued.
    C. When his blood sugar is low.
    D. At no specific times.

143. Positive Trousseau's and Chvostek's signs indicate

    A. Hyperthyroidism.
    B. Hypoparathyroidism.
    C. Hypopituitarism.
    D. None of these.

144. Which one of the following insulin preparations has the fastest onset and shortest duration of effect?

    A. Protamine zinc.
    B. Semilente.
    C. NPH.
    D. Regular.

145. Mr. Miller comes to the office with a boil on his neck. The technical term for boil is

    A. Bulla.
    B. Angioma.
    C. Furuncle.
    D. Macule.

146. Patients prone to digitalis toxicity include

    A. The elderly.
    B. Those receiving diuretics.
    C. Those with impaired hepatic function
    D. All of the above.

147. The *primary* purpose of giving digitalis to a patient with congestive heart failure is to

    A. Slow the heart rate.
    B. Speed the heart rate.
    C. Increase strength of myocardial contraction.
    D. Enhance kidney function.

148. Nursing measures to prevent thrombophlebitis include

    A. Providing footboard walking.
    B. Frequent massaging of calfs.
    C. Gatching knee of bed.
    D. Supporting popliteal area with pillows.

149. When heparin therapy is utilized for treatment of thrombophlebitis, it should be administered

    A. Intramuscularly.
    B. Subcutaneously.
    C. Intradermally.
    D. Intravenously.

150. Methods utilized to avoid postural hypotension associated with antihypertensive drug therapy include

    A. Forcing fluids to maintain blood volume.
    B. Changing position slowly.
    C. Keeping lower extremities elevated at all times.
    D. All of the above.

151. Paralytic ileus is a complication of abdominal surgery. Which of the following would *not* be carried out for a patient with paralytic ileus?

    A. Placed on oral fluids only.
    B. Insertion of nasogastric tube.

256

C. Administration of Prostigmin.
D. Placement of a rectal tube.

152. The drug most commonly used to treat juvenile diabetics is

A. Glucagon.
B. Orinase.
C. Insulin.
D. Adrenalin.

153. Herpes simplex is caused by

A. A virus.
B. A staphylococcus.
C. A streptococcus.
D. An allergy.

154. Mr. John Barr is a sixty-five-year-old farmer. He has been a heavy smoker for the past 40 years. He has just returned from surgery with a left lobectomy due to cancer. A lobectomy is defined as

A. The surgical removal of a lobe of the lung.
B. The surgical removal of an entire lung.
C. A surgical inspection of the lung.
D. The insertion of a drainage tube.

155. A chest tube was inserted at the time of surgery. The purpose of this tube is to

A. Supply oxygen to the thoracic cavity.
B. Remove fluid from the alveolar sacs.
C. Provide a means of instilling medication into the thoracic cavity.
D. Provide for removal of air and fluid from the pleural space.

156. This chest tube is connected to a water-seal suction. The purpose of this water is to

A. Provide humidity for the oxygen.
B. Maintain a closed system so air cannot enter the pleural space.
C. Provide a sterile environment for drainage.
D. Provide for an accurate means to measure drainage.

157. Mr. Barr is encouraged to cough and deep breathe. The reason for this is

A. To promote chest-tube drainage.
B. To increase oxygen intake.
C. To maintain respiratory function.
D. All of these.

158. To assist the patient with "dumping syndrome," it is important to decrease the chance of postoperative feeding complications by teaching the patient to

A. Increase fluid intake with meals.
B. Exercise moderately following meals.
C. Decrease sodium and carbohydrate intake.
D. Increase carbohydrate intake at meals.

159. Mr. Gannon's doctor ordered a Foley catheter. The catheterization was performed

A. With surgical asepsis.
B. Only by professional nurses with specialty training.
C. Under the supervision of the physician.
D. With medical asepsis.

160. Daily care of the Foley catheter will include

A. Providing routine irrigation to maintain patency.
B. Disconnecting the catheter to allow ambulation without embarrassment.
C. Clamping the catheter every four hours.
D. Cleansing the area around the urinary meatus.

161. After the patient's condition improved, the Foley catheter was removed, and he experienced frequent urination of small amounts. The physician ordered measurement of the residual urine. After the patient voided, the nurse should

A. Send a specimen to the laboratory.
B. Catheterize the patient and record the amount obtained.
C. Measure the voiding and notify the physician.
D. Send the patient to radiology for examination.

162. Emergency treatment for compound fractures should consist of

A. Reducing the fracture if possible.
B. Leaving the wound open to allow fluid to escape and to prevent a hematoma.
C. Immobilizing the fracture.
D. Immobilizing the fracture only after you clean out the wound.

163. Mrs. Godfrey was admitted with complaints of suprapubic tenderness with palpation and urinary urgency with dysuria. Her admitting diagnosis was cystitis. The practical nurse would expect her nursing care to include all of the following except

A. Urine culture and routine examination.
B. Adequate fluid intake.
C. Intake and output.
D. Seizure precautions.

164. The practical nurse teaches Mrs. Godfrey the importance of

A. Restricting her activity.
B. Maintaining good perineal hygiene to avoid fecal contamination of the urinary meatus.
C. Remaining in the same position for long periods of time to decrease the bladder irritation.
D. Limiting her oral fluids.

165. When the report of the urine examination was returned, the practical nurse was surprised to find

    A. RBC present in the urine.
    B. Glucose negative.
    C. Specific gravity 1.015.
    D. No WBC or RBC reported.

166. The reaction of the nurse would be to

    A. Notify the physician immediately.
    B. Check to determine that an error was not made in identification of the specimen.
    C. Tell the patient her tests are fine.
    D. Assume that the physician had made the wrong admitting diagnosis.

167. An important aspect of treatment of a patient with lupus erythematosus is

    A. Absolute bed rest in the early stages of the disease.
    B. Avoidance of sunlight, which spreads the disease.
    C. Increased dietary bulk to prevent constipation.
    D. Alcohol sponges to decrease temperature.

168. Mrs. Johnson, twenty-three years old, was admitted to the hospital at 8:00 P.M. with a diagnosis of appendicitis. On admission she stated that she had been vomiting and experiencing pain all day. Which of the following signs and symptoms are indicative of appendicitis?

    A. High fever.
    B. Anorexia.
    C. Tenderness localized in the lower left quadrant.
    D. Nausea and vomiting only when eating.

169. Nursing interventions for Mrs. Johnson during the preoperative period will include

    A. Keeping her flat in bed.
    B. Allowing only sips of water.
    C. Using a heating pad on the tender area to decrease pain.
    D. Using an ice bag on the tender area to decrease pain.

170. Preoperative care for any surgical patient should include all of the following except

    A. Increasing the protein intake to help prevent postoperative protein depletion.
    B. Providing for adequate elimination.
    C. Ensuring that the patient is psychologically prepared for surgery.
    D. Making sure that a nurse explains the surgical procedure before performing the skin prep.

171. Following a hypophysectomy, the nurse would observe signs for all of the following except

    A. Adrenal insufficiency.
    B. Acute thyroid crisis.
    C. Hypoglycemia.
    D. Hypertension.

172. When teaching the patient safe self-administration of steroid therapy, which of the following would the nurse *not* include?

    A. The medication should never be stopped abruptly.
    B. The medication should be taken with a meal or snack.
    C. The patient should take precautions against contracting infections.
    D. The patient may need to increase salt intake.

173. Alice is admitted to the hospital with a diagnosis of mitral stenosis. As part of a diagnostic work-up, the doctor orders a phonocardiogram. This study is a

    A. Graphic recording of the movement of the body generated with each heart beat.
    B. Recording of heart sounds translated into electrical energy.
    C. Measurement of the velocity of blood flow through the arterial system.
    D. Graphic recording of the pressure of blood in the right atrium.

174. Alice undergoes a cardiac catheterization. What is the method that will confirm the diagnosis of mitral stenosis?

    A. Right side of the heart catheterization.
    B. Left side of the heart catheterization.
    C. Both sides of the heart catheterization.
    D. Entry at right atrium into right ventricle.

175. Following a cardiac catheterization the patient should be instructed to

    A. Maintain Fowler's position for 24 hours.
    B. Withhold food and fluid for 6 hours.
    C. Maintain bed rest for 24 hours.
    D. Exercise the involved extremity(ies).

176. Mr. Jacks, a thirty-six-year-old truck driver, came to the emergency room with complaints of severe right-flank pain which radiated to the inguinal and testicular area. He was pallored, diaphoretic, and nauseated. His physician ordered an analgesic, routine urinalysis, and admission to the hospital. The nurse recognized these symptoms as suggestive of

    A. Nephritis.
    B. Acute appendicitis.
    C. Prostatic hypertrophy.
    D. Renal lithiasis.

177. Mr. Jacks was scheduled for an immediate IVP, and the nurse placed him on

   A. NPO regimen.
   B. Forced fluids.
   C. Enemas until clear.
   D. 24-hour urine collection.

178. The nurse instructed Mr. Jacks to do all of the following *except*

   A. Save his urine for measurement.
   B. Eat his supper when his nausea subsided.
   C. Notify the nurse of voidings, so the urine could be strained.
   D. Refrain from eating or drinking until further notice.

179. The charge nurse is especially interested in any allergies because

   A. The intravenous dye contains iodine.
   B. It is routine information.
   C. Mr. Jack will have to have antibiotic therapy.
   D. His symptoms suggest allergic reaction.

180. As the practical nurse is straining Mr. Jack's urine, Mr. Jack suddenly says he feels better and is hungry. The nurse finds a stone and knows to

   A. Save it for the physician to see.
   B. Record the incident and discard the stone.
   C. Page the physician STAT.
   D. Medicate the patient.

181. If removal of the stone had required surgery and a cystostomy resulted, the care of the suprapubic catheter would include

   A. Placing a urinal around the tube to collect urine.
   B. Clamping the tube and allowing the patient to void through the urinary meatus before removing the tube.
   C. Performing catheter irrigations every four hours to prevent infection.
   D. Limiting fluid intake to 1500 cc per day.

182. Which of the following skin cancers has the poorest prognosis because it metastasizes so rapidly and extensively via the lymph system?

   A. Basal cell epithelioma.
   B. Squamous cell epithelioma.
   C. Malignant melanoma.
   D. Sebaceous cyst.

183. Miss Crown has meningitis. She cannot extend her leg without pain while lying on her back with her thigh flexed on her abdomen. This symptom is called a positive

   A. Brudzinski's sign.
   B. Babinski reflex.

   C. Kernig's sign.
   D. Reflex action.

184. Specific postoperative nursing management for a lumbar laminectomy patient includes

   A. Coughing and deep breathing.
   B. Turning from side to side as a unit.
   C. Checking for tingling sensation in the fingers.
   D. Observing both surgical sites.

185. When oxygen is administered, it is passed through sterile distilled water before it reaches the patient. The reason for this is to

   A. Allow for accurate administration.
   B. Humidify the oxygen.
   C. Increase the concentration of the oxygen.
   D. Allow for the observation of the oxygen.

186. When a patient receives oxygen, the environment is kept free of all possible sources of sparks or fire because oxygen

   A. Supports combustion.
   B. Is highly combustible.
   C. Is explosive.
   D. Is in higher concentrations than normal.

187. Ben is admitted with first degree burns of his entire right arm and with second and third degree burns of his neck, abdomen, and back. His orders are for "open treatment." A symptom present in second degree burns that is not found in first degree is

   A. Erythema.
   B. Warmth.
   C. Vesicles.
   D. Deep tissue destruction.

188. "Open treatment" means

   A. Leaving Ben in an open ward.
   B. Leaving the windows of his room open.
   C. Opening his dressing at least bid.
   D. Placing him in reverse isolation.

189. According to the Rule of Nine, what percentage of Ben's body is burned?

   A. 1 to 18 percent.
   B. 19 to 33 percent.
   C. 34 to 49 percent.
   D. Over 50 percent.

190. Thrombophlebitis can occur following surgical intervention. A thrombus in the calf of the leg can be identified by which of the following signs?

   A. Doll's sign.
   B. Kernig's sign.
   C. Hegar's sign.
   D. Homan's sign.

191. Which one of the following medications would most likely be used to control postoperative nausea and vomiting?

    A. Compazine.
    B. Demerol.
    C. Talwin.
    D. Codeine.

192. Which of the following best describes the effect of the drug Orinase?

    A. Eliminates the need for diet therapy.
    B. Stimulates the pancreas to produce insulin.
    C. Stimulates the liver to release glycogen as glucose.
    D. Is a form of oral insulin.

193. Mrs. Marsh is admitted for urological surgery. Choose the one nursing objective that would *not* be appropriate at this time.

    A. Assess the functional status of the urinary tract with evaluation studies.
    B. Assess cardiopulmonary status of the patient.
    C. Give inhalation therapy to encourage deep respiratory movements.
    D. Recognize and try to relieve fear and anxiety.

194. The main complication following a nephrostomy that the nurse must be aware of is

    A. Bleeding from the site.
    B. Cardiopulmonary involvement following the procedure.
    C. Difficulty in restoring fluid and electrolyte balance.
    D. Contamination.

195. If hemorrhage does occur, the most immediate intervention of the nurse would be

    A. Notify the surgeon immediately.
    B. Treat the patient for shock while help is on the way.
    C. Go to the nearest nursing station and get help.
    D. Immediately place the patient in high Fowler's position.

196. All of the following factors would affect wound healing *except*

    A. Adequate nutrition through proper diet.
    B. Edema.
    C. Age.
    D. Iron.

197. Which of these is *not* a common complication of diabetes?

    A. Retinopathy.
    B. Cataracts.
    C. Hyperpnea.
    D. Neuropathy.

198. You use U80 insulin for Mr. Aim's injection. U80 means

    A. There are 80 units in a 10 ml vial.
    B. It is 80 percent pure.
    C. There are 80 units in each cc.
    D. None of these.

199. In order to perform range-of-motion exercises, it is necessary to understand joint movement. A freely movable joint is also known as

    A. Amphiarthrotic.
    B. Arthritic.
    C. Diarthrotic.
    D. Synarthrotic.

200. Trigeminal neuralgia results in severe recurrent paroxysms of pain on one side of the face. Which of the following nursing measures would probably *not* be helpful in preventing onset of pain?

    A. Provide small feedings of soft foods.
    B. Protect the patient's face from drafts.
    C. Place a cold compress on the affected side.
    D. Phrase questions that may be answered by gestures or short answers.

201. Joan Carolson was diagnosed as having cholelithiasis. She had been having several episodes of gallbladder attacks over the past year. Which one of the following symptoms would most likely bring Joan to the doctor?

    A. Chronic pain in lower right abdomen.
    B. Chronic pain in lower left abdomen.
    C. Fatty food intolerance while eating.
    D. Fatty food intolerance several hours after eating.

202. The major postoperative complication following a cholecystectomy is

    A. Paralytic ileus.
    B. Thrombophlebitis.
    C. Pneumonia.
    D. Hemorrhage.

203. A T-tube was placed in the common bile duct at the time of surgery. Which of the following statements is correct concerning the T-tube?

    A. It prevents backflow of bile into the liver.
    B. Patient is positioned in prone position to promote bile drainage.
    C. The T-tube is connected to drainage bottle kept at the level of the bed.
    D. The T-tube is clamped and only released at intervals.

204. Roger Latimer is a twenty-year-old college student admitted through the emergency room with head and neck injuries following a motorcycle

accident. He developed dyspnea and cyanosis so a tracheostomy was performed. A tracheostomy is defined as

A. An opening into the trachea to facilitate breathing.
B. The insertion of a chest tube.
C. The removal of the trachea.
D. An opening into the respiratory tract for removal of a foreign object.

205. The doctor ordered a mist mask to be placed over the tracheostomy tube. The purpose of this mist is to

A. Keep the mucous membrane moist.
B. Assist in coughing.
C. Allow for easier removal of mucus.
D. Add moisture to the inspired air.

206. Tracheal suctioning was ordered prn. This will be done to

A. Observe the respiratory rate.
B. Maintain a patent airway.
C. Observe for bleeding.
D. Prevent bleeding.

207. When caring for Mr. Latimer, the nurse should be alert for

A. A sudden mood change.
B. Signs of allergy to the tracheostomy tube.
C. Signs of respiratory difficulty.
D. All of these.

208. Which of the following diets is appropriate for hyperinsulinism (hypoglycemia)?

A. High fat, high carbohydrate.
B. Low protein, high carbohydrate.
C. Low carbohydrate, high protein.
D. Low fat, low protein.

209. With a severely burned patient, the nurse must know that the major loss to the body is

A. Electrolytes.
B. Water.
C. Blood.
D. Skin.

210. The vertebral column is part of the

A. Appendicular skeleton.
B. Axial skeleton.
C. Ventral cavity.
D. Spinal cord.

211. The process of cartilage being replaced by bone is known as

A. Calcification.
B. Deposition.
C. Ossification.
D. Reabsorption.

212. Mr. Isaacs, a sixty-seven-year-old with diagnosed benign prostatic hypertrophy, is admitted for a transurethral resection (TUR). These postoperative patients are particularly prone to

A. Pneumonia.
B. Hemorrhage.
C. Fluid and electrolyte imbalance.
D. Cerebral vascular accidents.

213. A three-way retention catheter will accomplish all of the following except

A. Provide a route for sterile irrigation.
B. Provide a route for urinary drainage.
C. Maintain patent urinary outlet.
D. Establish proper urine production.

214. On the first postoperative day, Mr. Isaacs is concerned at the sight of the reddened color of his urine. The nurse will tell him

A. "I know. I'm concerned about it also and have reported it to the charge nurse."
B. "That is to be expected. Each day it will continue to clear until it is normal."
C. "Oh, that's nothing. Don't worry about it."
D. "I don't know why it's that color. You'd better ask your doctor."

215. Postoperative pain can be controlled by all of the following except

A. Avoiding unnecessary movement by having the patient positioned for at least four hours at a time.
B. Medicating for pain at least every four to six hours the first 24 hours postoperatively.
C. Keeping the bed linens free of wrinkles.
D. Keeping the environment quiet and restful.

216. Which one of the following nursing interventions will patients with retinal detachment have on their care plan for the first postoperative day?

A. Turn, cough, hyperventilate every two hours.
B. Up ad lib.
C. Remove eye patch during day.
D. Complete bed bath.

217. Preoperative nursing interventions for patients having cataract surgery will include

A. Instillation of mydriatic drugs.
B. Instillation of miotic drugs.
C. Instillation of topical anesthetics.
D. Instillation of cryogenic drugs.

218. Instructions given to patients following cataract surgery include the information that

    A. The eye patch will be removed in three to four days, and they will be able to use the eye without difficulty.
    B. They must use only one eye at a time to prevent double vision.
    C. They will be able to judge distances without difficulty.
    D. Contact lenses will be fitted before discharge from the hospital.

219. Which one of the following would indicate a possible wound infection?

    A. Increased temperature within the first 24 hours after surgery.
    B. Serosanguineous drainage on dressing.
    C. Erythema surrounding suture line three to four days postoperatively.
    D. Bright-red drainage on dressing the night of surgery.

220. Muscles that help in the movement of bones are classified as

    A. Branching.
    B. Involuntary.
    C. Smooth.
    D. Striated.

221. To better understand what part a skeletal muscle moves, you should know the muscle's point of origin and insertion. The point of insertion is defined as

    A. The more movable end of the muscle.
    B. The more fixed point of attachment.
    C. The distal end.
    D. The proximal end.

222. The practice of cautious administration of fluids to a burned patient who is hypovolemic is based on a major principle that

    A. Fluids by themselves do not contain the necessary electrolytes.
    B. Fluids are given to maintain kidney perfusion.
    C. When fluids move back into the vascular compartment, there is a danger of congestive heart failure from too much fluid.
    D. There is an extracellular fluid volume shift occurring after 24 hours.

223. What effect will infectious processes occurring in a person who is taking steroid replacements have on the medication dosage?

    A. Increased dosage needed.
    B. Decreased dosage needed.
    C. Decreased, then increased dosage needed.
    D. No change in dosage needed.

224. When irrigating the nasogastric tube, the nurse will use normal saline and

    A. Medical asepsis.
    B. Surgical asepsis.
    C. Sterile water.
    D. All of these.

225. Routine testing of the patient's urine for sugar and acetone is part of nursing care for all of the following conditions *except*

    A. Diabetes mellitus.
    B. Cushing's syndrome.
    C. Acromegaly.
    D. Diabetes insipidus.

226. A patient with gastric pain is advised to take any of the following antacids *except*

    A. Aluminum hydroxide.
    B. Amphojel.
    C. Maalox.
    D. Soda bicarbonate.

227. Mr. Calkins has just had a herniorrhaphy. Following oral Demerol for pain, the patient vomits and states that he feels he has to vomit again. You would carry out all of the following interventions *except*

    A. Have the patient take slow, deep breaths.
    B. Offer carbonated uncola beverages if not NPO.
    C. Administer IM Demerol to relieve his pain.
    D. Splint the incisional area.

228. Postoperative teaching for a person with a spinal fusion includes advising the patient

    A. Not to lift or stoop for long periods.
    B. To use leg weights to strengthen leg muscles.
    C. To use a sun lamp to alleviate soreness.
    D. To perform sit-up exercises every day.

229. Which of the following items constitutes one meat exchange on the ADA exchange diet?

    A. One cup of whole milk.
    B. Two ounces of cheddar cheese.
    C. One-fourth cup tuna fish.
    D. Ten small nuts.

230. A patient with peritonitis is placed in semi-Fowler's position in order to

    A. Decrease the pain from the infection.
    B. Localize the infection to the pelvic cavity rather than the diaphragm.
    C. Facilitate breathing, as the diaphragm is relieved of pressure.
    D. Make the patient more comfortable.

231. A patient with peritonitis may have an intestinal tube in place to remove flatus and secretions.

Which of the following is *not* an essential consideration of the nurse?

A. Provide frequent oral hygiene.
B. Observe the NG tube for patency.
C. Record the color and amount of drainage.
D. Pin tubing to patient's gown.

232. Mrs. Culley has otosclerosis and is scheduled for a stapedectomy. This condition chiefly involves the

A. Auditory canal.
B. Tympanic membrane.
C. Ossicles.
D. Auditory nerve.

233. All the following are appropriate nursing measures to maintain optimal positioning and function after a CVA *except*

A. Placing the patient in prone position 15 to 30 minutes 3 times a day.
B. Conducting passive ROM exercises four times daily.
C. Encouraging self-care activities as soon as possible.
D. Changing position between affected and unaffected side every two hours.

234. Mrs. Markin has some residual expressive aphasia. Which of the following would be the most therapeutic nursing action?

A. Anticipate her needs and requests.
B. Encourage communication by writing or using an alphabet board.
C. Encourage every attempt to communicate without correcting words or usage.
D. Use and encourage pantomime.

235. The nurse noted that Mrs. Markin seemed to be unaware of objects on her right side. Examination revealed a visual loss in the right half of each visual field. Which of the following is the most important in assisting the patient to compensate for this loss?

A. Place on the unaffected side those items that are used frequently.
B. Position the patient so that her unaffected side is toward the activity in the room.
C. Frequently encourage the patient to position and turn her head to scan the environment on the affected side.
D. Approach the patient on the unaffected side.

236. Mrs. Markin is due to be discharged from the rehabilitation center. She has regained partial use of her arm and almost full use of her leg. Home visits are being planned by the nurse for the primary purpose of

A. Assisting the patient in activities of daily living.
B. Assessing the home for safety hazards.
C. Assisting the patient in transferring learning from the hospital environment to the home.
D. Assisting the patient in performing prescribed physical therapy.

Answers and Rationale

1. (D) Angina pectoris is severe chest pain due to temporary inability of the coronary arteries to meet metabolic needs of the myocardium.

2. (A) Sublingual administration allows for rapid absorption, which is of prime importance in the treatment of angina. Sublingual administration of nitroglycerin relieves anginal pain in one to three minutes.

3. (D) Pruritus is the technical term for itching.

4. (A) Prednisone is a steroid.

5. (C) Recording preconvulsive signs will assist the physician in determining the location of the tumor. Restricting patient's movements may cause serious injury to her. It is best to move objects away from her. If the jaw is forcibly opened, you can actually break it.

6. (B) Moro reflex, also called the startle reflex, is present in normal newborn infants. The gag reflex can be absent, but it can be an indication of many other conditions, such as oversedation; it is certainly not the most important sign of neurological pathology. A positive Babinski is indicative of neurological disorder.

7. (B) A cleansing enema is usually not given because of the potential increase in intracranial pressure.

8. (D) Pulse deficit is the difference between an apical and radial pulse rate and is of no significance in a neurological exam.

9. (D) Hyperthermia is a complication of brain surgery, and since the patient probably is not fully oriented, a rectal temperature should be taken. Trendelenburg's position increases intracranial pressure; morphine may depress respirations or "made" reactions. Restraints are not routinely used; however, side rails are used for safety.

10. (D) Lethargy is the earliest sign of increased intra-cranial pressure. It is due to compression of the brain from edema or hemorrhage (or both).

11. (A) Hypertonic solutions are administered because they are relatively impermeable to the blood-brain barrier. The solution reduces edema by a rapid movement of water out of the ventricles into the blood. Corticosteroids also reduce pressure but have a much slower action. Corticosteroids assist in sustaining the initial action of the IV fluids when used in conjunction with them.

12. (D) These methods will help to prevent the spread of microorganisms.

13. (A) With the head of the bed elevated, the dia-phragm drops down and allows the lungs to expand.

14. (A) Until the gag reflex returns, the patient can-not handle foods or liquids, and may aspirate.

15. (C) A *scope* refers to an "instrument used for vis-ual examination," and *broncho* refers to "bronchi."

16. (C) Allows patient an opportunity to ventilate her fears which may easily be relieved by education from the nurse regarding the exam.

17. (C) Patient swallows contrast medium, usually barium, and the route is observed by fluoroscopy and documented with x-ray. The radiologist ob-serves the structures as well as their function.

18. (C) Occult blood is "hidden" and is not easily detected by the naked eye. The small specimen is collected in a clean container.

19. (A) Anal irritation is more accurately associated with diarrhea than constipation.

20. (A) As the name implies, direct visualization of the sigmoid colon by the use of an endoscope allows the physician to inspect the mucosa and obtain a biopsy if desired. The barium studies can-not give this information.

21. (C) Neomycin suppresses normal bacterial flora, thereby "sterilizing" the bowel preoperatively to decrease possibilities of postoperative infection.

22. (A) With confirmed diagnosis of carcinoma of the lower bowel, permanent colostomies are most com-mon due to the lack of remaining distal bowel for future anastomosis.

23. (B) Daily narcotics should not be required at this stage of the disease. A mild analgesic may be pre-scribed to manage the discomfort after abdominal surgery.

24. (B) By neutralizing excessive gastric acid often created by stress, the epigastric burning and dis-comfort are relieved.

25. (A) Critical reduction of blood supply to the myo-cardium for a prolonged period results in sustained oxygen deprivation. As a result, cardiac muscle is destroyed.

26. (A) Myocardial infarction results from a sustained interruption in the blood flow to the myocardium. Administering oxygen helps in the relief of pain, the prevention of arrhythmias, and the minimiza-tion of myocardial necrosis. Caution must be used if the patient has chronic obstructive lung disease.

27. (B) A soft diet decreases bulk and enhances elimi-nation of solid wastes. Ease in defecation prevents straining and an increased workload on the heart.

28. (B) Anticoagulants are administered to decrease the occurrence of venous thrombosis and emboli as well as to prevent the extension of a clot that has already formed.

29. (C) Polycythemia vera is an overproduction of red cells and hemoglobin. Phlebotomy means "making an opening into a vein"; in this disease excess blood is removed from the vascular system by taking it from a vein.

30. (B) Gamma globulin is a plasma protein, as are serum albumin and fibrinogen.

31. (D) Patients with leukemia often have a decreased resistance to infection for many reasons. One rea-son is that they receive large doses of steroids. These patients are placed in reverse isolation to protect them from exposure to disease-producing microorganisms.

32. (B) Sugar and acetone content of the urine should not be a factor in the other conditions.

33. (C) Due to increased sugar and bacteria content with aging of the urine, the nurse will have the pa-tient void the urine which has been collecting in the bladder for the past hours, and collect another specimen in 30 to 40 minutes to obtain urine that reflects the current urine content of sugar and ace-tone. This is known as "second voided specimen collection."

34. (B) Because of low solubility in urine, which may lead to crystalluria and renal damage, adequate fluid intake must be accomplished when the patient is receiving sulfa derivatives.

35. (A) Leucocytosis is the increased production of WBC's. Histoplasmosis is a respiratory disease;

phagocytosis, the process of destruction of bacteria; and erythropoiesis, the process of production of RBC's.

36. (A) A consistently quiet position leads to, among other complications, urinary stasis and infection. Without tiring the patient, range-of-motion exercises linked with adequate fluid intake decrease the incidence of urolithiasis or cystitis.

37. (C) Hemodialysis is the only procedure that can function as the kidney.

38. (C) *Epi* means "up on" or "on top of," and *dermis* is "true skin."

39. (A) A normal pH of the skin (4.2 to 5.6) must be maintained to slow the growth of bacteria that are normally present.

40. (B) The oversecretion in an adult causes excessive growth in the short, flat bones.

41. (B) Patients with diabetes insipidus excrete large amounts of dilute urine. Normal urine has a specific gravity of 1.010 to 1.030; Mr. Adams's urine has a lower specific gravity.

42. (C) Vasopressin has an antidiuretic action.

43. (B) Fracture is defined as a break but does not describe the severity or type of damage to the bone.

44. (D) Deformity, loss of function, and pain are all likely to occur due to the loss of alignment. There is no reason for a foul odor since decomposition of tissue has not occurred yet.

45. (D) A cast is rigid and used to maintain alignment. If it is too tight, it will press on blood vessels. The color and temperature of the toes will change with decreased blood supply, and as the blood is slowed through the walls of the vessels, edema will occur.

46. (A) Since the patient cannot feel sensory stimuli, a blockage of the nerves between the central nervous system and the peripheral system would be indicated.

47. (B) If a wet cast is handled with the fingers, indentations in the cast will occur. This can cause pressure on the patient and cause weakness in the cast.

48. (C) Due to liver destruction, portal hypertension occurs. Vitamin K will not stop hemorrhage at this point as the problem is directly related to the distended and dilated veins which have ruptured.

49. (C) A Sengstaken-Blakemore tube provides pressure in both the upper cardiac portion of the stomach and the esophagus by means of a double lumen balloon.

50. (B) Cerebral anoxia occurs frequently in severe trauma to the brain. A blood clot or edema can cause an interruption of the blood circulation, which leads to anoxia.

51. (C) Blood pressure is increased with a wide pulse pressure (the difference between the systolic pressure and the diastolic pressure). The cerebrospinal fluid pressure may cause elevated blood pressure by reducing oxygen supply to the hypothalmic vasomotor center. The excess of carbon dioxide which then forms will stimulate the center and cause an increase in the blood pressure.

52. (D) Glucagon is one of the principal hormones controlling carbohydrate metabolism. It promotes a rise in blood sugar. It would not be used in a patient with a head injury. Mannitol is an osmotic diuretic, and so it decreases cerebral edema. Solu-Cortef, a corticosteroid, will assist in decreasing cerebral edema through its antiinflammatory effect. Dilantin is used to prevent seizure activity.

53. (D) All of these are important objectives as well as psychological support and careful observation.

54. (A) Until a condition is specifically diagnosed, the treatments described in answers B, C, and D can exacerbate the disease and cause disfigurement and/or spreading of dermatoses.

55. (D) Pneumonia is an acute inflammation of the lung tissues.

56. (C) The patient's energy should be conserved to enable the body to use all of its resources for fighting the disease.

57. (B) Pneumonia may be caused by a virus, bacteria, or fungi, which would be present in the secretions.

58. (D) The bag can be closed without touching the inside or the contents in order to prevent the spread of microorganisms.

59. (B) Skin traction is defined as the application of tape or sponge rubber to the skin with weights attached to the tape.

60. (D) All of these points must be checked to maintain traction. The weights must not touch anything because that lessens the pull. If the rope is not on the pulley, the alignment is poor. When the foot plate rests on the pulley, the amount of traction is lessened.

61. (B) If the affected leg is elevated, flexion of the hip occurs which could cause dislocation of the hip.

62. (D) The nurse should not give the bath, but assist the patient as necessary. In this way the patient exercises joints, blood flow is stimulated, and some independence is maintained.

63. (B) An ileostomy. Ulcerative colitis progresses from the anal area backward through the colon. Indications for surgery include no improvement with continued deterioration in the patient's condition. The operation of choice is usually a total colectomy and an ileostomy. Any procedure more limited will prove to be of only temporary benefit in most cases.

64. (B) Due to constant irritation of the colon, the stools are frequent, bloody, and often contain mucus and pus. Constipation would not be a likely symptom.

65. (B) High protein diet will aid in tissue repair. The low residue diet prevents the need for excessive peristalsis. A bland diet is less irritating to the tissue.

66. (A) Ileostomy patients do not have irrigations performed, as the contents are liquid and contain few formed stool particles. Fluids would be forced to combat dehydration. Meticulous skin care and appliance fit are necessary because the contents are extremely caustic to the skin.

67. (C) Ms. Jones's medication therapy includes steroids; she needs protection from infections and potential infections.

68. (A) Answer B is associated with Cushing's syndrome; answer C is associated with diabetes mellitus; answer D is associated with acromegaly.

69. (B) Highly specialized tissue in the cerebral cortex is most sensitive to a lack of oxygen.

70. (C) Respiration is controlled by many different areas of the brain.

71. (B) A patent airway is always a priority need, particularly in the patient with a head injury, because hypoxia and hypercapnia cause cerebral edema with increasing intracranial pressure.

72. (D) Blood in the CSF, within the subarachnoid space, is irritating to the meninges.

73. (B) Gonadotropic, or sex gland, hormones are made by the anterior pituitary.

74. (C) Oxytocin and vasopressin are made by the posterior lobe, and ACTH by the anterior lobe of the pituitary.

75. (D) The pituitary gland because it directly affects the functioning of the other endocrine glands.

76. (A) Congestive heart failure results when the heart is unable to pump adequate amounts of blood. The cardiac workload and activity should be reduced to allow the heart to rest.

77. (A) In left-sided heart failure there is increased pulmonary pressure and congestion. Fluid accumulates in the alveoli, and the patient develops dyspnea, orthopnea, and cough.

78. (D) Fowler's position allows for good lung expansion as well as decreasing venous return from the lower extremities.

79. (D) Acute pulmonary edema is excessive quantities of fluid in the pulmonary interstitial spaces or in the alveoli usually following severe left ventricular failure.

80. (C) Rotating tourniquets reduces the workload of the heart by temporarily interfering with venous return to the heart.

81. (C) When rotating tourniquets are utilized they may be applied clockwise or counterclockwise. Making a diagram ensures that the tourniquets are always rotated in the same direction at 15-minute intervals.

82. (C) The prefix *erythro* means "red," and the suffix *cyte* means "cell."

83. (B) The disease may be so mild that it is discovered through a routine urinalysis, which shows hematuria, proteinuria, and casts.

84. (B) Bed rest would protect the poorly functioning kidneys (activity may increase urinary abnormalities) as well as facilitate diuresis.

85. (C) Patients in early stages of renal failure are hypertensive due to poor kidney perfusion and function, probably caused by renal ischemia.

86. (D) Lasix actually increases blood flow to the kidney, thereby increasing the production of urine. Answer B is wrong because intrarenal resistance is decreased, and answer C is wrong because Lasix is not antimicrobial.

87. (C) A low protein diet is important because damaged kidneys may not be able to eliminate protein digestion waste products.

88. (C) Daily weight should reflect fluid loss and is another method to evaluate the diuresis desired.

89. (A) Recognizing that these symptoms may also represent infectious hepatitis, which is communicable by excreta, the nurse will protect patients and personnel by observing enteric precaution isolation until diagnosis is confirmed.

90. (B) Gallbladder and liver functions are stimulated by ingestion of fats.

91. (B) Gallbladder disease is considered familial but not inherited. Statistics show higher incidence among aging females with history of obesity, diabetes, and pregnancy.

92. (B) The first emergency measure, regardless of potential trauma, is checking for and maintaining an open airway. If patient is not adequately oxygenated, other measures are of little or no value.

93. (C) Twisting or bending can cause spinal cord trauma.

94. (A) Persons with hyperthyroidism are hyperactive, nervous, and irritable; provision for adequate rest is a major nursing challenge.

95. (C) The eyes protrude, or bulge, due to fluid collecting around the eye sockets.

96. (D) Common postoperative complications are laryngeal nerve damage, tetany or hypocalcemia, as well as respiratory distress.

97. (C) The primary causative factor in asthma is an inherited allergic tendency.

98. (B) Asthma is defined as recurrent paroxysms of dyspnea with a characteristic wheezing.

99. (A) Bronchodilators tend to reduce bronchospasms by relaxing the smooth muscles of the bronchi, which relieves dyspnea and wheezing.

100. (D) The asthmatic patient may be very anxious and looks to the nurse for support and reassurance.

101. (B) Rheumatoid arthritis is thought to be an autoimmune disease. Osteoarthritis is the process of aging.

102. (A) There is no scientific proof that exercise that provides stress or copper bracelets help arthritis in any way. A soft mattress would cause greater strain on joints, but heat increases circulation of the area.

103. (B) Fixation of a joint is called arthrodesis. Insertion of a prosthesis is the replacement of only the head of the femur. There is usually no plastic surgery involved when the head and the neck of the femur are amputated.

104. (D) All are important to prevent complications.

105. (A) Acetylsalicylic acid relieves pain in muscles. In arthritis much of the pain comes from muscle spasms.

106. (B) Eczema is an allergic disorder that may be triggered by food or other allergies.

107. (A) The vaccine can cause vaccinia which can superimpose the pustular eruptions of the viral infection on the eczema.

108. (B) Contusion of brain means "bruising"; concussion means "jarred."

109. (B) Chlorpromazine reduces peripheral vasoconstriction and prevents shivering. This is important since shivering increases CSF pressure and oxygen use.

110. (B) Pain is reduced upon eating when patient has duodenal ulcer. When the duodenum is empty, about two to three hours after eating, the pain returns.

111. (C) Bright-red bloody stools indicate a bleeding problem low in the gastrointestinal tract. A bleeding duodenal ulcer would have tarry stools.

112. (C) Atropine is administered to reduce tracheobronchial secretions which results in dry mucous membranes. This aids in preventing postoperative respiratory complications.

113. (D) Sedatives, which are usually administered with anticholinergic drugs, are responsible for decreased responsiveness.

114. (A) The other interventions, even though carried out preoperatively, need to be done much earlier than one hour prior to surgery.

115. (D) All the other reports are within normal range. The ketonuria indicates a problem suggestive of diabetes mellitus or other metabolic disorder.

116. (A) Nasogastric intubation leads to electrolyte imbalance through the suctioning out of the gastric contents. Large amounts of sodium and potassium are lost through the suctioning and, if not replaced by IV fluids, can lead to serious electrolyte imbalance.

117. (D) Since an incision has been made into the stomach organ itself, hemorrhage is occasionally a complication of gastric resection.

118. (C) As increased amounts of food, particularly those high in carbohydrate, enter the jejunum, the patient becomes weak, nauseated, dizzy, and perspires profusely. Symptoms are due to a form of hypoglycemia.

119. (C) Corneal drying occurs first, since blinking causes moisture spread across the eyeball. The degree of drying may eventually lead to scarring and blindness.

120. (D) Aura occurs first, then cry, then fall.

121. (B) The primary nursing goal during a seizure is to protect the patient from physical injury and to maintain a patent airway if possible.

122. (B) Regular physical activity tends to inhibit seizure activity.

123. (C) Positioning the patient on this side will reduce pain by helping to splint the chest and will encourage the expansion of the other side of the chest.

124. (A) Sit-up exercises help tone the abdominal muscles. In this instance it would be more beneficial to Mr. Levin to strengthen his arm muscles to help him when walking with crutches.

125. (B) The possibility exists that Mr. Levin could hemorrhage from the stump. The dressing is not changed unless ordered, and the prone position is usually not indicated until first day postoperative.

126. (A) When the prosthesis is in place immediately following surgery the patient can stand up several hours postoperative and walk the next day. The operative site is closed to outside contamination and benefits from improved circulation due to ambulation.

127. (C) The only response with all correct components. Steroids are not given for Cushing's syndrome treatment; potassium depletion and sodium and water retention occur.

128. (A) Vesicles are like blisters and are filled with clear, serous fluid.

129. (C) Erythematous is the adjective for erythema and means "red."

130. (C) Multiple inflammation of an area will cause thickening of that tissue.

131. (B) Force of gravity in postural drainage will facilitate the drainage of the bronchial tree.

132. (C) Myxedema is hypothyroidism in adults.

133. (B) Autoimmunity and a specific virus are being investigated as possible causes of multiple sclerosis.

134. (D) Patches of sclerotic tissue and nerve degeneration occur in the area of myelin sheath destruction.

135. (D) Pain is rarely seen as a primary symptom of this disorder.

136. (C) By reducing symptoms, this steroid hastens remission of her disease.

137. (C) The electroencephalogram records electrical activity of the brain and is used to determine "brain death." Pneumoencephalogram, ventriculogram, and myelogram involve the use of air, gas, or dye to outline the brain or spinal cord on x-ray.

138. (D) Aspirin is an antipyretic and also an analgesic.

139. (C) Impetigo is a contagious disease caused by a staphylococcus or streptococcus and is easily spread to other areas of the patient or to other people.

140. (B) Physical activity is necessary to maintain function and to prevent deformities in relation to immobility of muscles. Independent function also fosters self-esteem.

141. (A) *Pill-rolling* is the descriptive term since the movement of fingers and thumb resembles this action.

142. (B) Stress and fatigue seem to increase tremors, while purposeful acts or sleep seem to decrease them.

143. (B) These signs indicate an acute hypocalcemia as seen in severe hypoparathyroidism.

144. (D) Regular insulin has the fastest action—about one hour.

145. (C) A furuncle is a boil; a carbuncle is a larger, more deeply rooted boil.

146. (D) The use of potassium-depleting diuretics may result in digitalis toxicity. Impaired hepatic function interferes with the metabolism of the drug. Elderly and debilitated patients are prone to digitalis toxicity.

147. (C) The chief effect of digitalis is increased strength of contraction by direct action on the myocardium. With congestive heart failure, digitalis increases cardiac output, decreases heart size, and improves circulation.

148. (A) Footboard walking and tightening and relaxing of leg muscles promote venous return. Gatching the knee of the bed and supporting the popliteal area interfere with venous return. Massaging of calfs is contraindicated as this may dislodge small clots that may have formed.

149. (B) Heparin is usually given deep subcutaneously into the fatty layer of abdomen or above the iliac crest. Intramuscular route is usually contraindicated because of the danger of hematoma and hemorrhage.

150. (B) Changing position slowly allows the body to adjust to changes in gravitational force.

151. (A) The patient will be kept NPO until bowel sounds are present, abdominal distention relieved, and flatus is passed.

152. (C) Juvenile diabetics will probably need insulin therapy the rest of their lives since often they do not produce it.

153. (A) Herpes simplex, or cold sore, is caused by a virus as is herpes zoster.

154. (A) *Lobe* refers to a lobe of a lung. *Ectomy* is a suffix which means the surgical removal of a part.

155. (D) Air enters the chest cavity when it is opened, and fluid collects during surgery. A tube is placed in the pleural space to drain this collection and to allow for the reexpansion of the lung.

156. (B) The end of the drainage tube is kept under water, and this water seals the tube so air cannot enter the tube and be drawn back into the pleural space.

157. (C) This will help to prevent the accumulation of fluids in the lungs.

158. (C) Dumping syndrome can be prevented by decreasing fluid intake at meal times, taking in six small feedings per day, lying down following meals, and decreasing carbohydrates and salt intake. The hypoglycemic state which causes the syndrome arises from the pancreas responding by increasing the insulin output when large amounts of carbohydrates are introduced into the jejunum.

159. (A) Practical nurses are prepared to catheterize patients observing surgical asepsis because of the sterility of the system being entered.

160. (D) Whether the hospital or nursing care facility uses soap and water or an antibacterial procedure, the Foley catheter should be cleansed regularly to decrease the incidence of infection from the retention catheter which connects the environment with the internal sterile urinary bladder.

161. (B) Proper procedure to measure the residual urine, which is the amount retained in the bladder after voiding, is to catheterize the patient immediately after voiding to obtain the residual. It need not be analyzed unless the physician suspects infection.

162. (C) You should cover the wound with a sterile dressing and immediately immobilize it. Do not attempt to clean out the wound or to reduce the leg.

163. (D) Cystitis, inflammation of the bladder, should not cause central nervous system irritation leading to seizures. The urine culture will determine the causative organism if infection is present; the amount of output will help evaluate the function of the kidneys; and adequate fluid intake will decrease the irritation of the bladder mucosa.

164. (B) One of the most common causative organisms is *Escherichia coli*, which is normal bowel flora. Restricting her activity and fluids may lead to calculi formation, and failure to change positions more frequently than every four hours will increase the bacterial content of the urine from stasis.

165. (D) White blood cells and red blood cells are usually present in urine samples from patients with cystitis. White blood cells respond to the inflammation, and the irritation of the mucosa and irritation of the urethra cause bleeding.

166. (B) The nurse should evaluate the possibility of a nursing or lab identification error, and repeat the test.

167. (B) Sunlight spreads lesions and aggravates the patient's photophobia (sensitivity to light).

168. (B) Patients will have a low-grade temperature, tenderness in lower right quadrant, and nausea and vomiting without reference to eating. Pain starts in the upper abdomen and progresses to the right quadrant.

169. (D) Semi-Fowler's position relieves abdominal pain and tension. Mrs. Johnson is NPO to decrease peristalsis. Heat is never used because it could cause the appendix to rupture, thus causing peritonitis.

170. (D) The physician is the one who should initially instruct the patient in the surgical procedure. The nurse only reinforces teaching and explains areas which were unclear to the patient. The surgical preparation should not be carried out until the physician has discussed the procedure with the patient.

171. (D) Hypotension is most likely to occur.

172. (D) The patient may need to decrease salt intake.

173. (B) A phonocardiogram is a diagnostic test in which heart sounds are translated into electrical energy by a microphone and recorded.

174. (B) Both sides of the heart can be studied during cardiac catheterization. In the situation given, the left side of the heart would be catheterized since the mitral valve is located between the left atrium and ventricle.

175. (C) Maintaining bed rest for 24 hours following a cardiac catheterization reduces the possibility of hemorrhage or hematoma formation at insertion sites.

176. (D) Characteristic symptoms of urolithiasis.

177. (A) Realizing that the patient could require surgical removal of an existing stone, the nurse places him NPO as a precautionary measure.

178. (B) If surgery is anticipated, the patient will be maintained NPO regardless of the status of his nausea.

179. (A) Anaphylactic reactions have occurred with the intravenous dye used for the pyelogram in patients with hypersensitivity to iodine derivatives.

180. (A) Realizing the passage of the stone is important but not an emergency situation, the nurse saves it for the physician to examine. The nurse also realizes that with passage of the stone, the patient will not require analgesia unless another stone creates pain.

181. (B) Patency of the urethra and meatus should be established before the removal of the suprapubic catheter, which is ensuring urine elimination.

182. (C) Basal cell epithelioma and squamous cell epithelioma are both superficial, easily excised, slow-growing tumors. A sebaceous cyst is a benign (nonmalignant) growth.

183. (C) This is a description of Kernig's sign and is caused by meningeal irritation.

184. (B) Twisting the patient's back while turning will place strain on the operative site and cause pain. The patient must be turned as a unit or "log" to avoid this result.

185. (B) Oxygen can dry out mucous membrane if it is not humidified before administration.

186. (A) Oxygen itself does not burn, but if it is present it will allow a small fire to spread rapidly.

187. (C) First degree burns involve the epidermis so redness and warmth is present. Second degree involves the dermis, and vesicles form between epidermis and dermis. Third degree involves deep tissue with destruction or charring.

188. (D) Open method for burns involves placing the patient in reverse isolation. In this method all equipment brought into the patient is sterile to protect the patient from the environment, not to protect others from the patient.

189. (C) According to the Rule of Nine, Ben's right arm would be 9 percent, his abdomen 9 percent, and his back 18 percent, for a total of 36 percent. Burn degree is not taken into account.

190. (D) On dorsiflexion of the foot, the patient will experience upper posterior pain in the calf if a clot is present. This is termed Homan's sign.

191. (A) Compazine is a psychotropic drug, but in small doses it tends to control nausea and vomiting. The other drugs are central nervous system depressants.

192. (B) Orinase is often used in conjunction with other therapy and stimulates insulin secretion by the pancreas.

193. (C) IPPB therapy would be used postoperatively to increase respiratory movement and aid in the expectoration of secretions.

194. (A) While all of the other conditions may be complications, bleeding from the site is the main concern. The procedure is done to relieve urinary stasis which may have resulted in kidney congestion.

195. (B) The patient should not be left unattended to notify the surgeon or to get help. The nurse should treat for shock, summon help by the room call light, and reassure the patient.

196. (B) Postoperatively, some edema would be expected and should not affect the healing process, as would malnutrition, anemia, and advanced age.

197. (C) Diabetes causes complications in the nervous system and the vascular system but *not* in the respiratory.

198. (C) *U80* indicates that each ml or cc of insulin contains 80 units.

199. (C) Amphiarthrotic is an articulation that permits little movement (the term *arthr* refers to joint). Synarthrotic means the articulation is joined by fibrous tissue so it is immovable.

200. (C) Sensitive trigger zones are present in the cheek and may be stimulated by cold temperatures or even washing.

201. (D) Pain is due to contraction of the gallbladder, which has stones present. The gallbladder empties when fat is present in the stomach. The gallbladder is located in the upper right side of the abdomen along the side of the liver.

202. (C) Patients with high abdominal incisions tend to splint and do not like to cough and deep breathe because of associated pain.

203. (A) Patients are positioned in a semi-Fowler's position to assist in drainage. The T-tube can be clamped before meals to accumulate enough bile for digestion. The drainage bottle is positioned below the level of the bed to facilitate drainage.

204. (A) *Trache* refers to trachea, and *ostomy* is a suffix which means "opening into."

205. (D) Moisture is necessary because the inspired air no longer enters through the normal route, which would help to moisten the inspired air.

206. (B) The tube will become blocked with mucus and prevent the movement of air in and out of the lungs.

207. (C) Respiratory complications could occur because of the area of the injuries and the insertion of the tracheostomy tube, which could easily become blocked.

208. (C) This diet tends to inhibit stimulation of insulin release.

209. (B) Water loss occurs from fluid moving from vascular compartment in burned area to interstitial tissues surrounding the burned area, causing edema.

210. (B) The vertebral column is part of the central axis of the body known as axial.

211. (C) Ossification is the formation of or conversion into bone.

212. (B) Because the procedure leaves a raw surface, the nurse will realize that hemorrhage in TUR patients is much more likely.

213. (D) Regardless of what kind of catheter is used, urine production depends upon kidney function, not elimination of the urine already produced.

214. (B) Understanding the technique for performing transurethral resection, the nurse expects hematuria the first postoperative day, clearing as each day passes. False reassurance, such as "Don't worry" or "Ask your physician," is suggestive that the nurse does not know either.

215. (A) Realizing that the other measures are suggested comfort measures, the nurse also knows that infrequent position changes leads to cardiopulmonary stasis and increases the incidence of pneumonia and thrombophlebitis postoperatively.

216. (D) Patient is to be kept at rest to prevent possible complications such as hemorrhage or further detachment. Patients should be kept on bed rest for several days. They are turned according to physician's orders. They are not allowed to cough, as this can cause increased intraocular pressure which could lead to hemorrhage.

217. (A) Mydriatric drugs are used to dilate the pupils in order to facilitate easy removal of the lens. Cryogenic just refers to low temperature; it is not a classification of drugs. Topical anesthetics would be instilled at the time of surgery, not preoperatively by the nurse.

218. (B) The function of the lens is that of accommodation, the focusing of near objects on the retina by the lens. Therefore, only the remaining lens will function in this capacity, dependent on whether a cataract is present.

219. (C) Erythema is usually one of the first signs of a possible wound infection. An increased temperature the first 24 hours is usually indicative of dehydration or possible pulmonary complications.

220. (D) The myofibrils of striated or skeletal muscles have alternating dark and light stripes, thus giving the appearance of striations.

221. (A) In order to predict what body part a skeletal muscle moves, you must know which end of the muscle is the point of insertion. At that point the most movement occurs.

222. (C) After 48 hours, fluids from interstitial tissues around the burned area start to move back into the vascular compartment, and an overload can result in congestive heart failure.

223. (A) Infectious processes increase the body's need for steroids.

224. (A) Since the GI tract is not considered a sterile system, the nurse will introduce sterile saline with medical asepsis to prevent introduction of pathogenic organisms.

225. (D) The sugar content of urine in diabetes insipidus is not of concern.

226. (D) Soda bicarbonate is absorbed into the system and destroys acid balance; it can lead to acidosis.

227. (C) There is a good possibility that the vomiting was caused by an allergic reaction to Demerol, so it should not be administered again.

228. (A) A fusion is done to stabilize several vertebra so these patients must try to keep their back straight. They can begin to lift items and stoop but not for long periods.

229. (C) All other responses are incorrect. Milk is from the milk exchange; nuts are from the fat exchange; one ounce of cheese is equivalent.

230. (B) The patient may be placed in semi-Fowler's position or have the head of the bed elevated four to six inches on blocks to promote the flow of drainage to the lower pelvic region, where it can localize in an abscess and be drained or be resolved by body defenses.

231. (D) Frequent oral hygiene is important to promote the patient's comfort. Abdominal distention, nausea or vomiting would indicate obstruction of the nasogastric tube. The intestinal tube should remain free to facilitate passage by peristalsis. Turning the patient from side to side will also facilitate advancement. A record of the color and amount of drainage should be maintained.

232. (C) The stapes, an ossicle in the middle ear, becomes fixed and immovable.

233. (D) Prolonged pressure on the affected side contributes to contractures, deformities, and decubitus ulcers due to loss of motor tone and circulation.

234. (C) Recovery of language is related to frequent attempts to communicate with a responsive listener. Allowing the patient to use his jargon to express his needs encourages further attempts to communicate.

235. (C) Homonymous hemianopsia is a common visual deficiency associated with hemiplegia. Loss of the visual field must be compensated for by the patient's increased conscious awareness of hazards to personal safety.

236. (C) Patients with brain damage following a CVA may have difficulty with new learning and generalization. Home visits may be necessary to aid in the transfer of learning from the hospital to the home.

Emergency Nursing

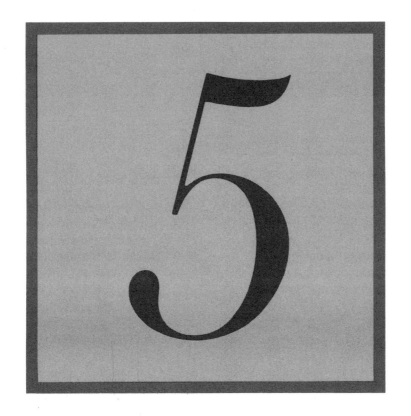

Emergency and First Aid Nursing

Disasters

Definition: A catastrophe which may be either natural or man-made in origin.

A. General guidelines: keep calm, take time to think, then take appropriate action.

B. First steps to take in a disaster—gather the following items:
   1. Water.
   2. Canned or sealed packaged foods that do not require refrigeration or cooking.
   3. Medicines needed by family members.
   4. First aid kit.
   5. Blankets or sleeping bags.
   6. Flashlights.
   7. Battery-powered radio.
   8. Covered containers for toilet and/or garbage.

C. Precautions after a disaster.
   1. Use caution in entering a building or working indoors.
   2. Check for gas leaks.
   3. Stay away from fallen or damaged electrical wires.

Water, Food, and Sanitation Principles

A. Care and use of water.
   1. Allow one quart of water per day per person.
   2. Strain rusty water through a paper towel or several thicknesses of clean cloth.
   3. Methods of purifying water.
      a. Boil 3 to 5 minutes.
      b. Add four purifying tablets per gallon of water.
      c. Add eight drops chlorine to one gallon of water, and let stand for 30 minutes.
      d. Add ten drops bleach to one gallon of water, and let stand for 30 minutes.
      e. Use 12 drops tincture of iodine per one gallon of water.

B. Care and use of food.
   1. One-half normal intake is adequate except for growing children and pregnant women.
   2. Store in covered containers.

C. Sanitation.
   1. Emergency toilet facility can be made by using a watertight container with snug-fitting cover.
   2. After each use, pour or sprinkle household disinfectant to decrease odor and germs.

D. Garbage—dispose of garbage by wrapping in newspaper and placing in air-tight container.

E. Insect control.
   1. Maintain cleanliness.
   2. Spray with insect repellant if available.

First Aid Care

Definition: Immediate care given to a person who has been injured or suddenly taken ill, when medical assistance is not available.

A. First aid training can mean the difference between life and death, temporary and permanent disability, and rapid recovery and long hospitalization.

B. General directions for giving first aid.
   1. Decisions and actions vary according to:
      a. Circumstances.
      b. Number of persons involved.
      c. Immediate environment.
      d. Availability of medical assistance.
      e. Availability of equipment and supplies.
   2. Improvise—make do with what is available.
   3. Set priorities.
      a. Sorting of casualties.
         (1) Sorting is done by most responsible person.
         (2) Rapid initial evaluation of the victims general condition to determine most seriously injured person.
      b. Priorities of treatment.
         (1) First priority is victim needing immediate attention in order to survive.
         (2) Second priority is victim needing immediate surgery.
         (3) Third priority is victim who re-

quires surgery but can tolerate a delay.

4. Cardinal rules.
   a. Establish airway.
   b. Stop bleeding.
   c. Treat for shock.
   d. Preserve function of injured area.
   e. Give comfort.
   f. Preserve cosmetic appearance.

5. When calling for assistance, give following information.
   a. Identify problem.
   b. Relate what is currently being done.
   c. Give your name and name of victim.
   d. Give location of accident.
   e. Relate number of persons involved.
   f. Give phone number you are calling from.

6. Once first aid is begun, remain with victim until qualified persons arrive or victim is able to care for self.

7. Do not make a diagnosis.

C. Dressings—applied over wounds.

1. Function.
   a. Assist in controlling bleeding.
   b. Absorb blood and wound secretions.
   c. Prevent additional contamination.
   d. Ease pain.

2. Sterilizing dressings.
   a. Place in moderate oven (350°) for three hours.
   b. Press clean cloth with iron.

D. Bandage—used to hold dressing or splint in place.

1. Material used.
   a. Usually gauze, cloth, or elastic.
   b. Emergency—handkerchief, belt, tie.

2. General principles for applying bandages.
   a. Snug but not so tight as to interfere with circulation.
   b. Leave fingertips and toes exposed when splint or bandage applied.
   c. Check for swelling, color changes, and coldness in extremities.

Common Emergencies

Wounds

Definition: Break in the continuity of the tissue of the body, either internal or external.

A. Classification.
   1. Open—break in the skin or mucous membrane.
   2. Closed—injury to underlying tissues without a break in the skin or mucous membrane.

B. Types of open wounds.
   1. Abrased. - bruise
   2. Incised. - cut.
   3. Lacerated. - tearing cut.
   4. Punctured. -.
   5. Avulsed. -tear away apart.

☆C. First aid for open wounds.
   1. Stop bleeding immediately.
   2. Protect wound from contamination and infection.
   3. Provide shock care.
   4. Obtain medical attention.

☆D. Techniques to stop severe bleeding.
   1. Direct pressure.
   2. Elevation.
   3. Pressure on supplying artery.
   4. Tourniquet.

E. Characteristics of closed wounds.
   1. No break in skin.
   2. Blood loss may be from outer openings of body cavities.
   3. Usually caused by an external force.
   4. Victim demonstrates signs of internal bleeding. or shock-↑ pulse

F. First aid for closed wounds.
   1. Check for fractures and other internal injuries.
   2. Treat for shock.
   3. Do not give fluids by mouth if internal injuries are suspected.

4. Apply ice to small areas of closed wounds.
G. Measures to prevent contamination or infection of wounds.
   1. Do not remove cloth pad initially placed on wound.
   2. Do not cleanse deep wounds which require medical attention.
   3. Use sterile dressing or cleanest dressing available. (dip)
   4. Do not remove deeply embedded objects.

Shock States

Definition: An abnormal physiological state in which there is insufficient circulating blood volume for the size of the vascular bed, thereby resulting in circulatory failure and tissue anoxia.

Classifications of Shock States

A. Hypovolemic.
   1. Definition: decreased intravascular fluid volume.
   2. Etiology.
      a. Blood loss (hematogenic)—from trauma, surgery, etc.
      b. Plasma and/or fluid loss.
         (1) Plasma loss—burns.
         (2) Fluid loss—diarrhea, vomiting, diabetes.
B. Neurogenic.
   1. Definition: massive vasodilation and pooling of blood due to failure of sympathetic nerve impulses to produce vasoconstriction.
   2. Etiology.
      a. Drug overdose, especially narcotics.
      b. Severe pain.
      c. Damage to medulla.
      d. Deep anesthesia.
C. Vasogenic.
   1. Definition: massive vasodilation and pooling of blood due to failure of peripheral vessels to react to neural stimuli.
   2. Etiology.
      a. Antigen—antibody reaction causes anaphylactic shock.
         (1) Insect stings.

(2) Allergies to drugs, particularly antibiotics.
(3) Blood transfusions.
(4) Vaccines.
   b. Bacterial invasion causes gram negative sepsis (septic shock).
      (1) Following urinary tract instrumentation.
      (2) Overwhelming bacterial invasion of an "at risk" patient.
D. Cardiogenic.
   1. Definition: left ventricular pump failure which results in circulatory inadequacy.
   2. Etiology.
      a. Myocardial infarction.
      b. Congestive heart failure.
      c. Cardiac arrest.

Early Shock

A. Early stages, regardless of cause.
   1. Decreased tissue perfusion.
   2. Cellular hypoxia.
   3. Increased sympathetic nervous system activity.
B. Oliguria—usually the first sign of shock.
   1. Decreased blood volume through kidneys.
   2. Decreased urine output; hyperkalemia can be a problem.
C. Hypotension.
   1. Due to compensatory peripheral vasoconstriction (not evident initially, but it does appear in late shock).
   2. Narrowing pulse pressure—due to systolic pressure falling and diastolic pressure being maintained.
   3. Traditional criteria—systolic blood pressure below 70 mm Hg.
D. Tachycardia—due to heart's responding to increased sympathetic activity.
E. Tachypnea.
   1. Medulla is stimulated by buildup in lactic acid through anaerobic metabolism.
   2. As blood pH is lowered, the respiratory rate increases in an effort to blow off excess car-

bon dioxide and return body to acid-base balance.

F. Cool, dry or moist skin is present.
   1. Caused by peripheral vasoconstriction.
   2. Blood is supplied to vital organs rather than to skin.

G. Sensorium changes—due to brain cell hypoxia.
   1. Restlessness.
   2. Apprehension and anxiety.
   3. Lethargy.
   4. Confusion.
   5. Semiconsciousness to coma.

H. Excess thirst is present due to loss of fluids or blood volume as well as peripheral vasoconstriction, which decreases salivary secretions.

I. Fatigue and muscle weakness—result of shift from aerobic to anaerobic metabolism leading to lactic acid buildup.

Severe Shock

A. Blood pressure: below 70 mm Hg and narrowing of pulse pressure (body loses ability to compensate and blood pressure drops rapidly).

B. Shallow, irregular respirations.

C. Tachycardia.

D. Level of unconsciousness: progresses to coma as blood supply to brain cell decreases.

E. Dilated, fixed pupils due to decreased oxygen to brain.

F. Anuria as blood supply to kidneys decreases sharply.

G. Cyanotic skin, mucous membranes, and nailbeds.

Hypovolemic Shock

Degrees of Shock

A. Slight: approximately 20 percent of blood volume is lost.

B. Moderate: approximately 35 percent of blood volume is lost.

C. Severe: approximately 45 percent of blood volume is lost.

Treatment and Nursing Care

A. Monitor patency of IV for drug (vasodilator), plasma expanders, IV fluid, or blood replacement.

B. Start IV fluid with D_5W. When adequate kidney function is assessed, Ringer's lactate (more isotonic) is used.

C. Place in supine position with feet and/or head slightly elevated (Trendelenburg's position compromises venous return as well as respirations).

D. Provide oxygen via nasal catheter, mask, or cannula.

E. Record vital signs every fifteen minutes. Changes take place slowly except in massive hemorrhage.
   1. Blood pressure.
      a. Decreased BP is usually late sign of shock.
      b. Orthostatic hypotension develops before systemic hypotension.
      c. Systolic BP below 80 mm Hg indicates inadequate coronary artery blood flow.
      d. Progressive drop in BP with a thready, increasing pulse indicates fluid loss.
      e. Decreased BP with strong, irregular pulse indicates heart failure.
   2. Respirations.
      a. Become rapid and shallow early in shock (compensation for tissue anoxia).
      b. Slow breathing (below four per minute) appears late in shock after compensatory failure.
      c. Emergency respiratory equipment (ventilator, trach tubes, etc.) should be available.
   3. Temperature.
      a. Below normal with hemorrhagic shock.
      b. Gradually increasing temperature indicates sepsis.
   4. Central venous pressure.

F. Insert Foley catheter for hourly urine volumes.
   1. Record intake and output.
   2. Notify physician if total urine output is below 30 cc/hour.

G. Monitor skin changes.
   1. Change in skin temperature and color reflect

changes in tissue oxygenation and perfusion.

    a. Cold, clammy skin indicates peripheral vascular constriction.

    b. Flushing and sweating reflects overheating, which indicates increased metabolic rate and the need for oxygen.

    c. Pallor and cyanosis indicate tissue hypoxia.

  2. Observe for restlessness—indicates hypoxia.

H. Place enough light covering over patient to prevent chilling, but not enough to cause vasodilatation.

I. Treat the cause of the shock (stop bleeding, prepare for surgery, etc.).

Cardiogenic Shock

Assessment

A. Cardiac arrhythmias leading to cardiac arrest.

B. Heart failure symptoms.
1. Orthopnea.
2. Cyanosis.
3. Dyspnea.
4. Pitting edema.
5. Distended neck veins.
6. Pulmonary congestion.

C. Acidosis.

D. Hypokalemia.

Treatment and Nursing Care

A. Administer digitalis preparation in addition to diuretics.

B. Watch for hypokalemia and arrhythmias.

C. Administer vasodilators or vasopressors, as ordered.

D. Check arterial blood gases frequently.

E. Monitor intra-aortic balloon.

F. Follow interventions for hypovolemic shock for additional nursing care.

Vasogenic Shock

Septic Shock (Toxic Shock)

A. Mortality—60 to 82 percent.

B. Caused by bacterial toxins (gm − or +); leads to vasodilatation.

C. Conditions leading to septic shock.
1. Peritonitis.
2. Urinary tract manipulations.
3. Gas gangrene.

Signs and Symptoms

A. Mild infection.
1. Fever; warm, pink face.
2. Perspiration.
3. Weakness, generalized aching.

B. Severe infection.
1. High temperature (over 104°) and sudden violent chills.
2. Hemorrhage into tissue.
3. Muscular pain.
4. Rapid, deep respirations.
5. Confusion and disorientation is present.
6. Warm, dry skin.

Nursing Care

A. Administer broad spectrum antibiotics and then organism specific antibiotics.

B. Provide systemic supportive nursing management.

Anaphylactic Shock

A. Caused by hypersensitivity to allergen (allergic reaction to medication, bee sting, etc.).

B. Antigen—antibody reaction.

C. Increased cell membrane permeability—histamine is released, causing marked vasodilatation.

D. Bronchiolar constriction.

E. Pooling of blood, causing decreased venous return.

F. Decreased cardiac output and hypoxia.

Signs and Symptoms.

A. Local edema.

B. Urticaria (occasional).

C. Flushed face.

D. Apprehension is present.

E. Dyspnea, respiratory difficulty, cyanosis, wheezing.

F. Vertigo, decreased blood pressure, increased pulse.

Treatment and Nursing Care

A. Identify causative agent.

B. Position for optimal cerebral perfusion (flat or 30-degree elevation if dyspneic).

C. Maintain patent airway.

D. Administer epinephrine, sub q.
   1. Dilates bronchioles and constricts arterioles.
   2. Side effects: tachycardia, CNS stimulation.
   3. Rapid acting.

E. Administer oxygen.

F. Administer antihistamine (Benadryl).
   1. Relieves itching, wheals, congestion of nasal mucosa.
   2. Side effect: dries mucous membranes.

G. Maintain IV of D_5W—as much as 2000 cc in one hour.

H. Administer corticosteroids.
   1. Reduce formation of cellular proteins and decrease edema.
   2. Side effects: same as any steroids.

I. Administer aminophylline—bronchodilator; controls bronchospasms.

Snake Bite

Signs and Symptoms

A. Assess extent of envenomation: Rattlesnakes, copperheads, cottonmouths (pitvipers) are responsible for 98 percent of venomous bites.

B. Signs:
   1. Blood oozing from wound.
   2. One or two distinct puncture wounds.
   3. Edema and discoloration.
   4. Numbness around bite within 5 to 15 minutes.
   5. Painful and enlarged lymph nodes.

C. Reactions to poisonous snakes occur within 30 to 60 minutes.

D. Advanced signs indicating shock.
   1. Nausea, vomiting.
   2. Ecchymosis, blebs, blisters.
   3. Bleeding.
   4. Weakness, vertigo, clammy skin.

Treatment and Nursing Care

A. Emergency treatment: within 30 to 60 minutes of medical help.
   1. Immobilize area with support or sling.
   2. Apply tourniquet.
   3. Do not allow patient to physically exert self as this hastens spread of venom.
   4. Seek medical help immediately.

B. Emergency treatment: when medical help is not available within 30 to 60 minutes.
   1. Apply nonocclusive tourniquet or constriction band 5 to 13 cm above wound.
      a. Adjust to allow for venous and lymphatic flow restriction but allow for arterial flow.
      b. Loosen, but do not remove, for 1½ minutes every 15 minutes.
   2. Wash around bite with alcohol, hydrogen peroxide, or soap and water.
   3. Sterilize knife with match flame, alcohol, or soap and water, make longitudinal incision (not cross marks) 0.3 to 0.6 cm long and no more than 0.3 cm deep through each fang mark.
   4. Apply suction over incision site.
   5. Procedure must be done within 10 minutes of bite. After 30 to 60 minutes, little venom will be extractable.

C. In-hospital treatment.
   1. Within 30 to 60 minutes, make incisions and use suction intermittently for at least one hour.
   2. Test for sensitivity to horse serum.

3. Judge severity of envenomation before giving antivenin.
   a. Minimal pitviper bite: 1 to 5 ampules of antivenin (Crotalid) IM.
   b. Moderate bite: 5 to 9 ampules IV drip.
   c. Severe bite: 9 ampules IV drip immediately and up to 20 ampules over next 4 to 24 hours, until edema ceases and symptoms improve.
4. Administer tetanus toxoid.
5. Administer analgesics for pain.
   a. ASA for mild pain.
   b. Codeine or Demerol for severe pain.
6. Administer antibiotics.
   a. Initial dose: ampicillin, erythromycin, or tetracycline 500 mg.
   b. Maintain 250 mg every 4 hours for 24 hours.

Bee Sting

Signs and Symptoms

A. Generalized itching.
B. Erythema and hives.
C. Feeling of heat throughout body.
D. Weakness, vertigo.
E. Nausea, vomiting, abdominal cramps.
F. Tightness in chest, difficulty swallowing or breathing.

Treatment and Nursing Care

☆A. Remove stinger with tweezers or by scraping motion with fingernail. Do not squeeze venom sac.
B. Immediately administer epinephrine 1:1000 solution sub q. as ordered.
   1. Adult: 0.25 to 0.3 ml at sting site and same amount in unaffected arm.
   2. Child: 0.01 ml/kg (maximum 0.25 ml at each site).
C. Repeat injections as ordered one to three times at 20-minute intervals until blood pressure and pulse rise toward normal.
   1. Adult: 0.3 to 0.4 ml.

2. Child: less than 20 kg, 0.10 to 0.15 ml; over 20 kg, 0.15, to 0.3 ml.
D. Apply tourniquet above sting on an extremity. Loosen every three to five minutes to allow venom to slowly enter circulation.
E. Cleanse sting area and apply ice to relieve pain and edema.
F. Administer pressor agents as ordered if blood pressure does not stabilize following 2 to 3 sub q injections of epinephrine.
   1. Aramine or Levophed drugs of choice.
   2. Administer IV drip at 30 to 40 drops per minute.
G. Monitor IV solution of D_5W with 250 mg aminophylline and 30 to 40 mg Solu-Cortef to support circulation and prevent shock.
H. Observe for signs of laryngospasm or bronchospasm. Be prepared to assist with a tracheostomy.
I. Keep patient warm and positioned supine with head and feet slightly elevated.
J. Administer rapid-acting antihistamine: Benadryl 50 mg IM as ordered.

Choking

Definition: Temporary or permanent asphyxia due to obstruction of the airway.

A. Signs and symptoms.
   1. Violent choking.
   2. Alarming attempts at inhalation.
   3. Cyanosis of face, neck, and hands.
   4. Cessation of breathing.
   5. Inability to speak.
   6. Unconsciousness.
B. First aid measures.
   1. Remove object if possible.
   2. Allow victim to assume position of comfort.
   3. Encourage coughing.
   4. Heimlich maneuver.
   5. Artificial respirations if breathing ceases.
   6. Obtain medical assistance.

Poisoning

Definition: Introduction into the body or onto the skin surface of any solid, liquid or gas that tends to impair health or to cause death.

A. First aid treatment.
1. Call doctor or poison control center. Give the following information.
    a. Age of victim.
    b. Name and amount of poison taken.
    c. Whether or not victim vomited.
2. If victim is conscious, give antidote, if known.
3. Induce vomiting if material ingested is not strong acid or petroleum product.
4. If inhaled gases, remove victim to fresh air.
5. If contact poison, wash exposed areas.
B. Follow-up treatment as prescribed.

Frostbite and Cold Exposure

A. Signs and symptoms.
1. White or grayish-yellow skin.
2. Pain.
3. Blisters.
4. Area cold and numb.
5. Mental confusion.
B. First aid treatment.
1. Cover area.
2. Rewarm area quickly.
3. Do not rub.
4. Elevate affected area.

Heat Exhaustion

Definition: Response to heat characterized by fatigue and weakness; occurs when intake of water cannot compensate for loss of fluids through sweating.

A. Signs and symptoms.
1. Pale, clammy skin.
2. Profuse perspiration.
3. Headache.
4. Nausea.
5. Dizziness.
6. Fainting.
B. First aid treatment.
1. Offer victim sips of salt water—½ glass every 15 minutes for one hour.
2. Have victim lie down and elevate feet.
3. Place in cool environment.
4. Apply cool, wet cloths.

Heat Stroke

Definition: Response to heat characterized by extremely high body temperature due to disturbance in sweating mechanism.

A. Signs and symptoms.
1. High body temperature—104 or higher.
2. Hot, red, dry skin.
3. Rapid, strong pulse.
B. First aid treatment—cool body quickly.

Burns

Definition: Injury of the skin, subcutaneous tissue, muscle, and/or bones caused by heat, chemical agent, or radiation.

A. Classification of burns.
1. First degree—red skin, mild swelling and pain, rapid healing.
2. Second degree—red or mottled skin, blisters, considerable swelling, wet appearance due to loss of plasma, and severe pain.
3. Third degree—deep tissue destruction, white or charred appearance, complete loss of all layers of skin. Skin graft needed for healing.
☆B. First aid treatment for first degree burn.
1. Apply cold water or submerge in cold water.
2. Prevent contamination.
3. Avoid greasy substances.
C. First aid treatment for second degree burn.
1. Immerse burn, if fairly small area, in cold water for 1 to 2 hours.
2. Apply clean cloths.

3. Blot area dry.
4. Do not break blisters.
5. Do not apply antiseptic preparations or home remedies.
6. Elevate affected extremities.
7. Seek medical attention.

D. First aid treatment for third degree burns.
1. Do not attempt to remove clothing from burned area.
2. Cover burn with sterile dressing.
3. Elevate involved extremities.
4. Do not immerse burn in water or apply ice water to it.
5. If medical help is not quickly available, and victim is conscious and not vomiting, give victim, at 15 minute intervals, a solution of ½ teaspoon of salt and ½ teaspoon of soda in a quart of water.

Fracture

Definition: A break or crack in a bone.

A. Types of fractures.
1. Open—bone ends protrude through skin.
2. Closed—bone cracked or broken but does not protrude through skin.

B. Signs and symptoms.
1. Victim heard or felt bone snap.
2. Abnormal or false motion in body area.
3. Differences in shape and length of corresponding bones.
4. Obvious deformities.
5. Swelling.
6. Discoloration.
7. Pain or tenderness to touch.

C. First aid measures.
1. Prevent motion of injured parts and adjacent joints. (even if uncure its broke)
2. Elevate involved extremities.
3. Apply splints.

☆ D. Splinting—device used to immobilize extremity or trunk when a fracture is suspected.

1. Purpose.
a. Immobilize part.
✳ b. Decrease pain. (muscle spasm
c. Reduce chance of shock.
d. Protect against further injury during transportation.

2. Principles.
a. Ensure splint is long enough to extend past joint on either side of suspected fracture.
b. Place pad between splint and skin.
c. Immobilize joints above and below location of suspected fracture.
d. Apply splint to extremity; do circulation checks to fingers/toes.

Sprain

✳ *Definition*: Injury to a joint ligament or a muscle tendon in region of a joint.

A. Signs and symptoms.
1. Swelling.
2. Tenderness.
3. Pain on motion.
4. Discoloration.

B. First aid measures.
1. Do not allow walking if ankle or knee sprained.
2. Elevate limb for twenty-four hours.
3. Apply ice first twenty-four hours.
4. If swelling and pain persist, seek medical attention.

Strain

Definition: Injury to a muscle as a result of overstretching.

A. Signs and symptoms.
1. Pain on motion.
2. Discoloration.

B. First aid measures.
1. Bed rest.
2. Heat.
3. Bed board (with back sprain).

Dislocation

Definition: Injury to capsule and ligaments of a joint that results in displacement of a bone end at a joint.

A. Signs and symptoms.

1. Swelling.

2. Obvious deformity.

3. Pain upon motion.

4. Tenderness to touch.

5. Discoloration.

B. First aid measures.

1. Splint and immobilize affected joint in position as found.

2. Do not reduce dislocation or correct deformity near a joint.

3. Apply sling if appropriate.

4. Elevate affected part if possible.

Emergency Treatments

Cardiopulmonary Resuscitation (CPR)

Suspect Unconsciousness

A. Call out for help.
B. Quickly approach victim.
C. Check responsiveness.
   1. Shake shoulders.
   2. Shout "Are you OK?"
D. Obtain proper position.
   1. Victim: flat on firm surface.
   2. Rescuer: next to victim at approximately the same level.

Respiratory Management

A. Airway obstruction.
☆1. Food or other foreign body aspirant (if known cause of unconsciousness).
   a. Tilt head—hyperextend neck and chin forward.
   b. One attempt to ventilate will not be successful if obstructed.
   c. If not successful, reposition head and reattempt to ventilate.
   d. If not successful, presence of foreign body is assumed.
   e. Turn patient to one side and finger-probe for obstruction.
   f. If unsuccessful, roll patient to side and administer four sharp blows to the back between scapulas with back of the hand.
   g. Return patient to back and repeat finger-probe.
   h. Then repeat mouth-to-mouth breathing and evaluate condition of patient.
   i. If this method proves unsuccessful institute Heimlich maneuver.
☆2. Heimlich maneuver—abdominal thrust.
   a. Place patient in sitting or standing position. Stand behind and place arms around waist of patient.
   b. Make a fist and place it halfway between xiphoid and umbilicus.

   c. Place other hand on top of fist and perform a quick upward thrust.
   d. Repeat this maneuver three more times before returning to first method of removing a foreign body.
   e. Repeat entire procedure until open airway is obtained or advanced life support service is available.
   3. Oral airway obstructants that are blood, emesis, mucus or water.
   a. Turn head to side.
   b. Suction (if available).
   c. Finger swoops.
B. Open airway.
   1. Adult.
   a. Apply head-tilt method.
   b. Apply jaw-thrust or chin-lift method (if neck injury even remotely possible).
   2. Infant or toddler.
   a. Tilt head back without hyperextension.
   b. Use normal, horizontal alignment, flat surface.
C. Evaluate respiratory function.
   1. Maintain open airway.
   2. Observe for respiratory activity.
   a. Put ear down near mouth.
   b. Look for chest movement.
   c. Feel for air flow with cheek.
   d. Listen for exhalation.
☆D. Procedure.
   1. Maintain open airway.
   2. Form tight seal.
   3. Adult management.
   a. Replace victim's dentures (if any).
   b. Pinch off nostrils.
   c. Fit mouth-to-mouth seal.
   4. Infant or toddler management.
   a. Encircle nose and mouth.
   b. Maintain tight seal.
   5. Administer four quick, full breaths.
   a. Give breaths as fast as you can.
   b. Between breaths, release seal for exhalation.
   c. Take fresh breath; do not allow completion deflation of lungs (stairstep volume).
   d. Maintain position.

e. Assess volume: adult—800 cc minimum; infant—cheek full puffs.

Circulatory Management

A. Take major pulse.
   1. Adult: carotid preferably and femoral as alternate.
   2. Palpate one side, with two fingers, for five seconds.
☆B. Procedure (if pulseless).
   1. Precordial thump (on adults monitored by EKG only).
      a. Place hands on midline, lower half of sternum, two finger-widths above xiphoid process.
      b. Apply single sharp blow 8 to 12 in above sternum.
      c. Use fleshy side of fist.
      d. Evaluate effectiveness immediately on EKG and confirm with pulse, or proceed with CPR as indicated.
   2. Cardiac compressions (firm surface or cardiac board needed).
   3. For adults.
      a. Place hand on midline, lower half of sternum, two finger-widths above xiphoid.
      b. Place heel of one hand on sternum, other hand superimposed.
      c. Interlace fingers or extend off rib cage.
      d. Rate 80 per minute, depth 1½ to 2 in.
      e. Contraindicated when abdominal pain is present.
      f. Release pressure between compressions for cardiac refilling.
      g. Do not take hands off chest between compressions.
   4. For children.
      a. Place hand on midline sternum, midway between xiphoid process and cricothyroid notch.
      b. Use heel of one hand only.
      c. Rate 80 per minute, depth ¾ to 1½ in. for small child, 1 to 2 in. larger child.
   5. For infants.

      a. Place fingers on midline sternum, midway between xiphoid process and cricothyroid notch.
      b. Use two fingers only.
      c. Rate 100 per minute, depth ½ to ¾ in.
      d. Count compressions: one, two, three, four, five.

Interpolation (Compressions: Ventilations)

A. Lone rescuer: (15:2 for adults; 5:1 for infants).
B. Two rescuers: (5:1 adults).
☆C. Changing roles.
   1. Compressor sets pace (one, one thousand, two, one thousand, three, one thousand, four, one thousand, breath).
   2. Compressor observes for need and institutes change.
   3. Compressor states, "Change, one-thousand; two, one-thousand."
   4. Rescuer giving breaths gets into position to give compressions.
   5. Rescuer giving compressions moves to victim's head after fifth compression, counts pulse for five seconds.
   6. If no pulse, rescuer checking pulse states, "No pulse, start CPR," gives a breath, and CPR is begun again.

CPR Evaluation

☆A. In process.
   1. Check major pulse after one minute of CPR.
      a. Equal to 4 sets of 15:2 by one rescuer.
      b. Equal to 12 sets of 5:1 by two rescuers.
   2. Check major pulse every four to five minutes thereafter.
   3. Check pupil every four to five minutes; optional if third trained person present (not always a conclusive indicator).
   4. Observe for abdominal distention (all age groups).
      a. If evident, reposition airway and reduce force of ventilation.
      b. Maintain a volume sufficient to elevate ribs.
   5. Ventilator must check carotid pulse fre-

quently between breaths to evaluate perfusion.

6. Ventilator must observe each breath for effectiveness.

7. If respiratory arrest only, check major pulse after each minute (12 breaths) to ensure continuation of cardiac function.

B. After termination.

1. Diagnosis made (no pulse, no respirations) and intervention instituted within one minute after unconsciousness.

2. Assistance summoned and entry into Emergency Medical System done promptly and efficiently.

3. Proper CPR performed until acceptable termination.

4. No delay in CPR longer than five seconds (except extraordinary circumstances).

5. No delay in CPR longer than fifteen seconds for extraordinary circumstances (intubation, transportation down stairs).

6. Victim outcome.

a. Condition.

b. Potential for cardiac rehabilitation.

c. Secondary complications (fractured ribs, ruptured spleen, lacerated liver, etc.).

Termination of CPR

A. Successful resuscitation.

1. Spontaneous return of adequate life support.

2. Assisted life support.

B. Transfer to emergency vehicle (other trained rescuers assume care).

C. Pronounced dead by physician.

D. Exhaustion of rescuer(s).

Review Questions

1. The main function of a pressure dressing would be to

   A. Assist in the control of bleeding.
   B. Support a body part.
   C. Absorb blood.
   D. Ease pain.

2. To prevent shock, immediate treatment should include

   A. Apply ice to lower body temperature.
   B. Elevate lower extremities and prevent loss of body heat.
   C. Elevate upper extremities and apply blankets to raise body temperature.
   D. Maintain patent airway and prevent vomiting.

3. Mr. Kulick needs a whole blood transfusion immediately, and his type and cross match is not completed. Which of these types of blood would he most likely receive?

   A. O.
   B. A.
   C. AB.
   D. B.

4. The complication that can develop if a victim vomits after ingesting a strong acid is

   A. Burns of the mouth, esophagus, and stomach.
   B. Heart attack.
   C. Pneumonia.
   D. Stroke.

5. You arrive at an accident and find the victim bleeding profusely from a deep laceration on his left lower forearm. Your choice of action would be to

   A. Apply a tourniquet just below the elbow.
   B. Apply pressure directly over the wound.
   C. Call for the emergency squad.
   D. Treat the victim for shock.

6. How far do you depress the chest of an adult when doing external cardiac compressions?

   A. 1/2 to 3/4 inches.
   B. 1/2 to 1 inch.
   C. 1 to 1½ inches.
   D. 1½ to 2 inches.

7. If you are eating in a restaurant and someone yells, "Help! My husband is choking," as a first aider, the first thing you should do is

   A. Give an abdominal thrust.
   B. Give a back blow.
   C. Establish an airway.
   D. Ask the victim, "Can you talk?"

8. An open fracture is defined as a

   A. Break or crack in a bone.
   B. Fracture not related to open wounds on surface of body.
   C. Fracture associated directly with an open wound with bone ends protruding through the skin.
   D. Injury to a joint ligament.

9. The first aid measures which should be done before a victim is transferred include all the following *except*

   A. Establish or maintain airway.
   B. Dress wounds.
   C. Splint fractures.
   D. Provide fluids to prevent shock.

10. You are supporting a young woman who is in active labor. She is full term, and this is her first pregnancy. Because of a blizzard, you are unable to get her to the hospital. What is the most important thing for you as the first aider to do?

    A. Time contractions for frequency and duration.
    B. Remain calm and let nature take its course.
    C. Boil all the equipment you will need for the delivery.
    D. Provide her with a light meal so she can maintain her strength.

11. Characteristics of a second-degree burn include

    A. Reddening of the skin.
    B. Damage to but not through the epidermis, with resultant blisters.
    C. Damage to but not through the dermis, with resultant blisters.
    D. Damage to and including the subcutaneous layer, appearing white or brown in color.

12. Thirty-year-old Jim Brown has burns on the front and back of both his legs and arms. Approximately what percentage of his body has been involved?

    A. 27%.
    B. 36%.
    C. 45%.
    D. 54%.

13. Two-year-old Chris Brown has been pulled from the same fire in which his father was involved. He has burns on his head and back. What approximate percentage of the child's body surface has been burned?

    A. 18%.
    B. 27%.

C. 36%.
D. 45%.

14. Lisa, an 18-year-old, has burned both of her arms while trying to put out a grease fire. She has reddening and blisters on each arm. She arrives in the hospital five minutes later. The initial care will most likely be

A. Cover her arms with dry, sterile dressings.
B. Immerse her arms in cold water for a couple of minutes before dressing.
C. Apply copious amounts of petroleum jelly to relieve pain.
D. Apply silver nitrate to her burns and cover with sterile dressings.

15. Immediate care for burns caused by a liquid chemical should include

A. Irrigation after the clothing has been removed.
B. Use of a powerful stream of water to irrigate burned tissue.
C. Use of a garden hose to irrigate large affected areas.
D. Use of neutralizing solution prior to irrigation with water.

16. Heat exhaustion typically presents with

A. Weakness, dizziness, and cool skin.
B. Weakness and flushed, hot skin.
C. Muscle cramps, wet skin, and thirst.
D. Dizziness and hot, dry skin.

17. Proper care for frostbitten extremities includes

A. Gentle rubbing with snow to increase peripheral circulation.
B. Warm-water immersion, with water temperature between 105°F and 115°F.
C. Protection from further damage by removing the patient to a warmer environment but not allowing thawing to occur.
D. Slow rewarming in room air or warm water at less than 105°F.

18. Choose the group of signs and symptoms that best describes the condition of a person experiencing heat stroke.

A. Pale, moist skin; rapid pulse; and slow, deep respirations.
B. Hot, dry skin; rapid pulse; and slow, deep respirations.
C. Hot, dry skin; normal pulse; and normal respirations.
D. Pale, moist skin; weak pulse; and rapid respirations.

19. Shock can be caused by all of the following conditions *except*

A. Heart damage.
B. Blood vessel constriction.
C. Loss of blood volume.
D. Blood vessel dilation.

20. Which of the following conditions is usually present when a person is in shock?

A. High urinary output.
B. Slow pulse.
C. Slow respirations.
D. Fall in blood pressure.

21. General signs of shock can include

A. Diaphoresis.
B. Cherry-red skin color.
C. Slow, shallow respirations.
D. Lustrous eyes and constricted pupils.

22. Additional signs of shock include

A. Nausea and vomiting.
B. Restfulness.
C. Hot, dry skin.
D. Lack of thirst.

23. A common sign or symptom present during anaphylactic shock is a

A. Stable blood pressure.
B. Cherry-red skin color.
C. Bounding pulse.
D. Wheezing sound during exhalation.

24. The most effective means of controlling external bleeding of an extremity is the use of

A. Direct pressure.
B. Pressure points.
C. Tourniquets.
D. Elevation.

25. Tourniquets are used only as a last resort to control bleeding because they

A. Are difficult to apply.
B. Must be released every 20 minutes.
C. Can only be used below the elbow or knee.
D. Cause considerable nerve and tissue damage.

26. Care for a patient with a piercing foreign object should include

A. Applying direct pressure on the object to control bleeding.
B. Using minimal dressings in order to allow constant observation.
C. Cutting the object off as close to the skin as possible.
D. Leaving the object in place and immobilizing it.

27. Choose the signs which best represent a patient who has reached the level of irreversible shock

    A. Pale skin, rapid and weak pulse.
    B. Cyanotic skin, rapid and weak pulse.
    C. Pale skin, slow and weak pulse.
    D. Cyanotic skin, rapid and strong pulse.

28. CPR may be discontinued when

    A. You are instructed to do so by the RN.
    B. You are instructed to do so by a physician.
    C. The patient is not breathing.
    D. The patient becomes deeply cyanotic.

29. Unconsciousness can be established by observing a patient's appropriate response to

    A. Verbal stimuli.
    B. Pupillary reaction to light.
    C. Pinching the lobe of the ear.
    D. Opening the airway.

30. An unconscious patient's airway may first be cleared by performing any of the following except

    A. Forceful mouth-to-mouth ventilation.
    B. Head tilt.
    C. Head tilt—neck lift.
    D. Jaw–thrust maneuver.

31. The best maneuver for opening an airway in a patient with a suspected neck injury is the

    A. Head tilt.
    B. Head tilt—chin lift.
    C. Head tilt—neck lift.
    D. Jaw–thrust maneuver.

32. How many times per minute should artificial ventilation be performed?

    A. 12 times in an adult.
    B. 20 times in an adult.
    C. 8 times in a child.
    D. 14 times in an infant.

33. The period of time allowed for checking unresponsiveness in a patient who appears to be unconscious should be

    A. Less than four seconds.
    B. Four to ten seconds.
    C. Five to eight seconds.
    D. Ten to twelve seconds.

34. After the airway has been opened, you should

    A. Ventilate two times.
    B. Palpate the pulse.
    C. Ventilate four times.
    D. Observe three to five seconds for respiration.

35. During mouth-to-mouth ventilation, you should

    A. Keep your mouth on the patient's mouth.
    B. Feel no resistance when the patient's lungs are expanded.
    C. Look straight down at the patient's face after each breath for reaction.
    D. Hear air escaping after each ventilation.

36. The period of time used to establish pulselessness in a nonbreathing adult is

    A. Less than five seconds.
    B. Five to ten seconds.
    C. Ten seconds or more.
    D. Four to eight seconds.

37. Two nurses are performing proper CPR on an adult. Their ratio of compression to ventilation will be

    A. 15:2.
    B. 5:2.
    C. 3:1.
    D. 5:1.

38. Which of the following is a correct statement regarding CPR?

    A. CPR can be performed in bed.
    B. Artificial ventilation must be performed with external chest compressions.
    C. Pressure on the ziphoid can lacerate the stomach.
    D. CPR produces 50% of the normal blood flow.

39. When performing adult CPR alone, you should

    A. Use 15:2 ratio.
    B. Use 5:1 ratio.
    C. Compress at a rate of 60 per minute.
    D. Allow total exhalation after each breath.

40. If you need to interrupt CPR, you should

    A. Never interrupt CPR for more than five seconds.
    B. Interrupt CPR for the time it takes to transport.
    C. Never interrupt CPR for more than 15 seconds.
    D. Interrupt CPR only when you are tired.

Answers and Rationale

1. **(A)** Pressure causes constriction of vessels and aids in control of bleeding.

2. **(B)** To prevent shock, the victim should be placed in "shock position" (lying flat with legs raised higher than head) and covered with a blanket to

prevent loss of body heat, as shock victims lose body heat through perspiration. In head injury, victim is positioned with head elevated.

3. (A) Blood type O is considered universal donor. It has no antigens in the red cells that could be destroyed by antibodies in the recipient's blood.

4. (A) Strong acid substance will burn tissue of the mouth, esophagus and stomach when swallowed. If the victim vomits, the acid will further damage the tissue as it passes through the tissue in the vomitus. Pneumonia is a complication of vomiting a petroleum product.

5. (B) First choice of action is to stop the bleeding with direct pressure over the wound. If that is not successful you then have the option to use elevation, pressure on supplying artery; last resort — tourniquet.

6. (D) 1½ to 2 inches is recommended by the American Heart Association to provide adequate pressure within the chest cavity to provide stimulation to the heart.

7. (D) By asking, "Can you talk?" you can establish that victim has something in his airway. If victim is able to answer, he is not choking. A victim is unable to talk when choking.

8. (C) Simple definition of an open fracture; need to be able to recognize the fact that an open fracture requires the bone ends to protrude through the skin.

9. (D) To prevent shock in this situation, the first aider would utilize positioning. The concern here is to safely move injured victim, and you would also want to consider controlling the hemorrhage.

10. (B) Most important is to remain calm and let nature take its course — do not rush things. The mother may be offered fluids but no solid foods, since digestion stops when labor begins.

11. (C) A second-degree burn includes damage to the epidermis and dermis and often results in blisters. This burn does not damage tissue below the dermis. A first-degree burn appears as reddening of the skin. A third-degree burn involves tissue below the dermis and may appear white or charred.

12. (D) Mr. Brown's burns cover approximately 54% of his body surface. Each arm is 9% (18%) and each leg is 18% (36%).

13. (C) Chris Brown has burns involving his head

(18%) and back (18%), for a total of 36% body surface involvement. The head of a small child represents a much larger surface than an adult's head; therefore, it is considered 18% instead of 9%.

14. (B) Lisa has first- and second-degree burns on both of her arms. The rule of cooling applies in the first 15 minutes after a burn if less than 20% of the body surface has been involved. Lisa has 18% involvement. Immersion in cold water for 3-5 minutes will reduce pain and further burn damage.

15. (C) Immediate care for almost all liquid chemical burns should be irrigation with water. Irrigation should be done as soon as possible, with clothing removed after irrigation of the area has begun. Burned tissue is delicate, and powerful streams of water could cause tearing of the skin. Do not attempt to neutralize chemicals prior to copious water irrigation.

16. (A) Heat exhaustion typically presents with the patient complaining of weakness or vertigo. The skin is cool and wet. Heat stroke presents with hot, often dry skin and body weakness, rapidly progressing to unconsciousness.

17. (D) Proper care of frostbitten extremities is done by rewarming in warm room air or by immersing in warm water. The water temperature should be monitored constantly and kept between 100°F and 105°F. Do not rub frostbitten or frozen areas, as this will increase tissue damage.

18. (B) A person experiencing heat stroke will most likely have hot, dry skin; a rapid pulse; and slow, deep respirations.

19. (B) Constriction of blood vessels reduces the size of the cardiovascular container and thus increases available volume. This action would be desirable for a patient in shock and is often accomplished through the use of drugs.

20. (D) Falling blood pressure generally indicates shock. Urinary output is reduced due to poor perfusion. The pulse rises in rate and becomes weak in quality (thready). Respiration rate increases as the respiratory system tries to adjust for the hypoxia present.

21. (A) Diaphoresis is common in shock. The skin color will first be pale or ashen, later changing to cyanosis. Respirations will normally be deep and rapid. The eyes will be lusterless and dull.

22. (A) As nerve control over the blood vessels is lost, the blood vessels in the abdomen dilate, causing nausea and vomiting. The patient will also be

restless and thirsty and have cool, clammy skin.

23. (D) Wheezing sounds during exhalation are common during anaphylactic shock. This is due to the constriction of the smaller bronchi. The skin may be flushing, itching, or covered with hives. The pulse will be weak and the blood pressure may fall drastically.

24. (A) Direct pressure is the most effective way of controlling bleeding. It can be augmented by elevating the wound above the level of the heart. Pressure points only slow bleeding, as collateral circulation is almost always present. Tourniquets are seldom needed.

25. (D) Tourniquets are used only as a last resort because they oftentimes crush a considerable amount of tissue beneath them, causing permanent damage. Once applied, they should not be removed until the physician does so. Tourniquets should not be used below the elbow or knee, due to the additional potential of damage to these tissues, as nerves are closer to the surface of the skin. Seldom is bleeding so profuse that direct pressure and elevation cannot control it in these regions.

26. (D) A piercing object should be left in place and immobilized unless it is penetrating the skin less than one millimeter. Large, bulky dressings can help to stabilize the object. Direct pressure around the object will help to control bleeding.

27. (B) A patient in shock who starts to exhibit cyanosis of the skin, nailbeds, or lips has probably reached a state of irreversible shock. That is not to say he or she cannot be saved through vigorous resuscitative efforts. The vessels themselves are no longer adequately perfused and thus dilate and exhibit cyanosis. The pulse will be weak and rapid, perhaps not even perceptible.

28. (B) CPR may be discontinued if a physician assumes responsibility. Discontinuing CPR is a medical decision and should not be ceased even though police may instruct you to do so. Once you begin, you may cease CPR only if you become exhausted and cannot continue, or if you are relieved by another BLS provider.

29. (A) Verbal stimuli and a patient's response or lack thereof is the best indicator of unconsciousness. An unconscious patient's pupils may continue to react to light; opening the airway is not an appropriate stimulus. Pinching the lobe of the ear offers little in the way of pain stimuli.

30. (A) Forceful mouth-to-mouth ventilation should only be used as a last resort in clearing an airway obstruction. This action may blow an obstruction past the narrow point of the airway (larynx and epiglottis) and provide a partial airway.

31. (D) The jaw-thrust maneuver would be the best choice for opening an airway in a patient with a suspected neck injury. This can be done with the patient's neck and head in a neutral position, thus not further endangering the spine.

32. (A) An adult should be artificially ventilated at least 12 times per minute; a child should be ventilated even more often.

33. (B) You should take four to ten seconds to check unresponsiveness in a patient who appears to be unconscious. Give the patient a chance to awaken and respond.

34. (D) After the airway is opened, allow three to five seconds for the patient to ventilate on his or her own. After five seconds, ventilate four times if respiration is not present.

35. (D) During mouth-to-mouth ventilation, you should hear air escaping after each ventilation. Remove your mouth after each ventilation. You should feel resistance (reduced compliance) as the lungs fill during your ventilation.

36. (B) Five to ten seconds should be used to establish pulselessness after ventilating a non-breathing adult four times. This interval will allow time for proper location of the carotid pulse and for planning what to do next.

37. (D) Two-person CPR, performed on an adult, is performed at a ratio of five compressions to one ventilation.

38. (B) Artificial ventilation must be performed when external chest compressions are done. CPR should only be done on a firm surface. The stomach is in the upper left quadrant and probably would not be lacerated by the xiphoid. Proper CPR will produce between 25-33% of the normal flow of blood.

39. (A) In one-person CPR on an adult, you should deliver 15 compressions and then two breaths, all in a period of 15 seconds.

40. (C) CPR may be interrupted for up to 15 seconds in order to move a patient downstairs or out of a hazardous location. Generally, five seconds is the limit. Keep in mind that each time CPR is stopped, blood pressure falls to zero.

Geriatric Nursing

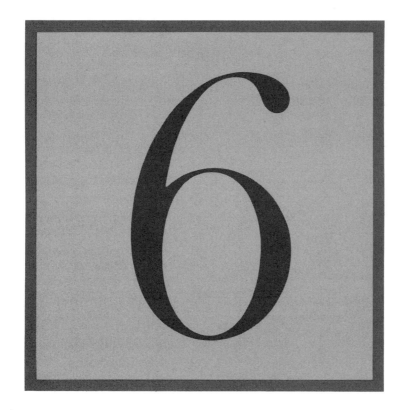

General Concepts

General Principles

Terminology

A. Geriatrics—concerned with the diseases and care of patients with diseases of old age.

B. Gerontology—study of the normal aging process.

C. Aging—natural continuous process.
   1. Begins at birth.
   2. Is common to all living organisms.

D. Old age.
   1. Over 65 years of age.
   2. After retirement.

E. Frail elderly—75 years or over.

F. Ageism—negative attitude toward elderly.

Profiles

A. Those over 65 in 1980.
   1. Make up about 10% of the population.
   2. Most live in urban or rural settings.
   3. Yearly income of 15%-25% is at or below the poverty level.
   4. About 50% are high school graduates.
   5. About 50% have convenient access to senior service centers but a low number use these centers.
   6. 2-10% are alcohol abusers.

B. Cost of health care for the aged.
   1. Only 5% are institutionalized.
   2. 25% of all prescription drugs are for the elderly.
   3. Diseases may be multiple and chronic (over 40% have more than one illness concurrently).
   4. Disability results more readily when an aging person becomes ill.
   5. Response to treatment is diminished.
   6. Resistance is lower due to the aging process so person is more susceptible to disease.
   7. The aged have less resistance to stressors: mental, environmental, and physical.

8. Poor health care is prevalent.
   a. Less than one third have annual checkups.
   b. Many see health care as a service to be used only during life crisis.
   c. Many see more than one doctor, so care is fragmented.

C. Increased life expectancy.
   1. Advanced health care.
   2. Decreased infant/child mortality.
   3. Improved nutrition and sanitation.
   4. Increased infectious disease control.

D. Causes of death.
   1. Heart disease is major cause.
   2. Cancer is second.
   3. Stroke/CVA is third.

E. Major fears of the aged.
   1. Physical and economic dependency.
   2. Chronic illness.
      a. Arthritis 44%.
      b. Hypertension 39%.
      c. Hearing deficit 28%.
      d. Heart disease 27%.
   3. Loneliness
   4. Boredom resulting from not being needed.

Aging Process

Theories of Aging

A. Individualized process.
   1. Each person ages at a different rate.
   2. Each person ages in a different manner.
   3. No single factor has been found to cause or prevent aging.

B. Biological theories.
   1. Genetic programming and/or mutations.
   2. "Wear and tear"—overexertion and stress cause body cells to wear out.
   3. Accumulation of age pigments or lipofuscin in body structures.
   4. Increased amounts of collagen in tissue.
   5. Exposure to radiation, pathogens, nutritional deficiencies.
   6. Autoimmune reactions.

C. Psychosocial theories.
   1. Activity.

a. Aging will increase in direct proportion to decrease in activity.

b. Optimum pattern is to continue in lifestyle of middle age.

2. Personality-continuity—basic personality or behavior patterns are unchanged by aging.

3. Disengagement—society and individual withdraw from each other.

Factors That Influence Aging

A. Heredity.

B. Nutrition.

C. Health status.

D. Life experiences.

E. Environment.

F. Stress.

Physiological Changes

A. Cells.

1. Fewer in number.

2. Larger in size.

3. Decreased total body fluid due to decreased intracellular fluid.

B. Nervous system.

1. Decreased speed of nerve conduction.

2. Delay in response and reaction time, especially with stress.

3. Diminution of sensory faculties.

a. Decreased vision.

b. Loss of hearing.

c. Diminished sense of smell and taste.

d. Greater sensitivity to temperature changes with low tolerance to cold.

C. The ear.

1. Presbycusis.

a. Progressive hearing loss in inner ear.

b. High frequency tones are lost first.

c. Sounds are distorted; difficulty understanding words when other noises in background.

d. 50% of those over age 65.

2. Tympanic membrane atrophic, sclerotic.

3. Cerumen accumulates; may impact due to increased amount of keratin.

D. The eye.

1. Pupil sphincter sclerosis with loss of light responsiveness.

2. Cornea more spherical.

3. Lens more opaque.

4. Increased light perception threshold.

a. Adapt to darkness more slowly.

b. Difficult to see in dim light.

5. Loss of accommodation.

6. Decreased visual field; less peripheral vision.

7. Decreased color discrimination on blue/green end of scale.

E. Cardiovascular system.

1. Heart valves thicken and become rigid.

2. **Cardiac output decreases 1% per year after age 20 due to decreased heart rate and stroke volume.**

3. Vessels lose elasticity.

a. Less effective peripheral oxygenation.

b. Position change from lying to sitting or sitting to standing can cause blood pressure to drop up to 65 mm Hg.

4. Blood pressure increases due to increased peripheral vessel resistance.

a. Systolic may normally be 170.

b. Diastolic may normally be 95.

F. Respiratory system.

1. Respiratory muscles lose strength and become rigid.

2. Ciliary activity decreases.

3. Lungs lose elasticity.

a. Residual capacity increases.

b. Larger on inspiration.

c. Maximum breathing capacity decreases; depth of respirations decreases.

4. Alveoli increases in size, reduced in number.

5. Arterial blood oxygen $_pO_2$ decreases to 75 mm Hg.

6. Arterial blood carbon dioxide $_pCO_2$ unchanged.

7. Coughing ability is reduced.

G. Gastrointestinal system.

1. Tooth loss.

a. Periodontal disease major cause of loss after 30 years of age.

b. Other causes include poor dental health, poor nutrition.

2. Taste sensation decreases.

   a. Chronic irritation of mucous membranes.

   b. Atrophy of up to 80% of taste buds.

   c. Lose sensitivity of those on tip of tongue first: sweet and salt.

   d. Lose sensitivity of those on sides later: salt, sour, bitter.

3. Esophagus dilates.

4. Stomach.

   a. Hunger sensations decrease.

   b. Secretion of gastric acid decreases.

   c. Emptying time decreases.

5. Peristalsis weakens and constipation is common.

6. Absorption function is impaired.

   a. Body absorbs less nutrients due to reduced intestinal blood flow and atrophy of cells on absorbing surfaces.

   b. Decrease in gastric enzymes affects absorption.

7. Liver.

   a. Smaller with decreased storage space.

   b. Decreased blood flow.

H. Genitourinary system.

1. Kidneys.

   a. Smaller due to nephron atrophy.

   b. Renal blood flow decreases 50%.

   c. Glomerular filtration rate decreases 50%.

   d. Tubular function diminishes.

      (1) Less able to concentrate urine; lower specific gravity.

      (2) Proteinuria 1+ is common.

      (3) Blood urea nitrogen BUN increases to 21 mg%.

   e. Renal threshold for glucose increases.

2. Bladder.

   a. Muscle weakens.

   b. Capacity decreases to 200 ml or less causing frequency.

   c. Emptying is more difficult, causing increased retention.

3. Prostate enlarges in some degree in 75% of men over 65.

4. Vulva atrophies.

5. Vagina.

   a. Mucous membrane becomes dryer.

   b. Elastic tissue decreases so surface is smooth.

   c. Secretions become reduced, more alkaline.

   d. Flora changes.

6. Sexuality.

   a. Older people are sexual beings also.

   b. There is no particular age at which a person's sexual functioning ceases.

   c. Frequency of genital sexual behavior (intercourse) may tend to decline gradually in later years, but capacity for expression and enjoyment continue far into old age.

I. Endocrine system.

1. Production of most hormones is reduced.

2. Parathyroid function and secretion are unchanged.

3. Pituitary.

   a. Growth hormone present but in lower blood levels.

   b. Reduced ACTH, TSH, FSH, LH production.

4. Reduced thyroid activity.

   a. Decreased basal metabolic rate.

   b. Reduced I^{131} uptake.

5. Reduced aldosterone production.

6. Reduced gonadal secretion of progesterone, estrogen, testosterone.

J. Integumentary system.

1. Wrinkles due to loss of subcutaneous fat.

2. Scalp hair thins and grays.

3. Hair in nose and ears thickens.

4. Skin pigmentation increases due to clustering of melanocytes.

5. Elasticity lessens due to decreased hydration and vascularity.

6. Fingernails become hard and brittle.

7. Toenails become overgrown and horny.

8. Sweat glands decrease in number and function.

K. Musculoskeletal system.

1. Bone loses density and brittleness increases.

2. Kyphosis with backward tilt of head occurs.
3. Hips, knees, wrists flex.
4. Discs thin so height decreases.
5. Joints enlarge and stiffen.
6. Tendons shrink and sclerose with decrease in tendon jerks.
7. Muscle fibers atrophy.
   a. Person moves more slowly.
   b. Muscle cramps and/or tremors occur.

Psychological Changes

A. Factors that influence these changes.
   1. Physiological changes primarily, especially those of the sense organs.
   2. General health.
   3. Educational level.
   4. Heredity.
   5. Environment.
B. Drastic personality change is rare.
   1. More often honest expression of how one feels.
   2. "Rigidity" may be due to other factors such as diseases.
C. Memory.
   1. Old memory unchanged.
   2. Long term memory.
      a. Hours to days ago.
      b. Some change.
   3. Short term or recent memory.
      a. 0–10 minutes.
      b. Poor.
D. IQ.
   1. Unchanged with information, mathematics, and verbal expressions.
   2. Reduced performance on spatial perceptions and psychomotor skills.
      a. Changes in vision.
      b. Pressures of time factor.

Psychosocial Changes/Adjustments

A. Retirement.
   1. Worth often judged by productivity.
   2. Identity tied up with job role.
B. Sense or awareness of mortality.
C. Alteration in living style, i.e., nursing home, moving in with children.

D. Economic deprivation.
   1. Increased cost of living on a fixed income.
   2. Increased need for costly medical care.
E. Chronic disease and disability.
F. Social isolation loneliness.
G. Sensory deprivation (blindness and deafness).
H. Nutritional deprivation.
I. Series of losses, i.e., relationships, friends, family.
J. Loss of physical strength and agility.
   1. Body image altered.
   2. Self-concept altered.

Nursing Care

Assessment

A. Purpose.
   1. Determine patient's self-care capacities/limitations.
   2. Provide basis for individualized nursing care plan.
   3. Aid in avoiding stereotyping and labeling patient.
   4. Give patient time to answer.
B. Baseline assessment.
   1. Temperature.
      a. May be as low as 95°F.
      b. Sublingual most accurate.
   2. Pulse.
      a. Rate, rhythm, volume.
      b. Apical, radial, pedal, other sites as indicated by disorder.
   3. Respirations.
      a. Rate, rhythm, depth.
      b. Irregularity common.
   4. Arterial blood pressure.
      a. Lying, sitting, standing.
      b. Postural hypotension common.
   5. Weight—gradual loss in late years.
   6. Orientation level.
   7. Memory.
   8. Sleep pattern.
   9. Psychosocial adjustment.

C. Nervous system.
   1. Facial symmetry.
   2. Level of alertness—presence of organic brain changes.
      a. Not all persons become senile.
      b. Most people have memory impairment.
      c. The change is gradual.
   3. Eyes: movement, clarity, presence of cataracts.
   4. Pupils: equality, dilation, construction.
   5. Visual acuity—decreases with age.
      a. Do not test facing window.
      b. Use hand-held chart.
      c. Check condition of glasses.
   6. Sensory deprivation.
   7. Hearing acuity
      a. Hearing aid.
      b. Tinnitus.
      c. Cerumen in outer ear—do not clean.
   8. Presence of pain.
D. Cardiovascular system.
   1. Peripheral circulation, color, warmth.
   2. Auscultate apical pulse.
   3. Check for jugular vein distention.
   4. Dizziness.
   5. Fainting.
   6. Edema.
E. Respiratory system.
   1. Chest excursion.
   2. Auscultate chest/lung/breath sounds.
   3. Describe cough, if present; describe sputum.
   4. Rib cage deformity.
F. Gastrointestinal system.
   1. Nutritional status.
   2. Dietary intake.
   3. Anorexia, indigestion, nausea, vomiting.
   4. Chewing, swallowing.
   5. Condition of teeth, gums, buccal cavity.
   6. Auscultate bowel sounds.
   7. Palpate for distention, dilated colon.
   8. Constipation, diarrhea.
G. Genitourinary system.
   1. Urine: appearance, color, odor.
   2. Bladder distention, incontinence.
   3. Frequency, urgency, hesitancy.
   4. Fluid intake, output.
   5. Dysuria.
   6. Sexuality.
      a. Lack of opportunities for expression.
      b. Social stigma toward activity.
H. Integumentary system.
   1. Skin.
      a. Temperature, degree of moisture.
      b. Intactness, open lesions, tears.
      c. Tugor.
      d. Pigmentation alterations.
   2. Bruises, scars.
   3. Condition of nails.
   4. Condition of hair.
   5. Infestations.
I. Musculoskeletal system.
   1. Contractures.
      a. Muscle atrophy.
      b. Tendon shortening.
      c. Lack of adequate joint motion.
   2. Mobility level.
      a. Ambulate with or without assistance or devices.
      b. Limitations to movement.
      c. Muscle strength.
      d. Gait.
   3. Range of motion of joints.
   4. Paralysis.
   5. Kyphosis.
J. Psychosocial.
   1. Exhibits increasing dependency.
   2. Concerns focus increasingly on self.
   3. Displays narrower interests.
   4. Needs tangible evidence of affection.
K. Life story.
L. Immunization history.

Planning

A. Involve the patient and his family in planning.
B. Enlist cooperation of other health care professionals.

C. Set priorities.

   1. Patient may be content with situation as it is.

   2. Encourage change, but do not force it.

   3. Safety is a major concern.

D. Prevent problems.

E. Afford patient adequate time for input.

F. Write out all plans and schedules.

Nursing Actions

A. Provide adequate lighting.

   1. Natural lighting best.

   2. Avoid glare.

   3. Night light at all times in bathrooms, halls.

B. Encourage sensory stimulation.

   1. Large print books.

   2. Changes in environment.

   3. Colors patient can see.

C. Maintain reality orientation.

   1. Calendars.

   2. Clocks.

   3. One-to-one visits.

D. Provide circulatory care.

   1. Avoid tight/restrictive clothing.

   2. Change position, especially from horizontal to vertical.

   3. Provide warmth by applying blankets and clothing.

   4. Encourage activity to increase circulatory stimulation.

   5. Provide support and use safety measures during transfer.

   6. Use gentle friction during bath.

E. Provide respiratory care.

   1. Clean nares if nasal passages are clogged

   2. Protect from draughts.

   3. Promote respiratory activity with exercises.

     a. Deep breathing.

     b. Forced expiration.

     c. Coughing.

     d. Inflatable toys.

   4. Oxygen therapy caution: check for carbon dioxide narcosis.

     a. Confusion.

     b. Profuse perspiration.

     c. Visual disturbance.

     d. Muscle twitching.

     e. Hypotension.

     f. Cerebral dysfunction.

F. Provide gastrointestinal care.

   1. Stimulate appetite.

     a. Small, frequent feedings of high quality.

     b. Attractive meals.

     c. Wine if allowed.

     d. Female, 1600 calories; male, 2200.

     e. Hot foods hot; cold foods cold.

     f. Preferred foods if possible; ethnic choices.

   2. Lessen/prevent indigestion.

     a. Fowler's position for meals.

     b. Antacids contraindicated.

     c. Smaller meals without gas formers.

     d. Adequate fluids.

   3. Prevent constipation.

     a. Ensure adequate bulk and fluid in diet.

     b. Encourage activity.

     c. Ensure regular and adequate time for bowel movement.

     d. Provide privacy and normal positioning.

     e. Administer laxative or suppository if above not effective.

G. Provide genitourinary care.

   1. Adequate fluid intake: 2000–3000 ml daily.

   2. Incontinence prevention.

     a. Offer opportunity to void every two hours.

     b. Keep night light in bathroom to prevent falls.

     c. Schedule diuretics for maximum effect during daylight hours.

     d. Limit fluids near and at bedtime.

   3. Sexuality.

     a. Provide counseling if desired.

     b. Provide opportunity for desired sexual expression.

     c. Encourage touching and companionship, which are important for older people.

H. Provide integumentary care.

1. Bathing.

   a. Have patient take complete bath only twice a week due to dryness of skin.

   b. Use superfatted soap or lotions to aid in moisturizing.

2. Clip facial hairs for female patients if desired.

3. Handle gently to prevent skin tears.

4. Cut toenails unless contraindicated.

   a. Mycosis of nails.

   b. Medical/surgical disorder.

I. Provide musculoskeletal care.

1. Ambulate within limitations.

2. Alter position every two hours; align correctly.

3. Prevent osteoporosis of long bones by providing exercises against resistance.

4. Provide active and passive exercises.

   a. Rest periods necessary.

   b. Paced throughout the day.

5. Provide range-of-motion exercises to all joints three times a day.

6. Educate family that allowing the patient to be sedentary is not helpful.

7. Encourage walking, which is best single exercise for the elderly.

J. Provide psychosocial care.

1. Encourage psychological activity to aid sense of normality.

2. Encourage life review.

3. Assist in selecting and attending activities.

4. Foster touching, which is a very useful tool in establishing trust.

5. Provide dignity and the feeling of worth.

6. Foster the wellness approach to life.

K. Maintain safety.

1. Siderails when in bed.

   a. Often awaken disoriented for various reasons.

   b. Fall easily due to weakened muscles.

   c. Orthostatic hypotension.

2. Bed in low position when not giving direct patient care.

3. Handrails in bathrooms and halls.

4. Uncluttered rooms and floors.

5. Adequate, nonglare lighting.

6. Restraints when necessary.

Medications and the Aged

Overview

A. Twenty five percent of all prescription drugs are for those 65 and over.

B. Multiple chronic diseases often present.

1. May have several physicians for care.

2. Use of over-the-counter drugs.

3. Drug interactions are altered in the aged.

4. Drug profile imperative.

C. Increased number of side effects to medications.

☆ Administration

A. Oral route.

1. Check for mouth dryness.

   a. Drug may stick and dissolve in mouth.

   b. Drug may irritate mucous membrane.

2. Place patient in sitting position.

3. Crush tablets if they are very large.

4. Do not open capsules.

5. Do not crush enteric-coated tablets.

6. Check with pharmacy for liquid preparations if patient has difficulty swallowing tablets.

B. Suppository.

1. Position for comfort.

2. May take longer to dissolve due to decreased body core temperature.

3. Do not insert suppository directly from refrigerator.

C. Parenteral.

1. Site may ooze medication or bleed due to decreased tissue elasticity.

2. Do not use immobile limb.

3. Danger of overhydration with IV.

D. Self-administration.

1. Check compliance with amounts and times.

2. Color code to facilitate proper administration.

Drug Action

A. Absorption may be lessened.
1. Fewer cells on absorbing surfaces.
2. Diminished GI blood flow.
3. Increased gastric pH.
4. Increased gastric emptying time.
5. Decreased intestinal mobility.

B. Distribution may be altered.
1. Circulatory changes.
2. Decreased body temperature.
3. Smaller body size.
4. More fat to lean body mass.
5. Decreased plasma albumin—drug binds to albumin; what does not bind is active.

C. Metabolism, decreased liver function.
1. Decreased blood flow through liver.
2. Decreased hepatic mass.
3. Decreased enzyme activity.

D. Excretion.
1. Renal system changes, primarily responsible for excretion on drugs.
2. Biological half-life of drugs increased up to 40%.

Delirium, Depression and Dementia

Delirium

Definition: Acute brain syndrome that interferes with cerebral functioning.

Etiology

A. Metabolic, circulatory, endocrine disorders.
B. Drugs, systemic intoxication.
C. Infection.
D. Sensory changes.

Characteristics

A. Abrupt onset, usually reversible.
B. Course can fluctuate hourly.
C. Vivid hallucinations, delusions.
D. When oriented denies confusion, tries to make "what happened" make sense.
E. Tries to answer mental status examination questions.
F. Severe, bizarre behaviors.

Nursing Care

A. Supportive
B. Identify etiology and remove or treat.
1. First step is often to discontinue all medications.
2. Provide nutritional and fluid intake.

Depression

Definition: State of mind where person loses interest in life and finds no pleasure in activities; feels hopeless and sad.

Etiology

A. Reaction to life event.
B. Reaction to environment.

Characteristics

A. Course usually 2 weeks to 6 months, varies day to day.
B. Often aware of event and date that triggered depression.
C. Mental status examination.
1. Often can answer correctly.
2. Can spell "world" backward.
3. May not try to answer.
D. Symptoms.
1. Difficulty in remembering and concentrating.
2. Poor task performance.
3. Alterations in appetite and weight, sleep patterns.

4. Feels worthless, self-reproach.
5. Loss of motivation, lethargic.

Nursing Care

A. Supportive.
B. Antidepressants.
  1. Check cautions regarding drug use in the elderly.
  2. Few manufacturers have included geriatric dose in literature; start small.

Dementia

Definition: Acquired impairment of memory and other intellectual abilities secondary to structural brain damage; this damage may be microscopic.

Characteristics

A. Diagnostic criteria—must meet one criteria numbered 1 through 5.
  1. Sufficiently severe loss of intellectual abilities to interfere with social or occupational functioning.
  2. Memory impairment, usually short-term memory.
  3. Impairment of abstract thinking or impaired judgement or disturbance of higher cortical function or personality change.
  4. Cloudy state of consciousness.
  5. Presence of a specific organic etiology or presumed presence.
B. Onset slow, insidious, unrelated to specific situation.
C. Gradual degeneration.
D. Mental status examination.
  1. Early in the disease will attempt to find the right answer.
  2. Later will not understand question.
  3. The more severe the dementia, the more errors.
E. Symptoms.
  1. Paranoid accusations.

2. Personality changes, withdrawn.
3. Confusion noted by others but not by the patient.
4. Unaware of memory loss.
  a. Begins with recent memory loss.
  b. Later problem with coding and retrieving information.
5. Oblivious to failures.

Alzheimer's Disease

Definition: Degeneration of all layers of the cortex and atrophy of the cerebrum.

A. Etiology is unknown.
B. Most common dementia in the elderly (50%).
C. Incidence in U.S. is 1.2 million over 65.
D. Diagnosis by exclusion.
  1. No other diagnosis applicable.
  2. Specific data from brain autopsy.
    a. Neurofibrillary tangles.
    b. Neuritic plaques.
    c. Amyloid clusters.
E. Possible predisposing factors.
  1. Genetic.
  2. Familial history of Down's Syndrome.
  3. Enzyme deficiency.
  4. Immune system deficiency.
  5. Slow growing virus.
  6. Aluminum toxicity.
  7. Head trauma.
  8. Acetylcholine deficiency, a neurotransmitter.
F. Symptoms.
  1. Physically health appears good.
  2. Onset slow, progressive decline.
  3. Restless, irritable.
  4. Aphasia, can produce words but not sentences.
  5. Intellectual impairment.
  6. Disoriented to person, place and time.
  7. Motor ability declines.
  8. Incontinent.
  9. Doesn't recognize staff or family.

Nursing Care

A. Supportive.

B. Verbal communication

1. Short words, simple sentences, verbs and nouns.

2. Call patient by name and identify yourself.

3. Speak slowly, clearly; wait for response.

4. Ask only one question, give one direction at a time.

5. Repeat do not rephrase.

C. Nonverbal communication.

1. Use gestures, move slowly.

2. Stand directly in front of patient, maintain eye contact.

3. Move or walk with patient; don't try to stop.

4. Listen actively; show interest.

5. Chart all phrases and nonverbal techniques used and use those that "work."

6. Maintain the patient's physical activity within limits of safety.

   a. Walk outside if grounds are fenced, alarmed or if accompanied.

   b. Dance.

   c. Exercises with simple commands.

   d. Active games.

   e. Balance activities.

   f. Activities of daily living.

7. Mental stimulation.

   a. Simple hobbies.

   b. One-to-one contact.

   c. Reality orientation.

   d. Play word, number games.

8. Encourage self-care, give cues. Pantomime brushing teeth instead of brushing patient's teeth.

9. Put families in touch with support groups such as Alzheimer's Disease and Related Disorders Assoc., Inc. chapters. (ADRDA).

Associated Degenerative Diseases

A. Multi-infarct Dementia.

1. Second most common dementia in the elderly.

2. Focal neurological signs and symptoms.

3. History of significant cerebrovascular disease.

B. Korsakoff's syndrome.

1. Varied symptoms associated with chronic alcoholism.

2. Often associated with Wernicke's encephalopathy.

C. Pick's disease.

1. Rare heredogenerative process not associated with the normal aging process.

2. Similar to Alzheimer's but involvement does not include parietal lobes.

D. Huntington's chorea—genetically transmitted disorder.

1. Characterized by onset of symptoms after the age of thirty.

2. Progressive mental and physical deterioration is inevitable.

E. Arteriosclerosis—a generic term referring to localized degeneration caused by vascular changes.

1. Sudden onset.

2. Occurs in forty to fifty age group.

F. Paresis—central nervous system degeneration caused by invasion of brain cells from *Treponema pallidum* (syphilis).

1. Infection may have occurred much earlier but remained untreated by penicillin.

2. Symptoms reflect general brain disorder deterioration.

Psychological Reactions to OBS Disorders

A. Changes in self-concept.

B. Anger and frustration as reactions to forced changes in various life roles.

C. Denial used as a defense.

D. Depression.

E. Limitations accepted.

F. "Sick" role assumed.

1. Becomes dependent.

2. Lacks motivation.

Nursing Care

A. Meet both physical and psychological needs.

B. Help client maintain contact with reality.
1. Give feedback.
2. Avoid small chatter.
3. Personalize interaction.
4. Supply stimulation to motivate client.
5. Keep client from becoming bored and distracted.

C. Assist client in accepting the diagnosis.
1. Be supportive.
2. Maintain good communication.
3. During denial phase, listen and accept; do not argue.
4. Assist development of awareness.
5. Help client develop the ability to cope with his or her altered identity.

D. Focus of interactions with client.
1. Conduct short, frequent contacts with client.
2. Use concrete ideas in communicating with the client.
3. Maintain a reality orientation by allowing the client to talk about his or her past and to confabulate.
4. Acknowledge the client as an individual.

E. Provide a safe, stable, consistent environment.

F. Assess the client's disabilities, and help develop a nursing plan to deal with them.

G. Become a member of the rehabilitation team.

Review Questions

Mrs. Adamms, aged 79, is admitted to the acute hospital following a fall. Her past medical history is "normal"; she has presbycusis. She is scheduled for surgery to repair a fractured hip. The evening of admission her vital signs are T. 97.8 F; P 82; R 16; BP 155/90.

1. Presbycusis involves

   A. Sclerosis of the tympanic membrane.
   B. Sclerosis of the middle ear.
   C. Inner ear abnormalities.
   D. Otic nerve hypertrophy.

2. The earliest sign/symptom of presbycusis is

   A. The inability to discriminate voices.
   B. The inability to hear high frequency sounds.
   C. Ringing in the ears.
   D. Dizziness.

3. The chief treatment for presbycusis involves

   A. Surgery to repair the defect.
   B. Utilization of an approved hearing aid.
   C. Specific long term drug therapy.
   D. Patient and family education.

4. The morning of surgery you note that Mrs. Adamms' oral temperature is 97.2 F. You would

   A. Wrap her in warm blankets to increase her core temperature.
   B. Report her temperature to the anesthesiologist immediately.
   C. Take her temperature by the rectal route and report the findings to her doctor.
   D. Record the temperature as obtained and do nothing more.

5. Before surgery Mrs. Adamms' blood pressure is 170/90. You would consider

   A. This dangerously high and report it immediately.
   B. It normal and simply record it.
   C. Her slightly hypotensive for her age.
   D. Her condition hypertensive and a candidate for the hospital's education program on hypertension.

6. Which of these laboratory values could be considered normal for Mrs. Adamms but abnormal for a 20-year-old patient

   A. Urine specific gravity 1.020.
   B. Proteinuria 1+.
   C. Straw colored urine.
   D. Urine sugar negative.

7. Her preoperative medication order includes Meperedine 25 mg. IM at 7:30 A.M.

   A. You should call the anesthesiologist to double check the dosage, since it is in the lower range of normal.
   B. You should use the Z tract method of injection to prevent the medication from oozing at the injection site.
   C. You should follow orders and give that drug, in that dose, by that method, at that time.
   D. You would delay the injection up to ½ hour because you realize the dosage is lower than normal.

8. Mrs. Adamms develops hypostatic pneumonia postoperatively. Which of these assessments would you most likely make?

   A. Altered breath sounds on auscultation.
   B. Temperature above 100 F.
   C. Chest pain especially on expiration.
   D. Shallow, irregular respirations.

9. You encourage Mrs. Adamms to deep breathe and cough; this helps prevent

   A. Formation of decubiti.
   B. Constipation.
   C. Collection of fluid in the lungs.
   D. Progressive muscle weakness.

10. The doctor asks you to get Mrs. Adamms out of bed and into a wheelchair. Before positioning her in the wheelchair the nurse should *always*

    A. Take her vital signs and record them.
    B. Dangle her on the edge of the bed.
    C. Make certain that she wants to get up.
    D. Get another licensed nurse to help.

Mr. Plees, aged 70, is admitted to a skilled nursing facility (SNF) with the diagnosis of organic brain syndrome and orthostatic hypotension.

11. Which of the following is/are considered necessary for his comfort and safety?

    A. Handrails in halls and by toilets.
    B. Light blue walls for a calming effect.
    C. Floors with wall-to-wall carpeting.
    D. Room humidity of 15%.

12. Mr. Plees complains that his food "has no taste" and asks for more seasoning. Which of these would he be least able to "taste"?

    A. Vinegar.
    B. Sugar.
    C. Salt.
    D. Pepper.

13. He is disoriented at times. This is most likely to occur

    A. When he first gets out of bed after breakfast.
    B. After he ambulates in the hall.
    C. After his family visits.
    D. When he awakens, especially at night.

14. Mr. Plees complains that he is "falling apart." He has no teeth and wears full dentures; he uses glasses and bilateral hearing aids. Which of the following is preventable with proper care?

    A. Tooth loss due to periodontal disease.
    B. Eye accommodation loss.
    C. Presbycusis or deafness.
    D. Prostate enlargement.

15. The best nursing action to lessen the severity of Mr. Plees' orthostatic hypotension is

    A. Turning him from side to side every two hours.
    B. Limiting his visitors with respiratory infections.
    C. Changing his position especially from horizontal to vertical.
    D. Encouraging him to cough and deep breathe.

16. Miss Smite is frequently constipated and takes two tablespoons of mineral oil every day but doesn't like the taste. You should discourage the use of mineral oil chiefly because it

    A. Can cause nutritional deficiency.
    B. Is habit forming.
    C. Is unpleasant to taste.
    D. Is an expensive laxative.

17. When using a soft vest restraint for a patient it should be

    A. Released every eight hours to check the patient's circulation.
    B. Applied directly against the skin to prevent slipping.
    C. Used only with doctor's orders or on unit/floor policy.
    D. Made of mesh and not solid cloth to encourage air circulation.

18. Exercise is best done

    A. In the early morning when the person is rested.
    B. Morning and evening.
    C. Only at specific times as ordered by the physician.
    D. Throughout the day with the time gradually increased.

19. On IQ tests the aged do less well on

    A. General information.
    B. Psychomotor skills.
    C. Verbal comprehension.
    D. Math problems.

20. Which of these is not a true statement about the musculoskeletal system?

    A. Discs thin and the patient becomes shorter.
    B. Movement is slower due to joint stiffness.
    C. Muscle tremors are common.
    D. Bone increases in density.

21. The vagina

    A. Is moist.
    B. Has increased acidity.
    C. Has flora change.
    D. Is more elastic.

22. The best single exercise for the elderly is

    A. Bicycling.
    B. Walking.
    C. Passive range of motion.
    D. Swimming.

23. Blood urea nitrogen is often elevated in the elderly chiefly due to changes in the

    A. Liver.
    B. Kidney.
    C. Diet.
    D. Level of exercise.

24. Diabetes is a common disorder in the elderly. Which of the following would be accurate and the "least expensive" diagnostic tool?

    A. Urine test for sugar.
    B. Urine test for acetone.
    C. Blood test for sugar.
    D. Family history and subjective symptoms.

25. Mr. David Drown, age 70, was brought to the psych unit by his son and daughter and admitted with the tentative diagnosis of organic brain syndrome, dementia type. Mr. Drown had become increasingly difficult to deal with at home—he would become irrationally angered, only occasionally follow directions, make poor judgments, was labile, and, at times, seemed to forget events that had just occurred. In assessing Mr. Drown's condition, which one of the following statements is true?

    A. Prognosis is good, because the organic condition usually tends to be reversible.
    B. Symptoms are not closely related to the patient's basic personality.
    C. Patients display reduced intellectual capacity, emotional stability, memory, judgment, and social sensitivity.
    D. The onset is abrupt and rapidly progressive.

26. All the following are causative factors associated

with organic brain disorder *except*

A. Korsakoff's psychosis.
B. Alzheimer's disease.
C. Keratolytic syndrome.
D. Pick's disease.

27. General nursing care of patients with organic brain syndrome would include

A. Establishing a calm, supportive environment.
B. Providing physical care specific to the cause.
C. Establishing reality orientation.
D. All of the above.

28. The best nursing approach to Mr. Drown would be

A. Short, concrete, reality-oriented interactions.
B. A complete explanation to Mr. Drown about his problems.
C. A flexible therapy schedule.
D. Confrontation of the patient whenever he loses contact with reality.

29. In assessing Mr. Drown, the nurse is likely to observe a loss of Mr. Drown's ability to

A. Learn and make good judgments.
B. Verbalize.
C. Physically mobilize.
D. Participate in ADL.

30. The nurse assigned to orient Mr. Drown to the unit would demonstrate her knowledge of organic brain syndrome best by which of the following interventions?

A. Give the patient a complete orientation to the unit and its rules.
B. Limit the orientation to small, specific amounts of essential information.
C. Ask Mr. Drown questions to see if he understands.
D. Only show Mr. Drown his room as all else will confuse him.

31. The best example of reality orientation for Mr. Drown is

A. "Good morning, Mr. Drown. Do you know where you are?"
B. "Mr. Drown, breakfast is in the dining room in a few minutes."
C. "Good morning, Mr. Drown. I'm Mrs. Meyer, your nurse for today. This is your first morning at Washington Hospital."
D. "Good morning, Mr. Drown. Did you sleep well? What would you like to have for breakfast? Do you know where the dining room is?"

32. Late one night Mr. Drown is found wandering around the halls. He says he is looking for his wife. It is important that the nurse use which of the following approaches?

A. Matter-of-fact attitude as you help him back to his room.
B. Remind him about staying in his room.
C. Remind him of where he is and assess why he is having difficulty sleeping.
D. Allow Mr. Drown to sleep in the dayroom so he will not disturb the other patients.

33. Barbiturates are not ordered for Mr. Drown's insomnia for which of the following reasons?

A. Potential liver damage.
B. Habituation and dependence.
C. Delirium and paradoxical excitement.
D. Central nervous system depression.

34. In planning for Mr. Drown's activities of daily living, it is essential that the nursing staff

A. Encourage Mr. Drown to do as much of his own care as possible.
B. Assume that Mr. Drown needs to have the staff take care of him.
C. Make Mr. Drown responsible for his own care.
D. Assign another patient to assist Mr. Drown and socialize with him.

35. The nurse should encourage Mr. Drown to participate in activities which provide him a chance to

A. Interact with other patients.
B. Compete with others.
C. Succeed at something.
D. Succeed at long term projects to give him a sense of continuity.

36. Mr. Drown is assigned to a reminiscence group. The purpose of this type of group is to

A. Orient him to reality.
B. Obtain feedback and encouragement from other patients.
C. Decrease his isolation and loneliness.
D. Provide the nurse with more information about his memory gaps.

Answers and Rationale

1. (C) The problem is in the inner ear.

2. (B) The earliest symptom is the inability to hear high frequency/pitch sounds/tones; later mid pitch is lost and the ability to discriminate between voices and room noises.

3. (D) The patient and family need to be taught the importance of voice modulation and to speak more

slowly and clearly. A hearing aid is not useful.

4. (D) A temperature of 97.2 is normal for the elderly. Her baseline temperature was 97.8. The rectal route is not felt to be reliable in the elderly due to decreased blood flow.

5. (B) This is within the normal range.

6. (B) Protein is frequently found in the urine due to altered kidney filtration and reabsorption.

7. (C) Preoperative drugs must be given at the time stated. A tract injection is traumatic and is only used when necessary for drugs like Imferon.

8. (A) The elderly frequently do not have an elevated temperature or pain with pneumonia. Shallow, irregular respirations are normal.

9. (C) Hypostatic pneumonia is caused by the collection of secretions in the lungs. Deep breathing and coughing aid in the movement of these secretions.

10. (B) Unless contraindicated, all patients should always be dangled for a few minutes prior to getting them out of bed. This gives the blood flow a chance to stabilize and often prevents dizziness and/or fainting.

11. (A) Mr. Plees should be encouraged to use these rails for support. Carpeting has been found to hold unpleasant odors and is difficult to clean.

12. (B) The taste buds for sweet are on the tip of the tongue. Some taste buds for salt are on the tip but others are on the sides. The taste buds on the tip of the tongue are lost first.

13. (D) Mr. Plees is most likely to be disoriented if he awakens in the dark because of the elderly's slowness in adapting to dim light.

14. (A) Tooth loss due to periodontal disease may be prevented by proper diet and dental health. The others may be lessened by therapy but not prevented.

15. (C) Orthostatic hypotension occurs more frequently with a shift in body position and can be lessened by routinely altering the patient's position.

16. (A) Fat soluble vitamins bind with mineral oil and therefore could be excreted with the stool.

17. (C) The elderly's circulation is poor and thus restraints should be released every two hours to check the circulation and change position.

18. (D) Exercise should be paced throughout the day with a stimulating type in the morning and a relaxing type in the evening.

19. (B) This is probably due to their diminished vision and the pressure of time they feel in testing.

20. (D) Bone decreases in density and becomes more brittle.

21. (C) The vagina becomes smooth, dry, alkaline and the flora changes.

22. (B) Walking provides exercise for all the muscles. Distances should be increased gradually.

23. (B) The kidney filtration rate decreases so fewer waste products are removed from the blood.

24. (C) Blood tests would be the best indicator of sugar level. (A) is incorrect because many elderly patients with an elevated blood sugar have a negative urine sugar. Glucose threshold in the kidney is increased in the elderly.

25. (C) Senile psychosis has a poor prognosis, is usually progressive and irreversible, and the symptoms are closely related to the patient's basic personality. All of the characteristics in (C) fit the picture of senile psychosis.

26. (C) Keratolysis is the normal shedding of skin at regular intervals.

27. (D) In addition to the principles listed, the nurse should use a firm, friendly approach.

28. (A) Organic brain syndrome patients need a safe, consistent environment and reality orientation. Confrontation and environmental instability further confuse the patient by increasing his anxiety level.

29. (A) The patient's decreased ability to learn and make good judgments is central to assessing and planning his care. His ability to verbalize, be mobile, and participate in ADL is not necessarily impaired.

30. (B) The orientation should be limited to small, specific amounts of essential information as the patient's immediate recall is impaired. Questioning him may further confuse him and add to his anxiety.

31. (C) This response orients the patient to reality by establishing the time of day, who he is, who the nurse is, and where he is. The other responses do not orient him and add to his confusion by not being specific or overwhelming him with questions.

32. (C) This answer orients the patient to time and place in addition to assessing the underlying cause of his sleep disturbance. Answer (B) is only a short term solution and (D) does not focus on his problem but on other patient needs.

33. (C) In organic brain disorder barbiturates commonly cause delirium, confusion, and paradoxical excitement.

34. (A) The nursing care plan needs to be based on the patient level of functioning and to reinforce independence and self-care as appropriate. Answer (B) creates an atmosphere of dependence while (C) totally ignores Mr. Drown's realistic dependence needs. Answer (D) places the responsibility for the patient's care onto another patient.

35. (C) It is essential that Mr. Drown be encouraged to participate in activities that provide him with immediate success which increases his self-esteem. Interaction with others is important but is secondary to improving his self-esteem. Answers (B) and (D) are contraindicated as they are detrimental to the patient as he does not have the ability to compete with others or succeed at long term projects.

36. (C) The purpose of reminiscence is to allow the patient to interact with others in a way that is easy and comfortable for him. Answers (B) and (D) may be true but are not the major focus of this type of group.

Maternity and Gynecological Nursing

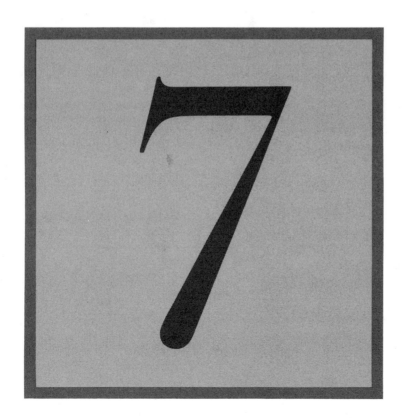

Anatomy and Physiology of Female Reproductive System

Anatomy

External Genitalia

A. Collectively called the vulva.

B. Visible structures.
   1. Mons veneris (mons pubis).
   2. Labia majora.
   3. Labia minora.
   4. Clitoris.
   5. Vestibule.
   6. Urethral meatus.
   7. Skene's and Bartholin's glands.
   8. Hymen.
   9. Perineum.

Internal Organs

A. Located in pelvic cavity.

B. Reproductive structures.
   1. Uterus—muscular organ with central cavity.
      a. Functions.
         (1) Structure of fetal development.
         (2) Site of menstrual shedding.
      b. Sections.
         (1) Corpus (body)—lies below tubal insertion and composed of three layers.
            (a) Perimetrium—external layer.
            (b) Myometrium—middle layer.
            (c) Endometrium—internal layer.
         (2) Fundus—lies above tubal insertion.
   2. Cervix—canal located between internal and external os.
      a. Internal os opens into body of uterine cavity.
      b. External os opens into vagina.
   3. Fallopian tubes.
      a. Two slender muscular tubes extending laterally from the cornu of uterine cavity to ovaries.
      b. Passageways through which ova reach uterus.
   4. Ovaries.
      a. Flat, oval-shaped organs.
      b. One ovary located on each side of uterus.
      c. Functions.
         (1) Develop and expel ova.
         (2) Secrete certain hormones.
   5. Vagina.
      a. Canal extending from lower part of vulva to cervix.
      b. Functions.
         (1) Allows for passage of menstrual blood.
         (2) Allows for passage of fetus.
         (3) Provides site for copulation.

Support Structure (Pelvis)

A. Important in obstetrics.
   1. Passage through which baby passes at birth.
   2. Disproportions between fetus and size of pelvis make vaginal delivery difficult or impossible.

B. Bone formations.
   1. Two innominate bones.
   2. Sacrum.
   3. Coccyx.

C. Pelvic cavities.
   1. False pelvis—shallow extended portion above brim that supports abdominal viscera.
   2. True pelvis—portion that lies below pelvic brim; divided into three sections.
      a. Pelvic outlet.
      b. Mid-pelvis.
      c. Pelvic inlet.

D. Pelvic types.
   1. Gynecoid—nearly round or blunt; typical of normal female.

2. Android—wedge-shaped; typical of male.
3. Anthropoid—oval-shaped.
4. Platypelloid—oval-shaped, transversely.

E. Measurements of the pelvis.
   1. Diagonal conjugate (CD)—distance between sacral promontory and lower margin of symphysis pubis. Measurement greater than 11.5 cm adequate.
   2. True conjugate, or conjugate vera (CV)—distance from upper margin of symphysis to sacral promontory. Measurement greater than 11 cm adequate.
   3. Tuberischial diameter (TI)—transverse diameter of outlet. Measurement greater than 8 cm adequate.
   4. Size determination.
      a. X-ray pelvimetry is most accurate means of determining size of pelvis.
      b. X-ray pelvimetry is contraindicated to avoid undue exposure of mother and infant unless pelvic contraction is suspected.

Physiology

Menstruation and the Menstrual Cycle

A. Menstruation.
   1. Culmination of menstrual cycle.
   2. Discharge of blood, mucus, and epithelial cells from the uterus.

B. Menstrual cycle.
   1. Occurrence—usually between ages of twelve and forty-five.
   2. Duration—about twenty-eight days but varies from twenty-one to thirty-five days; ovulation occurs about fourteen days before beginning of menstruation.

C. Menstrual cycle regulated primarily through phasic hormonal control of pituitary, ovaries, and uterus.
   1. Proliferative phase.
      a. Follicle stimulating hormone (FSH), released by anterior pituitary, stimulates the development of the graafian follicle.
      b. As graafian follicle develops, it produces increasing amounts of follicular fluid containing a hormone called *estrogen.*
      c. Estrogen stimulates build-up or thickening of the endometrium.
      d. As estrogen increases in the bloodstream, it suppresses secretion of FSH and favors the secretion of the luteinizing hormone (LH).
      e. LH stimulates ovulation and initiates development of the corpus luteum.
   2. Secretory phase.
      a. Follows ovulation, which is the release of mature ovum from the graafian follicle.
      b. Rapid changes take place in the ruptured follicle under the influence of LH.
      c. Cavity of the graafian follicle is replaced by the corpus luteum (mass of yellow-colored tissue).
      d. Main function of the corpus luteum is to secrete progesterone and some estrogen.
      e. Progesterone acts upon the endometrium to bring about secretory changes that prepare it for pregnancy. Also, progesterone maintains the endometrium during the early phase of pregnancy, should a fertilized ovum be implanted.
   3. Menstrual phase.
      a. Corpus luteum degenerates in about eight days unless the ovum is fertilized.
      b. There is a cessation of progesterone and estrogen produced by corpus luteum and blood levels drop.
      c. Endometrium degenerates and menstruation occurs.
      d. The drop in blood levels of estrogen and progesterone stimulate production of FSH and a new cycle begins.

D. Discomforts associated with menstruation.
   1. Breast tenderness and feeling of fullness.
   2. Tendency toward fatigue.
   3. Temperament and mood changes—because

of hormonal influence and decreased levels of estrogen and progesterone.

4. Discomfort in pelvic area, lower back, and legs.
5. Retained fluids and weight gain.

E. Abnormalities of menstruation.

1. Dysmenorrhea (painful menstruation).
   a. May be caused by psychological factors: tension, anxiety, preconditioning (menstruation is a "curse" or should be painful).
   b. Physical examination is usually done to rule out organic causes.
2. Treatment.
   a. Oral contraceptives—produce anovulatory cycle.
   b. Mild analgesics such as aspirin.
   c. Urge patient to carry on normal activities to occupy her mind.
   d. Dysmenorrhea may subside after childbearing.
3. Amenorrhea (absense of menstrual flow).
   a. Primary—over the age of seventeen and menstruation has not begun.
      (1) Complete physical necessary to rule out abnormalities.
      (2) Treatment aimed at correction of underlying condition.
   b. Secondary—occurs after menarche—does not include pregnancy and lactation.
      (1) Causes include psychological upsets or endocrine conditions.
      (2) Evaluation and treatment by physician is necessary.
4. Menorrhagia (excessive menstrual bleeding)—may be due to endocrine disturbance, tumors, or inflammatory conditions of the uterus.
5. Metrorrhagia (bleeding between periods)—symptom of disease process, benign tumors, or cancer.

F. Counseling guidelines.

1. Assist with providing education about the physiology of normal menstruation and correct misinformation.
2. Assist with providing education about abnormal conditions associated with menstruation—absence of menstruation, bleeding between menstrual periods, etc.
3. Assist with providing education related to normal hygiene during menstruation.
   a. Importance of cleanliness.
   b. Use of perineal pads and tampons.
   c. Continuance of normal activities.

Development of the Fetus

Fertilization

Definition: A gamete is a matured sex cell (ovum or spermatozoon) that has undergone maturation and is ready for fertilization.

A. Fertilization takes place when two essential cells (sperm and ovum) unite; usually occurs in outer third of fallopian tube.

B. Each reproductive cell (one gamete) carries 23 chromosomes.

C. Each sperm carries two types of sex chromosomes, X and Y; when united with female, X chromosome determines the sex of the child (XY–male; XX–female).

D. After fertilization the fertilized egg descends to the uterus within three days.

Table A. Multiple Pregnancies

Double Ovum	Single Ovum
Dizygotic or fraternal twins	Monozygotic or identical twins
Ova from same or different ovaries	Union of a single ovum and a single sperm
Same or different sex	Same sex
Brother or sister resemblance	Identical genetic pattern
Two placentas but may be fused	One placenta
Two chorions and two amnions	One chorion and two amnions

Fetal Development

A. Embryo is the fertilized ovum during the first two months of development.

B. Fetus is product of conception from two months to time of birth.

C. Implantation occurs about the seventh day after fertilization.

D. During embryonic development, cells arrange themselves into three layers.

E. Fetal membranes and amniotic fluid.

1. Fetal membranes (those which surround the fetus) are composed of two layers.
   a. Amnion (glistening inner membrane) forms early, about the second week of embryonic development; encloses the amniotic cavity.
   b. Chorion is the outer membrane.

2. Amniotic fluid forms within the amniotic cavity and surrounds the embryo. Usually consists of 500 to 1000 ml of fluid at the end of pregnancy.
   a. Amniotic fluid contains fetal urine, lanugo from fetal skin, epithelial cells, and subaqueous materials.
   b. Function of the fluid is to provide an optimum temperature and environment for fetus and provide a cushion against injury; fetus also drinks the fluid, probably as much as 450 ml a day near term.
   c. Source is uncertain; replaced continuously at a rapid rate.

F. Placenta and fetal circulation.

1. Placenta—organ that provides for the exchange of nutrients and waste products between mother and fetus and acts as an endocrine organ. The placenta provides oxygen and removes carbon dioxide from the fetal system because its respiratory system is not yet functioning.
   a. Placenta develops by the third month.

(1) Formed by union of chorionic villi and decidua basalis.

(2) Fetal surface smooth and glistening.

(3) Maternal surface red and fleshlike.

(4) Exchange takes place between mother and fetus through diffusion.

(5) Materials passed through placenta in addition to nutrients are drugs, antibodies to some diseases, and certain viruses. Large particles such as bacteria cannot pass through barrier.

(6) Hormones produced by the placenta.
   (a) Chorionic gonadotropin can be detected in the urine about fifteen days after implantation. This hormone stimulates the corpus luteum to maintain endometrium.
   (b) Estrogen and progesterone.

b. The umbilical cord extends from the fetus to the center of the fetal surface of the placenta.

(1) Main vessels in the umbilical cord are two arteries and one vein.

(2) The umbilical cord is protected by mucoid connective tissue termed Wharton's jelly.

(3) Its length is twenty inches; its width is one inch.

2. Fetal circulation.
   a. Vein carries oxygenated blood.
   b. Arteries carry venous blood.
   c. There are three bypasses in fetal circulation.
      (1) Two bypasses exist because the lungs are not functioning.
         (a) Ductus arteriosus, between pulmonary artery and aorta.
         (b) Foramen ovale, between right and left atrium.

(2) Ductus venosus bypass exists because the fetal liver is not used for exchange of waste.

    d. Bypasses must close following birth to allow blood to flow through the lungs for respiration and through the liver for waste exchange.

G. A multiple pregnancy is one in which two or more embryos are contained in the embryo. May be the result of fertilization of a single ovum or two separate ova.

H. Calculation of expected date of delivery or confinement (EDC).

    1. Nägele's rule—count back three months from first day of last menstrual period (LMP) and add seven days.
       Example: LMP July 18, 1979.
              EDC April 25, 1980.

    2. Pregnancy usually does not terminate on the exact EDC. It may vary from one week before to two weeks after the expected date.

Table B. Fetal Growth

Age	Development
End of one month or four weeks	Form of embryonic disc No clearly defined features Body systems rudimentary form Cardiovascular system functioning
End of two months or eight weeks	Head greatly enlarged, about the size of rest of body Some fetal movement as a result of beginning neuromuscular development Facial features becoming distinct Body covered with thin skin
End of three months or twelve weeks	Teeth forming under gums Center ossification appearing in most bones Fingers and toes are differentiated and bear nails Kidneys able to secrete Eyes have lids which are fused shut until six months Fetus swallows Sex distinguishable Fetal heart heard with ultrasonic equipment
End of four months or sixteen weeks	Lanugo appears over body Meconium in intestines Face has human appearance Size about 6 in. long; weight about 3.5 oz
End of five months or twenty weeks	Skeleton begins to harden Buds of permanent teeth develop Vernix caseosa makes appearance Fetal movements stronger and felt by mother Fetal heart rate heard with fetoscope Size about 10 in. long; weight about 11 oz
End of six months or twenty-four weeks	Fat beginning to deposit beneath skin Body and head better proportioned Eyebrows and eyelashes appear Size about 12 in. long; weight about 1½ lbs

Age	Development
End of seven months or twenty-eight weeks	Skin reddish and covered with vernix Size about 14 in. long; weight about 2½ lbs May be viable if born at this time, though still immature
End of eight months or thirty-two weeks	Nails are firm and extend to end of digits Lanugo begins to disappear Size about 16 in. long; weight about 4 lbs Increased chance for survival if born at this time
End of nine months or thirty-six weeks	Increased fat deposits under skin Increased development Size about 18 in. long; weight about 5 lbs Chances for survival are good
End of ten months or forty weeks	Full term Little lanugo Smooth skin Size about 20 in. long; weight 7–7½ lbs Optimum time for survival

Maternal Changes During Pregnancy

Physiological Changes

Reproductive Organs

A. Uterus increases in weight from two ounces to about two pounds at the end of gestation and increases in size five to six times.
   1. Changes in tissue.
      a. Hypertrophy of muscle cells and development of new muscles.
      b. Development of connective and elastic tissue, which increases contractility.
      c. Increase in the size and number of blood vessels.
      d. Hypertrophy of the lymphatic system.
      e. Growth of the uterus is brought about by the influences of estrogen during the early months and the pressure of the fetus.
   2. Other changes.
      a. Contractions occur throughout pregnancy, starting from very mild to increased strength.
      b. As the uterus grows, it rises out of the pelvis displacing intestines and may be palpated above the symphysis pubis.
B. Ligaments.
   1. Broad ligaments located in the pelvis.
   2. They become elongated and hypertrophied to help support and stabilize uterus during pregnancy.
C. Cervix.
   1. Becomes shorter, more elastic, and larger in diameter.
   2. Marked thickening of mucous lining and increased blood supply.
   3. Edema and hyperplasia of the cervical glands and increased glandular secretions.
   4. Mucous plug expelled from cervix as cervix begins to dilate at onset of labor.
D. Vagina.
   1. Increased vascularity, deepening of color to dark red or purple (Chadwick's sign).
   2. Hypertrophy and thickening of muscle.
   3. Loosening of connective tissue.
   4. Increased vaginal discharge.
   5. Secretions have high pH.
E. Perineum.
   1. Increased vascularity.

2. Hypertrophy of muscles.
3. Loosening of connective tissue.

F. Ovaries and tubes.
1. Usually one large corpus luteum present in one ovary.
2. Ovulation does not take place.

Breasts

A. Changes in tissue.
1. Extensive growth of alveolar tissue, necessary for lactation.
2. Montgomery's glands enlarge.

B. Other changes.
1. Increase in size and firmness; become nodular.
2. Nipples become more prominent, and areolae deepen in color.
3. Superficial veins grow more prominent.
4. At the end of third month, colostrum appears.
5. After delivery, anterior pituitary stimulates production and secretion of milk.

Abdomen

A. Contour changes as the enlarging uterus extends into the abdominal cavity.

B. Striae gravidarum usually appear on the abdomen as pregnancy progresses.

Skin

A. Pigmentation increases in certain areas of the body.
1. Breasts—primary areolae deepen in color.
2. Abdomen—linea nigra, dark streak down the midline of the abdomen, especially prominent in brunettes.
3. Face—chloasma, the "mask of pregnancy" pigmentation, distributed over the face; usually disappears after pregnancy.
4. Face and upper trunk—occasionally spider nevi or palmar erythema develops with the increase in estrogen.

B. Pigmented areas on abdomen and breast usually do not completely disappear after delivery.

Circulatory System

A. Considerable increase (about 50 percent) in volume of blood as a result of:
1. Increased metabolic demands of new tissue.
2. Expansion of vascular system, especially in the reproductive organs.
3. Increased steroid hormones which cause retention of sodium and water.

B. Increase in plasma volume is greater than increase in red blood cells and hemoglobin, although dilution is not sufficient to cause anemia (low hemoglobin in pregnancy usually caused by iron-deficiency anemia).

C. Heart increases in size and cardiac output is increased 25 to 50 percent.

D. Blood pressure *should not* rise during pregnancy.

E. Fibrinogen concentration increases until term.

F. Iron requirements are increased to meet demands of increased blood supply and growing fetus (need cannot be met by diet alone; supplement usually given).

G. Palpitations may be experienced during pregnancy due to sympathetic nervous disturbance and intraabdominal pressure caused by enlarging uterus.

Respiratory System

A. Thoracic cage is pushed upward and the diaphragm is elevated as the uterus enlarges.

B. Thoracic cage widens to compensate so that vital capacity remains the same or is increased.

C. Oxygen consumption is increased 15 percent to support fetus and tissue.

D. Shortness of breath may be experienced in latter part of pregnancy due to pressure upon diaphragm caused by enlarging uterus.

Digestive System

A. Nausea, vomiting, and poor appetite are present in early pregnancy because of a decreased gastric motility.

B. Constipation is due to a decrease in gastrointestinal motility, reduced peristaltic activity, and the pressure of the uterus; it may be present in latter half of pregnancy.

C. Flatulence and heartburn may be present as a result of decreased gastric acidity and decreased motility of the gastrointestinal tract.

Urinary System

A. Kidneys.
   1. Kidney and renal function is increased.
   2. Renal blood flow and glomerular filtration is increased.
B. Bladder and ureters.
   1. Blood supply to the bladder and pelvic organs is increased.
   2. Pressure of the uterus on the bladder causes frequent urination during early pregnancy.
   3. Atonia of smooth muscles during pregnancy leads to dilatation of ureters and renal pelvis; may cause urine stasis.
   4. A decrease in bladder tone is caused by hormonal influences; a decrease in bladder capacity occurs because of crowding. Such decrease may lead to complications during pregnancy and in the postpartum period.

Joints, Bones, Teeth and Gums

A. Softening of pelvic cartilages occurs, probably due to the relaxin hormone.
B. Postural changes occur as upper spine is thrown forward to compensate for increased abdominal size.
C. Demineralization of teeth does not occur as a result of normal pregnancy but may be related to poor dental hygiene.
D. Increased vascularity of gums due to hormonal changes with tendency to bleed easily.

Endocrine System

A. Placenta produces the hormones human chorionic gonadotropin (HCG) and placental lactogen (HPL).
   1. Production of estrogen and progesterone is taken over from the ovaries by the placenta/fetal unit after the second month.
   2. Normal cycle of production of estrogen and progesterone is suspended until after delivery.
B. Anterior lobe of pituitary gland enlarges slightly during pregnancy.
C. Adrenal cortex enlarges slightly.
D. Thyroid enlarges slightly and thyroid activity increases.
E. Aldosterone levels gradually increase beginning about the fifteenth week.

Metabolism

A. Increase in body weight (a twenty-five-pound weight gain is usually recommended).
B. Some of the weight gain is caused by retention of fluid and by deposits of fatty tissue.
C. Water metabolism.
   1. Tendency to retain fluid in body tissues, especially in the last trimester.
   2. Reversal of fluid retention usually takes place in the form of diuresis in the first twenty-four hours postpartum.
D. Basal metabolic rate increases.

Emotional Changes

Altered Emotional Characteristics

A. Quick mood changes and a certain amount of emotional lability is common.
B. Emotional reactions may change during pregnancy; may range from early rejection of pregnancy to that of elation.
C. Pregnant women may become more passive and introverted in second trimester.
D. A woman may be puzzled by changes in her feelings and needs reassurance from the nurse that these are normal reactions about which one need not feel guilty.
E. Father of the baby needs to be informed that the woman's emotional lability, attitudes, and feelings toward sex are emotional reactions of pregnancy and will pass.

F. The woman may have fears and worries about the baby and herself and needs to be able to express her feelings to the nurse.

Taking on the Maternal Role

A. Pregnant woman may fantasize or daydream to "experience" the role of mother before the actual birth occurs.
B. Takes on adaptive behaviors that are best suited to her own personality and situation.
C. Experiences a "letting go" of her former role (e.g., as a career woman).
   1. May experience ambivalence about letting go of her old role to take on the new one.
   2. Desire to have a baby influences adjustment and acceptance of the maternal role.

Childbirth Preparation

Theories of Childbirth

A. Factors that influence pain in labor.
   1. Preconditioning by "old wives' tales," fantasies, and fears. Accurate information about the childbirth process can often alleviate effects of preconditioning.
   2. Pain produces stress, which in turn affects the body's functioning. Interpretations of and reactions to pain can be altered by a refocusing of attention and by conditioning.
   3. Feelings of isolation. Social expectations and tension may also increase feelings of pain.
B. Childbirth education classes.
   1. Read method (original natural childbirth movement).
      a. Its purpose is to eradicate negative attitudes of mother through education.
      b. A basic principle establishes that childbirth is a natural occurrence and should not be painful.
      c. Presents a thorough understanding of anatomy, physiology of pregnancy, labor, and delivery.

   d. Encourages exercise to foster relaxation and prepare woman for physical work of labor; breathing (diaphragmatic, abdominal) and panting.
   2. Lamaze method (psychoprophylactic method).
      a. Basic thrust is education and training.
      b. Instruction in anatomy, the physiology of the reproductive system; an extensive study of labor and delivery; replacement of misinformation and superstition with facts.
      c. Training that consists of controlled breathing and neuromuscular exercises.
      d. Husband, family member, or a friend is included in the class and serves as coach.
   3. LeBoyer technique (used in delivery room to reduce stress of birth upon infant).
      a. Room temperature is increased to a comfortable level for infant, lights are dimmed, noise is controlled.
      b. Infant is placed in skin-to-skin contact on mother's abdomen and gently stroked; cord clamping is delayed until pulsation stops.
      c. Infant is submerged up to head in a bath of warm water until it appears relaxed, then is dried and wrapped snugly in a warm blanket.

Nutritional Guidelines for Pregnancy

A. Influences upon dietary habits and nutrition.
   1. Food—many emotional connotations originating in infancy.
   2. Eating habits influenced by:
      a. Emotional factors.
      b. Cultural factors.
      c. Religious beliefs.
      d. Nutritional information.
      e. Age—especially adolescent and aged.
      f. Physical health.
      g. Personal preferences.
B. Nutritional needs in pregnancy.
   1. Influenced by above factors.

2. Must supply caloric and nutritional needs of mother as well as promote optimum fetal growth.
3. May be complicated by:
   a. Poor maternal nutrition before pregnancy.
   b. Medical complications prior to pregnancy (diabetes, anemia).
   c. Complications resulting from pregnancy (toxemia, anemia).
   d. Pica (cravings).
C. Weight gain in pregnancy.
   1. Average weight gain recommended (even for obese patients)—24 pounds.
      a. 1st trimester—3 to 4 pounds
      b. 2nd trimester—10 pounds.
      c. 3rd trimester—10 pounds.
   2. Weight gain accounted by:
      a. Product of conception.

Fetus—average size	7.5 pounds
Placenta	1.5
Amniotic fluid	2
Uterus	2.5
Breasts	1
Extracellular fluid	3
Blood volume	3
	20.5 pounds

      b. Rest of weight gain deposited as fat stores or fluid representing energy stored for lactation.
D. Revised daily food guide.
   1. Iron and folacin—cannot be ingested in sufficient quantities by dietary means. Must be supplemented during pregnancy.
   2. 300 additional calories needed to meet recommended allowances.
   3. Protein intake includes both animal and vegetable protein.
      a. Vegetable protein may be omitted in those whose income will allow by increasing animal servings to three 3-oz. servings.
      b. One serving at least should be red meats.
   4. Whole grain items are better choices than enriched breads and cereals. They contain more magnesium, zinc, folacin, and vitamin B_6.

5. At least two tablespoons of fat or oils should be consumed daily for vitamin E and essential fatty acids.
E. Special diets.
   1. Adolescents
      a. Have high proportion of low-birth-weight infants.
      b. Dietary habits often poor.
      c. Plan menu to include necessary items around foods they like.
      d. Stress balanced diet—avoid empty calories.
   2. Low sodium.
      a. Presently sodium restriction is *deemphasized.*
      b. Sodium essential in maintaining increased body fluids needed for adequate placental flow, increased tissue requirements, and renal blood flow.
      c. If moderate salt intake is necessitated, avoid highly salted foods such as canned soups, potato chips, soda pop.
   3. Weight control.
      a. Presently, weight loss in pregnancy is discouraged.
      b. Even obese client should gain 24 pounds to insure adequate nutrition for fetal growth.
      c. Strict dieting may lead to ketosis which has proven harmful to fetal brain.
      d. Stress careful dietary planning to include essential nutrients and avoid empty calories.
      e. Weight reduction program should begin *after* lactation only.

Signs and Discomforts of Pregnancy

Signs of Pregnancy

Presumptive Signs

A. Cessation of menstruation (amenorrhea).
B. Breasts increase in size with feeling of fullness; nipples more pronounced, areola darker.

C. Nausea and vomiting ("morning sickness") appear in about 50 percent of pregnant women and usually disappears at the end of the third month.

D. Frequent urination (desire to void) usually occurs in the first three to four months. Pressure on the bladder from an enlarged uterus gives the sensation of a distended bladder.

E. Quickening (first perception of fetal movement) occurs between sixteenth and eighteenth week.

F. Increased pigmentation of skin, chloasma, linea nigra, and striae gravidarum.

G. Fatigue with periods of drowsiness and lassitude during first three months.

Probable Signs

A. Enlargement of the abdomen, which usually occurs after the third month when the fetus rises out of the pelvis into the abdominal cavity.

B. Changes in internal organs.
1. Change in shape, size, and consistency of the uterus.
2. Hegar's sign—softening of the isthmus of the uterus, occurs about sixth week.
3. Goodell's sign—softening of the cervix, occurs beginning of the second month.

C. Braxton Hicks contractions—slight, irregular contractions usually not felt by the woman until seven months, but contractions begin in the early weeks of pregnancy and continue through gestation.

D. Ballottement—pressure on an organ giving a sudden push to the fetus and feeling it rebound in a few seconds to the original position; usually possible in the fourth to fifth month.

E. Outline of the fetus by abdominal palpation (a probable sign, because a tumor may simulate fetal parts).

F. Positive pregnancy test is based upon the secretion of chorionic gonadotropin in the urine of a pregnant woman; it is usually detectable ten days after the first missed period.

Positive Signs

A. Apparent after eighteenth to twentieth week.

B. Auscultation of fetal heart rates (120–160) with stethoscope or ultrasonic equipment. (Note: with ultrasonic equipment, fetal heart rate may be heard at twelve weeks.)

C. Active fetal movements are perceptible by the physician.

D. X-ray or sonogram examination showing fetal outline. X-ray not visible until fourteenth week or later, when bone calcification occurs.

Pseudocyesis (Pseudopregnancies)

A. The emotional control of physiological functioning that is psychological in origin; woman believes she is pregnant when she is not.

B. Clinical manifestations.
1. Amenorrhea, breast changes, and secretion of colostrum.
2. Enlargement of abdomen.
3. Reports of quickening.
4. Appears any age, but more common in older women.

C. Treatment.
1. Uncover underlying emotional problem.
2. Offer continued emotional support as this is important.

Physical Examination

A. Initial examination.
1. Complete history is recorded (past pregnancies, medical history, and family history).
2. Physical examination of pelvis, breasts, and abdomen.
3. Blood pressure, urinalysis, blood work including Rh factor, rubella titer, pap smear, slide for gonorrhea and VDRL.
4. Diet and health instructions are given to patient.

B. Subsequent examinations are usually done once a month until the last trimester, then more frequently.
  1. Weight and blood pressure taken; urine tests for protein and sugar content made.
  2. Palpation of abdomen.

3. Auscultation of fetal heart tones.
4. Observation for untoward signs and symptoms.
5. Continuing health care and instructions.

C. See Table B for pregnancy discomfort and relief measures.

Table B. Major Discomforts and Relief Measures

Discomfort	Trimester Most Prominent	Relief Measures
Nausea and vomiting	1st	Instead of three large meals daily, have five or six small, frequent meals In between meals, have couple of crackers or a piece of toast without fluid Avoid foods high in carbohydrates, with a strong odor, or fried and greasy Plan rest period after meals If nausea occurs at regular intervals when stomach is empty, plan ahead by eating twenty to thirty minutes earlier Antinausea drug may be prescribed
Urinary frequency	1st and 3rd	Wear perineal pads if there is leakage
Heartburn	2nd and 3rd	Avoid fatty, fried, and highly spiced foods Have small frequent feedings Use an antacid
Abdominal distress	1st, 2nd, and 3rd	Eat slowly, chew food thoroughly, take smaller helpings of food
Flatulence	2nd and 3rd	Maintain daily bowel movement Avoid gas-forming foods Take antiflatulents as prescribed by physician
Constipation	2nd and 3rd	Drink sufficient fluids Eat fruit and foods high in roughage Exercise moderately Take stool softener if prescribed by physician
Hemorrhoids	3rd	Apply ointments, suppositories, warm compresses Avoid constipation Rest
Insomnia	3rd	Exercise moderately to promote relaxation and fatigue Change position while sleeping If severe, take medication as prescribed by physician

Backaches	3rd	Rest Improve posture Use a good abdominal support and wear comfortable shoes Do exercises such as squatting, sitting, and pelvic rock
Varicosities, legs and vulva	3rd	Avoid long periods of standing or sitting with legs crossed Sit or lie with feet and hips elevated Move about while standing to improve circulation Wear support hose
Edema of legs and feet	3rd	Elevate feet while sitting or lying down Avoid standing or sitting in one position for long periods
Cramps in legs	3rd	Extend cramped leg and flex ankles, pushing foot upward with toes pointed toward knee Increase calcium intake
Pain in thighs or aching of perineum	3rd	Alternate periods of sitting and standing Rest
Shortness of breath	3rd	Sit up Lie on back with arms extended above bed
Supine hypotensive syndrome	3rd	Change position to left side to relieve pressure of uterus on inferior vena cava
Vaginal discharge	3rd	Practice proper cleansing and hygiene Avoid douche unless recommended by physician Observe for signs of vaginal infection common in pregnancy

Complications of Pregnancy

Danger Signals

A. Bleeding from vagina.
B. Escape of amniotic fluid denoting premature rupture of membranes.
C. Abdominal pain.
D. Dizziness or blurring of vision.
E. Persistent headache.
F. Edema of face and fingers.
G. Persistent and severe vomiting.
H. Chills and elevated temperature.

Abortion

Definition: Abortion is the expulsion of the fetus before it is viable; abortion may be spontaneous or induced.

Categories of Abortion

A. Threatened—some loss of blood and pain without loss of products of conception.
B. Imminent—bleeding profuse, contractions severe, bearing down sensation; without intervention, products of conception will be lost.
C. Inevitable—bleeding, contractions, ruptured membranes, and cervical dilatation.

D. Incomplete—portion of products of conception remain in uterine cavity.

E. Complete—all products of conception expelled.

F. Habitual—abortion in three or more succeeding pregnancies.

G. Therapeutic—medically terminated for woman's physical or emotional health.

H. Criminal—termination of pregnancy outside medical or approved facilities.

Etiology

A. Abnormalities of fetus.

B. Abnormalities of reproductive tract.

C. Injuries—physical and emotional shocks.

D. Endocrine disturbances.

E. Acute infectious diseases.

F. Maternal diseases.

G. Psychogenic problems.

Signs and Symptoms

A. Vaginal bleeding.

B. Intermittent contractions and pain which usually begin in the small of the back; abdominal cramping.

Treatment

A. Notification of physician immediately.

B. Endocrine therapy (usually progesterone if deficiency).

C. Correction of abnormalities or disturbances of reproductive tract.

D. Avoidance of stress and exertion during early pregnancy.

E. Bed rest and sedation; avoid climbing stairs and coitus until at least two weeks after bleeding stops.

F. Oxytoxic drug may be given to hasten process of abortion, if it is inevitable, and to promote contraction of uterus after abortion.

G. Medication for pain if necessary.

H. Blood available for transfusion.

I. Dilatation and curettage may be necessary in an incomplete abortion.

J. Administration of RhoGAM in Rh-negative women.

K. Maintain sterile technique in all examinations and treatments.

Nursing Care

A. Offer emotional support and comfort; do not say, "Everything will be all right," if there is loss of the fetus.

B. Save all perineal pads and expelled tissue for examination.

C. Observe for and report signs of shock.

D. In criminal abortions, observe for serious complications such as septic shock, thrombophlebitis, and renal failure.

Habitual Abortion

Definition: Habitual abortion is the condition in which the patient has spontaneously aborted three or more consecutive times.

Etiology

A. Endocrine disturbances.

B. Blood incompatibilities.

C. Incompetent cervical os.

D. Chromosomal abnormalities.

E. Abnormalities of reproductive tract.

F. Fibromas of uterus.

G. Psychological.

Treatments

A. Hormone therapy (estrogen and progesterone) and thyroid therapy for endocrine disturbances.

B. Shirodkar procedure (internal os constricted by encircling suture which is removed when labor begins) for incompetent cervical os.

C. Surgical correction of abnormalities, if possible, and removal of fibromas.

D. Psychotherapy for psychological cause.

Hydatidiform Mole

Definition: Benign neoplasm of the chorion in which chorionic villi degenerate, become filled with a clear viscid fluid, and assume the appearance of grapelike clusters involving all or parts of the decidual lining of the uterus.

Incidence

A. Rare, occurs once in every two thousand pregnancies except in the Orient, where it is far less rare.
B. Usually there is no fetus found.

Etiology

A. May be pathological ova.
B. High incidence in the Orient may be due to a protein deficiency in diet.

Signs and Symptoms

A. Pregnancy appears normal at first.
B. Bleeding varies from spotting to profuse.
C. Rapid enlargement of the uterus.
D. Nausea and vomiting appear earlier; usually are more severe and last longer.
E. Severe preeclampsia may develop in the early part of the second trimester.
F. Hypertension may occur with the rapid expansion of the uterus.
G. Characteristic vesicles may be passed.

Diagnosis

A. Test for increased titer of chorionic gonadotropin. It is best to collect a 24-hour specimen for the total daily output.
B. Sonography which will give positive diagnosis in the first trimester.
C. Amniography—x-ray following injection with contrast dye.

Treatment and Nursing Care

A. Evacuation of uterus as soon as positive diagnosis is made (by dilatation and curettage or vacuum curettage suction).
B. Follow-up visits to physician for examination, because hydatidiform mole may lead to choriocarcinoma of uterus.
C. Observe for hemorrhage.
D. Provide emotional support for there may be fear of malignancy or patient may feel the loss of the baby.

Extrauterine (Ectopic) Pregnancy

Definition: A pregnancy that develops outside the uterus.

Process of Pregnancy

A. Although the fertilized ovum usually attaches to the uterine lining, it may become implanted at any point between the graafian follicle and the uterus.
B. Tubal pregnancy is the most common form (95 percent) but the ovum may attach to an ovary, the abdomen, or interligaments.
C. Implantation.
   1. Ovum attaches to tube and erodes into mucosa wall, as it would to the endometrial lining of the uterus.
   2. Tube increases in size and stretches.
   3. Pregnancy usually terminates during the first three months by:
      a. Spontaneous tubal abortion.
      b. Tubal rupture.
      c. Death and disintegration of products of conception within the tube.

Etiology

A. Progress of ovum through tube is delayed for some reason.
B. Tubal deformities that are either congenital or due to disease such as gonorrhea.
C. Tumors pressing against the tube.
D. Adhesions from previous surgery.

E. Tubal spasms.

F. Migration of ovum to opposite tube.

Signs and Symptoms

A. Woman may or may not know she is pregnant.

B. May have history of missed periods and "spotting."

C. May have slight abdominal pain.

D. Early signs of pregnancy may be present.

E. Uterus enlarges and decidua develops due to hormonal influence.

F. Often first symptom is a sudden excruciating pain in lower abdomen.

G. May feel faint and have signs of shock as a result of hemorrhage into the peritoneal cavity.

H. May have little external bleeding.

Treatment and Nursing Care

A. Immediate removal of the affected tube.

B. Blood transfusions may be necessary.

C. Observe for signs of shock and give treatment for shock as necessary.

D. Provide emotional support; patient may be frightened and feel the loss of the pregnancy.

Placenta Previa

Definition: A placenta develops so that it partially or completely covers the internal os when ovum implants low in the uterus towards the cervix. Occurs once in every 150 deliveries.

Types

A. Complete—os entirely covered.

B. Partial—only part of os covered.

C. Marginal—margin overlaps os.

Etiology

A. Occurs more often in multiparas.

B. Occurs more often with increased age of woman.

Signs and Symptoms

A. Painless vaginal bleeding after the seventh month without precipitating cause.

B. Bleeding may be intermittent.

C. As internal os begins to dilate, the part of placenta that overlies the os separates and leaves gaping vessels so that bleeding occurs.

D. Uterus usually remains soft and flaccid.

Diagnosis

A. History of painless bleeding begins late in pregnancy.

B. Localization of placenta by ultrasound.

C. Sterile vaginal or pelvic examinations are usually not done as part of diagnosis until adequate preparation has been made.

Treatment and Nursing Care

A. Immediate hospitalization.

B. Usually placed on bed rest.

C. Blood is typed and crossmatched for possible transfusion.

D. Treatment depends upon type of placenta previa, condition of woman, and viability of baby.

   1. Mechanical pressure applied to placental site by bringing down baby's head and occluding blood vessels; usually accomplished by the rupture of membranes.

   2. Delivery by cesarean section.

E. If baby is small and bleeding stops, delivery is usually postponed.

F. Count perineal pads.

G. Observe for hemorrhage.

H. Give emotional support, explain procedures, and help allay fears.

I. Carefully monitor fetal heart tones.

Abruptio Placentae

Definition: A separation of the placenta from the normal implantation site in upper segment of uterus before birth of baby. Occurs once in five hundred deliveries.

Types

A. Complete separation—placenta becomes completely detached from uterine wall.
B. Partial separation—portion of placenta adheres to uterine wall.
C. External—blood escapes from the vagina.
D. Concealed—blood is retained in uterine cavity.

Etiology

A. Trauma.
B. Chronic vascular renal disease.
C. High parity.

Signs and Symptoms

A. Vaginal bleeding accompanied by abdominal pain is chief external sign.
B. Concealed signs.
   1. Intense, cramplike uterine pain.
   2. Uterine tenderness and rigidity.
   3. Lack of alternate contraction-relaxation of uterus.
   4. Fetal heart tones indicate bradycardia or are absent.

Treatment and Nursing Care

A. Depends upon severity and extent of labor.
B. Treatment for blood loss and shock.
   1. Moderate bleeding—rupture membranes to hasten delivery and help control bleeding.
   2. Severe—immediate cesarean section.
C. Keep patient on bed rest.
D. Observe for signs of shock.
E. Carefully monitor contractions, fetal heart tones, and vital signs.
F. Maintain record of intake and output.
G. Nursing actions after delivery.
   1. Observe closely for hemorrhage.
   2. Carefully record intake and output; observe for anuria or oliguria. Anuria may develop as a result of acute tubular necrosis.

Hyperemesis Gravidarum

Definition: Pernicious vomiting during pregnancy.

Signs and Symptoms

A. Usually develops during the first three months of pregnancy.
B. Persistent nausea and vomiting.
C. May have abdominal pain and hiccups.
D. Considerable weight loss.
E. May become severely dehydrated.
F. May have depletion of essential electrolytes because of unreplaced loss of sodium chloride and potassium.
G. Metabolic acidosis may develop.
H. Blood urea nitrogen increases.

Causes

A. May be caused by the addition of new substances to the body system such as a toxicity or maladjustment of the maternal metabolism.
B. Psychological disturbances may be the underlying cause, or it may be a combination of psychological and toxic factors.

Treatment and Nursing Care

A. Aimed at reducing the severity of symptoms.
B. Give frequent small feedings in small amounts every two hours; dry foods preferred.
C. Avoid giving spicy or fried foods.
D. Give antiemetics as prescribed along with a tranquilizer or a sedative.
E. If vomiting is persistent:
   1. Patient is usually hospitalized.
   2. Dehydration and starvation is treated by administration of parenteral fluids.
   3. Rest and sedatives are prescribed.
F. Use tact and understanding of the patient's problem.
G. Carefully record intake and output; maintain IV's.
H. Observe for acetone odor on breath.

Pregnancy Induced Hypertension

Definition: A group of conditions (formerly called toxemias) that usually appear after the twentieth week. The major symptoms, hypertension, proteinuria, and edema, most frequently occur in young or elderly primigravidas, women with deficient diets, multiple pregnancies, polyhydramnios, and in long-standing diabetes.

Preeclampsia

Definition: An acute, hypertensive disease peculiar to pregnancy that may be mild or severe.

Signs and Symptoms

A. Usually appears after the twenty-fourth week.
B. Major symptoms are hypertension, proteinuria, and edema, which may appear separately or together. Two of the three symptoms are usually needed for diagnosis.
C. Mild.
    1. Blood pressure above 140/90 or systolic 30 mm Hg and diastolic 15 mm Hg above normal.
    2. Edema.
    3. Proteinuria (1 gm in twenty-four hours).
D. Severe.
    1. Blood pressure 160/110 or above, or systolic 50 mm Hg above normal.
    2. Massive edema with excessive weight gain.
    3. Proteinuria (5 gm or more in twenty-four hours).
    4. Oliguria (400 cc or less in twenty-four hours).
    5. Visual disturbances.
    6. Headache.

Treatment and Nursing Care

A. Mild.
    1. Patient usually remains at home.
    2. Extra rest is prescribed.
    3. Adequate fluid intake is maintained.
    4. Highly salted food is avoided.
    5. Weight is checked daily.
    6. Physician should be notified if further symptoms occur.
    7. Physician may order antihypertensive drugs.
B. Severe.
    1. Antihypertensive drugs.
    2. Increased protein diet; sodium intake is usually not restricted, but patient should avoid use of highly salted foods. (Note: This is a recent trend. The use of low-sodium diet may still be included on state board exams.)
    3. Efforts to increase diuresis (diuretics may or may not be given).
    4. Maintain bed rest.
    5. Administer sedatives if ordered.
    6. Observe for signs of central nervous system irritability and hyperactivity.
    7. Take and record vital signs.
    8. Measure and record intake and output.
    9. Check weight at same time each day.
    10. Test urine for protein; record.
    11. Limit visitors.
    12. Maintain seizure precautions.
    13. Provide diversional activities.

Eclampsia

Definition: A more severe form of toxemia usually accompanied by convulsions and even coma.

Signs and Symptoms

A. Severe edema with tremendous weight gain.
B. Scanty urine.
C. Urine may contain red blood cells, varied casts, and protein.
D. Blood pressure may rise to 200/110.
E. There may be visual disturbances, blurring, or even blindness caused by edema of the retina.
F. Severe epigastric pain.
G. Convulsions (both tonic and clonic).
H. Labor may begin; fetus may be born prematurely or die.

Treatment and Nursing Care

A. Prevent and/or control convulsions.
   1. Quiet, dark room.
   2. Have mouth gag available.
   3. Have suction available.
   4. Use padded side-rails.
B. Promote diuresis; measure and record intake and output.
C. Take and record vital signs.
D. Provide oxygen as necessary.
E. Maintain IV; give fluid if ordered.
F. Monitor fetal heart tones.
G. Observe carefully for anuria and convulsions after delivery.
H. See Appendix 1 for drugs normally used during toxemia.

Polyhydramnios

Definition: An excessive amount of amniotic fluid. Usual normal amount is 500–1000 ml. In polyhydramnios there is over 2000 ml, which is excessive.

Etiology

A. Actual cause is unknown. Occurs frequently in:
   1. Fetal malformations.
   2. Diabetes.
   3. Erythroblastosis.
   4. Multiple pregnancies.
   5. Toxemias.
B. Diagnosis usually made through clinical observation of the greatly enlarged uterus.

Signs and Symptoms

A. Related to pressure of the enlarged uterus or adjacent organs.
B. Edema of the lower extremities.
C. General abdominal discomfort.
D. Occasional shortness of breath.

Treatment

A. Amniocentesis offers only temporary relief.
B. Delivery.

Fetal Demise (Death)

Signs and Symptoms

A. Cessation of fetal movement.
B. Absence of fetal heart tones.
C. Failure of uterine growth.
D. Low urinary estriol.
E. Negative pregnancy test that may remain positive for a few weeks due to elevated human chorionic gonadotropin.
F. X-ray (overlapping of skull bones).
G. Uterus feels smaller.

Treatment and Nursing Care

A. Labor usually begins spontaneously a few weeks after death of fetus.
B. Labor may be induced if it does not occur spontaneously.
C. Watch patient closely for signs of disseminated intravascular disease from prolonged retention of the dead fetus.
D. Provide emotional support to parents.
E. Guide parents in planning future pregnancies.
F. Observe for hemorrhage.
G. Observe for psychological disturbances; refer for psychological counseling.

High Risk Pregnancy

Definition: A pregnancy that refers to any condition that may interfere with the normal development or delivery of the fetus; or, to any preexisting maternal disease that may increase the risk of pregnancy.

Predisposing Factors

A. Age of under 17, of over 35, or unmarried.
B. Parity (having borne five or more pregnancies).
C. Previous conditions.
   1. Previous infant death, premature birth, or congenital malformations.
   2. History of cardiac disease, diabetes, renal disease, or other maternal conditions.
   3. Difficulty in conceiving.
   4. Narcotic or alcohol addiction.
   5. Less than a year since last pregnancy.
   6. Rh incompatibility and sensitization.

Conditions Leading to High Risk

A. During pregnancy.
   1. Infection.
   2. Bleeding.
   3. Pregnancy Induced Hypertension.
B. Intrapartum Conditions
   1. Premature labor.
   2. Abnormal fetal positions.
   3. Premature rupture membranes.

Cardiovascular Disease

Characteristics

A. Classification.
   1. Class I—no alteration of activity.
   2. Class II—slight limitation of activity.
   3. Class III—marked limitations of activity.
   4. Class IV—symptoms present at rest.
B. Pregnancy expands plasma volume, increasing cardiac output and load on heart.
C. Most deaths are caused by cardiac failure, when blood volume is at a maximum in the last weeks of the second trimester.
D. Heart failure occurs infrequently in labor.
E. Over age thirty-five, there is an increase in the incidence of heart failure and death.

Management During Pregnancy

A. With proper management, mortality is minimal.
B. Patient should avoid acute infections, especially respiratory infections.
C. Patient should rest frequently.
D. Strenuous activities such as stair climbing, heavy cleaning, and straining should be avoided.
E. Patients in Class III and over may be hospitalized before labor for controlled rest and diet.
F. If patient decompensates or has distress symptoms with exertion, she should remain on bed rest or in a chair.
G. Salt intake may or may not be restricted. Diuretics may be prescribed if signs of heart failure occur. The use of highly salted foods is discouraged.
H. Iron supplement is important.
I. Digitalis treatment when indicated.
J. Emotional stress should be avoided.

Management During Labor

A. Observe for signs that cardiac function is deteriorating such as pulse rate over 110 or respiratory rate over 24.
B. Relieve pain and anxiety.
C. Vaginal delivery usually preferred.
D. Patient may decompensate in early postpartum phase.

Nursing Care

A. Educate about special needs and danger signals during pregnancy and postpartum.
B. Be alert for signs of decompensation during pregnancy, especially in the second trimester.
C. During labor:
   1. Check vital signs every fifteen minutes or more often as needed.
   2. Keep patient in bed and preferably lying on one side or in semirecumbent position.
   3. Administer oxygen as necessary.
   4. Provide calm atmosphere and emotional support to alleviate fears.

5. Administer pain medications as ordered to reduce discomfort during labor.
6. Be alert for signs of impending heart failure.
7. Monitor fetal heart tones.

D. Careful observation during postpartum period.

E. Counsel during postpartum to have help at home and planned rest periods.

Diabetes

Definition: Diabetes is a chronic metabolic disease due to a disturbance in normal insulin production.

Characteristics

A. White's Classifications.
   1. Class A—abnormal glucose tolerance test, indicative of latent or gestational diabetes.
   2. Class B—diabetes beginning after age twenty.
   3. Class C—diabetes at ages ten to nineteen years, or beginning in adolscence after age ten.
   4. Class D—diabetes of long duration, or onset in childhood before the age of ten.
   5. Class E—evidence of pelvic vascular disease.
   6. Class F—nephropathy, including capillary glomerulosclerosis.
   7. Class R—malignant retinopathy.

B. Implications of Diabetes in Pregnancy
   1. Diabetes is more difficult to control.
   2. There is a tendency to develop acidosis.
   3. Patient is prone to infection.
   4. Toxemia, hemorrhage, and polyhydramnios are more likely to develop.
   5. Latent diabetes may develop into full-blown diabetes.
   6. Insulin requirements are increased.
   7. Premature delivery is more frequent.
   8. Infant may be overgrown but have functions related to gestational age rather than size.
   9. Infant is subject to hypoglycemia, hyperbilirubinemia, respiratory distress syndrome, and congenital anomalies.
   10. Stillborn and neonatal mortality rates are high, but may be reduced by proper management and control of diabetes.

Nursing Care

A. Reinforce teaching the effects of diabetes on the mother and fetus during pregnancy and the reasons for frequent testing of blood sugar and urine for sugar and acetone.

B. Emphasize good nutrition and health practices.

C. If hospitalized:
   1. Maintain insulin on regular schedule.
   2. Test urine for sugar and acetone as ordered.
   3. Provide adequate diabetic diet as prescribed by physician.
   4. Provide for diversion.
   5. Monitor fetal heart tone.
   6. Check vital signs, especially blood pressure q.i.d. and p.r.n.
   7. Weigh daily at the same time.
   8. Keep accurate records of intake and output.
   9. Provide support and explanations to help allay fears and reduce anxiety.
   10. Watch for symptoms of hyperglycemia or hypoglycemia.

D. In labor:
   1. Same as above.
   2. Carefully regulate insulin and provide I.V. glucose as labor depletes glycogen.

E. Postpartum.
   1. Close observation for insulin reaction—precipitous drop in insulin requirements usual—hypoglycemic shock may occur.
   2. Close observation for early signs of infection.
   3. Close observation for postpartum hemorrhage.

Anemia

A. Usually caused by iron deficiency.
B. Symptoms.

1. Patient tires easily and looks pale.
2. Hemoglobin values are usually checked routinely in antipartum care.
3. Usually treated by diet and an iron supplement.

Urinary Tract Infection

A. Usually occurs after the fourth month or in early postpartum—affects 10 percent of maternity patients.
B. Causes.
   1. Pressure on ureters and bladder.
   2. Hormonal effects on tone of ureters and bladder.
   3. Displacement of bladder.
C. Kidneys as well as ureters may be involved.
D. Symptoms.
   1. Frequent micturition.
   2. Paroxysms—pain in kidney.
   3. Fever and chills.
   4. Catheterized urine specimen contains bacteria and pus.
E. Treatment.
   1. Bed rest.
   2. High fluid intake.
   3. Antibiotic treatments.
   4. Urinary antispasmodics and analgesics.

Infectious Diseases

Rubella

A. In the first trimester rubella may cause congenital anomalies.
B. Vaccine is available and should be given to children from age one to puberty or to the mother in early postpartum, while she is still hospitalized. (Vaccine should not be given if pregnancy is suspected.)
C. Titer is usually checked on first prenatal visit.

Acute Infectious Diseases

A. Diseases such as influenza, scarlet fever, toxoplasmosis, and cytomegalovirus may be transmitted to the fetus.
B. Diseases may cause abortions or malformations in early pregnancy or premature labor or infant death in later pregnancy.

Venereal Disease

A. Syphilis.
   1. May cause abortion or premature labor.
   2. Infection is passed to the fetus after the fourth month of pregnancy as congenital syphilis.
   3. VDRL test for syphilis on first prenatal visit. (May repeat at a later date as disease may be acquired after initial visit.)
   4. Treatment—during pregnancy, procaine penicillin G with 2 percent aluminum monostearate, I.M. normally in divided doses.
   5. All cases of syphilis must be reported to health authorities for treatment of contacts.
B. Gonorrhea.
   1. Common contagious bacterial disease.
   2. Incidence has been steadily rising as a result of increase in premarital sex.
   3. May be mildly symptomatic in women and may persist unsuspected.
   4. May cause salpingitis after third month if left untreated.
   5. Slide for gonorrhea usually done on first prenatal visit.
   6. Important to treat sexual partner, as patient may become reinfected.
   7. Infection may be transmitted to baby's eyes during delivery, causing blindness.
   8. Soon after birth all newborns have prophylactic treatment of one percent silver nitrate or an antibiotic preparation.
   9. Treatment—same as for syphilis. Other antibiotics may be used for sensitivity to penicillin.
C. Herpes simplex type 2—genital herpes.
   1. Involves external genitalia, vagina, cervix.
   2. Development and draining of painful vesicles.

3. Treatment—symptomatic—no specific cure identified. Safe use of Acyclovir has not been established for pregnant women.
4. Virus is lethal to fetus if innoculated during vaginal delivery. Usual mode of delivery is C-section.

Adolescent Pregnancy

A. Risk to mother and fetus is increased.
   1. Crisis of pregnancy compounds the crises of adolescence related to physical, social, emotional, social development.
   2. Patient may be unwed, which may cause additional problems.
   3. Physical development may not be complete.
   4. High incidence of prematurity and toxemia.

B. Nursing care.
   1. Encourage early antepartum care.
   2. Provide health instruction on pregnancy, nutrition, and hygiene.
   3. Observe for complications frequently.
   4. Provide emotional support and counseling.

Labor and Delivery

Definition of terms

A. Labor is the process by which the products of conception are expelled from the body.

B. Delivery refers to the actual birth.

C. Adaptive processes.
   1. During latter months of pregnancy, the fetus adapts to the maternal uterus enabling it to occupy the smallest space possible.
   2. The term *attitude* refers to the posture the fetus assumes in utero.
   3. *Fetal lie* is the relationship of the long axis of the baby to the long axis of the mother.

Presentation

A. A term used to describe that part of the fetus which lies closest to the true pelvis.

B. Cephalic—presentation of any part of fetal head.
   1. May be vertex, face, or brow.
   2. Vertex most common and most favorable for delivery. Head is sharply flexed in the pelvis with chin near chest.

C. Breech—presentation of buttocks or lower extremities.
   1. Types.
      a. Complete or full—buttocks and feet present (baby in squatting position).
      b. Frank—buttocks only present, or legs are extended against anterior trunk with feet touching face.
      c. Incomplete—one or both feet or knees presenting, footling single or double, or knee presentation.
   2. May rotate to cephalic during pregnancy but possibility lessens as gestation nears term.
   3. May be rotated by physician but usually returns to breech position.

Position

A. A term used to describe the relationship of the fetal presenting part to the maternal bony pelvis.

B. Position is determined by locating the presenting part in relationship to the pelvis.

C. Woman's pelvis is divided into four imaginary quadrants (right anterior, right posterior, left anterior, and left posterior).

D. Most common positions (abbreviations usually used).
   1. LOA (left occiput anterior)—occiput on left side of maternal pelvis and toward front, face down, favorable for delivery.
   2. LOP (left occiput posterior)—occiput on left side of maternal pelvis and toward rear or face up.
      a. Usually causes back pain during labor.
      b. May slow the progress of labor.
      c. Usually rotates before delivery to anterior position.
      d. May be rotated in delivery room by physician.
   3. ROA (right occiput anterior)—occiput on right of maternal pelvis, toward front, face down, favorable for delivery.
   4. ROP (right occiput posterior)—occiput on right side of maternal pelvis, face up. Same problems as LOP.

E. Means of assessing fetal position during labor.
   1. Leopold's maneuver—method of abdominal palpation to determine information about the fetus such as presentation, engagement, and rough estimate of fetal size.
   2. Vaginal examination.
   3. Rectal examination (rarely done at this time).

Engagement

A. Largest diameter of presenting part has passed into the inlet of the maternal pelvis. Usually takes place two weeks before labor in primiparas, but not until labor in multiparas.

B. May be assessed by Leopold's maneuver or vaginal or rectal examination.

Station

A. Degree to which presenting part has descended into pelvis is determined by the station (the relationship between the presenting part and the ischial spines).
B. Assessed by vaginal or rectal examination.
C. Measured in numerical terms.
   1. At level of spines: 0 station.
   2. Above level of spines: $-1, -2, -3$ cm.
   3. Below level of spines: $+1, +2, +3$ cm.
D. Other terms used to denote station.
   1. High—presenting part not engaged.
   2. Floating—presenting part freely movable in inlet of pelvis.
   3. Dipping—entering pelvis.
   4. Fixed—no longer movable in inlet but not engaged.
   5. Engaged—biparietal plane passed through pelvic inlet.

Premonitory Signs of Labor

Physical Signs of Impending Labor

A. Premonitory signs—physiologic changes that take place the last several weeks of pregnancy, indicating that labor is near.
B. Lightening—descent of the uterus downward and forward which takes place as the presenting part descends into the pelvis.
   1. Time in which it takes place varies from a few weeks to a few days before labor. In multigravida, it may occur during labor.
   2. Sensations.
      a. Relief of pressure on diaphragm, and breathing is easier.
      b. Increased pelvic pressure leading to leg cramps, frequent micturition, and pressure on rectum.
C. Braxton Hicks contractions.
   1. May become quite regular but do not effectively dilate cervix.
   2. Usually are more pronounced at night.
   3. May play a part in ripening the cervix.

D. Decrease in weight—there is usually a decrease in water retention due to hormonal influences.
E. Cervical changes—cervix usually becomes softer, shorter, and somewhat dilated. May be dilated 1 to 2 cm by the time labor begins.
F. Bloody show.
   1. Tenacious mucous vaginal discharge, usually pinkish or streaked with blood, which is expelled from the cervix as it shortens and begins to dilate.
   2. Labor usually begins within twenty-four to forty-eight hours.
G. Rupture of membranes.
   1. May break any time before labor or during labor. Occasionally, they remain intact and are ruptured by the physician during labor (amniotomy).
   2. May gush or trickle.
   3. Patient usually advised to come to the hospital as labor may begin within twenty-four hours.
   4. If labor does not begin spontaneously, it is induced to avoid intrauterine infections.

Nursing Care

A. Test vaginal secretions for alkalinity with Nitrozine paper—normal vaginal pH is acidic.
B. Keep patient on bed rest if ordered.
C. Watch for signs of infection.
D. Watch for signs of labor.
E. Watch for prolapse of cord.
F. Monitor fetal heart rate regularly.
G. Observe amniotic fluid for foul odor or signs of fetal distress (meconium staining); record time, amount, color, and odor, if present.

Assessment of Fetal Maturity and Placental Function

Studies for Delivery Capability

A. Estriol excretion.
   1. Estriol level increases as the fetus grows and decreases when growth ceases.

2. Provides guide to placental functioning and fetal well-being.

B. Amniocentesis
1. Introduction of a needle through the abdominal and uterine wall and into the amniotic cavity to withdraw fluid for examination.
2. Preparation of patient.
   a. Have patient empty bladder.
   b. Take fetal heart rate.
   c. Make patient comfortable.
   d. Explain and give reassurance that the procedure will not harm the baby.
   e. Prepare abdomen with antiseptic solution.
   f. Have necessary equipment available.
3. Indications:
   a. Sex of baby.
   b. Certain congenital defects such as mongolism.
   c. State of fetus affected by Rh isoimmunization.
   d. Fetal maturity.

C. Creatinine level.
1. Progressive rise as fetus approaches term.
2. Excreted in fetal urine; measures increasing muscle mass.
3. Values of 2 mg/100 ml amniotic fluid correlates with gestation of about thirty-six weeks.

D. Bilirubin level.
1. Amount of bilirubin in amniotic fluid decreases near term of normal fetus. Usually disappears during the last month of gestation.
2. Exposure of blood sample to light for a period greater than a few seconds invalidates the test.

E. Cytological studies—percentage of lipid globules present gives indication of fetal age (sebaceous glands of fetus begin to function and shed near term).

F. Sonography.
1. Used to measure biparietal diameter of the fetal skull after sixteen weeks (should be measured weekly when growth retardation is suspected).

2. Can determine position of placenta.

G. X-ray measure.
1. Gives evidence of total fetal length.
2. Can indicate ossification in epiphyseal centers.
3. Gives evidence of size of fetal skull.
4. Should not be taken before sixteen weeks gestation.

H. Oxytocin challenge text.
1. Test designed to measure the fetus reaction to uterine contractions.
2. Performed on high risk patients (postmature diabetes).
3. If placental flow is normal, fetus remains oxygenated during uterine contractions.
4. Placental insufficiency produces characteristic late deceleration pattern during contraction. Fetal bradycardia is less than 120 beats per minute.
☆ 5. Procedure.
   a. Measured dosage of oxytocin by infusion pump; piggybacked into main IV line.
   b. Dosage is increased q 15–20 minutes until patient has three uterine contractions in ten minutes.
   c. Oxytocin is then discontinued.
   d. Patient is monitored with external fetal monitor. Baseline fetal heart rate is established prior to beginning the test.
   e. Apply external monitor and obtain baseline fetal heart rates.
   f. Observe for complications.
      (1) Fetal heart rate below 120.
      (2) Sustained uterine contractions.
      (3) Supine hypotensive syndrome.

Induction of Labor

Oxytocin Infusion

A. Indications for use.
1. Patient overdue (two weeks or more); placental functions reduced.
2. Toxemia.
3. Diabetes.

4. Premature rupture of membranes (should deliver within twenty-four hours).
5. Uncontrolled bleeding.
6. Rh sensitization (rising titer).
7. Excessive size of fetus.
B. Prerequisites for successful induction.
   1. Fetal maturity.
   2. Cervix amenable to induction (at times, patient may be induced for several days consecutively with rest at night to ripen cervix, if it is desirable to deliver fetus because of complications).
   3. Normal cephalopelvic proportions.
   4. Fetal head engaged.
C. Danger signals.
   1. Prolonged uterine contractions (over 90 seconds with less than 30 seconds rest period between).
   2. Sustained uterine contractions.
   3. Fetal heart tones above 160 or below 120; change in heart rhythm.
   4. Hemorrhage and shock.
   5. Elevated blood pressure.
   6. Abruptio placentae.

Buccal Pitocin

A. Usually oxytocin linquet placed in parabuccal space at approximately thirty-minute intervals until labor is well established.
B. May be promptly removed should adverse reactions occur.

Nursing Care

A. Nursing procedures.
   1. Maintain patient on bed rest.
   2. Provide normal care of patient in labor.
   3. Monitor IV fluids.
   4. Auscultate fetal heart tones.
B. Emergency measures.
   1. Check patient frequently.
   2. *Immediately* report abnormalities in contractions or fetal heart tones.

Process of Labor and Delivery

Theories Pertaining to Cause of Labor

A. Absolute causes unknown.
B. Alterations in hormonal balance of estrogen and progesterone increases uterine contractility.
C. Degeneration of the placenta so that it no longer provides necessary elements to fetus.
D. Overdistention of uterus incites a stimulus which triggers release of oxytocin and initiates contractions.
E. High levels of prostaglandins near term may stimulate uterine contractions.
F. It may be a combination of several of these physiological occurrences that produce the type of contraction necessary for true labor.

Forces that Produce Labor

A. Muscular contractions originate primarily in muscles of uterus and secondarily in abdominal muscles.
B. Uterine muscles contract during first stages and bring about effacement and dilatation of the cervix.
C. Abdominal muscles come into play after complete cervical dilatation and help to expel the baby.

Duration of Labor

A. Varies according to individual.
B. Average.
   1. Primipara—up to eighteen hours; some may be shorter, others longer.
   2. Multipara—up to eight hours; some may be shorter, others longer.
C. Length of labor depends on:
   1. Effectiveness of contractions.
   2. Amount of resistance baby must overcome to adapt to the pelvis.
   3. Stretching ability of soft tissue.
   4. Preparation and relaxation of mother (fear and anxiety can retard progress).

Uterine Contractions

A. Characteristics.
1. Involuntary—cannot be controlled by will of mother.
2. Intermittent—periods of relaxation between contractions. Intervals allow mother to rest and also allow adequate circulation of uterine blood vessels and oxygenation of fetus.
3. Regular—occur once true labor is established.
4. Discomfort in back usually starts low and radiates around to abdomen).
5. Increase in discomfort from intensity, frequency, and duration of contractions as labor progresses.

B. Methods for monitoring contractions.
1. Place finger lightly on the fundus of the uterus (the most contractile portion), and relate what you feel in your fingers to seconds and minutes on a clock. Uterus becomes firm, then hardens, and then decreases in hardness.
2. Use electronic monitoring device; external (less accurate) or internal (catheter inserted into uterine cavity which measures internal pressures); relay information to a graph.

C. Contractions are monitored for frequency, duration, and intensity.
1. Frequency—measure by timing contractions from the beginning of one contraction to the beginning of next.
2. Duration—measure time at beginning of contraction to beginning of period of decreasing intensity. Cannot be measured exactly by feeling with the hand.
3. Intensity—measure by internal fetal monitoring device; cannot be measured by feeling.
4. Contractions may be described as mild, moderate, or intense.

D. Purpose of contractions.
1. To propel presenting part forward.
2. To bring about effacement and dilatation of the cervix.

Effacement and Dilatation

A. Effacement—process by which cervical canal is progressively shortened to a stage of complete obliteration. Progresses from a structure of 1 to 2 cm in length to almost complete obliteration.
B. Dilatation—process by which external os enlarges from a few millimeters to approximately 10 cm.
C. All that remains of the cervix after effacement and dilatation is a paper-thin circular opening about 10 cm in diameter.
D. Effacement and dilatation may be measured by vaginal or rectal examination.

Changes in the Uterus

A. Uterus usually becomes differentiated in two distinct portions as labor progresses.
1. Upper portion is contractile and becomes thicker.
2. Lower portion is passive, becomes thinner and more expanded.
B. Boundary between the two segments is termed the *physiologic retraction ring*.

False Labor

A. Signs.
1. Irregular contractions.
2. Contractions that may cause discomfort.
3. Discomfort is usually located in abdomen.
4. Labor usually does not intensify.
5. Discomfort may be relieved by walking.
6. Contractions do not bring about appreciable changes in cervix.
B. Sometimes difficult to differentiate false labor from true labor until woman is observed for several hours in the hospital.

Signs of Imminent Delivery

A. Increase in bloody show.
B. Nausea, vomiting, and shaking.
C. Pressure on rectum, and woman feels the urge to push (involuntary bearing down).

D. Deep grunting sound from woman.

E. Woman states she is ready to deliver.

F. Bulging of the perineum.

Four Stages of Labor

Stage One

A. Stage one begins with first true labor contraction and ends with complete cervical dilatation.

B. Latent (effacement) phase.

1. Begins with onset of regular contraction pattern.

2. Dilatation 0 to 1 to 4 cm; membranes usually intact.

3. Contractions are mild and become well established.

4. Contractions are 5 to 15 minutes apart and last about 30 to 45 seconds.

5. Cervix thins.

6. Usually some bloody show.

7. Station is anywhere from −2 cm to +1 cm in multipara; at 0 in primigravida.

8. Woman may be quite comfortable, talkative, alert, and cheerful.

9. Woman has lots of energy and feels she can cope with labor.

C. Active (dilatation) phase.

1. Dilatation 4 to 7 cm.

2. Dilatation is more rapid.

3. Contractions are 3 to 5 minutes apart, last 30 to 45 seconds.

4. Increase in bloody show.

5. Station varies from −1 to 0 cm.

6. Woman becomes tired and less talkative and shows lack of energy.

7. Woman may need coaching on breathing techniques, or analgesia (anesthesia).

D. Transitional phase.

1. Dilatation 7 to 10 cm.

2. Contractions are intense and close (2 to 3 minutes apart, lasting 50 to 90 seconds).

3. Station +3 or +4 cm.

4. Copious bloody show.

5. Desire to bear down or defecate.

6. Membranes may rupture spontaneously if they have not done so previously; physician may rupture them artificially.

7. Woman's attention and feelings are inner-directed; she feels exhausted and no longer able to cope.

8. Signs of restlessness, shaking, nausea, vomiting, trembling, burping, or crying may be present.

Stage Two

A. Stage two begins with complete dilatation and ends with birth of baby.

B. Mechanism of labor and delivery.

1. Sequence of movements of presenting part through birth canal. Head usually enters transverse and must rotate LOA or ROA for birth.

2. Engagement—head enters pelvis.

3. Descent—movement which occurs simultaneously with passage of head through pelvis.

4. Flexion—occurs as head descends and meets with resistance. In extreme flexion the smallest diameter of the head presents.

5. Internal rotation—head usually enters with long diameter conforming to long diameter of inlet (usually transverse position) and must be rotated before it can emerge from outlet (head rotates so that smallest diameter presents to conform to pelvis).

6. Extension—follows internal rotation. The head, which is flexed as it passes through birth canal, must extend for birth.

7. External rotation or restitution—soon after birth, the head rotates to either mother's right or left side (fetal position before birth).

8. Expulsion—with delivery of shoulders, rest of body is expelled spontaneously.

C. Stage of expulsion.

1. Expulsion brought about by contractions of uterine and abdominal muscles.

2. Contractions are every 2 to 3 minutes, last 60 to 90 seconds.

Stage Three

A. Stage three, or placental stage, begins with birth and ends with delivery of placenta.

B. Phase of placental separation.
1. Usually takes place with next few contractions after birth.
2. Usually begins at center but may begin at edges.
3. Some bleeding usually accompanies separation of placenta.

C. Phase of expulsion.
1. May be expulsed spontaneously by mother, but is usually expressed manually by the physician after separation is complete.
2. Mechanisms.
   a. Schultze (most common)—placenta is inverted on itself, and the shiny fetal surface appears; 80 percent separate in center.
   b. Duncan—descends sideways and the maternal surface appears.

Stage Four

A. Stage four begins with delivery of placenta and ends when postpartum condition of the mother is stabilized.

B. First hour after birth is critical.

Nursing Care in Labor and Delivery

Latent Phase

Admission

A. Details of care vary from hospital to hospital.

B. Check vital signs—temperature, pulse, respirations, and blood pressure.

C. Check fetal heart tones (FHT).

D. Determine intactness of membranes.

E. Give prep (perineal shave) and enema (if ordered by physician).

F. See that appropriate forms are completed.

G. Encourage woman to void; check urine for sugar and acetone.

H. Determine frequency, intensity (mild, moderate, severe), and duration of contractions.

I. Determine amount and character of bloody show.

J. Determine amount of cervical dilatation and effacement.

K. Keep bell cord within easy reach.

After Admission (Dilatation—3 cm)

A. Maintain bed rest if membranes have ruptured. (In some hospitals the patient may be allowed out of bed with ruptured membranes if the baby's head is well engaged and the patient is otherwise all right.)

B. Note frequency, duration, and strength of contraction every 30 minutes or prn.

C. Auscultate FHT every 15 minutes or prn.

D. Check blood pressure every 30 minutes or prn.

E. Check vital signs once per shift or more often if needed.

F. Periodic vaginal examination as indicated.

G. Observe for ruptured membranes and take FHT immediately if membranes rupture.

H. Reinforce breathing techniques or teach breathing techniques if woman has had no classes.

I. Keep family informed of progress.

J. Encourage the presence of patient's husband or a significant other person.

K. Provide support based upon woman's knowledge of the labor process.

L. Reduce stimuli if woman wants to rest.

M. Start IV if ordered; usually NPO.

Active Phase (Dilatation 4 to 7 cm)

A. Encourage breathing techniques.

B. Maintain IV fluids.

C. Encourage voiding.

D. Auscultate FHT every 15 minutes or prn.

E. Monitor contractions.

F. Take blood pressure every 30 minutes or prn.

G. Periodic vaginal examination to determine progress.

H. Observe amount and character of show.

I. Urge mother to stay off back, avoid supine hypotensive syndrome, and to lie on side.

J. Administer medications as ordered. Tranquilizing drugs may be given in early labor, but analgesics are not usually given until labor is well established.

K. Assist with anesthesia, if given, and monitor blood pressure and FHT.

L. Continue giving patient support and information.

Transitional Phase (Dilatation 7 to 10 cm)

A. Continue with care listed above.

B. Explain progress to patient and encourage her to continue with breathing and relaxing techniques.

C. Discourage bearing down efforts until dilatation is complete.

D. Encourage deep ventilation prior to and after each contraction.

E. Monitor contractions lightly with fingers as abdomen is sensitive.

F. Accept irritable behavior and aggression; continue supportive care.

G. Help patient to push when ready.

H. Observe for signs of imminent delivery, and transfer patient to delivery room when ready.

Assessment of the Fetus

Fetal Distress

A. Signs.
   1. FHT above 160 or below 120 beats per minute.
   2. Meconium-stained fluid (during hypoxia, bowel peristalsis increases, and meconium is likely to be passed).
   3. Fetal hyperactivity.

B. Immediate nursing interventions.
   1. Turn patient to left side; if no improvement, turn to right side. This procedure relieves pressure on umbilical cord during contractions and pressure of uterus on the inferior vena cava.
   2. Report findings immediately.

Signs of Complications of Labor

A. Fetal distress.

B. Fetal tachycardia—persistent fetal heart rate above 160 or an increase in the basal rate, 20 to 30 beats/minute.

C. Fetal bradycardia—below 120 beats/minute.

D. Absent, minimal, or irregular FHT.

E. Foul smelling or meconium-stained amniotic fluid.

F. Fetal hyperactivity.

G. Elevated temperature in woman.

H. Dehydration.

I. Hemorrhage.

J. Inadequate uterine relaxation between contractions—over 90 seconds and less than 30 seconds between contractions.

K. Anxiety in woman.

L. Distended bladder.

Nursing Responsibilities

Delivery Room Care

A. Transfer woman carefully from bed to delivery table; place in lithotomy position.

B. Pad stirrups to avoid pressure to popliteal veins and pressure areas. Gently raise both legs simultaneously into stirrups to avoid ligament strain. Adjust stirrups and drape patient.

C. Provide patient with handles to pull on as she pushes.

D. Cleanse vulva and perineum using sterile technique, commonly referred to as perineal "wash down."

E. Auscultate FHT every 5 minutes or after each push—transient fetal bradycardia not unusual due to head compression.

F. Check blood pressure and pulse every 15 minutes prn.

G. Allow baby's father in room, and position him at the head of the delivery table.

H. Encourage patient and keep her informed of advancement of baby.

I. Encourage patient to take a deep breath before beginning to push with each contraction and to sustain push as long as possible (long pushes are preferable to frequent short pushes).

Postpartum Care

A. Palpate fundus every 15 minutes and prn for first hour.

B. Massage fundus gently if it is not firm.

C. Check TPR and blood pressure upon admission; check blood pressure every 15 minutes and prn for first hour.

D. Encourage voiding and measure amount.

E. Check lochia for color, consistency, and amount.

F. Inspect perineum and episiotomy for signs of bleeding, unusual redness, or swelling.

G. Weigh pads if unusual bleeding noted.

H. Allow mother and baby's father the privacy to talk.

I. Encourage mother to rest.

J. Provide medications for pain as ordered and needed.

K. Chart all pertinent data.

L. Maintain intake and output the first twenty-four hours or until patient is voiding a sufficient quantity.

Operative Obstetrics

Obstetrical Procedures

Episiotomy

A. An incision made into the perineum during delivery to facilitate the birth process.

B. Types.
  1. Midline—incision from the posterior margin of the vaginal opening directly back to the anal sphincter.
     a. Healing is less painful.
     b. Incision is easy to repair.
  2. Mediolateral—incision made at 45-degree angle to either side of the vaginal opening.
     a. Healing process is quite painful.
     b. Incision is harder to repair.

C. Purpose.
  1. To spare the muscles of perineal floor from undue stretching and tearing (lacerations).
  2. To prevent the prolonged pressure of the baby's head on perineum.

D. Method.
  1. Generally done during contraction when the baby's head pushes against perineum and stretches it.
  2. Blunt scissors are used.
  3. Mother is usually given an anesthetic (regional, local, or inhalation).

Forceps Delivery

A. Baby is extracted from the birth canal by the physician with the use of a specially designed instrument; cervix must be fully dilated.

B. Types.
  1. Low forceps—presenting part on perineal floor.
  2. Midforceps—presenting part below or at the level of the ischial spine.
  3. High forceps—presenting part not engaged (rarely if ever used today).

C. Indications.
  1. Fetal distress.
  2. Poor progress of fetus through the birth canal.
  3. Failure of the head to rotate.
  4. Maternal disease or exhaustion.
  5. Woman unable to push (as with regional anesthesia, caudal or epidural).

D. Complications.
1. Lacerations of the vagina or the cervix; there may be oozing or hemorrhage.
2. Rupture of the uterus.
3. Intracranial hemorrhage and brain damage to the fetus.
4. Facial paralysis of the fetus.

Cesarean Delivery

A. Incision into abdominal wall and uterus to enable the delivery of an infant.
B. Types.
1. Classical—vertical incision through the abdominal wall and into the anterior wall of the uterus.
2. Low segment transverse—transverse incision made into lower uterine segment after abdomen has been opened.
   a. Incision made into part of uterus where there is less uterine activity and blood loss is minimal.
   b. Less incidence of adhesions and intestinal obstruction.
3. Cesarean hysterectomy—abdomen and uterus are opened, baby and placenta are removed, and then the hysterectomy is performed. Conditions indicating hysterectomy.
   a. Presence of diseased tissue or fibroids.
   b. An abnormal pap smear.
   c. Ruptured uterus.
   d. Uncontrolled hemorrhage, abruptio placentae, uterine atony, or other disorders.
C. Indications.
1. Fetal distress unrelieved by other measures.
2. Uterine dysfunction.
3. Certain cases of placenta previa and premature separation of placenta.
4. Prolapsed cord.
5. Diabetes or certain cases of toxemia.
6. Cephalopelvic disproportion.
7. Malpresentations such as transverse lie.

Nursing Management

Postoperative Care

A. Take vital signs (blood pressure, pulse and respiration) every fifteen minutes for two to three hours.
B. Observe site of incision for bleeding every fifteen minutes for two to three hours.
C. Palpate fundus for location and tone every fifteen minutes for two to three hours.
D. Check lochia for amount and color every fifteen minutes for two to three hours.
E. Reinforce abdominal dressing as necessary.
F. Observe drainage from Foley catheter (amount, color, pressure of blood, and other aspects).
G. Check level of consciousness.
H. Measure intake and output.
I. Assist patient to deep breathe, cough, and turn.
J. Change perineal pad as needed.
K. Reassure the patient that the delivery is over, and give her information regarding the condition of the baby. (If something is wrong with the baby, usually the physician will first discuss this with parents.)
L. Help ambulate patient (usually the first postpartum day).
M. Give stool softener as ordered and needed.
N. Encourage patient to talk about delivery and baby.
O. Reinforce physician's teaching about care at home.
1. Planned rest periods.
2. Avoidance of heavy lifting for four to six weeks.
3. Signs of infection.
4. Care of the breasts.
5. Avoidance of constipation.
6. Nutritive diet.
7. Arrangements for postpartum checkup in four to six weeks.

Complications of Labor and Delivery

Dystocia

Definition: Prolonged and difficult labor and delivery, i.e., it extends for twenty-four hours or more after the onset of regular contractions.

Classification

A. Dystocia may be classified in several ways; although the divisions are artificial, they are useful in looking at the processes involved.
   1. Dysfunctions of powers or forces with respect to the uterus and abdominal muscles.
   2. Abnormalities of the passengers (the fetus and placenta).
   3. Abnormalities of the passages (bony and soft tissue).
   4. May be a combination of two or more dysfunctions and abnormalities.
B. Characteristics.
   1. True labor begins but fails to progress.
   2. Dystocia may occur during latent or active phase of labor.
   3. It is important to look at the rate of progress as well as the overall length of labor, i.e., is the patient slowly progressing or is she arrested at one spot?

Dysfunctional Labor

A. Prolonged latent phase—time required to dilate cervix to 4 cm is prolonged; primipara over twenty hours, multipara fourteen hours.
   1. Causes or contributing condition.
      a. Oversedation.
      b. "Unripe" cervix.
      c. False labor.
      d. Uterine dysfunction or abnormalities.
   2. Treatment and nursing care.
      a. Encourage rest as woman is usually exhausted.
      b. Narcotic agent is given to stop labor and promote rest.
      c. Vaginal examination is made to determine fetal position and station.
      d. X-ray pelvimetry is made to determine the disorder.
      e. Performance of amniotomy (artificial rupture of membranes) if conditions are favorable for vaginal delivery.
      f. Oxytocin is given as a stimulant.
      g. Labor usually progresses normally after rest and stimulation by oxytocin.
B. Prolonged active phase—dilatation slower than 1.2 cm per hour for primigravida; dilatation slower than 1.5 cm per hour for multigravida.
   1. Causes.
      a. Cephalopelvic disproportion (CPD).
      b. Malpositions.
      c. Excessive sedation or anesthesia.
      d. Unknown causes.
   2. Treatment and nursing care.
      a. Usually no active treatment is given if dilatation is regular unless labor will be prolonged over twenty-four hours; then give supportive therapy.
      b. Cesarean section may be indicated in CPD or for labor over twenty-four hours.
C. Arrested active phase—lack of progress.
   1. Causes.
      a. CPD.
      b. Malposition of the fetus.
      c. Excessive sedation and anesthesia.
      d. Uterine abnormalities.
   2. Medical treatment and nursing care.
      a. Vaginal examination to determine position and station of fetus.
      b. X-ray pelvimetry to determine CPD.
      c. Provide rest for exhausted patient.
      d. Cautious use of oxytocic stimulation if malposition, CPD, and other abnormalities are ruled out.
      e. Cesarean section if appropriate.
D. Complications of prolonged labor (see Tables C and D).

Other Causes of Dysfunctional Labor

A. Tetanic uterine contractions—contraction lasting over ninety seconds. May lead to fetal aphyxia or uterine rupture.

B. Precipitate delivery—labor of three hours or less duration. May lead to injury of mother and fetus due to trauma.

C. Rupture of the uterus—splitting of the uterine wall accompanied by extrusion of all or part of uterine contents into the abdominal cavity. Baby usually dies and mortality rate in mothers is high due to blood loss.

   1. Signs of rupture.

      a. Acute abdominal pain and tenderness.

      b. Presenting part no longer felt through cervix.

      c. Feeling in patient that something has happened inside her.

      d. Cessation of labor pains (no contractions).

      e. Bleeding usually internal; may be some external bleeding.

      f. Signs of shock (pale appearance, pulse weak and rapid, air hunger, and exhaustion).

   2. Treatment.

      a. Laparotomy to remove fetus.

      b. Hysterectomy, although uterus may be sutured and left in.

      c. Blood transfusions.

      d. Antibiotics to prevent infection from traumatized tissues.

Nursing Care

A. Promote rest (darken room, reduce noise level).

B. Position patient for comfort.

C. Give patient a back rub.

D. Provide clean linen and gown; allow patient to bathe or shower if permissible.

E. Promote oral hygiene.

F. Give patient reassurance and support.

G. Explain procedures to the patient.

H. Let mother express feelings and emotions freely.

I. Watch for signs of exhaustion, dehydration, and acidosis.

J. Monitor vital signs.

K. Monitor FHT.

L. Monitor contractions for frequency, intensity, and duration.

M. Watch for signs of excessive bleeding and fetal distress.

N. Administer medications as ordered.

Abnormalities of the Passengers

Abnormal Presentations and Positions

A. Occiput posterior position.

   1. Usually prolongs labor because baby must rotate a longer distance (35 degrees or more) to reach symphysis pubis.

   2. Possible results.

      a. Persistent occiput posterior (head does not rotate).

      b. Deep transverse arrest (head arrested in transverse position).

   3. Treatment.

      a. Head usually rotates itself with contraction.

      b. Rotation may be done by physician manually or with forceps.

B. Breech prolongs labor because soft tissue does not aid cervical dilatation as well as the fetal skull.

C. Face presentation is rare; results in increased prenatal mortality.

   1. Chin must rotate so it lies under symphysis pubis for delivery.

   2. If baby is delivered vaginally, the face is usually edematous and bruised, with marked molding.

   3. Cesarean section is indicated if face does not rotate.

D. Transverse lie.

   1. Long axis of fetus at right angles to long axis of mother.

   2. Spontaneous version may occur. Cesarean section is the usual method of delivery.

Excessive Size of Fetus

A. Disproportion between the size of the fetus and the size of the pelvis when fetus is ten pounds or over.
B. Head is usually large and less moldable.
C. Size of shoulders may also complicate delivery.
D. Causes.
   1. Multiparity—birth weight may progress with each pregnancy.
   2. Maternal diabetes.
E. Size may be determined by sonography and x-ray.
F. Treatment.
   1. Vaginal delivery if disproportion is not too great. Usually there are fetal injuries—brachial plexus, dislocated shoulder.
   2. Cesarean section indicated if proportion too great.
G. Fetal abnormalities.
   1. Hydrocephalus.
   2. Tumors.

Abnormalities of Passage

Cephalopelvic Disproportion

A. Disproportion may be in inlet, mid-pelvis, or outlet.
B. Pelvis is considered contracted if it is reduced enough in size to interfere with normal delivery.
C. Trial labor may be done in borderline cases.
D. Determined by x-ray of pelvis (pelvimetry).
E. Cesarean delivery is the usual method of treatment.

Other Complications of Labor

Premature Labor and Delivery

A. Occurs when pregnancy terminates after the period of viability but usually before the end of the thirty-sixth week.

B. Betamethasone or some other drug is administered to the mother to hasten fetal maturity by stimulating development of lecithin when membranes are ruptured and premature labor cannot be arrested.

Prolonged Pregnancy

A. Pregnancy of over forty-two weeks gestation.
B. Complications.
   1. Amniotic fluid decreases and vernix caseosa disappears; infant's skin appears dry and cracked.
   2. Infant may weigh less.
   3. Chronic hypoxia due to placental dysfunction.
   4. Infant may pass meconium due to hypoxia.
C. Determination of gestational age usually made to ascertain actual duration of pregnancy by means of estriol studies, sonography.
D. Oxytocin challenge test to determine fetus's ability to tolerate labor.
E. Labor stimulated with oxytocin.
F. Cesarean section if induction contraindicated.

Prolapsed Umbilical Cord

A. Descent of prolapsed cord through cervical canal along side of the presenting part; may even protrude from the vagina.
B. Causes.
   1. Ruptured membranes before engagement.
   2. Abnormal presentations.
   3. Premature infant—presenting part does not fill the birth canal and allow for more space.
   4. Polyhydramnios.
C. Symptoms.
   1. Abnormal fetal heart pattern.
   2. Cord may be palpated or seen on vaginal examination.
D. Complications—cord is compressed between presenting part and pelvis resulting in fetal asphyxia.
E. Immediate treatment and nursing care.
   1. Presenting part elevated off umbilical cord.

2. Place patient in knee-chest position or exaggerated Trendelenburg's position.
3. Maintain patient on absolute bed rest.
4. Cover exposed cord with sterile dressing if available.
5. Auscultate FHT every two minutes.
6. Stay with patient and offer support.
7. Cesarean section is prescribed if cervix is not dilated enough to allow the baby to pass. Haste is important.

Fetal Distress

Signs and Symptoms

A. Fetal heart rate: above 160 or below 120 beats per minute indicates distress.
B. Meconium-stained fluid. During hypoxia, bowel peristalsis increases, and meconium is likely to be passed.
C. Fetal hyperactivity.
D. If labor is monitored, check:
    1. Variable deceleration pattern.
    2. Late deceleration pattern.
    3. Fetal pH below 7.2.

Nursing Care

A. Discontinue oxytocin if being infused.
B. Turn to left side; if no improvement, turn to right side. This procedure relieves pressure on umbilical cord during contractions and pressures of uterus on the inferior vena cava.
C. Administer oxygen via mask at 6 to 7 l/minute.
D. Correction of hypotension: elevate legs and increase perfusion of IV fluids.
E. Notify R.N. and physician.
F. Prepare for emergency cesarean delivery if no improvement.

Vena Caval Syndrome (Supine Hypotensive Syndrome)

Definition: Shocklike symptoms that occur when venous return to the heart is impaired by weight of gravid uterus causing partial occlusion of the vena cava.

Signs and Symptoms

A. Check for risk factors—multiple pregnancies, obesity, polyhydramnios.
B. Shock-like symptoms caused by reduced cardiac output.
    1. Hypotension.
    2. Tachycardia.
    3. Sweating.
    4. Nausea and vomiting.
    5. Air hunger.
C. Fetal distress; caused by reduced flow of blood to placenta from reduced cardiac output.

Nursing Care

A. Assist mother to turn to left side (using a wedge pillow) to shift weight of fetus off inferior vena cava.
B. Provide oxygen with tight mask if recovery is not immediate after positioning.
C. Monitor fetal heart rate to determine fetal status.

Table C. Complications and Signs of Distress in the Mother

Complication	Signs of Distress	Possible Nursing Care
Infection	Elevated temperature and pulse	Maintain sterile technique while doing vaginals Keep vaginals to a minimum Administer antibiotics as ordered
Exhaustion	Loss of emotional stability Lack of cooperation	Provide supportive therapy and comfort measures to promote relaxation and relieve tension Encourage rest Administer sedation as ordered
Dehydration	Dry tongue and skin Concentrated urine Acetonuria	Monitor IV fluids Place a wet cloth to the patient's mouth Make a frequent check of bladder elimination

Table D. Complications and Signs of Distress in the Fetus

Complication	Signs of Distress	Possible Nursing Care
Asphyxia	Irregular heart rate Heart rate above 160 or below 120 Passage of meconium in the vertex position	Administer oxygen to the mother Constantly observe and monitor FHT Check for prolapse of the cord Prepare delivery room equipment for possible resuscitation of the baby at birth
Generalized infection	Irregular heart rate Heart rate above 160 or below 120	Administer antibiotics to the mother Keep vaginals to a minimum Follow same care (except cord check) as asphyxia

Obstetric Anesthesia and Analgesia

Anesthesia During Labor

General Characteristics

A. No optimum anesthesia exists.
B. Ranks fourth as the cause of maternal death; other three include hemorrhage, infection, and toxemia.
C. History and physical should be obtained before administering anesthesia.
D. Should be NPO before use.
E. Should be administered by trained personnel.
F. Choice of the type of anesthesia in obstetrics is determined by the specific patient situation and condition.

General Inhalation Anesthetics

A. Advantages.
    1. May anesthetize patient rapidly.
    2. Depth and duration can be controlled.
    3. Effects are rapidly dissipated in both infant and mother.
    4. These anesthetics cause uterine relaxation when necessary for manipulation.
    5. Inhalation anesthetics are preferred in hypovolemic patient and in patient whose condition prohibits the use of regional anesthetics.
B. Disadvantages.
    1. Woman is not awake for delivery.
    2. Brings about respiratory depression of the infant.
    3. May cause emesis and aspiration in the patient.
    4. May be flammatory.
C. Common types.
    1. Ether—seldom used.
    2. Halothane—used in selected cases only.
    3. Penthrane—analgesia and light anesthesia; it may be used as a self-administered analgesic.
    4. Thiopental (Pentothal)—IV anesthesia usually used as an adjunct in induction of anesthesia.
    5. Trichloroethylene (Trilene) is often used in self-administration by mask during labor and delivery. Never leave patient alone when she is using self-administered anesthesia.

Regional Analgesia and Anesthesia

A. Drugs given to block the nerves carrying sensation from the uterus to the pelvic region.
B. Some common agents used.
    1. Novocaine.
    2. Xylocaine.
    3. Pontocaine.
    4. Carbocaine.
C. Vasoconstrictor agents (e.g., epinephrine) are commonly used in conjunction with regional anesthetics.
    1. Slow absorption and prolong the effect of the anesthetic.
    2. Prevent secondary hypotension.
D. Two principle types of regional anesthesia are nerve root block and peripheral nerve block.
E. Nerve root block.
    1. General considerations.
        a. Usually relieves pain completely if administered properly.
        b. Provides vasodilation below the anesthetic level which may be responsible for a decrease in blood pressure.
        c. Does not depress the respiratory center, and therefore does not harm the patient unless hypotension in the patient is severe enough to interfere with uterine flow.
        d. May cause postspinal headache.
        e. Contraindicated in a hypovolemic patient or in the case of central nervous system disease.
        f. Drug may impede labor if given too early (before 5 to 6 cm dilatation).

g. Special skill of anesthesiologist required to administer drug.

h. Infant may need forceps delivery because the mother usually cannot push effectively due to level of anesthesia.

2. Types.

a. Caudal.

b. Lumbar epidural.

c. Saddle block.

d. Spinal.

3. Nursing Care.

a. Assist patient to a knee-chest position over a bolster or on her left side with head flexed and knees drawn up.

b. Monitor blood pressure every 3 to 5 minutes until stabilized; then every 30 minutes or prn.

c. Auscultate FHT.

d. If hypotension does occur:

(1) Turn mother to one side, off the inferior vena cava.

(2) Give oxygen by mask.

(3) Notify physician.

e. Watch for signs of dizziness, nausea, faintness, and palpitations.

C. Peripheral nerve block.

1. General considerations.

a. May be done by attending physician (does not require an anesthesiologist).

b. Local injection of anesthetic to block peripheral nerve endings.

c. Less effective in relieving pain than nerve root block.

d. May cause transient bradycardia in fetus, possibly due to rapid absorption of the drug into fetal circulation.

e. Usually there are no maternal side effects.

f. Needle guide such as Iowa trumpet usually used.

2. Types.

a. Paracervical.

b. Pudendal block.

3. Nursing management.

a. Measure vital signs.

b. Auscultate FHT.

c. Assist patient to a dorsal recumbent position.

d. Offer reassurance and support during procedure.

e. Auscultate FHT every 5 minutes for 15 to 30 minutes and every 30 minutes thereafter.

Postpartum Period

Physiology of the Puerperium

Definition: Period of four to six weeks following delivery in which the reproductive organs return to the normal, nonpregnant state.

Uterus

A. Involution—rapid diminution in the size of the uterus as it returns to the nonpregnant state.

B. Lochia—discharge from the uterus, consisting of blood from vessels of the placental site and debris from the decidua.

C. Placental site—blood vessels of the placenta become thrombosed or compressed.

Cervix and Vagina

A. Cervix—remains soft and flabby the first few days, and the internal os closes.

B. Vagina—usually smooth walled after delivery. Rugae begin to appear when ovarian function returns and estrogen is produced.

Ovarian Function and Menstruation

A. Ovarian function depends upon the rapidity in which the pituitary function is restored.

B. Menstruation—usually returns in four to six weeks in a nonlactating mother.

Urinary Tract

A. May be edematous and contain areas of submucosal hemorrhage due to trauma.

B. May have urine retention due to loss of elasticity and tone and loss of sensation from trauma.

C. Diuresis—mechanism by which excess body fluid is excreted after delivery. Usually begins within the first twelve hours after delivery.

Breasts

A. Proliferation of glandular tissue during pregnancy due to hormonal stimulation.

B. Usually secrete colostrum the first two to three days postpartum.

C. Pituitary stimulates secretion of prolactin after placental hormones inhibiting the pituitary are no longer present.

D. In three to four days breasts become firm, distended, tender, and warm (engorged), indicating production of milk.

E. Milk usually produced in response to sucking of infant.

Blood

A. White blood cells increase during labor and early postpartum period and then return to normal in a few days.

B. Decrease in hemoglobin, red blood cells, and hematocrit usually return to normal in one week.

C. Elevated fibrinogen levels usually return to normal within one week.

Nursing Care of the Postpartum Patient

Assessment

A. Check vital signs every 8 hours and prn—decreased blood pressure, increased pulse, or temperature over 100.4°F.

B. Check fundus for consistency and level. Massage fundus lightly with fingers if it is relaxed.

C. Check lochia for amount, color, consistency, and odor. Watch for hemorrhage.

D. Check perineum for redness, discoloration, or swelling.

E. Check episiotomy for healing; check for drainage.

F. Check breasts for engorgement and cracking of nipples.

G. Check emotional status of new mother for depression or withdrawal.

H. Check for problems with flatus or elimination and bladder or bowel retention.

Other Nursing Considerations

A. Administer drug to inhibit lactation (if ordered and if it has not been given immediately postpartum).

B. Apply breast binder or bra after twenty-four hours for seven days.

C. Administer RhoGAM as ordered within seventy-two hours postpartum to Rh-negative mother who is not sensitized.

D. Maintain intake and output until patient is voiding a sufficient quantity without difficulty; usually the first two voids are measured.

E. Teach mother perineal care and give perineal care until mother is able to do so.

F. Encourage ambulation as soon as ordered and as patient is able to tolerate it, giving assistance the first time.

G. Encourage verbalization of mother's feelings about labor, delivery, and baby.

H. Give perineal light as ordered.

I. Give warm sitz baths as ordered.

Emotional Aspects of Postpartum Care

The Maternal Role as Outlined by Rubin

A. Taking-in phase (the first two to three days).
  1. Mother's primary needs are her own; she needs sleep and food.
  2. Mother usually is quite talkative. She wants to discuss labor and delivery. She is assimilating and appropriating experience.
  3. Nurse can listen and help the patient interpret events to make them more meaningful.
  4. Important for nurse to interpret future mother-child relationship at this important time.

B. Taking-hold phase (from the third postpartum day to about two weeks); the phase varies with each individual.

1. Emphasis is on present.
2. Mother is impatient and wants to get on with reorganization of her life.
3. Less passive and more in control of situation.
4. Begins to take hold of "mothering" task, which takes priority over all else.
5. May be unsure of herself. It is important for nurse to reassure mother and not make her feel awkward.
6. Success at this time is important for the future mother-child relationship.
7. Important time for nurse to share information without making mother feel inadequate.

C. Letting-go phase—usually occurs after discharge from hospital.

1. Mother may feel a deep loss over the separation of the baby from part of her body; she may grieve over this loss.
2. Mother may be caught in dependent-independent role; she wants to feel safe and secure yet wants to make decisions. Teenage mother needs special consideration because of the conflicts taking place within her as part of adolescence.
3. Mother may feel resentful and guilty about the baby causing so much work.
4. May have difficulty adjusting to the mothering role.
5. May feel conflict between the roles of mother and wife.
6. May feel upset and depressed at times (postpartum blues).
7. May be concerned about her other children.
8. Important for nurse to encourage vocalization of these feelings and give positive reassurance.

Role of the Baby's Father

A. Encourage the father to hold and care for the baby.

B. Encourage parents to take turns caring for the baby at night so that the mother can rest once she is home.

C. Explain the feelings that are normal to the mother at this time, e.g., tension, fatigue, insecurity in the mothering role, and her need to be dependent and independent.

Breast Feeding

Nursing Management

A. Conditions of breast when breast feeding should be postponed.

1. Tenderness and hardness.
2. Pain and redness.
3. Cracking of nipples.

B. Feeding procedure.

1. Put baby to breast as soon as mother's and baby's conditions are stable (on the delivery table in some hospitals, or within six to twelve hours in others).
2. Have mother assume comfortable position sitting or lying down.
3. Guide baby to breast.
4. Gently press breast away from baby's nose.
5. Usually the baby is nursed two to three minutes at each breast the first time, gradually building to ten minutes or so on each side in later feedings.
6. Release suction by inserting a finger into the baby's mouth (the breast will become sore if baby is pulled off it).
7. Burp baby after feeding at each breast.
8. Stay with mother each time she nurses until she feels secure or confident with the baby and feedings.
9. Baby should not nurse more than every two hours.

C. Instruction.

1. Explain to the mother that the baby's stool will be yellow and watery; that it is not uncommon for nursing infants to have three to four stools each day or even one for each feeding.
2. Dry the breast after feeding and allow it to air occasionally, especially if it is sore.

3. Use general hygiene and wash the breast once daily.

4. Encourage the mother to eat a well-balanced diet and drink 3000 cc of fluid daily.

5. Explain to the mother that she may offer sterile water but not formula to the baby between feedings. (The baby will not be hungry if given formula then and will not nurse well later.)

6. Formula may be given at feeding time, or the mother may express milk manually and put it in a bottle if she plans to be away during feeding time.

7. Breasts may leak between feedings or during coitus. Place a washcloth or pad in brassiere.

8. Uterine cramping may occur the first few days after delivery while nursing as oxytocin stimulation causes the uterus to contract.

9. Medications or drugs should be avoided unless specified by the physician (drugs are passed to infant through breast milk).

10. Some foods such as cabbage or onions may alter the taste of milk or cause gas in the infant.

11. Birth control pills are usually avoided while nursing as they decrease milk production and are passed to the infant in the milk.

Clinical Problems in Puerperium

Postpartum Hemorrhage

Definition: A blood loss of 500 ml or more during or after delivery.

Causes

A. Lacerations of the cervix or of the high vaginal walls, with oozing from blood vessels.

B. Retained placental tissue or incomplete separation of the placenta. This is the most frequent cause of late postpartum hemorrhage. (May occur from twelve to twenty-one days after delivery.)

Signs and Symptoms

A. Uterine atony.
   1. Boggy, relaxed uterus.
   2. Dark bleeding.
   3. Passage of clots.
B. Lacerations.
   1. Firm fundus.
   2. Oozing of bright red blood.
C. Retained placental tissue.
   1. Boggy, relaxed uterus.
   2. Dark bleeding.
D. Shock.
   1. Air hunger (difficulty in breathing).
   2. Restlessness.
   3. Weak rapid pulse.
   4. Rapid respirations.
   5. Decrease in blood pressure.

Treatment and Nursing Care

A. Recognize abnormal bleeding and determine source.

B. Monitor intravenous solutions, blood, or volume expanders.

C. Administer oxytocin if uterus is boggy.

D. Assist with laceration repair.

E. Assist with removal of retained placental tissue.

F. Prevent infection.

G. Hysterectomy may be indicated if bleeding cannot be controlled.

H. Check for clotting defect.

I. Monitor vital signs every 15 minutes or until stable.

J. Palpate fundus every 15 minutes or prn while bleeding continues; then every 2 to 4 hours.

K. Gently massage fundus until firm. Be careful not to overmassage.

L. Weigh pads and linen.

M. Provide for warmth.

N. Measure intake and output.

Puerperal Infection

Definition: An infection in genitalia as a consequence of abortion or labor and delivery.

Causes

A. Organisms that were introduced during labor and delivery.
B. Bacteria normally present in vaginal tract.

Predisposing factors

A. Weakened resistance due to prolonged labor and dehydration.
B. Traumatic delivery.
C. Excessive vaginal examinations during labor.
D. Premature rupture of membranes.
E. Excessive blood loss.
F. Anemia.
G. Intrauterine manipulation.
H. Retained placental fragments.

Signs and Symptoms

A. Elevated temperature of 100.4°F or more.
B. Discomfort in the abdomen and tenderness.
C. Burning on urination.
D. Foul-smelling lochia or discharge; decreased amount.
E. Pelvic pain.
F. Chills.
G. Rapid pulse.
H. Malaise.

Endometritis

Definition: An inflammation of the lining of the uterus.

General Considerations

A. Most frequent site of infection.
B. Uterus may be boggy, relaxed, and tender.
C. If untreated, may spread through lymphatic system to whole body causing septicemia.

Treatment and Nursing Care

A. Antibiotics.
B. May have pelvic examination.
C. Establish adequate drainage of uterus.
D. Monitor IV fluids if ordered.
E. Encourage fluid intake (3000–4000 cc) if not contraindicated.
F. Administer medications as ordered.
G. Provide high-calorie nutritive diet.
H. Place patient in Fowler's or semi-Fowler's position as ordered. Position of patient may impede extension of infection from moving upward in pelvis.
I. Provide emotional support to mother, who is usually in isolation and unable to see baby.

Thrombophlebitis

Definition: Development of a thrombi at placental site which becomes infected, causing inflammation of the deep pelvic veins. Thrombophlebitis may be confined to blood vessels in uterine wall, or it may extend to ovarian, hypogastric, or femoral veins. Femoral thrombophlebitis, commonly called "milk leg," may originate in a leg vein.

Signs and Symptoms

A. Discomfort in abdomen and pelvis.
B. Tenderness localized on one side of the pelvis.
C. Femoral symptoms usually do not appear until the second week or later.
  1. Edema and pain in affected leg.
  2. Chills and fever.

Treatment and Nursing Care

A. Administer antibiotics until temperature is stable.
B. Give anticoagulants.
C. Provide bed rest and diversion.
D. Apply warm compresses as ordered (for fifteen to twenty minutes).
E. Bed cradle—keep bed clothes off leg.
F. Antiembolic stockings.
G. Elevate affected leg.

H. Never massage leg and teach patient not to do so.

I. Teach patient to watch for signs of excessive bleeding.

J. Allow patient to express fears and concerns.

K. Watch for signs of pulmonary embolism.

Cystitis and Pyelitis

Definition: Cystitis is an inflammation of the bladder; pyelitis is an inflammation of the renal pelvis.

Signs and Symptoms

A. Usually begin several days into the postpartum.

B. Suprapubic or perineal discomfort.

C. Frequent urination.

D. Burning sensation on urination.

E. Elevated temperature.

F. Urine contains pus, bacteria, and red blood cells on microscopic examination.

G. Pain in flank area.

Treatment and Nursing Care

A. Observe patient closely postpartum for full bladder or residual urine.
   1. Palpate bladder for distention.
   2. Palpate fundus (full bladder displaces fundus upward and to the sides).

B. Institute measures to help patient void.

C. Insert catheter as ordered, using sterile technique.

D. Force fluids.

E. Administer drugs as ordered: antibacterials, antispasmodics.

F. Obtain urine specimens for microscopic examination.

G. Provide emotional support to patient, and allow her to express feelings about her illness and the baby.

Mastitis

Definition: An infection in breast tissue due to invading organisms, usually staphylococcus.

Causes

A. Infected hands of mother or attendants.

B. Bacteria normally present in lactiferous glands.

C. Fissure in nipples.

D. Bruising of breast tissue.

E. Stasis of milk or overdistention may injure tissue, but does not cause infection in itself.

F. Infected baby.

Signs and Symptoms

A. Chills.

B. Fever 103°F or above.

C. Elevated pulse rate.

D. Lobe may become hard to the touch, red, and painful.

E. May progress to abscess if untreated.

Treatment and Nursing Care

A. Administer medications as ordered.

B. Apply ice pack as ordered.

C. Make sure mother is wearing snug-fitting, supportive brassiere.

D. Teach mother to empty breast if nursing is to be continued.

E. Wash hands before touching patient's breast.

F. Teach mother careful handwashing and care of the breast.

G. May require incision and drainage if abscess develops.

H. Some physicians recommend breast feeding be stopped; others favor discontinuance with artificial removal of milk for a few days.

Newborn

Immediate Care of the Newborn

Principles of Maintenance

A. Maintain body temperature.
   1. Place infant in heated incubator or crib with radiant heat.
   2. Wipe off fluid, mucus, and excessive vernix.
   3. Avoid excessive exposure.
   4. Wrap infant in warm blankets.
   5. Transfer to the nursery as soon as possible, after parents have seen and held infant.
B. Maintain respiration.
   1. Place infant on side, in modified Trendelenburg's position, to facilitate drainage of mucus.
   2. Suction mucus as needed with bulb or suction catheter attached to mucus trap.
   3. Provide oxygen as needed.
C. Prevent infection.
   ☆ 1. Eye care—apply two drops of one percent silver nitrate in conjunctival sacs. Flush eyes with water in about two minutes; apply antibiotic ointment to prevent eye infection in the infant if the mother was infected with gonorrhea.
   2. Cord care—use sterile gauze to cover.
   3. Carry out proper hand washing before receiving baby or wear sterile gloves.

General Observations

A. Apgar scoring, one and five minutes (see Table E); based on the scoring method developed by Virginia Apgar.
B. Congenital malformations.
C. Umbilical cord—two arteries and one vein.
D. Meconium staining—skin, nails.
E. Abnormal cry or no cry.
F. Injuries caused by birth trauma—dislocated shoulder, edema of scalp, lacerations.
G. Respiratory—nasal flaring, retractions, expiratory grunt.
H. Neurological status—reflexes, tremors, and twitching.

Nursing Care

A. Clamp the cord if so requested by the physician; should be clamped one inch from the base or left longer if the mother is Rh negative (in case of possible blood exchange).
B. Identify the baby with bands.
C. Show the baby to the parents and allow them to hold the infant with help (if not contraindicated).
D. Observe the mother's reactions to baby.
E. Transfer the baby to the admitting nursery with appropriate data.

Table E. Apgar Scoring

Sign	0	1	2
Heart tone	Absent	Slow (less than 100)	Over 100
Respiratory effort	Absent	Slow, irregular	Good, crying
Muscle tone	Flaccid	Some flexion of extremities	Active motion
Reflex irritability	No response	Cry	Vigorous cry
Color	Blue, pale	Body pink, extremities blue	Completely pink

Care in the Nursery

A. Care at admission and during the first twelve hours.
1. Check rectal temperature.
2. Weigh and measure—total length and head circumference.
3. Place in heated crib.
4. Check respiratory rates every hour for four to five hours and prn.
5. Check for nasal flaring, retractions, expiratory grunt, breath sounds.
6. Check apical pulse every hour for two to three hours; watch for above 180 or below 100.
7. Keep bulb syringe available and suction as needed.
8. Administer vitamin K as ordered.
9. Bathe and dress baby when his or her temperature is stable.
10. Place in an open crib when baby's temperature is stable.
11. Administer feeding as ordered; usually water is given every four to six hours.
12. Assess baby for congenital defects.

B. Routine nursing care.
1. Assessment.
   a. Observe for jaundice—check general skin color, blanching, sclera of the eyes.
   b. Check for respiratory difficulty—mucus, flaring of nostrils, grunting, and other signs.
   c. Note tremors, twitching, muscle tone, and reflexes.
   d. Take baby's temperature each shift.
   e. Check baby's weight daily.
   f. Note amount voided and number of stools.
   g. Check for signs of infection on the skin and cord.
2. Apply alcohol to cord daily prn.
3. Circumcision care.
   a. Observe for bleeding.
   b. Change petroleum gauze as necessary.
   c. Keep area clean to prevent infection.
4. Check to see if the test for phenylketonuria has been done.
5. Provide for nutrition and hydration.
6. Teach mother how to hold and burp the baby.
7. Use proper hand-washing between babies to prevent spreading infection.
8. Isolate babies with known or suspected infections.
9. Be sure that the mother understands the doctor's orders regarding care of the infant before she goes home and plans follow-up visits to the physician.

Physical Characteristics

Respiratory Status

A. Infant's respiratory system must function immediately after loss of placental function; adequate maturation at birth is necessary.
B. Normal respiration is about 30–40; over 60 or below 30 may indicate a problem. Respiration may be slightly elevated during crying episodes or shortly afterwards.

Circulatory Status

A. Ductus arteriosus, ductus venosus, and foramen ovale should close (may not be complete for one or two days).
B. Peripheral circulation may be sluggish (there may be mottling, acrocyanosis).
C. Pulse may be variable—normal 120–160; it may be as high as 170 with crying or below 120 when resting.
D. Anemia is common in early months because of the decrease in erythropoiesis and breakdown of red blood cells. Baby may need an iron-supplemented formula.
E. Physiologic jaundice—normal level less than 1 mg/100 ml blood.
1. Jaundice visible in the skin, sclera.
2. Does not become visible until the second or third day after birth.

3. Caused by impairment in the removal of bilirubin—deficiency in the production of glucuronide transferase, which is needed to convert indirect insoluble bilirubin to direct water soluble bilirubin and then excreted.

4. Jaundice begins to decrease by the sixth or seventh day.

5. It may require treatment, although it usually does not if watched carefully. If needed, usual treatment is phototherapy.

F. Transitory deficiency in the ability of the blood to clot. Bacteria in the intestines are necessary for the production of vitamin K. Bacteria are not present in the intestines during the first few days after birth. Vitamin K IM usually given after birth to aid in blood coagulation.

Ability to Maintain Body Heat

A. The baby suffers a large loss of heat because he is wet at birth and because of the coolness of the delivery room. The infant should be placed immediately in a warmer and dried off.

B. Temperature may be taken by rectum or axilla (usually taken by rectum the first time to check for patent anus).

Weight

A. Infants usually lose between 5 to 10 percent of their body weight the first few days because of low fluid intake and loss of excess fluid from tissue.

B. They usually regain weight lost within seven to fourteen days.

Head

A. Head or face may be asymmetrical due to birth trauma.

B. Molding of head may be present (elongation of head as it passes through birth canal to accommodate pelvis); usually disappears in about a week.

C. Caput succedaneum—diffuse swelling of soft tissues of scalp caused by an arrest in circulation in those tissues present over the cervix as it dilates.

D. Cephalohematoma—extravasation of blood beneath periosteum of one of the cranial bones because of a ruptured blood vessel during the trauma of labor and delivery.

E. Anterior and posterior fontanel.
1. Should be open.
2. Should neither bulge (may indicate intracranial pressure) nor be depressed (may indicate dehydration).

F. Ears well formed and cartilage present.

Gastrointestinal System

A. Salivary glands immature.

B. May have Epstein's pearls (white raised areas on palate caused by an accumulation of epithelial cells).

C. May have transient circumoral cyanosis.

D. Infant stools.
1. Meconium plug—thick gray-white mucus passed before meconium.
2. Meconium—sticky, black, tarry looking stools, consisting of mucus, digestive secretions, vernix caseosa, and lanugo; usually passed during the first twenty-four hours after birth.
3. Transitional stool passed second to fifth day; greenish, yellow color, and loose (partly meconium and partly milk).
4. Number of stools varies. Breast-fed infants usually have more bowel movements.
5. Stools should be observed for color, frequency, and consistency.

E. Regurgitation following feeding is common. It may be reduced by frequent burping during feedings.

Genitourinary System

A. Check presence of voiding.

B. Uric acid crystals (pink or reddish spots) may appear on diaper due to high uric acid secretion.

C. Genitalia.
1. Female.
   a. May have heavy coating of vernix between labia.
   b. Usually has mucus discharge. Mucus may be blood-tinged due to elevated hormonal levels in mother (pseudomenstruation).
2. Male.
   a. Size of penis and scrotum vary.
   b. Testicles should be descended or in inguinal canal.
   c. Circumcision—surgical removal of the foreskin of penis by physician.
      (1) Usually performed by the second or third day.
      (2) Observe for bleeding from postoperative site.
      (3) Observe for postoperative voiding.

Skin

A. Should be pinkish color.
B. Acrocyanosis (cyanosis of extremities) may be present for the first hour or two after birth. Persistent blueness may indicate complications such as heart disease.
C. Lanugo and vernix caseosa may be present.
D. Petechiae may be present because of the trauma of birth.
E. Milia—secretions of sebaceous materials in obstructed sebaceous glands (may be present and will disappear).
F. Hemangiomas may be present on nape of neck or upper eyelids.
G. Skin may appear dry or cracked.
H. Mongolian spots—bluish pigmented areas present on the buttocks of babies of Oriental, Negro, or Mediterranean heritage.

Effects of Maternal Hormones

A. Maternal hormones may cause enlargement of breast in both male and female infants, and "witches" milk, a milk-like substance, may be excreted from the breasts.
B. Vaginal bleeding in female infant.
C. Hypertrophy of vulva or prostate.

Neurological System

A. Muscle tone.
1. Fist usually kept clenched.
2. Baby should offer resistance when change in position is attempted.
3. Head should be supported when baby is lifted.
4. Muscles should not be limp.
B. Cry.
1. Cry should be loud and vigorous.
2. Baby should cry when hungry or uncomfortable.
C. Hunger.
1. Usually becomes fretful and restless at three to four-hour intervals.
2. May suck fingers or anything placed near mouth.
D. Sleep.
1. Sleeps about twenty out of twenty-four hours.
2. Often stirs and stretches while sleeping.
E. Senses.
1. Eyes.
   a. Eyelids may be edematous or have purulent discharge from the chemical irritation of silver nitrate.
   b. Light perception is present.
   c. Eye movement is uncoordinated.
   d. Usual color of eyes is blue-gray.
   e. May have subconjunctival hemorrhages, which disappear in a week or two.
2. Nose.
   a. Newborn breathes through nose.
   b. Sense of smell is present.
3. Ears—hearing is present at birth.
4. Taste is present at birth.
5. Touch is present at birth. Responds to stimuli and discomfort.
F. Immunity.
1. May receive from the mother some passive immunity to infectious diseases, such as measles, mumps, and diphtheria.
2. Capacity to develop own antibodies is slow during first few months.
3. Has little resistance to infection.

Feeding the Newborn

Schedules of Feeding

A. First feeding.
   1. May be breast fed on the delivery table.
   2. First feeding is usually within four to twelve hours after birth.
   3. Usually a test feeding of 5 to 10 drops of sterile water is made to determine baby's ability to swallow. Glucose is no longer given to prevent aspiration pneumonia.
B. Subsequent feeding.
   1. Routine schedule—three to four hour feedings.
   2. Self-demand—baby is fed according to his or her needs (when hungry) usually every three to six hours.

Calories and Fluid Needs

A. Fluid 150–200 ml/kg of body weight in twenty-four hours. More fluids should be given in hot weather or when the baby has an elevated temperature.
B. Caloric needs—approximately 110 C/kg of body weight or 50 C/lb of body weight.

High Risk Infants

Premature Infant

Definition: An infant born before a thirty-seven week gestation period, weighing less than 2500 gm and measuring less than 18½ inches (47 cm) long with a head circumference less than 13 inches (33 cm).

Characteristics

A. Skin is thin and capillaries are easily seen.
B. Lanugo is prominent; hair on the head is fine and fuzzy.
C. Little subcutaneous fat.
D. Body temperature is unstable and may be below normal.
E. Head is large in comparison to the rest of the body.
F. Poor muscle tone—muscles appear limp; baby assumes frog-like position when placed on abdomen.
G. Feeble cry.
H. Gagging and sucking reflexes may be weak.
I. Jaundice appears later than in the normal newborn, and it may be more severe and last longer (2 weeks).
J. Heightened capillary fragility and increased tendency towards hemorrhage.
K. Lack of immunity and lack of resistance to infection.
L. Poor ability to tolerate fats because of immaturity of digestive system.
M. Tendency towards periods of apnea because of immaturity of nervous system.
N. Tendency to develop respiratory distress, hypoglycemia, anemia, hypocalcemia.
O. High proportion of body surface to weight; leads to an increase in the loss of body fluids.
P. Immaturity of retina—leads to development of retrolental fibroplasia with increased levels of oxygen consumption.
Q. Immaturity of liver—difficulty detoxifying medications.
R. Renal function immature.
S. Reflexes—Moro's reflex is developed; grasp is feeble; rooting is present; sucking varies, although it is usually present at thirty-two weeks; poor coughing ability, gagging, and swallowing.

Nursing Care

A. Provide for family's needs to be met.
   1. Allow parents to visit baby frequently; as soon as possible, involve parents in infant care to promote parent-to-infant attachment.
   2. Answer questions openly, provide up-to-date information on baby's progress.
   3. Allow parents to talk freely about infant, give support as needed, and help parents to accept reality of situation.

4. Explain specialized care to parents. Have them report to pediatrician any of the following symptoms: diarrhea, vomiting, lack of appetite, or elevated temperature.

5. Allow mother to feel confident in caring for infant before discharge. Explain to mother infant's special needs.

B. Provide immediate care to infant.

1. Give immediate attention in delivery room and transport to nursery to maintain heat.

    a. Maintain skin temperature at about 36°C or 97.6°F in isolette or heated crib.

    b. Gradually wean infant from heated environment and watch temperature closely until stable.

    c. Warming infant too quickly may cause apneic spells.

2. Administer humidity (distilled water) usually between 40 to 70 percent as ordered.

C. Evaluate respiratory status.

1. Check respiratory rate—every hour and p.r.n.

2. Observe for the following signs of respiratory distress:

    a. Color of skin.

    b. Flaring of nares.

    c. Grunting retractions.

3. Auscultate breath sounds with stethoscope.

4. Analyze oxygen concentration one to two hours or as necessary to prevent retrolental fibroplasia and to ensure adequate oxygenation.

5. Observe for periods of apnea and stimulate by gently rubbing chest or tapping foot.

6. Percuss, vibrate and suction as ordered to remove mucus.

D. Reposition every two hours to promote aeration of all lobes of lung and facilitate drainage.

E. Monitor blood gases and electrolytes frequently; IV regulated by infusion pump to prevent circulatory overload.

F. Initiate feedings as ordered (usually begin with sterile water or breast milk); progress to dilute formula or breast milk to full strength as tolerated.

G. Give gavage feeding if respirations are about 60 breaths per minute.

1. Use premie nipple if bottle feeding.

2. Infants often require alternate feedings of gavage and bottle feeding.

H. Maintain intake and output including stool and weigh daily.

I. Organize care to conserve energy with rest periods after each feeding.

J. Measure head circumference and length at least once a week.

K. Maintain aseptic technique and strict isolation techniques with infected babies.

L. Prevent skin breakdown: change position, careful cleansing and handling.

M. Observe for signs of infection: vomiting, jaundice, lack of appetite and lethargy.

N. Check heart rate by apical pulse for a full minute every one to two hours.

O. Frequently check for bleeding from umbilical catheter.

1. Apply pressure to puncture site as necessary to prevent bleeding.

2. Administer vitamin K as ordered after birth to prevent hemorrhage.

3. Frequently check monitors if monitored electronically.

P. Gently stroke and talk to baby when giving care.

Q. Hang colorful mobiles or other nonharmful objects in crib.

R. Hold baby during feeding as soon as condition permits.

S. Encourage parents to hold, cuddle, feed, and diaper baby as soon as baby's condition permits.

Small for Gestational Age

Definition: Refers to infants who are significantly undersize for gestational age. Also called intrauterine growth retardation (IUGR).

Characteristics

A. Postmature infants.

B. Defective embryonic development.

C. Placental insufficiency.

D. Associated factors: diabetes, toxemia, maternal infection, maternal malnutrition, cigarette smoking, multiple gestation.

E. Infant appearance.
1. Little subcutaneous tissue.
2. Loose, dry, scaling skin.
3. Appears thin and wasted; old for size.
4. May be meconium staining of skin, nails.
5. Sparse hair on head.
6. Active, alert, seems hungry.
7. Cord dries more rapidly than normal infants.

Signs and Symptoms

A. Hypoglycemia: nervousness, cyanosis, apnea, temperature instability, weak cry.

B. Hypothermia: lethargy, poor feeding pattern, cold to touch, slow respiration.

C. Asphyxia: may have been deprived while in utero or aspirated amniotic fluid. Infant may require resuscitation at birth.

D. Polycythemia: usually asymptomatic but may have tachypnea, retractions.

Nursing Care

A. Provide care similar to premature infant until the infant is stabilized.

B. Protect from cold stress: keep warm, usually in isolette.

C. Perform tests for glucose levels.

D. Weigh daily and maintain intake and output.

Diseases Affecting the Newborn

Respiratory Distress Syndrome

Definition: A group of clinical symptoms signifying that the infant is experiencing problems with the respiratory system.

Etiology

A. Symptoms are the result of a decrease in the amount of surfactant in the infant's lungs as a result of one of the following conditions.
1. Prematurity—immaturity of lungs and inability to produce surfactant.
2. Hypoxia and acidosis.
3. Hypothermia.
4. High concentration of oxygen.

B. Respiratory distress syndrome is the most common cause of death in infants.

Signs and Symptoms

A. Increased respirations—60/min.

B. Retractions—subcostal followed by intercostal.

C. Cyanosis.

D. Expiratory grunting.

E. Lack of activity.

F. Inability to take in sufficient oxygen leading to low oxygen and hypoxemia.

G. Respiratory acidosis due to retention of carbon dioxide as a result of inadequate pulmonary ventilation.

H. Metabolic acidosis due to increased production of lactic acid.

I. Result of x-ray examination.
1. Atelectasis—collapsed portions of lung.
2. Fibrinous membrane that lines alveolar ducts and terminal bronchioles; membrane is formed by transudation of fluid from pulmonary tissue.

Nursing Care

A. Primarily supportive.

B. Maintain warmth—infant usually placed in isolette or open crib with overhead warmer. Skin temperature is maintained at 97.6°F.

C. Provide for nutrition and hydration—usually give IV glucose fluids during acute periods, then gradually increase feedings as tolerated.

D. Administer oxygen, warmed and humidified, in lowest concentration possible, via hood, nasal prongs, endotracheal tubes, or bag and mask. Oxygen may be given at atmospheric or increased airway pressure.

E. Apply continuous positive pressure to lungs during spontaneous breathing.

F. Apply positive pressure to lungs during expiratory cycle when using the mechanical ventilator.

G. Check and change nasal prongs frequently if used.

H. Loosely tape and check endotracheal tube frequently for correct placement and connection at adaptor site.

☆ I. Procedure for suctioning infant with endotracheal tube.

1. Disconnect from respirator at site of adaptor.

2. Instill few minims to 0.5 ml of sterile normal saline into tube to loosen secretions.

3. Suction no longer than five seconds using sterile catheter.

4. Ventilate infant as needed during procedure.

5. Reconnect tube to respirator; be certain it is in place and adaptor is secure.

6. Auscultate chest for breath sounds.

J. Provide postural drainage and percussion and suction as ordered.

K. Analyze oxygen concentration.

L. Keep parents informed of infant's progress.

M. Allow parents to visit child as much as possible and express their feelings about child's illness.

N. Gently stroke and talk with child while giving care.

Hyperbilirubinemia

Definition: An abnormal elevation of bilirubin in the newborn (above 13–15 mg/100 ml).

Etiology

A. Functional immaturity of the liver—usually appears after twenty-four hours and disappears after ten days.

B. Bacterial infections.

C. ABO and Rh incompatibilities—usually show up in the first twenty-four hours and may be severe.

D. Enclosed bleeding, such as hematoma, from trauma of delivery.

Signs and Symptoms

A. Jaundice, progressing from head to extremities.

B. Pallor.

C. Infant is lethargic and feeds poorly.

D. Urine is concentrated and stools are light in color.

E. If untreated, infant may progress to muscular rigidity or flaccidity, increased lethargy, high-pitched cry, respiratory distress, decreased Moro's reflex, and spasms.

Treatment and Nursing Care

A. Observe infant carefully for signs of increased jaundice.

B. Observe for and prevent acidosis/hypoxia and hypoglycemia, which decrease binding of bilirubin to albumin and contribute to jaundice.

C. Maintain adequate hydration and offer fluids between feedings as ordered.

D. Maintain temperature at 97.6°F to avoid cold stress.

E. Take measures to avoid infection.

☆F. Treatment with phototherapy—fluorescent light breaks down bilirubin into water soluble products.

1. Do not clothe infant.

2. Cover infant's eyes to prevent retinal damage.

3. Change baby's position every two hours to ensure adequate exposure.

4. Remove infant from light and remove eye patches during feedings.

5. Carefully examine eyes for signs of irritation from eye patches.

6. Keep an accurate record of hours spent under fluorescent lights.

G. Meet emotional needs of infant.

H. Reinforce physician's instruction to parents and allow parents to express concerns and feelings.

I. Exchange transfusion may be done; considered only when bilirubin reaches extremely high levels (20 mg/ml in full term infant and 16 mg/ml in premature infant).

Hemolytic Disease of the Newborn

Definition: Alteration, dissolution, or destruction of red blood cells.

Etiology

A. Rh incompatibility—Rh antigens from the baby's blood enter the maternal bloodstream through the placenta. The mother's blood does not contain Rh factor, so she produces anti-Rh antibodies. These antibodies are harmless to the mother but attach to the erythrocytes in the fetus and cause hemolysis.

1. Problem may begin in early pregnancy; it may be mild to severe and can cause the death of the fetus.

2. Sensitization usually does not occur with the first pregnancy.

3. Diagnosis of Rh incompatibility.

a. Begins in pregnancy, with discoveries of antibodies in an Rh negative mother's blood by means of indirect Coombs' test.

b. Titration is used to determine the extent to which antibodies are present.

c. Analysis of amniotic fluid for bilirubin determines the severity of the disease (the higher the bilirubin content, the more severe the disease).

d. Testing of cord blood (direct Coombs' test) determines the presence of maternal antibodies attached to baby's cells.

B. ABO incompatibility—usually less severe.

Signs and Symptoms

A. Anemia—caused by destruction of red blood cells.

B. Jaundice—develops rapidly after birth.

C. Edema—usually seen in stillborn infants or those who die shortly after birth, most likely due to cardiac failure.

Treatment

A. For mild forms, treat as for hyperbilirubinemia.

B. For severe, give exchange transfusion after birth or intrauterine.

Infants of Diabetic Mothers

General Considerations

A. May be delivered early to prevent intrauterine death (after thirty-six weeks).

B. Often delivered by cesarean section.

C. Children with diabetic mothers have a higher incidence of congenital anomalies than the general population.

D. High incidence of hypoglycemia, respiratory distress, hypocalcemia, and hyperbilirubinemia.

Signs and Symptoms

A. Baby is usually excessively large in size and weight due to excess fat and glycogen in tissues.
   1. High blood sugar levels in mother cross the placenta and enter the baby's bloodstream, elevating blood sugar levels.
   2. High blood sugar stimulates infant's metabolic system to store glycogen and fat and increase the production of insulin.
B. May have puffy appearance of face and cheeks.
C. Enlarged heart, liver, and spleen.
D. Lethargy.
E. Irregular respiration.

Nursing Care

A. Observe for signs of hypoglycemia—twitching, difficulty in feeding, lethargy, apnea, seizures, and cyanosis.
B. Observe for signs of respiratory distress—tachypnea, cyanosis, retractions, grunting, nasal flaring.
C. Care is the same as for a premature infant.
D. Initiate feedings with sterile water or glucose water within two to four hours after birth, as ordered by physician.

Infant Born to Mother with Drug Addiction

General Considerations

A. There is a direct relationship between the duration of the maternal addiction and dosage and the severity of symptoms in the infant.
B. Heroin and morphine addiction are common offenders.
C. Infants usually have low birth weight.
D. Symptoms usually occur in infants within forty-eight to seventy-two hours. May occur as late as one week with methadone-treated mother.

Signs and Symptoms

A. Irritability and tremors.
B. Vomiting.
C. High-pitched cry.
D. Sneezing, nasal stuffiness.
E. Respiratory distress.
F. Fever.
G. Diarrhea.
H. Excess sweating.
I. Increased muscle tone.
J. Poor feeding.
K. Sucking of fist.
L. Convulsions (rare).

Nursing Care

A. Monitor respiratory and cardiac rates every thirty minutes and prn.
B. Take temperature every four to eight hours and prn.
C. Maintain warmth and swaddle infant in blanket.
D. Reduce external stimuli and handle infant infrequently.
E. Hold firmly and close to body during feedings and when giving care.
F. Pad sides of crib to protect infant from injury.
G. Administer small, frequent feedings as ordered.
H. Suction if necessary.
I. Cleanse buttocks and anal area carefully.
J. Measure intake and output.
K. Keep mother informed of infant's progress.
L. Promote mother's interest in infant.

Fetal Alcohol Syndrome

Characteristics

A. Maternal alcohol abuse throughout pregnancy results in fetal alcohol syndrome.
   1. Most serious cause of teratogenesis.
   2. In affected infants, growth is retarded; they are microcephalic with severe mental retardation.

B. Lesser amount of alcohol ingested throughout pregnancy results in less severe symptoms.
   1. Prenatal and/or postnatal growth retardation.
   2. Developmental delay.
   3. May not be diagnosed until early childhood.

Signs and Symptoms

A. Respiratory distress and apnea.
B. Cyanosis.
C. Seizures.
D. Major brain dysfunction symptoms.

Nursing Care

A. Position on side to facilitate drainage of secretions.
   1. Keep resuscitation equipment at bedside.
   2. Have suction available, especially following feeding.
B. Administer small feedings and burp well.
C. Support family and assist to accept anomalies.

Gynecology

Examination

A. Pelvic exam.
   1. Inspection of external genitalia for signs of inflammation, bleeding, discharge, and epithelial cell changes.
   2. Speculum may be inserted for visualization of vagina and cervix.
   3. Bimanual examination is done—gloved fingers of one hand inserted into vagina while abdomen palpated with other hand.
   4. Rectal exam.
B. Breast exam may also be done when woman comes in for pelvic.
C. Papanicolaou smear.
   1. Diagnosis for cervical cancer.
   2. Vaginal secretions and secretions from posterior fornix are swabbed and smeared on a glass slide.

Conditions of the Vulva

Vulvitis

A. An inflammation of the vulva which usually occurs in conjunction with other conditions such as vaginal infections and venereal disease.
B. Signs and symptoms.
   1. Burning pain during urination.
   2. Itching.
   3. Red and inflamed genitalia.
   4. Discharge.
C. Treatment and nursing care.
   1. Apply soothing compresses and give colloidal baths.
   2. Administer medicated creams.
   3. Administer sedatives (antihistamines).

Cancer of the Vulva

A. Signs and symptoms.
   1. Long-standing pruritus (itching).
   2. Foul-smelling discharge.
   3. Bleeding.
   4. Pain.
B. Treatment and nursing care.
   1. Vulvectomy is the preferred treatment.
   2. Immediate postoperative care.
      a. Observe dressings for signs of hemorrhage.
      b. Check vital signs until stable.
      c. Assist patient to turn, cough, and deep breathe every two hours.
      d. Give pain medications as ordered.
      e. Observe drainage, and empty Hemovac as necessary.
      f. Record intake and output.
      g. Maintain IV.
      h. Maintain catheter care to reduce incidence of infection.
      i. Position for comfort.
   3. Convalescent care.
      a. Encourage patient to verbalize feelings related to change in body image.

b. Irrigate wound as ordered, using solution as prescribed (usual solution is sterile saline hydrogen peroxide), which cleans area and improves circulation.

Conditions of the Vagina

Vaginal Infections

A. Vagina normally protected from infection by acidic environment.

B. Leukorrhea (whitish vaginal discharge) normal in small amounts at ovulation and prior to menstruation.

C. Trichomoniasis vaginalis—overgrowth of protozoan normally present in vaginal tract due to normal pH alteration.

D. Moniliasis—fungal infection caused by Candida albicans.
   1. Thrives in carbohydrate-rich environment; common in poorly controlled diabetes.
   2. Antibiotic or steroid therapy reduces protective organisms normally present.

E. Treatment—medications and vaginal inserts as prescribed.

Conditions of Ovaries and Pelvic Cavity

Endometriosis

A. Abnormal growth of endometrial tissue outside the uterine cavity.

B. This condition is a common cause of infertility.

C. Etiological theories.
   1. Embryonic tissue that remains dormant until ovarian stimulation after menarche.
   2. Endometrial tissue transported from the uterine cavity through the fallopian tubes during menstruation.
   3. Endometrial tissue transported by lymphatic tissue during menstruation.
   4. Accidental transfer of endometrial tissue to pelvic cavity during surgery.

D. Signs and symptoms.
   1. Lower abdominal and pelvic pain during menstruation due to distention of involved tissue and surrounding area by blood (symptoms are acute during menstruation).
   2. Dysmenorrhea—usually steady and severe.
   3. Abnormal uterine bleeding.
   4. Pain during intercourse.
   5. Back and rectal pain.

E. Treatment and nursing care
   1. Pregnancy may delay growth of lesions but symptoms usually recur after pregnancy.
   2. Hormone therapy with oral contraceptives usually eliminates menstrual pain and controls endometrial growth.
   3. Surgical intervention; total hysterectomy may be indicated.
   4. Provide emotional support.

Pelvic Inflammatory Disease (PID)

A. An inflammatory condition of the pelvic cavity that may involve ovaries, fallopian tubes, vascular system, or pelvic peritoneum.

B. Etiology.
   1. Staphylococcus or streptococcus.
   2. Venereal disease.
   3. Tubercle bacilli.

C. Signs and symptoms.
   1. Elevated temperature.
   2. Nausea and vomiting.
   3. Abdominal and low-back pain.
   4. Purulent, foul-smelling vaginal discharge.
   5. Leukocytosis.

D. Treatment and nursing care.
   1. Take measures to control the spread of infection.
   2. Place patient in semi-Fowler's position for dependent drainage.
   3. Take and record vital signs every four hours.
   4. Administer antibiotics, douches, and abdominal heat as ordered.
   5. Note nature and amount of vaginal discharge.

6. Avoid use of tampons and urinary catherization to prevent the spread of infection.

7. Promote good nutrition and fluid intake.

8. Explain rationale for treatment.

Conditions of the Uterus

Displacements

A. Retroversion and retroflexion—backward displacement of the uterus.

1. May cause difficulty in getting pregnant.

2. Treatment consists of moving the uterus to the normal position by shortening its ligaments.

B. Prolapse (usually occurs in multiparas).

1. Weakening of uterine supports causes the uterus to slip down into the vaginal canal; the uterus may even appear outside the vaginal orifice.

2. Prolapse may cause urinary incontinence or retention.

3. Treatment.

   a. Pessary—instrument that keeps the uterus in place by exerting pressure on ligaments and usually used in patients of advanced age.

   b. Surgery to reposition uterus and shorten ligaments; or hysterectomy.

Tumors

A. Benign fibroid tumors.

1. Occur in 20 to 30 percent of all women between the ages of twenty-five to forty.

2. Symptoms include menorrhagia, back pain, urinary difficulty, and constipation.

3. Fibroid tumors may cause sterility.

4. Treatment.

   a. Removal of tumors, if they are small.

   b. Hysterectomy is performed when there are large tumors.

B. Malignant tumors of the reproductive system (second highest cause of death in the female).

1. Cancer of the cervix—most common type of cancer in the reproductive system.

   a. Usually appears in females between the ages of thirty to fifty.

   b. Signs and symptoms include bleeding between periods—may be noted especially after intercourse or douching; leukorrhea.

   c. May become invasive and include tissue outside the cervix, fundus of the uterus, and the lymph glands.

   d. Treatment depends upon extent of the disease.

      (1) Hysterectomy.

      (2) Radiation.

      (3) Radical pelvic surgery in advanced cases.

2. Cancer of the endometrium (fundus or corpus of uterus).

   a. Usually not diagnosed until symptoms appear; Pap smear inadequate for diagnosis.

   b. Progresses slowly; metastasis occurs late.

   c. Treatment.

      (1) Early—hysterectomy.

      (2) Late—radium and x-ray therapy.

Hysterectomy

Types

A. Total—removal of the entire uterus but retention of fallopian tubes and ovaries.

B. Panhysterectomy—removal of the entire uterus, ovaries, and fallopian tubes.

C. Radical hysterectomy—wide removal of vaginal, cervical, uterosacral and other tissue along with the uterus.

D. Cervical.

E. Abdominal.

F. Vaginal.

Postoperative Nursing Care

A. Immediate care.

1. Observe incisional site for bleeding and reinforce dressings as needed.

2. Monitor vital signs frequently.

3. If patient has nasogastric tube to suction,

maintain NPO and observe amount, color, and consistency of drainage.

4. Administer pain medications as ordered.
5. Monitor IV fluids as ordered.
6. Provide for hygienic care.
7. Catheter care to prevent infection (observe amount and color of drainage).
8. Assist patient to cough, turn, and deep breathe.
9. Promote methods for decreasing pelvic congestion.
    a. Apply antiembolic stocking.
    b. Avoid high-Fowler's position.
10. Measure intake and output.
11. Apply range-of-motion exercises.

B. Common complications.
1. Hemorrhage.
2. Infection.
3. Pneumonia.
4. Paralytic ileus.
5. Thrombophlebitis.
6. Changes in body image.

Anterior and Posterior Colporrhaphy

A. Purpose.
1. Repair of cystocele—downward displacement of the bladder towards the vaginal entrance caused by tissue weakness, injuries in childbirth, and atrophy associated with aging.
2. Repair of rectocele—anterior sagging of rectum and posterior vaginal wall caused by injuries to the muscles and tissue of the pelvic floor during childbirth.

B. General postoperative care of the patient with cystocele and rectocele repair.
1. Observe for foul-smelling discharge from vaginal area or operative site.
2. Two methods of caring for perineal sutures.
    a. Sutures left alone until healing begins; thereafter, daily vaginal irrigations with sterile saline.
    b. Sterile saline douches twice daily beginning with the first postoperative day.

3. Observe for urinary retention and catheterize as necessary.
4. Prepare patient for discharge with instruction in perineal hygiene (no douching or coitus until advised by physician), and in detection of signs of infection.

Pelvic Exenteration

A. A surgical procedure that is performed for widespread cancer that cannot be controlled by other means.

B. Three types of pelvic exenteration.
1. Anterior pelvic—the removal of the reproductive organs, pelvic lymph nodes, adnexa, pelvic peritoneum, bladder, and lower ureter. Ureters are implanted in the small intestines or the colon.
2. Posterior pelvic—removal of the reproductive organs, vagina, adnexa, colon, and rectum. Pelvic lymph nodes may also be removed.
3. Total pelvic—removal of the reproductive organs, pelvic floor, pelvic lymph nodes, perineum, bladder, rectum, and distal portion of sigmoid colon. A substitute bladder is made from a segment of the ileum. Patient will have a permanent colostomy.

C. Care of the patient undergoing pelvic exenteration.
1. Exercise general postoperative procedures.
2. Observe surgical site for drainage and reinforce dressings as necessary; patient may have drainage tubes connected to suction from incision area.
3. Apply antiembolic stockings.
4. Encourage patient to express feelings.

Patient Receiving Radiation Therapy

A. Radiation therapy is treatment with radioactive substance given to break down cancerous tissue.

B. Therapy procedure.
1. Radioactive cobalt, radium, or iridium inserted into endocervical canal by radiotherapist.
2. Supplemented by external radiation.

C. Nursing care.
  1. Provide low-residue diet to prevent bowel movement and dislodging of radium.
  2. Inspect catheter to make sure it is draining (distended bladder will be in the path of radiation).
  3. Observe for unusual or profuse vaginal discharge.
  4. Instruct patient to lie on side or on back with head slightly elevated on pillow.
  5. Administer skin care to prevent tissue breakdown.
  6. While giving nursing care, encourage patient to talk and express anxieties.
  7. Measure intake and output.
  8. Observe patient for side effects, e.g., nausea, vomiting, anorexia, and redness or blistering of skin in pelvic area.
  9. Check vital signs and observe for elevated temperature.

Tumors of the Breast

Clinical Findings

A. Nontender lump in breast, usually in upper outer quadrant.
B. Dimpling of breast tissue surrounding nipple.
C. Asymmetry with affected breast being higher.
D. Nipple bleeding or retraction.

Types of Surgery

A. Simple mastectomy—removal of breast with no lymph nodes removed.
B. Radical mastectomy—removal of the breast, muscle layers down to chest wall, and lymph nodes in axillary region.
C. Lumpectomy.

Nursing Care

A. Continue giving emotional support begun preoperatively during postoperative period.
  1. Patient will have altered body image.
  2. Patient may be extremely depressed.

B. Position in semi-Fowler's position with the affected arm elevated to prevent edema.
C. Turn, cough, and hyperventilate to prevent respiratory complications.
D. Turn only to back and unaffected side.
E. Hemovac placed frequently.
  1. Maintain suction.
  2. Record amount of drainage.
  3. Record drainage characteristics.
F. Prevent complications of contractures and lymph-edema by encouraging range-of-motion exercises early in postoperative period.
G. IV fluids should not be administered in affected arm.
H. Monitor vital signs for prevention of complications such as infection and hemorrhage. Take blood pressure on unaffected arm only.
I. Pressure dressings should be reinforced. Observe for signs of restriction from dressing.
  1. Impaired sensation.
  2. Color changes of skin.
J. If skin grafts were applied, treat as for any other graft.
K. Encourage visit from Reach for Recovery Group.

Therapeutic Abortion

General Considerations

A. Legality.
  1. Abortion is now legal in all states as the result of a Supreme Court decision in January 1973.
  2. It is regulated in the following manner.
    a. First trimester—decision between patient and physician.
    b. Second trimester—decision between patient and physician (state may regulate who performs the abortion and where it can be done).
    c. Third trimester—states may regulate and prohibit abortion except to preserve the health or life of the mother.

B. Indications for abortion.

1. Medical—psychiatric condition such as chronic hypertension or disease in the mother (e.g., nephritis, severe diabetes, cancer, or acute infection such as rubella); possible genetic defects in the infant or severe erythroblastosis fetalis.

2. Nonmedical—socio-economic reasons, unmarried, financial burden, too young to care for infant.

C. Preparation of the individual.

1. Advise patient of available sources of abortion.

2. Inform patient as to what to expect from the abortion procedure.

3. Provide emotional support during decision-making period.

4. Maintain an open, nonjudgmental atmosphere in which the individual may express concerns or guilt.

5. Encourage and support the individual after the decision is made and after surgery.

6. Give information about contraceptives.

D. Complications and effects.

1. Abortion should be performed before the twelfth week, if possible, because complications and risks are lower during this time.

2. Complications.
   a. Infection.
   b. Bleeding.
   c. Sterility.
   d. Uterine perforation.

Techniques

A. First trimester.

1. Dilatation and curettage (D & C).
   a. Cervical canal is dilated with instruments of increasingly large diameter.
   b. Fetus and accessory structure is removed with forceps.
   c. Endometrium is scraped with curette to assure that all products of conception are removed.
   d. Process usually takes fifteen to twenty minutes.

2. Vacuum aspirator.
   a. Hose-linked curette is inserted into dilated cervix.
   b. Hose is attached to suction.
   c. The vacuum aspirator lessens the chance of uterine perforation, reduces blood loss, and reduces the time of the procedure.

B. Second trimester abortion.

1. Intraamniotic injection or amniocentesis abortion.
   a. Performed after the fourteenth to sixteenth week of pregnancy.
   b. From 50 to 200 ml of amniotic fluid are removed from the amniotic cavity and replaced with hypertonic of 20 to 50 percent saline that is installed through gravity drip over a period of forty-five to sixty minutes.
   c. Increased osmotic pressure of the amniotic fluid causes the death of the fetus.
   d. Uterine contractions usually begin in about twelve hours, and the products of conception are expelled in twenty-four to thirty hours.
   e. Oxytocic drugs may be given if contractions do not begin.
   f. Complications.
      (1) Infusion of hypertonic saline solution into uterus.
      (2) Infection.
      (3) Disseminated intravascular coagulation disease may develop during procedure.
      (4) Hemorrhage.

2. Hysterotomy.
   a. Incision is made through abdominal wall into uterus.
   b. Procedure is usually performed between the fourteenth and sixteenth week in pregnancy.
   c. Products of conception are removed with forceps.
   d. Uterine cavity is curetted.
   e. Tubal ligation may be done at same time.

f. Patient usually requires several days of hospitalization.

g. Operation requires general or spinal anesthesia.

3. Prostaglandins.

a. These hormone-like acids cause abortion by stimulating the uterus to contract.

b. They may be administered IV into the uterine cavity through the cervical canal, into the posterior fornix of the vagina, or after twelve weeks into the amniotic cavity. The IV method is least effective and has many possible side effects.

C. Nursing care.

1. Administer preoperative medications.

2. Ensure that patient understands the procedure.

3. Offer emotional support and let patient express feelings.

4. Monitor IV.

5. Check vital signs postoperatively.

6. Check for excessive bleeding.

7. Administer pain medications as ordered.

8. Instruct patient to watch for signs of excessive bleeding (more than a normal menstrual period) and infection (elevated temperature), foul-smelling discharge, persistent abdominal pain).

9. Administer oxytocic drug as ordered.

10. Administer RhoGAM as ordered for an unsensitized Rh-negative patient.

11. Offer fluids as tolerated after vital signs are stable and patient is alert and responsive.

Control of Parenthood

Influences on Parenthood

A. Tendency toward smaller families.

B. Career-oriented women who limit family size or who do not want children.

C. Early sexual experimentation necessitating sexual education and contraceptive information.

D. Reasons for tendency toward postponement of children.

1. Completion of education.

2. Economic factors.

E. High divorce rates.

F. Alternate family designs.

1. Single parenthood.

2. Communal family.

Methods of Birth Control

Chemical

A. Foam, cream, jelly agents.

1. Agent acts by killing or paralyzing the sperm.

2. Combined with a compound which coats the vagina so that agent acts as a vehicle for spermicide as well as a mechanical barrier through which sperm cannot swim.

B. Oral contraceptives.

1. Biologic mechanism.

a. The pill artificially raises the blood levels of both estrogen and progesterone, thereby preventing the release of FSH from the anterior pituitary. Without FSH the follicle does not mature and ovulation fails to take place.

b. Endometrial changes.

c. Alteration in cervical mucus making it hostile to sperm.

d. Altered tubal function.

2. Types of birth-control pills.

a. Combined—contain both estrogen and progesterone.

b. Sequential (mimics normal hormonal cycle)—estrogen given alone 15–16 days, followed by combination of estrogen and progestin for the next five days.

3. Minor side effects (usually diminish within a few months).
   a. Breast fullness and tenderness.
   b. Edema, weight gain.
   c. Nausea and vomiting.
   d. Chloasma.
   e. Breakthrough bleeding.
4. More serious side effects.
   a. Thrombophlebitis.
   b. Pulmonary embolism.
   c. Hypertension.

Mechanical

A. Diaphragm.
   1. Mechanical barrier that functions by blocking external os and closing access to cervical canal by sperm.
   2. Must be used in conjunction with vaginal cream or jelly to be effective.
B. Condom.
   1. Acts as a mechanical barrier by collecting sperm which then are not allowed contact with vaginal area.
   2. It is relatively inexpensive and may be readily purchased in a drugstore.
C. Intrauterine devices (IUD).
   1. Methods of action (not completely clear).
      a. More rapid transport of ovum through tube reaching endometrium before it is "ready" for implantation.
      b. IUD may cause substances to accumulate in uterus and interfere with implantation.
      c. IUD may stimulate production of cellular exudate which interferes with the ability of sperm to migrate to fallopian tubes.
   2. Usually made of soft plastic or nickel-chromium alloy.
   3. There are many types of devices available on market such as Lippes' loop and Saf-T-Coil.

4. Complications.
   a. Perforation of uterus.
   b. Infection.
   c. Spotting between periods.
   d. Heavy menstrual flow or prolonged flow.
   e. Cramping during menstruation.

Biologic

A. Rhythm.
   1. Based upon three principles.
      a. Ovulation usually occurs fourteen days before period begins.
      b. An ovum may be fertilized twelve to twenty-four hours after release from ovary.
      c. Sperm usually survives no longer than twenty-four hours in the uterine environment.
   2. On these bases, if coitus is avoided during the fertile period, pregnancy should not occur.
B. Coitus interruptus.
   1. Early form of contraception.
   2. Requires withdrawal of penis before ejaculation.
C. Sterilization.
   1. General considerations.
      a. Should be considered permanent—no guarantee fertility can be restored.
      b. Requires written consent of responsible, fully-informed individual.
   2. Male sterilization (vasectomy)—severing of sperm duct from each testicle making it impossible for sperm to pass from testes.
   3. Female sterilization—may be accomplished by the removal of the uterus and the ovaries, or the destruction of ovum-conducting ability of fallopian tubes.

Appendix 1. Common Drugs in Obstetrics and Gynecology

Name of Drug, Action, Dosage	Uses and Side Effects	Nursing Implications
Oxytocin, Syntocinon/Pitocin Classification: oxytocic Produces rhythmic contractions of uterine musculature Dosage: varies with method and purpose of administration. IV 5–10 USP units in 500 or 1,000 ml 5 percent dextrose in VS infused at rate 0.5–0.75 ml/min with rate gradually increased until patient has three to four good quality contractions in 10 minutes	Used to induce labor, constrict uterus, and decrease hemorrhage after delivery and postabortion Stimulates contractile tissue in lactating breast to eject milk Side effects: water intoxication; allergic reactions; death due to uterine rupture; pelvic hematomas; bradycardia	Observe for signs of sensitivity and overdose Monitor strength and duration of uterine contractions Check FHT every 15 minutes and prn Take P and BP every hour
Methergine Classification: oxytocic Produces constrictive effects on smooth muscle of uterus (more prolonged constrictive effects as compared to rhythmic effects of oxytocin or ergotrate); also has generalized vasoconstrictive effect Usual IM dose 0.2 mg (may be repeated in 2–4 h); usual oral dose 0.2 mg 3–4 × a day for 2 days	Used primarily after delivery to produce firm uterine contractions and decrease uterine bleeding May be used to prevent postabortal hemorrhage Side effects include nausea, vomiting, dizziness, increased BP, dyspnea, and chest pain	Check BP and pulse before administration of medication and check vital signs frequently after administration Injectable form deteriorates rapidly when exposed to lights and heat—do not use if discoloration occurs

Name of Drug, Action, Dosage	Uses and Side Effects	Nursing Implications
Vasodilan (isoxsuprine) Classification: vasodilator Relaxing effects on circulatory and uterine smooth muscle Usual oral dose 10–20 mg; tablets 3–4 times daily	Treatment of premature labor or during labor when contractions are unusually frequent and not coordinated. Most effective when given in early latent phase of labor; rarely stops active labor Side effects include nausea, vomiting, dizziness, transient hypotension and tachycardia	Take BP and P frequently Observe for signs of tachycardia and hypotension
Ritodrine (improved analog of isoxsuprine)	Hydrate woman prior to infusion with IV solution of 1000 cc normal saline Continuous monitoring (Swan-Ganz) of mother and infant important as mother-infant deaths have occurred	Same as above
Terbutaline, B_2, receptor stimulant; sympathomimetic	Treatment of premature labor and requires hospitalization Side effects: tachycardia, palpitations, sweating, tremors, restlessness, lethargy, drowsiness, headache, nausea, vomiting	Same as above

Name of Drug, Action, Dosage	Uses and Side Effects	Nursing Implications
Magnesium sulfate Depressive effects on central nervous system, and smooth, skeletal, and cardiac muscle Produces peripheral vasodilation Given IV in preeclampsia and eclampsia; dosage varies Usual dosage: initial dosage 4 gm in 250 cc 5% D/W at 5 cc/30 sec (approximately 20 min) or in continuous infusion	Used to prevent convulsions in preeclampsia and eclampsia. Also counteracts uterine tetany after large doses of oxytocin Side effects: *Maternal:* extreme thirst, hypotension, flaccidity, circulatory collapse, depression of CNS and cardiac system. *Fetal:* crosses placenta, lethargy, hypotonia Antidote: Calcium Gluconate, Keep available at bedside	Observe carefully for signs of magnesium toxicity: extreme thirst, feeling hot all over; loss of patellar reflex Monitor respirations (greater than 12/min), BP (hypotension), and P closely in order to assess effect of drug. Never leave client alone Patellar reflex should be checked continuously Check urine output continuously (greater than 30 cc/hr)
Pergonal Classification: hormone, purified preparation of gonadotropic hormones Promotes follicular growth and maturation in women with secondary anovulation; must be given with human chorionic gonadotropin to induce ovulation Usual dosage: 75 IU of FSH and 75 IU of LH IM daily for 9–12 days, followed by 10,000 U of HCG one day after last dose	Treatment of sterility due to defective luteal function Side effects include nausea, vomiting, diarrhea, fever, possible multiple births	Inform patient of complications and hazards of multiple births

Name of Drug, Action, Dosage	Uses and Side Effects	Nursing Implications
Estrogen preparations Classification: hormones Development and maintenance of sexual characteristics throughout adult life Common preparations Estradiol, Tace, Premarin Dosage varies, depends upon purpose for giving	Given to replace deficiencies, to control conception, relieve breast engorgement when lactation is to be suppressed Side effects include nausea, vomiting, diarrhea, skin rash, edema Diethylstilbestrol no longer used as it causes incidence of cancer in female offspring	Encourage follow-up visits to physician
Progesterone preparations Classification: hormones Normal functions— preparation and maintenance of edometrium for pregnancy. Suppresses ovulation and pregnancy and decreases uterine irritability Dosage varies	Given to control conception, amenorrhea, abnormal uterine bleeding, threatened abortion Side effects include GI symptoms, dizziness, headache, allergic reactions	Encourage follow-up visits to physician
Demerol Classification: synthetic narcotic analgesic Onset of action 15 min peaks 1 h, depresses CNS probably at both cortical and subcortical levels Dosage: 25–50 mg IM every 3–4 h prn relief of postsurgical pain	Produces analgesia in labor, postoperative relief of pain Side effects include dizziness, nausea, vomiting, dry mouth, sweating, decrease in BP	Evaluate progress of labor carefully; if given too late in labor, infant may be depressed Check for level of consciousness before administration Observe for nausea and vomiting

Name of Drug, Action, Dosage	Uses and Side Effects	Nursing Implications
Morphine Classification: analgesic Combination of depressive and stimulative effects on CNS and smooth muscles of gut Raises pain threshold and produces euphoria and sedation Usual dose: 3–10 mg IM during labor; postoperative—10 mg	Produces analgesia during labor, relief of postoperative pain. Side effects include nausea, vomiting, constipation, depression of respiratory center and cough, allergic reactions such as urticaria	Check level of consciousness and respiratory rate before administration Careful evaluation of progress of labor; if given too late, infant may be depressed
Nisentil Classification: synthetic analgesic Action similar to Demerol and morphine, but acts more quickly than Demerol and over a shorter period of time Dosage: 20–40–60 mg subcutaneous or IM every 2–4 h	Analgesia during labor; relief of pain after abortion Side effects include nausea, vomiting, depression of respiratory center	Monitor progress of labor carefully; if given too late in labor, infant may be depressed Check respiratory rate before administration
Nalline Hydrochloride, Narcan, Lorfan Classification: narcotic antagonists Acts as an antagonist to morphine, Demerol, and related analgesics	Treatment of respiratory depression in newborn when narcotic effect has not worn off in the mother prior to delivery Nalline may be given to the mother shortly prior to delivery to prevent respiratory depression due to analgesic side effects Side effects include drowsiness, lethargy, sweating	Check respiratory rate and color and cardiac rate of infant to see if medication is having desired effect

Name of Drug, Action, Dosage	Uses and Side Effects	Nursing Implications
Diuril Classification: diuretic Brings about diminished reabsorption of sodium and chlorides Results in increased urinary output; potassium may also be excreted Usual dosage: 500 mg IGM one or two times daily	Diminish fluid retention in toxemia of pregnancy Side effects include allergic reactions, nausea, weakness, dizziness, and muscle cramps	Give drug early in day to avoid disturbing sleep Encourage addition of potassium foods in diet (orange juice) to avoid depletion
Phenobarbital Classification: barbiturate Slow acting in low doses—depression of sensory functions. In higher doses depression of motor functions Usual dosage for sedative effect: range 15–50 mg 3–4 times daily	Sedative and anticonvulsive effects in toxemia of pregnancy Side effects include listlessness, depression, nausea, skin rash, restlessness, emotional disturbances	Check level of consciousness and responsiveness before administration

Appendix 2. Drugs Adversely Affecting the Human Fetus

Drugs	Adverse Effect	Comments
Analgesics		
Heroin and morphine	Respiratory depression; neonatal death; addiction	Near term Fairly well documented
Salicylates	Neonatal bleeding; coagulation defects	Near term
Anesthetics		
Mepivacaine	Fetal bradycardia; neonatal depression	Near term More studies needed
Antibacterials		
Chloramphenicol	"Gray syndrome" and death	Near term Fairly well documented
Nitrofurantoin	Hemolysis	Near term More studies needed
Novobiocin	Hyperbilirubinemia	Near term More studies needed
Streptomycin	8th nerve damage; hearing loss; multiple skeletal anomalies	Throughout pregnancy Debatable, more studies needed
Sulfonamides (long acting)	Hyperbilirubinemia and kernicterus	Near term Fairly well documented
Tetracyclines	Inhibition of bone growth; discoloration of teeth	2nd and 3rd trimesters Fairly well documented
Anticarcinogens		
Amethopterin	Cleft palate; abortion	1st trimester Fairly well documented
Aminopterin	Cleft palate; abortion	1st trimester Known teratogen
Cyclophosphamide	Severe stunting; fetal death; extremity defects	1st trimester More studies needed
Anticoagulants		
Warfarin	Fetal death; hemorrhage	Throughout pregnancy More studies needed
Antidiabetics		
Chlorpropamide	Prolonged neonatal hypoglycemia	Throughout pregnancy More evidence needed before implication

Drugs	Adverse Effect	Comments
Tolbutamide	Congenital anomalies	Throughout pregnancy One reported case only; evidence lacking
Antimalarials 　Quinine	Deafness	More studies needed
Anti-mitotic agents 　Podophyllum	Fetal absorption; multiple deformities	More studies needed
Antithyroid agents 　Methimazole	Goiter and mental retardation	From 14th week on Fairly well documented
Potassium iodide	Goiter and mental retardation	From 14th week on Fairly well documented
Prophylthiouracil	Goiter and mental retardation	From 14th week on Fairly well documented
Radioactive iodine	Congenital hypothyroidism	From 14th week on Fairly well documented
Depressants 　Phenobarbital	Neonatal bleeding; increased rate of neonatal drug metabolism	In excessive amounts
Reserpine	Nasal block	Near term One report only More studies needed
Thalidomide	Phocomelia; hearing defect	28th–42nd day Known teratogen
Diuretics 　Ammonium chloride	Acidosis	
Thiazides 　　(Hydrochlorothiazide) 　　(Chlorothiazide) 　　(Methyclothiazide)	Thrombocytopenia; neonatal death	Latter part of pregnancy One report only; evidence lacking
Stimulants 　Dextroamphetamine	Transposition of great vessels	One report only More evidence needed
Phenmetrazine	Skeletal and visceral anomalies	4th–12th week One report only More evidence needed

Drugs	Adverse Effect	Comments
Sex Steroids		
Androgens, estrogens, and oral progestins	Masculinization and labial fusion (early in pregnancy); clitoris enlargement (later in pregnancy)	Fairly well documented
Miscellaneous		
Acetophenetidin	Methemoglobinemia	More studies needed
Cholinesterase inhibitors	Transient muscular weakness	Throughout pregnancy More studies needed
Hexamethonium Bromide	Neonatal ileus and death	Throughout pregnancy More studies needed
Iophenoxic acid	Elevation of serum protein-bound iodine	
Isonicotinic acid hydrazide (INH)	Retarded psychomotor activity	More studies needed
Lysergic acid diethylamide (LSD)	Chromosomal damage; stunted offspring	1st trimester More studies needed
Nicotine and smoking	Small babies	Throughout pregnancy More studies needed
Vitamin A	Congenital anomalies; cleft palate; eye damage, syndactyly	Throughout pregnancy In large doses only
Vitamin D	Excessive blood calcium; mental retardation	Throughout pregnancy In large doses only
Vitamin K analogues	Hyperbilirubinemia; kernicterus	Near term In large doses

Excerpted from "Drugs Adversely Affecting the Human Fetus," 1971, Ross Laboratories, Columbus, Ohio.

Appendix 3. The Premature Infant

Need	Nursing Care
Needs of Family	
Keep separation to a minimum	Allow parents to visit baby frequently; as soon as possible, allow parents to help care for infant.
Provide data on baby's progress	Answer questions openly, provide up-to-date information on baby's progress.
Express feelings and concerns	Allow parents to talk freely about infant, give support as needed and help parents to accept reality of situation.
Provide information	Explain specialized care to parents. Have them report to pediatrician any of following symptoms: diarrhea, vomiting, lack of appetite, or elevated temperature.
	Help mother to feel confident in care of infant before discharge.
Needs of Infant	
Warmth	Immediate attention in delivery room and transporting to nursery to maintain heat. Maintain temp. at about 36°C or 97.6°F in isolette or heated crib.
	Gradually wean infant from heated environment and watch temperature closely until stable.
Oxygen and humidity	Administer oxygen (should be warmed and humidified). Administer humidity (distilled water) usually between 40–70 percent as ordered.
	Check respiratory rate—1 × h and prn.
	Observe for signs of respiratory distress, color, flaring, grunting retractions, skin color, auscultate breath sounds with stethoscope. Analyze oxygen concentration 2–4 h or as necessary to prevent retrolental fibroplasia and to ensure adequate oxygenation. Observe for periods of apnea and stimulate by gently rubbing chest or tapping foot; percuss, vibrate and suction as ordered to remove mucus.
	Reposition q 2 h to promote aeration of all lobes of lung and facilitate drainage.
	Monitor blood gases and electrolytes frequently. (Oxygen administration is determined by blood gases.)

Need	Nursing Care
Nutrition and hydration	May require IV feedings through umbilical catheter until stabilized. IV regulated by infusion pump to prevent circulatory overload. Initiate feedings as ordered (usually begin with sterile water or glucose water). Progress to dilute formula or breast milk to full strength formula as tolerated.
	Usually gavage feeding if respirations are about 60 breaths per minute. Use premie nipple if bottle feeding. Infants often require alternate feedings of gavage and bottle feeding.
	Maintain intake and output including stool; weigh daily and organize care to conserve energy with rest periods after each feeding. Measure head circumference and length at least once a week.
Prevention from infection	Maintain aseptic technique.
	Strict isolation techniques with infected babies.
	Prevent skin breakdown—change position, careful cleansing and handling.
	Observe for signs of infection—vomiting, jaundice, lack of appetite, lethargy; cover IV sites.
Maintenance of circulatory functioning	Check heart rate by apical pulse for a full minute q 1–2 h.
	Frequently check for bleeding from umbilical catheter. Apply pressure to puncture site as necessary to prevent bleeding. Administer vitamin K as ordered after birth to prevent hemorrhage.
Mothering and physical stimulation	Gently stroke and talk to baby when giving care.
	Hang colorful mobiles or other nonharmful objects in crib.
	Hold baby during feeding as soon as condition permits.
	Encourage parents to hold, cuddle, feed and diaper baby as soon as baby's condition permits.

Appendix 4. Recommended Daily Dietary Allowances for Pregnancy and Lactation

	Pregnancy		Lactation		Function	Sources
	14 to 18	Adult	14 to 18	Adult		
Calories	2400	2300	2600	2500	Meet increased nutritional needs as well as body maintenance.	All foods. Important to emphasize food values of foods and avoid empty calories.
Protein	78	76	68	66	Augment maternal tissues—bust, uterus, blood. Growth and development of placenta and fetal tissue. Constant repair and maintenance of maternal tissue.	All essential amino acids may be found in milk, meat, eggs, and cheeses. Other sources, though not complete protein by themselves: tofu, whole grains, legumes, nuts, peanut butter.
Iron	+ 18 mg	+ 18 mg	18 mg	18 mg	Essential constituent of hemoglobin. Part of various enzymes. Fetal development and storage, especially later part of pregnancy.	Good sources: liver, kidney, heart, cooked dry beans, lean pork and beef, dried fruits such as apricots, peaches, prunes, and raisins. Fair sources: spinach, mustard greens, eggs.
Calcium	1200 mg	1200 mg	1200 mg	1200 mg	Skeletal tissue. Bones; teeth. Blood coagulation. Neuromuscular irritability. Myocardial function. Fetal stores, especially last months.	Good sources: milk, cheese, ice cream, yogurt. Fair sources: broccoli, canned salmon with bones, dried beans, dark leafy vegetables.
Phosphorus	1200 mg	1200 mg	1200 mg	1200 mg	90 percent compounded with calcium. Rest distributed throughout cells—involved in energy production, building and repairing tissue, buffering.	Whole grain items: cereals, whole wheat bread, brown rice; milk.
Sodium	0.5 g	0.5 g	0.5 g	0.5 g	Metabolic activities. Fluid balance and acid-base balance. Cell permeability. Muscle irritability.	Table salt, meat, eggs, carrots, celery, beets, spinach, salted nuts, carbonated beverages.

	Pregnancy		Lactation		Function	Sources
	14 to 18	Adult	14 to 18	Adult		
Iodine	125 ug	125 ug	125 ug	125 ug	Necessary for health: mother and fetus; prevents goiter in mother; decreases chance of cretinism in infants.	Iodized table salt, cod liver oil.
Vita-min A	5000 Iu	5000 Iu	6000 Iu	6000 Iu	Tooth formation and skeletal growth. Cell growth and development. Integrity of epithelial tissue. Vision—light/dark adaptation. Fat metabolism.	Good sources: butter, egg yolk, fortified margarine, whole milk, cream, kidney, and liver. Fair sources: dark green and yellow vegetables such as sweet potatoes, pumpkins, mustard greens, collards, kale, bok choy, carrots, cantaloupe, apricots.
Ribo-flavin	1.7 mg	1.5 mg	1.9 mg	1.7 mg	Enzyme systems. Tissue functioning. Tissue oxygenation and respiration. Energy metabolism. Excreted in breast milk.	Good sources: kidney, liver, heart, milk. Fair sources: cheese, ice cream, dark leafy vegetables, lean meat, poultry.
Thia-mine	1.4 mg	1.3 mg	1.4 mg	1.3 mg	Carbohydrate metabolism. Normal appetite and digestion. Health of nervous system.	Good sources: enriched and whole grain products—bread and cereals, dried peas, beans, liver, heart, kidney, nuts, potatoes, lean pork. Fair sources: eggs, milk, poultry, fish, vegetables.
Niacin	16 mg	15 mg	18 mg	17 mg	Cell metabolism.	Good sources: fish, lean meat, poultry, liver, heart, peanuts, peanut butter. Fair sources: enriched and whole grain cereals and bread, milk, potatoes.
Folic acid B_{12}	4.0 mg	4.0 mg	4.0 mg	4.0 mg	Cell growth. Reproduction and formation of heme. Enzyme activities in production of protein. Deficiency results in megaloblastic anemia.	Dark green and leafy vegetables.

	Pregnancy		Lactation		Function	Sources
	14 to 18	Adult	14 to 18	Adult		
Pyri-doxine B$_6$	2.5 mg	2.5 mg	2.5 mg	2.5 mg	Essential coenzyme with amino acids. Deficiency may lead to hypochromic micro-cytic anemia.	Animal and vegetable protein such as meat, fish, beans, nuts and seeds, milk and milk products.
Vita-min D	400 Iu	400 Iu	400 Iu	400 Iu	Influences absorption, retention and utilization of calcium and phos-phorus. Formation of bones, teeth and other tissue.	Good sources: fortified milk, butter, egg yolk, liver, fish oils.
Vita-min C Ascorbic acid	60 mg	60 mg	80 mg	80 mg	Production of intracellular substances necessary for development and main-tenance of normal con-nective tissue in bones, cartilage and muscles. Role in metabolic processes involving protein and tissues. Increases absorption of iron.	Good sources: citrus fruits and juice, broccoli, cantaloupe, collards, mustard and turnip greens, peppers. Fair sources: asparagus, raw cabbage, other melons, spinach, prunes, tomatoes, canned or fresh chilis.

Source of daily requirements: *Nutrition During Pregnancy and Lactation.* California Department of Health, 1975.

Appendix 5. Prenatal Instructions

Nutrition

A. It is important that adequate nutrition is maintained.

B. See Appendix 4 for specific guidelines.

Use of Drugs

A. All drugs can be expected to cross the placenta and affect the fetus.

B. Greatest danger occurs in first trimester, especially when organs are developing (organogenesis).

C. Many other effects of drugs on the fetus are unknown and may not be evident for years.

D. Pregnant women should refrain from taking drugs during pregnancy; even commonly used drugs such as aspirin should only be taken by physician's order.

E. Nicotine in cigarettes may retard the growth of fetus.
   1. Causes vasoconstriction of woman's vessels resulting in decreased placental flow.
   2. Increases carbon dioxide levels in blood and reduces oxygen-carrying capacity.

F. See Appendix 2 for an outline on drugs that adversely affect fetus.

Exercise, Relaxation, and Rest

A. Exercise in moderation is beneficial but should never be carried on past the point of fatigue.

B. Sports may be participated in if they are part of the woman's usual activity and there are no complications present.

C. Fatigue is common in early pregnancy.

D. Frequent rest periods, at ten- to fifteen-minute intervals, are helpful in avoiding needless fatigue.

Review Questions

1. Which of the following is true regarding the newborn's weight after birth?

   A. Weight usually remains constant the first few days, then drops when infant goes home.
   B. Infant usually loses between 5 to 10 percent of body weight during the first few days after birth, and then begins to increase in weight after the fourth day.
   C. Infant usually begins to gain weight the first day after birth, when put on bottle or breast.
   D. Infant normally loses between 15 to 20 percent of body weight after birth but regains it rapidly.

2. Of the following conditions which one is not a result of metabolic error in the fetus?

   A. Phenylketonuria.
   B. Maple syrup urine disease.
   C. Galactosemia.
   D. Pyloric stenosis.

3. Considering the conditions above that are caused by inborn errors of metabolism, the most frequent traumatic result in the baby of such a condition is

   A. Mental retardation.
   B. Fetal death.
   C. Retrolental fibroplasia.
   D. Hypoxia.

4. Mrs. Jorgensen has been in labor for four hours. After a vaginal examination her obstetrician tells her that she is at -1 station. She asks you what this means. You tell her that in station -1 the presenting part of the fetus is

   A. In the false pelvis.
   B. At the level of the ischial spines.
   C. One cm above the level of the ischial spines.
   D. One cm below the level of the ischial spines.

5. Hyperbilirubinemia occurs in Rh incompatibility between mother and fetus because

   A. The mother's blood does not contain the Rh factor, so she produces anti-Rh antibodies that cross the placental barrier and cause hemolysis of red blood cells in infants.
   B. The mother's blood contains the Rh factor and the infant's does not, and antibodies are formed in the fetus that destroy red blood cells.
   C. The mother has a history of previous yellow jaundice caused by a blood transfusion, which was passed to the fetus through the placenta.
   D. The infant develops a congenital defect shortly after birth that causes the destruction of red blood cells.

6. Baby King's condition continues to worsen, and he is given an exchange transfusion. Nursing care of the infant following the transfusion would include all of the following *except*

   A. Observe for bleeding from the umbilical cord.
   B. Take vital signs frequently.
   C. Give IPPB therapy.
   D. Observe for signs of hypoglycemia and sepsis.

7. The development of anti-Rh antibodies within the mother could have been prevented with the administration of RhoGAM postabortion. Which of the following is true about RhoGAM?

   A. It must be given on the sixth day post-delivery.
   B. It should be given to an unsensitized mother after each pregnancy or abortion.
   C. It may be given even after sensitization occurs.
   D. It may be given to the infant.

8. Signs of sepsis in the newborn would include all the following *except*

   A. Periods of apnea or irregular respiration.
   B. Poor sucking reflex and feeding.
   C. Constipation.
   D. Irritability.

9. Mrs. Johns, who delivered a baby boy the previous evening, is crying when you enter her room. When you ask her what is wrong, she tells you that the doctor told her that her baby has a functional heart murmur. The best nursing response in this situation would be to

   A. Tell her to ask the doctor what it means.
   B. Tell her everything will work out all right.
   C. Tell her that a functional murmur is normal and will last a few weeks.
   D. Tell her that this type of murmur may indicate heart damage but the baby will certainly survive.

10. Baby Parks, an 8 lb. 6 oz. baby girl, was born at 8:15 A.M. in a normal, spontaneous birth. Apgar score was 9/9 and no abnormalities were noted. The cord was clamped and the baby was placed in a heated crib in the Trendelenburg position. The infant was dried thoroughly and banded. Silver nitrate one percent was placed in both eyes and flushed. Baby Parks was then rewrapped and shown to her parents before being brought to the nursery. The Apgar scoring is done on this infant

   A. To determine the sex of the baby.
   B. To appraise the infant for congenital anomalies.
   C. As an immediate appraisal of the infant's cardiac and respiratory status.
   D. As an immediate assessment of the infant's Rh status.

11. Baby Parks was given an Apgar score of 9 sixty seconds after delivery because

   A. Her heart rate was over 100.
   B. She gave a good strong cry.
   C. She had active movement of her arms and legs.
   D. She demonstrated acrocyanosis of the hands and feet.

12. The infant is usually placed in a heated crib in the Trendelenburg position immediately after birth to

   A. Prevent loss of heat and facilitate drainage of mucus.
   B. Increase oxygen intake.
   C. Allow the parents to view the infant more closely.
   D. Place the infant in an environment similar to the uterus.

13. Silver nitrate one percent is inserted into the newborn's eyes to prevent

   A. Spirochete infection.
   B. Gonococcal infection.
   C. Toxoplasmosis.
   D. Thrush.

14. An injection of vitamin K was given to Baby Jackson in the nursery. Vitamin K is given to

   A. Help conjugate bilirubin.
   B. Prevent Rh sensitization in the infant.
   C. Reduce the possibility of hemorrhage in the infant.
   D. Increase the infant's resistance to infection.

15. Baby Jackson had a large caput succedaneum on her head. The mother is concerned and asks what the swelling is. You would tell her

   A. It is a collection of blood in the tissue caused by trauma from delivery.
   B. It will take a couple of weeks to disappear on its own.
   C. The infant may suffer brain damage as a result of the caput.
   D. It is a swelling of the soft tissues of the scalp due to pressure on the cervix during dilatation.

16. The normal respiratory rate in the newborn is between

   A. 16 and 20.
   B. 60 and 80.
   C. 80 and 100.
   D. 30 and 50.

17. The normal apical pulse rate on the newborn is between

   A. 120 and 160.
   B. 60 and 80.

   C. 80 and 100.
   D. 180 and 200.

18. Baby Jackson showed signs of jaundice, and her lab value for bilirubin showed a total bilirubin of 15.0. The physician ordered continuous bile light and force fluids between feedings. Physiologic jaundice is due to

   A. Rh incompatibility with the mother.
   B. Presence of staphylococcus infection within the newborn.
   C. ABO incompatibility.
   D. Inability of the newborn to break down bilirubin.

19. An important principle to consider when an infant undergoes phototherapy is to

   A. Cover the eyes with eye patches to prevent retinal damage.
   B. Dress the infant to prevent chilling.
   C. Isolate the infant to prevent cross-contamination.
   D. Avoid handling the infant so as not to interfere with the treatment.

20. After two days' treatment with phototherapy, Baby Jackson showed a steady decline in the level of indirect bilirubin. She was discharged by the physician on a demand feeding schedule with a formula of Similac 20. Physiologic jaundice usually appears

   A. Within the first 24 hours and disappears after 3 days.
   B. Within the first 24 hours and lasts 6 to 7 days.
   C. On the second or third day and lasts 48 hours.
   D. On the second or third day and begins to decrease on the sixth or seventh day.

21. Nursing care of the "addicted" infant includes all the following except

   A. Frequent handling of infant.
   B. Frequent monitoring of cardiac and respiratory rates.
   C. Padding side of crib to protect from injury.
   D. Cleansing buttocks carefully to avoid skin breakdown from diarrhea.

22. RhoGAM is given to Mrs. Kanes, who delivered a healthy baby 24 hours ago. In order for the globulin to be effective, which of the following conditions should not be present?

   A. Mrs. Kanes is Rh⁰.
   B. The baby is Rh⁺.
   C. Mrs. Kanes has no titer in her blood.
   D. Mrs. Kanes has some titer in her blood.

23. On April 16 at 3:45 P.M., Baby Larson, a thirty-four-week 1550 gm female infant, was delivered to a seventeen-year-old unmarried primigravida. The infant demonstrated nasal flaring, intercostal retractions, expiratory grunt, and slight cyanosis. An umbilical catheter was inserted with IV infusion of 5 percent dextrose and water 30 cc to run over a 10-hour period. Blood gases and electrolyte studies were ordered immediately. All the statements below are criteria for diagnosis of prematurity *except*

   A. Birth weight.
   B. Length of gestation.
   C. Skin color.
   D. Body length.

24. Baby Larson was placed in a heated isolette because

   A. The premature infant has a small body surface for his or her weight.
   B. Heat increases flow of oxygen to extremities.
   C. The infant's temperature control mechanism is immature.
   D. Heat within the isolette facilitates drainage of mucus.

25. Immediate assessment of the premature infant in the nursery by the nurse would include all the following *except*

   A. Hunger status.
   B. Cardiac status.
   C. Respiratory status.
   D. Congenital abnormalities.

26. An infant with respiratory distress will show all the following *except*

   A. Respiration between 30–40.
   B. Cyanosis.
   C. Expiratory grunt.
   D. Carbon dioxide between 35–45.

27. Blood gases and electrolyte studies were ordered immediately on Baby Larson to assess

   A. The infant's leukocyte count.
   B. The infant's oxygen, carbon dioxide, and pH levels.
   C. The infant's antibody titer for Rh.
   D. The infant's blood glucose level.

28. Baby Kelly was diagnosed as having respiratory distress syndrome. Premature infants are likely to develop respiratory distress. Which one of the following conditions is *not* considered a possible cause?

   A. Alveoli are immature and produce inadequate amounts of surfactant.
   B. Premature infants have not received adequate numbers of antibodies from their mothers before birth.

   C. Nerves and respiratory center are immature.
   D. The premature infant's thoracic cage and respiratory muscles are weak.

29. The air in Baby Kelly's isolette is humidified to

   A. Improve cardiac rhythm.
   B. Prevent hyperbilirubinemia.
   C. Increase the infant's temperature.
   D. Prevent drying of bronchial secretions.

30. The physician will carefully regulate the concentration of oxygen that Baby Kelly receives, based upon the infant's pO_2 and pCO_2 levels, because high levels of oxygen

   A. Produce kernicterus.
   B. Cause retinal spasms leading to the development of retrolental fibroplasia.
   C. Cause peripheral circulatory collapse.
   D. Cause cardiac damage, which is not permanent.

31. The nurses use careful handwashing techniques while caring for Baby Larson because they know premature infants are more susceptible to infection than full-term infants. Which of the following does *not* explain why premature infants are more likely to develop infection?

   A. Liver enzymes are immature.
   B. Antibody formation is immature.
   C. Premature infants receive few antibodies from the mother, because antibodies pass across the placenta during the last month of pregnancy.
   D. Cellular and white blood cell defense may be ineffective.

32. Nursing care of the premature infant in preventing infection includes all the following interventions *except*

   A. Cover IV sites and keep dressings clean.
   B. Avoid caring for the infant if you have an infection.
   C. Use tap water for suctioning.
   D. Prevent skin breakdown by careful skin cleansing and little use of tape.

33. The premature infant has a tendency toward hemorrhage and anemia. Nursing care of Baby Larson would include all the following *except*

   A. Administer vitamin C shortly after birth.
   B. Record all blood loss including blood tests.
   C. Use care in handling the infant.
   D. Secure all IV connections and look for backflow of blood in tubing.

34. The most important nutritional principle to consider for Baby Larson would be

   A. Bottle feeding using a regular nipple.
   B. Gavage feeding.

C. Bottle feeding using a premie nipple.
D. Milk high in fat.

35. The premature infant has difficulty concentrating urine and may have large amounts of fluid lost. The nurse caring for Baby Larson would

A. Force fluids every half hour.
B. Observe color and amounts of urine and check its specific gravity.
C. Administer only high protein fluids.
D. Warm fluids before administration.

36. Mrs. Norman, a thirty-two-year-old housewife with a three-year-old child, had been trying to get pregnant for several months. She had been troubled with spotting between periods and excessive bleeding at menstruation. She consulted her physician, who administered a pelvic exam and a Pap smear. The result of her Pap smear was Class V. Her physician scheduled her for an immediate hysterectomy. Which of the following was probably Mrs. Norman's *least* concern upon being told she needed a hysterectomy?

A. Loss of childbearing ability.
B. Not understanding what Class V meant.
C. Fear of mutilation.
D. Fear of the vaginal examination.

37. Mrs. Norman was admitted to the hospital and scheduled for a total abdominal hysterectomy and bilateral salpingo-oophorectomy. While passing her room the evening before surgery, the nurse heard her crying. The nurse went into the room and sat on the chair beside the bed. Mrs. Norman said, "I wanted another baby so badly, and now I will never have another child." Which of the following statements by the nurse would be most helpful to Mrs. Norman?

A. "It is all right to cry. I know how difficult it must be to know you will never be able to have another child. I'll sit here with you for a while."
B. "No, you won't be able to have another child, but you can always adopt a child."
C. "Maybe you could talk to your doctor about postponing surgery until you have another child."
D. "At least you were lucky enough to have one child before the surgery."

38. Preoperative care of Mrs. Norman on the evening before surgery would include all the following *except*

A. Insert an indwelling catheter.
B. Force fluids after midnight.
C. Teach Mrs. Norman to support her incisional area and deep breathe and cough.
D. Administer a cleansing enema.

39. Mrs. Norman asks you if she will have hot flashes after surgery. You would reply,

A. "No, there is no reason for you to have hot flashes."
B. "Yes, hot flashes may occur. Your physician will probably place you on some form of estrogen therapy after surgery to alleviate hot flashes and other symptoms of induced menopause."
C. "Yes, you will probably have hot flashes after surgery, but it is just one of those things you will have to live with."
D. "Yes, you will have hot flashes, but they disappear after the first month."

40. Mrs. Norman is worried about her relationship with her husband and says, "Will I ever be able to have sexual relations with my husband again?" You could best respond by saying,

A. "Yes, but it will be at least a year before you can resume sexual relations."
B. "No, unfortunately the nature of your surgery makes it impossible for you to ever have sexual relations again."
C. "Yes, you will be able to resume normal sexual relations with your husband about six weeks after surgery."
D. "Since you cannot have children, there is no need for you to have sexual relations with your husband."

41. Convalescent care of Mrs. Norman would include all the following *except*

A. Observe for signs of infection.
B. Listen for breath sounds.
C. Involve significant others in patient's care.
D. Give daily vaginal irrigations.

42. Barbara, a twenty-one-year-old female patient, who is eighteen weeks pregnant, is admitted to the hospital for a saline abortion. Care of the patient during the saline infusion would include which of the following?

A. Check urine for sugar and acetone.
B. Ask the patient to deep breathe at appropriate times.
C. Observe for signs of saline leakage within the patient's circulatory system.
D. Massage the fundus of the uterus.

43. Nursing care for the patient after a saline abortion would include all the following *except*

A. Administer RhoGAM to Rh-negative mothers who are unsensitized.
B. Check vital signs frequently.
C. Teach the patient careful perineal care.
D. Explain to the patient she will probably have bright red bleeding for about three weeks.

44. After the abortion, Barbara begins to cry and says, "I feel so guilty. I should never have killed my baby." You could be most supportive to Barbara by saying,

    A. "You should be more careful in the future and use a method of birth control."
    B. "It's natural to feel sad, but you'll be back to normal in a short time."
    C. "You are feeling very sad right now, Barbara. I'll sit with you for a while; it may help to talk about it."
    D. "Your friend will be here soon to pick you up. Why don't you tell her about it when she comes."

45. Which one of the following conditions is a known teratogen (causes physical defects in developing embryo)?

    A. Scarlet fever.
    B. Rubella.
    C. Coronary heart disease.
    D. Dental X-rays.

46. In an emergency delivery which of the following principles best explains why the nurse would not cut the cord?

    A. The physician is responsible for cutting the cord.
    B. Cutting the cord under emergency conditions might lead to hemorrhage.
    C. Cutting the cord under emergency conditions might lead to infection.
    D. The nurse was never trained in the proper procedure.

47. Mrs. Jackson, a sixty-three-year-old woman, is receiving radium therapy for cancer. Observations of Mrs. Jackson would include all the following *except*

    A. Nausea and vomiting.
    B. Onset of menstruation.
    C. Elevated temperature.
    D. Position of radium.

48. In preparing Mrs. Jackson for discharge, you would tell her that

    A. She can resume sexual intercourse as soon as she gets home.
    B. She will be radioactive for at least six weeks.
    C. She should report vaginal or rectal bleeding immediately to the physician.
    D. Persistent nausea and vomiting are not significant and will continue for a while after discharge.

49. Which of the following is not a rationale for doing an amniocentesis on a woman who is 30 weeks pregnant?

    A. To determine fetal maturity.
    B. To determine presence of Tay-Sachs disease.
    C. To determine L-S ratio.
    D. To determine placental sufficiency.

50. Marion comes to the clinic and says she is sexually active and would like some form of birth control. After discussing the various methods of contraception, she decides she would like to use the pill. You tell Marion that the physician will need to know

    A. A list of her contacts.
    B. A complete history of her sexual experiences.
    C. If she has a history of thrombophlebitis or migraine headaches.
    D. If her parents approve and will sign a written consent.

51. In explaining the side effects of the pill to Marion, you would tell her that

    A. There are no known side effects of the pill.
    B. The pill is so effective that Marion need not be concerned with the side effects.
    C. If side effects show up, she should skip the pill for a few days.
    D. Side effects such as weight gain, nausea, and vomiting may appear but these usually clear up within the first to third cycle.

52. In preparing a patient for an IUD, you would

    A. Explain how an IUD functions and where it is placed.
    B. Tell the patient that the IUD will probably interfere with coitus.
    C. Tell the patient she will no longer be able to wear tampons.
    D. Explain that it is impossible to expel the IUD once it is in place.

53. When discussing family planning methods with a couple, the nurse should

    A. Include only the female in the discussion.
    B. Ensure that the couple have a thorough understanding of the method they choose.
    C. Choose the method that would best suit the couple.
    D. Point out that all methods are 99.9 percent effective, so it makes no difference which method they choose.

54. Genetic counseling is highly recommended for which of the following groups?

    A. A couple who is just planning to start their family.
    B. Parents who have had one abnormal child.
    C. Two people who are not married but planning to have a child.
    D. All parents or potential parents.

55. The follicle-stimulating hormone FSH, which stimulates the development of the ovarian follicle, is produced by the

    A. Adrenal cortex.
    B. Graafian follicle.
    C. Anterior pituitary.
    D. Cerebral cortex.

56. Which of the following is not a physiologic function of estrogen?

    A. Acts as nourishment for the embryo.
    B. Stimulates hypertrophy of the endometrium.
    C. Suppresses secretion of the follicle-stimulating hormone.
    D. Is responsible for growth of myometrium after implantation.

57. The hormone progesterone has all the following physiologic effects *except*

    A. Acts upon endometrium to prepare it for pregnancy.
    B. Facilitates transport of the fertilized ovum through the fallopian tubes.
    C. Inhibits implantation.
    D. Inhibits uterine motility during pregnancy.

58. Fertilization usually takes place in the

    A. Corpus luteum.
    B. Outer third of the fallopian tube.
    C. Corpus of the uterus.
    D. Cervix of the uterus.

59. Each reproductive cell (gamete) carries how many chromosomes?

    A. 24.
    B. 46.
    C. 23.
    D. 21.

60. Implantation occurs on the

    A. Fifth day after fertilization.
    B. Eleventh day after fertilization.
    C. Third day after fertilization.
    D. Seventh day after fertilization.

61. Which of the following is *not* a characteristic of amniotic fluid?

    A. Is normally yellow-green.
    B. Contains fetal urine, fetal lanugo, and epithelial cells.
    C. Provides a cushion against injury to the fetus.
    D. Provides optimum temperature to the fetus.

62. The placenta produces which one of the following hormones?

    A. Follicle-stimulating hormone.
    B. Adrenalin.
    C. Human chorionic gonadotropin.
    D. Testosterone.

63. Which of the following is *not* a characteristic of the placenta?

    A. Is formed by a union of the chorionic villi and decidua basalis.
    B. Allows bacteria to pass to the fetus.
    C. Controls fetal nutrition, respiration, and elimination of waste.
    D. Allows exchange between mother and fetus to take place through diffusion.

64. Sarah, a twenty-four-year-old married female, comes to the maternity clinic of a local hospital because she suspects that she is pregnant. She gives her last menstrual period as 8/9/79, which was two months ago. On talking to Sarah, you learn her menarche began at thirteen and she has had no major illnesses during her childhood or adult years. Sarah says, "If I am pregnant, when will my baby be due?" According to Nägele's rule, you would tell her

    A. 5/16/80.
    B. 4/13/80.
    C. 1/12/80.
    D. 6/6/80.

65. Upon examining Sarah, the physician finds Chadwick's sign. Chadwick's sign is

    A. Wavy streaks which appear on the abdomen, breast, and thighs during pregnancy.
    B. Thin yellowish fluid present in the breasts during pregnancy.
    C. Separation of the muscles due to abdominal distention during pregnancy.
    D. Deep reddish or purplish discoloration of the vagina due to increased vascularity.

66. Changes in the uterus during pregnancy include all the following *except*

    A. Increase in size and number of blood vessels.
    B. Atrophy of muscle cells.
    C. Hypertrophy of lymphatic system.
    D. Development of elastic tissue increasing contractility.

67. Changes in the breast during pregnancy include all the following *except*

    A. Breasts increase in size and firmness.
    B. Superficial veins grow more prominent.
    C. Montgomery's glands decrease in size.
    D. Nipples become more prominent, and areolae deepen in color.

68. Sarah was instructed by the nurse to immediately report any visual disturbances she was experiencing. The best rationale for this instruction is that the symptom

    A. Is a forerunner to preeclampsia.
    B. Indicates increased intracranial pressure.
    C. Is indicative of malnutrition.
    D. Is indicative of renal failure.

69. Sarah says, "I feel so different since I am pregnant." Which of the following is an expected characteristic of the altered emotional changes that take place during pregnancy?

    A. Quick mood changes.
    B. Violent outburst.
    C. Complete rejection of pregnancy.
    D. Emotionally insecure.

70. Presumptive signs of pregnancy include all the following *except*

    A. Periods of drowsiness and lassitude.
    B. Increased pigmentation of skin.
    C. Increased levels of the follicle-stimulating hormone.
    D. Frequency.

71. Probable signs of pregnancy include all the following *except*

    A. Increased gastric motility.
    B. Enlargement of abdomen.
    C. Changes in internal organs.
    D. Positive pregnancy tests.

72. Which of the following would be a positive sign of pregnancy?

    A. Hegar's sign.
    B. Ballottement.
    C. Auscultation of fetal heart tones.
    D. Outline of fetus by abdominal palpation.

73. In instructing Sarah about her nutritional needs during pregnancy, you would tell her that she has an increased need for all the following *except*

    A. Calories.
    B. Protein.
    C. High fat, high carbohydrate foods.
    D. Iron.

74. In giving prenatal instructions to Sarah, you would tell her that

    A. It is all right to take drugs during pregnancy because they do not cross the placenta.
    B. Smoking has little effect on the developing fetus.
    C. Sports should be avoided during pregnancy.
    D. Frequent rest periods should be planned to avoid needless fatigue.

75. Danger signals in pregnancy would include all the following *except*

    A. Vaginal bleeding.
    B. Persistent headache.
    C. Edema of hands and face.
    D. Constipation.

76. During which stage of a woman's pregnancy is it most difficult to control diabetes?

    A. When she first discovers she is pregnant.
    B. Early postpartum period.
    C. During the delivery process.
    D. During labor.

77. During which stage of labor would the nurse expect a mucus plug to be expelled?

    A. Braxton Hicks contractions.
    B. Effacement of the cervix.
    C. Transitional stage.
    D. Before delivery of the placenta.

78. Characteristics of the patient during the active stage of labor would normally include all the following *except*

    A. Contractions 1/2 to 1 minute apart and lasting 90 seconds.
    B. Dilatation of 4–7 centimeters.
    C. Mother less talkative.
    D. Increase in bloody show.

79. In the delivery room Sarah has just delivered a healthy seven-pound baby boy. The physician instructs you to suction the baby. You would

    A. Suction the nose first.
    B. Suction the mouth first.
    C. Suction neither nose nor mouth until the doctor gives you further instructions.
    D. Turn the baby on his side so the mucus will drain out.

80. Sarah is transferred from the recovery room to the postpartum unit. Routine care of the postpartum patient would include all the following *except*

    A. Maintain intake and output until patient is voiding in sufficient quantities.
    B. Massage fundus firmly every 15 minutes.

C. Assess emotional status of new mother.

D. Check breast for engorgement and cracking of nipples.

81. Mrs. Lambert is admitted to the maternity unit in her 36th week of pregnancy in an effort to control the further development of eclampsia. She is placed in a private room. The best rationale for this room assignment is

A. Mrs. Lambert is financially able to afford it.

B. Mrs. Lambert would be disturbed to be placed in a room where another mother was in active labor.

C. A quiet, darkened room is important to reduce external stimuli.

D. A rigid regimen is an important aspect of eclamptic care.

82. An expected symptom of a ruptured ectopic pregnancy would be

A. Elevated blood glucose levels.

B. Sudden excruciating pain in lower abdomen.

C. No signs of shock.

D. Extensive external bleeding.

83. Signs and symptoms of placenta previa would include all the following *except*

A. Uterus remains soft and flaccid.

B. Bleeding may be intermittent.

C. Bleeding occurs as internal os begins to dilate.

D. Bleeding is accompanied by intense pain.

84. Which one of the following conditions does *not* necessarily indicate the need for a cesarean delivery?

A. Breech baby.

B. Baby with absence of flexion of the head.

C. Abnormally large sized baby.

D. Abnormally small sized baby.

85. One of the known complications in infants delivered by cesarean section is

A. Respiratory distress.

B. Renal impairment.

C. ABO incompatibility.

D. Kernicterus.

86. Treatment of the patient with mild preeclampsia would include all the following *except*

A. High sodium diet.

B. Adequate fluid intake.

C. Daily weight.

D. Planned rest periods.

87. Of the following conditions, which one is a cardinal symptom of toxemia of pregnancy?

A. Weight gain of one pound a week.

B. Concentrated urine.

C. Hypertension.

D. Feeling of lassitude and fatigue.

88. Nursing care of the patient during pregnancy with cardiac problems would include all the following *except*

A. Alert patient to special needs during pregnancy, such as avoiding overexertion, sore throats, colds.

B. Alert patient to signs of decompensation, especially during second trimester.

C. Stress importance of taking prescribed medication, such as digitalis, and of observing for side effects.

D. Maintain patient on complete bed rest.

89. Your patient has had a Friedmann test. The test determines if

A. The fallopian tubes are patent.

B. Ovulation is occurring.

C. The patient is pregnant.

D. The sperm count is adequate.

90. Mrs. Saich has untreated *Candida albicans* vaginal infection. Baby Saich will be observed for symptoms of

A. Ophthalmia neonatorum.

B. Thrush.

C. Rhinorrhea.

D. Congenital syphilis.

91. The highest priority nursing intervention for a patient with a prolapsed cord would be to

A. Cover exposed cord with sterile dressing.

B. Leave the room momentarily to obtain assistance.

C. Place patient in knee-chest or exaggerated Trendelenburg's position.

D. Monitor fetal heartbeats.

92. Nursing care of a mother receiving regional anesthesia would include

A. Walk the patient to ensure medication is evenly distributed.

B. Ask the mother every 15 minutes to turn from side to side.

C. Monitor blood pressure every three to five minutes until stabilized.

D. Give patient sips of water to swallow during procedure.

93. Signs and symptoms of infection as a complication of the postpartum period would include all the following *except*

   A. Foul-smelling lochia or discharge.
   B. Rapid pulse.
   C. Discomfort and tenderness of the abdomen.
   D. Generalized rash.

Answers and Rationale

1. (B)   The infant usually loses 5 to 10 percent of his body weight after birth due to excess loss of fluids from body tissues and relatively low fluid intake. Infant usually regains this weight in 10 to 14 days.

2. (D)   This is an example of a congenital abnormality and does not fall into the category of a disorder of protein (abnormal or missing enzyme which interferes with metabolism).

3. (A)   Metabolic errors are often associated with mental retardation as it is believed that the missing enzyme causes metabolic changes which lead to retardation. The exact cause of the retardation, however, is not known.

4. (C)   The false pelvis is the upper, shallow portion of the pelvis that supports the enlarging pregnant uterus. The level of the ischial spines is zero. The measurement is described in centimeters above the ischial spines (minus), or below the ischial spines (plus).

5. (A)   Rh antigens from the fetus enter the bloodstream of the mother, inducing the production of anti-Rh antibodies in the mother. These anti-Rh antibodies cross the placenta, enter the fetal circulation, and cause hemolysis. The red blood cells are destroyed and broken down faster than the products of hemolysis, including bilirubin, can be excreted. Serum bilirubin rises quickly.

6. (C)   Intermittent positive-pressure breathing (IPPB) therapy is prescribed in respiratory conditions when the infant is having difficulty with oxygen-carbon dioxide exchange.

7. (B)   RhoGAM should be given after an abortion, since fetal blood may enter the mother's circulation and set up a sensitization process.

8. (C)   Constipation is rarely a problem in the newborn. Diarrhea would more likely be the result of sepsis.

9. (C)   Your responsibility is to clarify the patient's understanding of the meaning of the term functional heart murmur and to allay her fears.

10. (C)   Apgar scoring indicates whether or not resuscitative measures are required. A score of 7-10 is vigorous, and these babies usually cry soon after birth; a score of 4-6 is depressed, some resuscitative measures required; 0-3, severely depressed, resuscitation required.

11. (D)   Apgar scoring is the evaluation of five vital signs: heart rate, respiratory rate, muscle tone, reflex irritability, and color. Scores of 0, 1, or 2 are given to each vital sign for a total of 10. Since the infant showed acrocyanosis, a score of 1 was given for color, for a total score of 9.

12. (A)   The infant is wet and delivery rooms are usually cool, resulting in heat loss in the infant through conduction, convection, and radiation. Placing her in a heated crib decreases heat loss, and the Trendelenburg position is used to facilitate drainage.

13. (B)   Silver nitrate is an anti-infective agent and is used to prevent development of gonorrheal conjunctivitis in the newborn.

14. (C)   Vitamin K is necessary for blood coagulation. The newborn has a transitory deficiency in the ability of the blood to clot. Bacteria are necessary for the production of vitamin K in the intestines, and bacteria are not present in sufficient numbers in the newborn until several days after birth.

15. (D)   Caput succedaneum is edema of the soft tissues of the scalp due to the difference in pressure on the scalp between those tissues directly against cervix and those which lie on the dilated portion of cervix.

16. (D)   Normal respiratory rate in infants is between 30-50. Above or below that indicates respiratory distress.

17. (A)   Normal cardiac rate in an infant is between 120-160. It may drop down to 100 when the child is resting and up to 180 when he is crying. Above or below that indicates a cardiac or circulatory problem.

18. (D)   The newborn's liver is immature; consequently, it cannot break down bilirubin in order to excrete it from the body.

19. (A)   The eyes of the infant are covered with patches during treatment because of the possibility of damage to the retina.

20. (D)   Physiologic jaundice shows up as the bilirubin level in the blood rises. As liver function

increases, bilirubin is excreted and blood levels of bilirubin go down.

21. (A) Infants born to mothers with drug addiction are hyperirritable and care should be planned so as not to constantly stimulate the infant. When held, the infant should be wrapped snugly in blankets and held close to the body.

22. (D) RhoGAM will not work if there is any titer in the blood; thus it is important to administer it within 72 hours after delivery or abortion if the mother shows no evidence of antibody production.

23. (C) Skin color is an indication of respiratory status. Diagnosis of prematurity is based on weight, length, length of gestation, and neurological and physical characteristics.

24. (C) The premature infant has poor body control of temperature and needs immediate attention to keep from losing heat. Reasons for heat loss include little subcutaneous fat and poor insulation, large body surface for weight, immaturity of temperature control, and lack of activity.

25. (A) It is important to provide nutrients to the infant and not deplete glucose stores, but other factors are more important in immediate assessment—cardiac, respiratory, temperature, neurological status, and the presence of congenital abnormalities.

26. (A) An infant with respiratory distress will have an elevated respiratory rate to try to increase the intake of oxygen in damaged lungs, which are not functioning properly. A respiratory rate between 30–40 is within the normal range.

27. (B) Blood gases are drawn to determine if the oxygen, carbon dioxide, and pH levels are within normal range. The treatment given to the infant depends to a great extent on these results. Normal values: pH 7.35–7.45, pO_2 40–60, pCO_2 35–45.

28. (B) Premature infants are prone to respiratory distress because they are unable to produce surfactant, which leads to atelectasis. The alveolar and the thoracic cage and respiratory muscles are weak, so the infant cannot take in enough air on inspiration.

29. (D) The infant has a weak cough and gag reflex and has difficulty removing mucus. Should the bronchial secretions become dry, they become tenacious and almost impossible for the baby to bring up and difficult to remove by suctioning. Oxygen is very drying to the mucous membranes and should always be humidified while being given (whether to an infant or adult).

30. (B) High blood levels of oxygen cause spasms of the retinal vessels, and the destruction of these vessels can cause retrolental fibroplasia and blindness.

31. (A) Immaturity of the liver is responsible for hyperbilirubinemia but is not directly related to the infant acquiring an infection.

32. (C) Sterile water should be used for suctioning and should be changed at least once during each shift.

33. (A) Vitamin K is administered after birth to aid in the clotting process.

34. (C) A regular nipple is too hard and will make it difficult for the infant to suck, causing unnecessary fatigue. A premie soft nipple should be used.

35. (B) It is important for the nurse to note the amount and color of urine excreted and to check its specific gravity when there is any question about the concentration. Fluids are usually administered at room temperature and include glucose (carbohydrate) as well as protein. The premature infant does not absorb fat well. Fluids are usually given routinely, but not on a force fluid basis because it would be too fatiguing.

36. (D) The fact that she had been trying to get pregnant and now, with a hysterectomy, could never have another child would be a major concern. Fear of cancer would also be a concern, but she would have been told what Class V meant.

37. (A) At this time the nursing intervention that would be most helpful to Mrs. Norman would be to be supportive by letting her cry and express her feelings about having the operation and never being able to have another child.

38. (B) Patients about to have surgery are usually kept NPO after midnight the day of surgery to prevent emesis and aspiration while under anesthesia and while recovering from anesthesia.

39. (B) Hot flashes are a common symptom after a hysterectomy and bilateral salpingo-oophorectomy because the ovaries are removed and estrogen and progesterone are no longer produced. A surgical menopause is induced.

40. (C) After a hysterectomy a patient is usually able to resume normal sexual relationships after six weeks providing healing has taken place and the physician says it is all right.

41. (D) Daily vaginal irrigations after a hysterectomy are usually contraindicated because of the danger of introducing microorganisms and infection into a new surgical area.

42. (C) A major complication of saline abortion is the introduction of the hypertonic saline solution into the patient's bloodstream during the saline infusion causing symptoms of thirst, flushed face, headache, tachycardia, numbness, and tingling in extremities.

43. (D) After an abortion there should be slight bleeding, similar to menstruation, for about seven days. After this time, any bright red bleeding would indicate that the products of conception were probably not completely expelled.

44. (C) Following an abortion the patient may have feelings of remorse and guilt. It is important for the nurse to allow the patient to express these feelings openly. The nurse should be an active listener and not pass judgment.

45. (B) Teratogen is a term denoting "monster-former," and rubella in the first trimester is known to produce monster babies. X-rays are also considered teratogens, but dental X-rays would not have high roentgens.

46. (C) Since Wharton's jelly expands as it hits the air, ligating blood vessels, there is no danger to the baby. Cutting the cord under emergency conditions could lead to infection.

47. (B) A patient who is sixty-three years old would most likely not be menstruating. If any bleeding is noted, it is most likely a sign of a complication.

48. (C) Any sign of vaginal or rectal bleeding during a radium implant should be reported immediately to the physician as it would indicate complications had developed.

49. (B) Thirty weeks is after the time period to perform a legal abortion. The procedure should be done before 20 weeks so the fetus with Tay-Sachs disease can be aborted if the mother chooses to do so.

50. (C) Since one of the suspected side effects of the pill is thrombophlebitis, it is important to know the patient's history. If it indicates a predisposition, the pill would not be the contraceptive method of choice.

51. (D) Side effects due to hormonal influence may appear during the first few months while taking birth control pills. These side effects usually disappear after the third month as the body adjusts.

52. (A) Since the IUD may cause cramping and heavy bleeding the first few months after insertion, the patient should be thoroughly instructed as to where the IUD is inserted, how it works, and common discomforts following its insertion. The patient should be shown how to feel the strings to determine if the IUD is in place and informed that these strings will in no way interfere with intercourse.

53. (B) Contraceptive methods must be thoroughly understood if they are to be used properly and prevent pregnancy. Both partners should be informed.

54. (B) The process of genetic counseling will give the parents with one abnormal child the necessary information (diagnosis of problem and risk figures for future pregnancies) upon which to base a decision about having more children.

55. (C) The basophilic cells of the anterior pituitary secrete the gonadotropic hormones, the follicle-stimulating hormone, and the luteotropic hormone.

56. (A) The embryo receives its nourishment from the egg until implantation, and thereafter from the chorionic villi, which later fuse into the placenta. Estrogen is responsible for growth of the myometrium but does not nourish the embryo.

57. (C) Progesterone inhibits uterine motility and favors implantation of the embryo. It also aids in preparing the endometrium for implantation.

58. (B) Fertilization usually takes place in the outer third of the fallopian tube.

59. (C) Each gamete carries 23 chromosomes, so that after union of the sperm and egg, there is a total of 46 chromosomes.

60. (D) Implantation usually occurs on the seventh day after fertilization.

61. (A) Amniotic fluid should be a clear fluid. Yellow-green amniotic fluid usually indicates that it is meconium stained and the fetus is stressed or has been recently stressed.

62. (C) The placenta takes over ovarian production of hormones and produces estrogen and progesterone as well as human chorionic gonadotropin (HCG).

63. (B) The placenta acts as the organ of respiration, excretion, and nutrition for the fetus. Drugs and small molecules such as viruses may pass the placental barrier, but the bacteria molecule is too large to pass through the placental barrier.

64. (A) Nägele's rule is to subtract three months and add seven days. Using this formula, Sarah would deliver on or around 5/16/80.

65. (D) With pregnancy, there is an increased vascularity and blood supply to the vaginal area causing tissue to appear deep red or purple.

66. (B) Hypertrophy of the uterine muscle during pregnancy occurs to allow for increased size.

67. (C) Montgomery's glands enlarge and become more visible during pregnancy.

68. (A) Visual disturbance is a symptom of preeclampsia, and the patient must immediately be put under a physician's care to prevent further development of eclampsia.

69. (A) Quick mood changes are expected and are the result of changes in hormonal balance in the body as well as the woman's attempt to adjust to the new life style necessitated by having a child.

70. (C) Follicle-stimulating hormone stimulates development of the graafian follicle, which then ruptures at ovulation, releasing a mature ovum. During pregnancy this cycle is interrupted until after delivery, when the menstrual cycle resumes.

71. (A) During pregnancy gastric motility is decreased, not increased, due to the physiological changes taking place during pregnancy.

72. (C) Auscultation of fetal heart tones, sonography, and X-ray are considered positive signs of pregnancy. Outlining the fetus by palpation is not always indicative of pregnancy as a tumor may feel like a baby.

73. (C) During pregnancy there is an increased need for calories, protein, iron, calcium, and other minerals and vitamins. A high fat, high carbohydrate diet is not recommended because it may cause excessive weight gain and fat deposits, which are difficult to lose after pregnancy.

74. (D) Fatigue is common during pregnancy, and rest periods should be planned during the day to maintain optimum health and functioning.

75. (D) Constipation is a discomfort associated with pregnancy but is not usually a complication of pregnancy. Signs of complications of pregnancy are vaginal bleeding, persistent headache, edema of hands and feet, and elevated blood pressure.

76. (B) Early postpartum is a crucial period because the placenta contains the hormone insulinase and the infant produces insulin. When the baby and placenta are removed, the mother's whole metabolism changes.

77. (B) The mucus plug occludes the pregnant cervix and is expelled as the cervix begins to efface or dilate. It is most often discharged prior to admission to the hospital.

78. (A) Contractions during the active stage of labor (dilatation 4 to 7 centimeters) are usually 2 to 3 minutes apart and last 35 to 45 seconds. Contractions every 1/2 to 1 minute do not allow for uterine resting period between contractions. This resting period is necessary to allow for adequate oxygenation of the uterus and the fetus.

79. (B) It is important to suction the mouth first as the delicate recepters on the nose may be stimulated and cause the infant to inhale the mucus in the mouth.

80. (B) The uterus should be massaged only when it feels boggy, and then it should be massaged very lightly with one hand over the symphysis pubis (to prevent inversion of the uterus) and the other placed lightly on the top of the fundus. To massage a contracted uterus firmly every 15 minutes could cause it to lose its tone.

81. (C) An important aspect of the treatment for preeclampsia is absolute quiet, and only a private room could accomplish this objective.

82. (B) In a ruptured ectopic pregnancy, there may be signs of shock, excruciating pain, and little bleeding. There should be no effect on blood glucose levels.

83. (D) Bleeding in placenta previa is usually not accompanied by pain. Bleeding accompanied by intense pain usually indicates abruptio placenta.

84. (D) A small baby could easily be delivered naturally if there were no abnormalities of the power or passage, while all the other conditions would require a cesarean delivery.

85. (A) During a normal birth the fetus passes through the birth canal, and pressure on the chest helps rid the fetus of amniotic fluid that has accumulated in the lung. The baby delivered by cesarean section does not go through this process.

86. (A) The patient with mild preeclampsia would more than likely be placed on a limited sodium diet or a normal diet that avoids highly salted foods. The preeclamptic patient has a tendency to retain sodium and fluids and become edematous.

87. (C) High blood pressure is one of the cardinal symptoms of toxemia, along with excessive weight gain, edema and albumin in the urine.

88. (D) Bed rest during pregnancy is not necessary for individuals with cardiac disease unless they are suffering from an extreme form of the disease. Bed rest may be advisable at certain times during pregnancy when the workload is especially hard on the heart or if signs of cardiac decompensation occur.

89. (C) The Rubin's test determines if the fallopian tubes are patent. The Friedmann test (rabbit test) is a modification of the A–Z pregnancy test. A sperm count is done as part of semen analysis.

90. (B) Ophthalmia neonatorum occurs in infants whose mothers have an untreated gonorrheal infection. Thrush is white patches on the infant's oral mucosa when the infant has come in direct contact with a contaminated maternal birth canal. Rhinorrhea occurs in the drug-dependent infant. Congenital syphilis occurs when the mother has untreated syphilis.

91. (C) Cord prolapse is a very serious complication. The danger to the fetus is great because compression on the cord leads to deprived oxygenation. Those patients should never be left alone, and the highest priority measure should be taken to relieve the pressure of the fetal body or head off the cord. This nursing action should be followed by administration of oxygen.

92. (C) Regional anesthesia, such as caudal or epidural, may cause vasodilatation by causing blood to pool in the extremities. This may lead to maternal hypotension. Immediate treatment is to elevate both legs for a few minutes in order to return the blood to the central circulation, and then turn the patient on her side to reduce pressure on the veins and arteries in the pelvic area.

93. (D) A generalized rash would not be a sign of postpartum infection but would indicate a virus infection, such as measles, or an allergic reaction to a medication or food. A rash should never be ignored; rather it should be charted and its cause investigated.

Pediatric Nursing

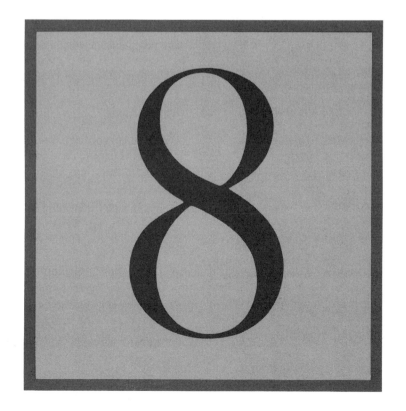

Growth and Development

Principles of Growth and Development*

Maturation

A. The process of maturation.
1. Process of attaining maximum growth and development.
2. Process of the unfolding of inherited tendencies, independent of any special practice or training.

B. Major principles of growth and development.
1. Occurs in an orderly sequence.
2. Continuous, but continuity may be interrupted by spurts of growth and periods of no growth.
3. Progresses at individualized rates.
4. Different ages vary for specific body structures.
5. Each individual has an inherent growth pattern.
6. Increases in structure (growth) are accompanied by increases in function (development).

C. Major influences on growth and development.
1. Genetic factors.
2. Environmental variations.

Profiles of Growth and Development

A. Physical development.
1. Growth rate.
   a. Rapid during infancy
   b. Slow and steady during childhood.
   c. Spurt during puberty.
   d. Decrease; maximum height attained during adolescence.
2. Height.
   a. Average length is 20 inches at birth.
   b. Increases ten inches in the first year.

For Growth and Development Milestones by age group, see Chapter One.

   c. Increases five inches in the second year.
   d. Increases three inches per year from the third to the sixth year.
   e. Increases by about two inches per year after sixth year.
   f. Peak reached by boys at about fourteen years of age.
   g. Peak reached by girls at about thirteen years of age.
3. Weight.
   a. Average weight is seven and a half pounds at birth.
   b. Doubles by the end of the fifth month, and triples by the end of first year.
   c. Increases by about five pounds per year until puberty, and then increases rapidly.
   d. Levels off with only little gain after puberty.
4. Body proportions.
   a. Striking changes from birth to maturity.
   b. At birth, head is one-fourth of the total body length; the adult head is only about one-eighth of the total body length.
5. Bone formation.
   a. What will later be bone begins as connective tissue, which gradually becomes cartilage, and finally, through the process of ossification, becomes bone.
   b. Bone formation complete in girls at about seventeen years of age.
   c. Bone formation is complete in boys at about nineteen years of age.
6. Teeth formation.
   a. First two lower central incisors appear between the fifth and seventh month followed by about one new tooth per month.
   b. The set of 20 deciduous teeth should be complete by the age of two and a half years. (For chart of dental development, see appendix 7.)

B. Motor development.
1. Includes learning, controlling, and integrating muscular responses.

2. Occurs in an orderly sequence, and is related to the maturation of the nervous system.
3. Begins at the head, moves downward, and proceeds from the center of the body toward the extremities.
4. Effective use of the hands for seizing and grasping objects (prehension) begins between the second and third month.
5. Ability to walk alone (locomotion) is attained gradually and begins with holding up the head; most infants have learned to walk alone between the ages of twelve and fourteen months.

C. Intellectual development.
1. Intelligence is the ability to think, to reason, to remember, and to imagine.
2. Intelligence develops gradually and continuously.

D. Emotional development.
1. Emotions begin to develop early.
2. Few individuals react to the same emotion in the same way.
3. Emotions of fear, excitement, anger, and joy are recognizable at one year of age.
4. Emotions are expressed by facial expressions, vocalization, and body movements.

Hospitalization

Stages of Separation Anxiety

A. Protest.
1. Characteristics: cries loudly, throws tantrums.
2. Nursing behaviors: stay close to the child to provide warmth and support.

B. Despair.
1. Characteristics: withdraws, shows no interest in eating, playing, or interacting; typical during extended hospitalization.

2. Nursing behaviors: recognize the anxiety and establish a relationship with the child; attempt to engage and involve the child in an activity.

C. Denial.
1. Characteristics: exhibits behavior that is often mistaken for happy adjustment; ignores mother and may regress.
2. Nursing behaviors: reassure the mother, develop a relationship with the child, and provide warmth and support to the child during long hospitalization.

Hospitalization of the Infant

Psychological Implications

A. Separation from the parent is threatening.
B. Decrease in sensory stimuli.
C. Causes of breakdown in mother-infant relationship.
1. Maternal guilt.
2. Hostile, cold hospital environment.
3. Lessened opportunity for mothering role; mother may feel inadequate.
4. Subordination of the parents by the staff.

Nursing Care

A. Take positive nursing action to prevent the detrimental effects of hospitalization.
B. Provide a prehospitalization nursing interview with the parents and give a tour of the pediatric unit.
1. Explain procedures, regulations, and the rationale behind the rules; arrange for parents to meet the staff.
2. Encourage parents to visit frequently and/or to possibly room in.
C. Counsel the parents regarding the infant's illness.
1. Elicit their understanding of the disease as well as its likely progressive course.
2. Correct any misconceptions and, if appropriate, reassure them that they are not the cause of the illness.

D. Encourage the parents to participate in the infant's care if they show an interest in doing so.
   1. Teach the parents procedures they are capable of doing.
   2. Show respect for superior knowledge of their infant in respect to likes, dislikes, and habits.
E. Assume role of the absent mother.
   1. Limit, initially, the number of people handling the infant; allow one person to become familiar with the infant and gradually introduce others.
   2. Provide closeness and warmth by cuddling.
   3. Avoid isolating the infant from sensory stimulation.
      a. Provide stimulation during feeding.
      b. Hang brightly colored mobiles within the infant's sight.
   4. Play with the infant.

Hospitalization of the Toddler and Preschool Child

Psychological Implications

A. Hospitalization is a very threatening experience for a child.
   1. Unfamiliar situations and procedures are experienced.
   2. Growing sense of identity and independence may be disrupted.
B. Experiences separation anxiety; child mourns the absence of the mother through protest, despair, and denial.
C. The loss of "body integrity" is feared.
   1. Does not realistically perceive how the body functions.
   2. May overreact to a simple procedure; some toddlers believe that drawing blood will leave a hole and that the rest of their blood will leak out.
D. Disruption of normal rituals and routines are resented; toddlers are often very rigid about those procedures that allow them a sense of security and control over otherwise frightening circumstances.

E. Loss of mobility is frustrating to a child.
F. Most recent acquired behaviors are frequently abandoned, and toddler reverts to safer, less mature patterns (regression).

Nursing Care

A. Introduce the child to hospital surroundings, preferably prior to hospitalization.
B. Explain all the procedures in simple terms and allow for further discussion, if desired.
C. Encourage parents to room in or to visit frequently once the child is hospitalized.
D. Suggest that the mother leave an object that the child associates with her for the child to "care for" until she can return. This procedure assures the child that his mother will return.
E. Encourage the parents to be honest about when they are going and coming. Do not tell the child they will stay all night and then leave when the child is asleep.
F. Paste family pictures to the crib.
G. Use puppet play to explain procedures and to gain an understanding of the child's perception of his hospitalization. Use puppets to work out anxiety, anger, and frustration.
H. When recording developmental history elicit exact routines and rituals that the child uses; attempt to modify hospital routine to continue these rituals.
I. Provide stretchers, wheelchairs, and carts for immobilized children.
J. Do not punish the child for reverting to less mature behavior patterns; explain the reasons for its occurrence to the parents.

Hospitalization of the School-Age Child

Psychological Implications

A. The school-age child needs to understand why things are happening as they are.
B. The child has a heightened concern for privacy.
C. The child is modest and fears disgrace.

D. Hospitalization interrupts busy school life, and child fears he or she will be replaced or forgotten by peer group.

E. Absence from peer group means a disruption of close friendships.

Nursing Care

A. Inform the child about his or her illness; take the opportunity to explain how the body functions.

B. Explain all procedures completely; allow the child to see special rooms (i.e., intensive care, cardiac catheter lab) prior to being sent to them for treatments.

C. Provide opportunities for the child to socialize with his or her peer group at meals and through team tournaments of cards, chess, and checkers.

D. Allow telephone privileges for calls to his or her home and friends.

E. Provide outlets (e.g., dart board and a boxing bag) for anger and frustration.

F. Give the child opportunity to make choices and exert independence.

G. Protect the child's privacy.

H. Provide tutors to prevent disruption of education.

I. Provide the opportunity to master developmental tasks of age group.

Hospitalization of the Adolescent

Psychological Implications

A. Concern with disruption of social system and peer group.

B. Fear of alteration of body image.

C. Fear of loss of independence.

D. Fear of change in future plans.

E. Concern with interruption in development of heterosexual relationships.

F. Resentment of loss of privacy.

G. The degree to which the young adult is affected depends on several factors.

1. Whether the illness is chronic or acute.

2. Whether the final prognosis necessitates a change in the young adult's future aspirations.

3. The number of changes which he or she must accept.

Nursing Care

A. Adolescents should be placed in rooms with their peers.

B. Allow telephone privileges with some limitations of time.

C. Enhance the adolescent's feeling of self-worth, and encourage as much independence as possible.

D. Allow reasonable heterosexual relationships to develop.

E. Provide for privacy.

F. Assist adolescent in role model identification.

G. Realistically discuss problems of the illness with the adolescent.

H. Always provide honest information.

I. Encourage the adolescent, if able, to accept reasonable responsibility for unit decorum.

General Assessment—Infant to Adolescent

General Principles

A. Maturational ability of the child to cooperate with the examiner is of major importance to adequate physical assessment.

B. When planning physical assessment of the child, the following points should be considered:

1. Establish a relationship with the child prior to the examination.
   a. Determine child's maturational level.
   b. Allow the child an opportunity to become more accustomed to the examiner.

2. Explain in terms appropriate to the child's level of understanding the extent and purpose of the examination.

3. Realize that the physical examination may be a stressful experience for the child, who is

helpless and depends on others for protection.

4. Limit the physical examination to what is essential in determining an adequate nursing diagnosis.

5. Proceed from the least to the most intrusive procedures.

6. Allow active participation of the child whenever possible.

Special Considerations for Each Age Group

The Infant

A. Accomplish as much of the examination as possible while the infant is sleeping or resting undisturbed.

B. Assess general condition.
   1. Symmetry and location of body parts.
   2. Color and condition of the skin.
   3. State of restlessness and sleeplessness.
   4. Adjustment to feeding regimen.
   5. Quality of cry.

C. Congenital anomaly appraisal.
   1. Neurological system.
      a. Reflexes: absent or asymmetrical (see Appendix 2).
      b. Head circumference: microcephaly, hydrocephaly.
         (1) 35 cm. at birth.
         (2) 40 cm. at 3 months.
         (3) 45 cm. at 9 months.
         (4) At birth, the head size is 2 cm. larger than the chest. Equals or exceeds chest until 2 years of age.
      c. Fontanels: closed, bulging.
         (1) Anterior measures 3.5 cm. by 3.5 cm. and closes by 18 months.
         (2) Posterior measures 1 cm. by 1 cm. and closes at 2 months.
      d. Eyes: cataracts, lid folds, spots on iris.
   2. Respiratory system.
      a. Breath sounds: signs of aspiration, asymmetry of lung expansion, retractions, grunting.
      b. Apnea.

3. Cardiovascular system.
   a. Color: cyanosis.
   b. Rate and rhythm: murmurs, tachycardia, bradycardia.
   c. Energy level: cannot suck for fifteen minutes without exhaustion or cyanosis.

4. Gastrointestinal tract.
   a. History of polyhydramnios.
   b. Patency: mucus, spitting, cyanosis, cannot pass nasogastric tube to stomach.
   c. Mouth: palate or lip not intact.
   d. Anus: not patent.

5. Genitourinary.
   a. Umbilical vessels: missing normal two arteries and one vein.
   b. Urine: abnormal stream.
   c. Masses: abdominal (Wilms' tumor).
   d. Boys: undescended testicles, hernia, urethra not opening at the end of the penis.
   e. Girls: labial adhesions.

6. Skeletal system.
   a. Fractured clavicle.
   b. Dislocated hip: asymmetric major gluteal folds, hip click.
   c. Legs and feet: clubbing, without straight tibial line.
   d. Spine: curved, inflexible, open.

D. Common Problems.

   1. Ear infections.
      a. Increased temperature, irritability.
      b. Rubbing or pulling ear.
      c. Change in eating habits.

   2. Upper respiratory infections.
      a. Duration of symptoms, severity.
      b. Wheezing, barking cough, anxiety, restlessness, use of accessory muscles.
      c. If throat is sore, check white patches on tonsils.

   3. Rashes.
      a. Onset, duration, description, location.
      b. Any event such as new food, exposure to animals.

   4. Contact dermatitis.
      a. Allergic problems.
      b. Diaper area rash: use of soap, lotions, powders; method of cleaning cloth diapers.

5. Hernias.
   a. Inguinal: lump in groin, with or without pain.
   b. Umbilical: can it be pushed back without difficulty or pain.
6. Scalp-cradle cap.
   a. Scalp scaling, crusted; method of washing hair.
   b. Application of any lotions or balms to hair.
7. Birth marks.
   a. Change in size, color, shape.
   b. Any bleeding or irritation.
8. Eye symmetry.
   a. Frequency of a problem with eye alignment: (time of day eyes wander).
   b. Light reflex symmetrical in both eyes.

E. Screening procedures.
   1. Developmental landmarks—DDST (Denver Developmental Screening Test).
   2. Vision.
   3. Hearing.
   4. Growth charts: head circumference, weight, length.

F. Nursing guidance areas.
   1. Growth and development changes.
   2. Stranger anxiety.
   3. Separation anxiety.
   4. Transitional objects.
   5. Accident prevention.

The Toddler and the Preschool Child

A. General considerations.
   1. Remember that separation anxiety is most acute at toddler age and body integrity fears most acute at preschool age.
   2. Involve the parent in examination as much as possible.
   3. Restrain child as much as necessary to protect the child from injury.
   4. Give careful explanation of each portion of the exam.
   5. Allow the child to handle the equipment and try out on doll.

B. Common Problems.
   1. Feeding and eating.
      a. Review food ingested in last 48 hours.
      b. Types of foods, adequate source of vitamins, minerals.
   2. Temper tantrums.
      a. Frequency, duration, precipitating event.
      b. Response of caretaker.
   3. Toilet training.
      a. Check ability to ambulate (indicating neuromuscular maturity).
      b. Bothered by wet diapers. Interested in toileting.
   4. Respiratory infections: see Infant section.
   5. Communicable diseases.
      a. Onset of symptoms, progression of disease, treatment of symptoms.
      b. Observation of complications.
   6. Gastrointestinal
      a. Onset, duration, intake and output.
      b. Signs of dehydration.

C. Screening procedures (same as Infant).

School Age Child

A. General considerations.
   1. Modesty important.
   2. Explain all procedures.
   3. Direct questions to child.

B. Common problems.
   1. School.
      a. Signs of school phobias, vomits before school, delays going.
      b. Increase in physical complaints.
   2. Nervous habits (stuttering, twitching, etc.).
      a. Onset, duration, precipitating event.
      b. Anxiety of child and parent over problem.
   3. Accidental trauma.
      a. Understanding of accident.
      b. Prevention, physical limitations.
   4. Respiratory infections: see Infant section.
   5. Gastrointestinal infections: see Preschooler section.

C. Screening procedures.
 1. Snellen vision testing.
 2. Sweep check audiometry.
 3. Height and weight measurement.
 4. Inspection of skin and teeth.

D. Nursing guidance areas.
 1. Need for autonomy.
 2. Toilet training.
 3. Imaginary friends.
 4. Fear of dark.
 5. Rituals and routines.

Adolescent

A. General considerations.
 1. Examine child alone if he wishes (privacy important).
 2. Note signs of puberty.
 3. Ascertain feelings about body image.

B. Common Problems.
 1. Acne.
  a. Existing skin care program.
  b. Personal hygiene.
 2. Dysmenorrhea.
  a. Degree of pain, missed school.
  b. Use of analgesics.
  c. Amount of exercise.
 3. Obesity.
  a. Eating patterns.
  b. Family concern.
  c. Amount of exercise.

C. Screening procedures (same as School Age).

D. Nursing guidance areas.
 1. Hazards of cigarette smoking and alcohol.
 2. Transmission and symptoms of venereal disease.
 3. Review sex education.
 4. Accident prevention—particularly automobile.
 5. Principles of nutrition.

The Newborn and Infant

Congenital Anomalies

Cleft Lip

Definition: Fissure or split in the upper lip resulting from failure of the two sides of the face to unite properly.

Treatment and Nursing Care

A. Preoperative care.
 1. Use a large holed, soft nipple for feedings.
 2. Prevent infections.
 3. Place nipple on side opposite defect.
 4. Bubble frequently.
B. Surgical procedure.
 1. Closure of lip.
 2. Performed at about three months of age or when infant is ten pounds.
C. Postoperative care.
 1. Observe for respiratory distress and swelling of tongue, nostrils, and mouth.
 2. Avoid circumstances that will cause crying.
 3. Watch for hemorrhage.
 4. Use elbow restraints and provide supervised rest periods to exercise arms.
 5. Feed with rubber-tipped medicine dropper on the side opposite the repaired cleft for three weeks.
 6. After feeding, clean suture line with half-strength hydrogen peroxide.
 7. Prevent crust formation on suture line by frequent cleansing and application of ointment.
 8. Lay infant on side or back with support to prevent rolling over on the abdomen.
 9. Prevent infections.

Cleft Palate

Definition: Fissure or split in the roof of mouth (palate) resulting from failure of two sides of face to unite. There may be involvement of both the hard and soft palate.

Signs and Symptoms

A. Poor sucking reflex so infant unable to form a vacuum in the mouth.
B. If able to talk, there may be a speech impediment.
C. Increased incidence of upper respiratory infections.

Treatment and Nursing Care

A. Preoperative care.
  1. Prevent infections.
  2. Give nothing by mouth.
B. Surgical procedure.
  1. May be performed in stages if the defect is bilateral.
  2. The repair is usually made after eighteen months of age.
C. Postoperative care.
  1. Apply hand restraints to prevent damage to the mouth.
  2. Provide good oral hygiene.
  3. Prevent infections.
  4. Provide safe toys with no small parts.
  5. Sedate and attempt to keep infant content.
  6. Feed liquids using a cup or spoon.

Esophageal Atresia

Definition: Closure of the esophagus during embryonic development; usually ends in a blind pouch.

Signs and Symptoms

A. Excessive amounts of saliva.
B. Drooling.
C. Respiratory distress with each feeding.

Treatment and Nursing Care

A. Preoperative care.
  1. Observe carefully.
  2. Clear airway.
  3. Elevate head of bed 30 degrees.
  4. Give nothing by mouth.
  5. Maintain sucking reflex.
B. Surgical procedure.
  1. Repair the esophagus.
  2. Gastrostomy for feeding access.
C. Postoperative care.
  1. Provide rest with infrequent handling.
  2. Keep gastrostomy tube open.
  3. Feed through gastrostomy tube.
  4. Maintain patent airway.
  5. Elevate head of bed 30 degrees.
  6. Maintain sucking reflex.

Hydrocephalus

Definition: Abnormal accumulation of spinal fluid within the brain causing an increase in intracranial pressure. Accumulation may be due either to blockage of the flow of spinal fluid or to the lack of proper absorption of the spinal fluid.

Signs and Symptoms

A. Increase in size and shape of head.
B. Suture lines separated with bulging fontanels.
C. Dilated scalp veins.
D. Strabismus and nystagmus.
E. "Sunset" eyes (sclera visible above the iris).
F. Projectile vomiting and anorexia.
G. Irritability and lethargy.
H. Poor neck control.

Treatment and Nursing Care

A. Preoperative care.
  1. Feed small amounts with care to prevent vomiting.
  2. Change position frequently to prevent pneumonia and pressure sores on the head.
  3. Support the infant's head when turning or moving.
  4. Prevent infection.
  5. Carefully observe vital signs.
  6. Observe for signs of increased intracranial pressure.
  7. Provide emotional support for both parents and infant.

B. Surgical procedure: ventriculovenous shunt performed to reduce the volume of spinal fluid within the ventricles.
C. Postoperative care.
 1. Maintain open airway.
 2. Carefully observe vital signs.
 3. Look for signs of increased intracranial pressure.
 4. Give nothing by mouth for four to six hours after surgery.
 5. Carefully begin to feed clear fluids.
 6. Meet the needs of the normal newborn.
 7. Measure head circumference.
 8. Position the head opposite the side of the shunt.
 9. Support the head when turning or changing the position.
 10. Prevent infection.
 11. Give emotional support to infant and parents.

Spina Bifida

Definition: Defect in the spinal column caused either by failure of the posterior part of the laminae of the vertebrae to fuse or by absence of part of the laminae. The defect usually occurs in the lumbosacral area, but it may occur at any level of the spine.

Types of Spina Bifida

A. *Spina bifida occulta:* Bony defect in the spine that may have a visible dimple or a small tuft of hair in the area.
B. *Meningocele:* Protrusion of meninges and cerebral spinal fluid through the opening in the spine which may be covered only by a thin membranous sac.
C. *Myelomeningocele:* Protrusion of meninges, cerebral spinal fluid, spinal cord, and nerves through the defect in the spine; there may be paralysis below the level of the defect.

Treatment and Nursing Care

A. Preoperative care.
 1. Prevent infection.
 2. Observe movement of the extremities.
 3. Observe bowel and bladder function.
 4. Provide normal newborn care.
B. Surgical procedure.
 1. Removal of the protrusion.
 2. Closure of the defect.
C. Postoperative care.
 1. Prevent infection.
 2. Use Credé method on the bladder.
 3. Provide range of motion exercises to lower extremities.
 4. Provide good skin care.
 5. Give emotional support to infant and parents.

Down's Syndrome

Definition: Physical malformation and degree of mental retardation resulting from a chromosomal defect.

Signs and Symptoms

A. Face characterized by rounded shape, flattened nose, thickened tongue, almond-shaped eyes, and flattened occiput.
B. Muscles flaccid; motor development will be slow.
C. Extremities characterized by short, fat hands with simian crease on the palms and little finger curved inward.
D. Mental capacity varies from mild to severe retardation. These children are usually very happy.

Nursing Care

A. Individualize according to needs of the infant and the family.
B. Give assistance in contacting community agencies that can assist the family with the infant's needs.
C. Encourage developmental activities initiated at the proper time.
D. Observe for other anomalies in the infant.

E. Alert the family of the necessity to take precautions against infection.

F. Refer the family to a geneticist.

Phenylketonuria (PKU)

Definition: Failure of the body to normally metabolize the amino acid phenylalanine. High levels of this amino acid in the blood can cause mental retardation. The condition is genetically transmitted; most state health departments mandate PKU testing before the infant's discharge from the hospital.

Signs and Symptoms

A. Brain development arrested by four months of age if left untreated.

B. Moderate to severe retardation by one year of age if left untreated. Retardation level correlates with high PKU levels and this condition is irreversible.

Treatment and Nursing Care

A. Restrict phenylalanine in the diet until about five years of age.

B. Eliminate foods high in protein, e.g., meat, poultry, fish, eggs, nuts, legumes, and milk products.

C. Observe for signs of phenylalanine deficiency, e.g., lethargy, anorexia, anemia, skin rashes, and diarrhea.

D. Suggest genetic counseling to the parents.

E. Gently remind parents to have all future children born to them screened for PKU.

Failure to Thrive

Definition: A syndrome characterized by an infant's failure to grow and develop with or without characteristic posturing or "body language." Etiology is nonspecific. May be organic or nonorganic.

Signs and Symptoms

A. History of infant includes feeding problems, vomiting, sleep disturbance, irritability, sucking ability, aversion to formula, and irregularity in daily activities.

B. Abnormal nutritional intake cause may be related to deficient intake, malabsorption, or poor assimilation.
   1. Number of calories, quality of calories, and feeding patterns.
   2. Weigh daily and observe reaction to nutritional program.

C. Nature of mother-child relationship.
   1. Relationship patterns.
   2. Ability of mother to perceive infant's needs.

Nursing Care

A. Priority—provide sufficient nutrients so that infant will grow.
   1. Develop a structured feeding routine.
   2. Weigh daily to assess weight gain.

B. Provide nuturing to infant.
   1. Ensure a warm, loving environment through holding, cuddling, and physical contact.
   2. Spend time talking to infant and building a trusting relationship.
   3. Maintain as much eye-to-eye contact as possible.

C. Provide a positive, quiet, nonstimulating environment to promote psychosocial growth.

D. Assist mother to develop a positive relationship with infant.

E. Document feeding behaviors and monitor infant progress.

Sudden Infant Death Syndrome (SIDS)

Definition: The sudden, unexplained death of an infant during sleep.

Characteristics

A. Largest single cause of death after neonatal

period.

B. Peak incidence 2 to 4 months; rare after 6 months.

C. Higher incidence in winter months, in low income groups, and in low birth weight infants.

D. Most deaths are unobserved and occur during sleep.

E. On autopsy, inflammation of upper respiratory tract is found.

F. Etiology unknown and controversial. Many theories involving CO_2 sensitivity, massive virus, poor response to stimulus.

Treatment

A. Support of parents—help work through feelings of guilt and loss.

B. Refer to National Foundation for Sudden Infant Death.

Congenital Heart Defects

Definition: A structural defect of heart or great vessels. The defects are present at birth. *Cyanotic* (with cyanosis) defects allow unoxygenated blood to circulate throughout the body. *Acyanotic* (without cyanosis) defects shunt blood previously oxygenated back to the lungs and allow oxygenated blood to go to the body.

Fetal Circulation

A. Major structures of fetal circulation.
1. Ductus venosus—a structure that shunts blood past the portal circulation.
2. Foramen ovale—an opening between the right and left atria of the heart that shunts blood past the lungs.
3. Ductus arteriosus—a structure between the aorta and the pulmonary artery that shunts blood past the lungs.

B. Changes in circulation at birth.
1. The umbilical arteries and vein and the ductus venosus become nonfunctional.
2. The lungs expand, reducing resistance, and greater amounts of blood enter the pulmonary circulation.
3. More blood in the pulmonary circulation increases the return of blood to the left atrium, which initiates the closure of the flap of tissue covering the foramen ovale.
4. The ductus arteriosus contracts and the blood flow decreases; eventually, the duct closes.

C. Two major clues to presence of heart disease.
1. Congestive heart failure.
   a. Begins before one year of age in majority of infants.
   b. Most infants are less than six months old.
2. Cyanosis.

Coarctation of Aorta

Definition: Stenosis or narrowing of the aorta.

Signs and Symptoms

A. Increased blood pressure in the arms.

B. Decreased blood pressure in the thighs; may have no femoral pulses that are palpable.

C. Headache and nose bleeds.

D. May have no audible murmurs.

Treatment and Nursing Care

A. Resection of the aorta or insertion of a graft.

B. Surgery delayed as long as possible, depending on the condition of the vessel.

Patent Ductus Arteriosus

Definition: Failure of the ductus arteriosus to close after birth.

Signs and Symptoms

A. Dyspnea on exertion.
B. Growth failure.
C. Loud murmur.

Treatment and Nursing Care

A. Closing of ductus.
B. Surgery usually performed between two and five years of age.

Atrial Septal and Ventricular Septal Defects

Definition: Failure of the septum in either the atrium or the ventricle to completely develop. The extent of severity of the defect is dependent on the size and location of the opening.

Signs and Symptoms

A. Frequent upper respiratory infections.
B. Cyanosis on exertion.
C. Loud murmurs.

Treatment and Nursing Care

A. Surgical closure to repair defect.
B. Surgery delayed as long as possible to allow child to grow.

Tetralogy of Fallot

Definition: Combination of four heart defects— ventricular septal defect, pulmonary stenosis, overriding of aorta, and hypertrophy of the right ventricle.

Signs and Symptoms

A. Cyanosis.
B. Growth failure.
C. Polycythemia.
D. Black-out spells.
E. Convulsions.
F. The child normally assumes a squatting position to facilitate breathing.

Treatment and Nursing Care

A. Surgical closure.
B. Surgery delayed as long as possible.

Transposition of the Great Vessels

Definition: Reversal of the position of the aorta and the pulmonary artery.

Signs and Symptoms

A. Cyanosis.
B. Dyspnea.
C. Tachycardia.
D. Increased respirations.

Treatment and Nursing Care

A. Preoperative care.
   1. Prevent infection.
   2. Encourage rest.
   3. Observe vital signs with care.
   4. Provide emotional support for the child and family.
   5. Prepare for surgery with the usual preoperative teaching of breathing exercises (e.g., cough and deep breathing; blow bottles).
B. Surgical procedure.
   1. Mustard procedure (delayed as long as possible).
   2. In infancy a shunt is usually necessary to get more oxygenated blood to the body.
C. Postoperative care.
   1. Maintain pulmonary function with suctioning, oxygen, deep-breathing, and/or care of the chest tubes.
   2. Observe vital signs, intake and output, and color.
   3. Provide good skin care.
   4. Provide adequate rest periods.
   5. Maintain patient comfort with medications and necessary positioning.
   6. Provide emotional support for the child and the family.

Disorders of the Infant

Otitis Media

Definition: Inflammation of the middle ear resulting from an infection-producing organism.

Signs and Symptoms

A. Pain in the ears.
B. Fever.
C. Irritability.
D. Headache.
E. Convulsions.

Treatment and Nursing Care

A. Antibiotics.
B. Myringotomy—incision that opens up the tympanic membrane.
C. Observe vital signs.
D. Take measures to reduce fever if present.
E. Provide good skin care; maintain cleanliness of the ear canal.
F. Irrigate ear if ordered.
G. Apply local heat to the ears if ordered.

Bronchiolitis

Definition: Inflammation of the bronchioles caused by thick mucus that traps air in the alveoli which leads to poor air exchange. Bronchiolitis usually occurs before eighteen months of age.

Signs and Symptoms

A. Dry, nonproductive cough.
B. Nasal discharge.
C. Dyspnea.
D. Cyanosis.
E. Dehydration.
F. Irritability.

Treatment and Nursing Care

A. Maintain patent airway.
B. Give nothing by mouth until dyspnea improved.
C. Maintain intravenous feedings as ordered.
D. Provide humidity and oxygen as necessary.
E. Elevate head of bed.

Pyloric Stenosis

Definition: Obstruction in the opening between the stomach and the intestine resulting from enlargement (hypertrophy) of the pyloric muscle. The condition is more common in the male infant and usually is diagnosed between four and six weeks of age.

Signs and Symptoms

A. Projectile vomiting soon after or during a feeding.
   1. Vomitus contains no bile.
   2. Formula appears to be almost the same as when ingested.
B. Weight loss and dehydration.
C. Constipation.

Treatment and Nursing Care

A. Preoperative care.
   1. Elevate head of bed 30 degrees.
   2. Give nothing by mouth.
   3. Maintain intravenous feedings as ordered.
   4. Adjust nasogastric tube to low suction.
B. Surgical procedure.
   1. Pyloromyotomy—the incision of pylorus muscles.
   2. Fredet-Ramstedt procedure.
C. Postoperative care.
   1. Adjust nasogastric tube to low suction for a few hours.
   2. Maintain intravenous fluids.
   3. Feed small amounts of clear liquids frequently, and increase them as tolerated.
   4. Elevate head of bed 30 degrees.
   5. Check dressing for bleeding.

Intussusception

Definition: Invagination or telescoping of one part of the bowel into another part below it. The condition occurs most frequently in boys between the ages of four and ten months.

Signs and Symptoms

A. Severe colic-like pain in the abdomen.
B. Progressive vomiting.
C. Bloody stools.
D. Shock.

Treatment and Nursing Care

A. Barium enema, which may be effective in reducing invagination.
B. Preoperative care.
  1. Adjust nasogastric tube to low suction.
  2. Give nothing by mouth.
  3. Maintain intravenous liquids.
  4. Provide emotional support.
C. Surgical procedure.
  1. May only need to manipulate the bowel back to its normal position.
  2. A resection may be required, depending on when the diagnosis was made.
  3. Excision of involved area with end-to-end anastomosis.
D. Postoperative care.
  1. Maintain intravenous fluids.
  2. Adjust nasogastric tube to low suction.
  3. Begin oral feeding of clear fluids.
  4. Observe vital signs.
  5. Check dressing for bleeding.

Hirschsprung's Disease (Congenital Megacolon)

Definition: Lack of normal nerve ganglia in the distal end of the colon. Length of colon involved varies with each individual. Condition is more common in males.

Signs and Symptoms

A. Newborn may or may not pass meconium.
B. Constipation is progressive as diet increases.
C. Progressive abdominal distention.
D. Anorexia.
E. Occasional vomiting.

Treatment and Nursing Care

A. Provide daily enemas, stool softeners, and a low residue diet.
B. Surgical procedure.
  1. Swenson's pull-through or variation of the procedure.
  2. Temporary colostomy above narrowed section.

Diarrhea

Definition: Frequent, watery bowel movements that result from an increased wave-like movement in the intestines.

Types of Diarrhea

A. Infectious—caused by either bacterial or viral organism.
B. Noninfectious—caused by an irritant in the intestinal tract, e.g., foods, drugs, laxatives, or other irritants.

Signs and Symptoms

A. May be mild to severe.
B. Frequent stools, usually foul smelling, greenish in color, watery, and expelled with force.
C. Abdominal distention.
D. Irritability.
E. Weight loss and dehydration.
F. Increased rate of peristalsis.

Treatment and Nursing Care

A. Replace electrolytes.
B. Give antibiotics if caused by an organism and/or to prevent secondary infection.

C. Give nothing by mouth. Desire for food will increase as stools decrease.
D. Isolate infant to prevent spread of diarrhea throughout the nursery.
E. Measure intake and output.
F. Weigh infant daily.
G. Maintain intravenous feedings if ordered.
H. Give good skin care.

Sickle Cell Anemia

Definition: Tendency of red blood cells to be crescent shaped when under low oxygen tension. The disorder results from the presence of abnormal type of hemoglobin and is transmitted as a recessive dominant trait, particularly among blacks.

Signs and Symptoms

A. In noncrisis state the infant experiences the following symptoms.
  1. Severe chronic anemia.
  2. Periodic crises with abdominal and joint pain.
  3. Enlarged spleen from increased activity.
  4. Jaundice from excessive red blood cell destruction.
  5. Widening of the marrow spaces of the bones.
  6. Gallstones.
B. In crisis state the infant experiences episodes with the following characteristics.
  1. Thrombotic crisis is the most frequent type and is caused by occlusion of the small blood vessels, which produces distal ischemia and infarction.
    a. Swelling of hands and feet.
    b. Large joints and surrounding areas may become painful and swollen.
    c. Severe abdominal pains.
  2. Sequestration crisis is less frequent and occurs only in young children; it is caused by pooling of blood in spleen.
    a. Enlargement of the spleen.
    b. Circulatory collapse.

Treatment and Nursing Care

A. Alleviate pain with analgesics.
B. Prevent dehydration with intravenous infusion if necessary and increased fluid intake.
C. Offer parents genetic counseling.
D. Counsel the family on physiology and prognosis of disease.

Cystic Fibrosis

Definition: Generalized dysfunction of the exocrine glands which produce excessive mucus and abnormal secretion of sweat. The changes in secretions eventually cause dysfunction of the pancreas and the lungs. The disorder is hereditary and is inherited as a recessive trait.

Signs and Symptoms

A. Pancreas involvement consists of copious, foul-smelling stools with large amount of fat but no trypsin. The infant has a good appetite but fails to gain weight.
B. Lung involvement consists of chronic cough and recurrent upper respiratory infections.
C. Sweat gland involvement consists of an increased sweat chloride test of over 60 mEq/liter.
D. An associated problem is the poor absorption of fat-soluble vitamin D; this may lead to osteoporosis.

Treatment and Nursing Care

A. Provide special nutritive foods.
  1. Pancreatic enzymes with meals and snacks.
  2. Water soluble vitamins.
  3. A moderately low fat and high protein diet; additional salt during summer.
B. Prevent respiratory infection.
  1. Keep the lungs clear of mucus.
  2. Provide mist tent at night to liquefy secretions.
  3. Provide aerosol therapy and postural drainage.
  4. Promote breathing exercises.

C. Provide good skin care to prevent irritation.

D. Educate the parents or interested others in proper care.

1. Teach at least two people the special procedures that are necessary for the infant's care.

2. Teach the proper care of the equipment, especially the cleaning process.

3. Encourage the responsible persons to participate in the infant's care while still hospitalized.

4. Refer the parents to the Cystic Fibrosis Foundation for additional help.

5. Refer parents to other community agencies if requested.

E. Give emotional support to child and family.

Celiac Disease (Gluten-Induced Enteropathy)

Definition: A chronic disease of intestinal malabsorption precipitated by ingestion of gluten or protein portions of wheat or rye flour.

Characteristics

A. A major cause of malabsorption in children, second only to cystic fibrosis.

B. Highest incidence occurs in caucasions.

C. Major problem is an intolerance to gluten, a protein found in most grains.

D. Basic defect is believed to be an inborn error of metabolism or an autoimmune response.

E. Inadequate fat absorption; as disease progresses it affects absorption of all ingested elements.

F. Long-term effects can be anemia, poor blood coagulation and osteoporosis.

G. Usually occurs when child begins to ingest grains. It may begin as early as six months and continue until fifth year.

Signs and Symptoms

A. Diarrhea or loose stools: bulky, foul smelling, pale, and frothy.

B. Failure to gain weight after a bout of diarrhea.

C. Abdominal distention.

D. Anorexia.

E. Irritability and restlessness.

F. Celiac crisis.

1. Vomiting and diarrhea.

2. Acidosis and dehydration.

3. May be precipitated by respiratory infection.

4. Excessive perspiration.

5. Cold extremities.

Nursing Care

A. Monitor appropriate diet.

1. Wheat and rye gluten as well as barley and oats are eliminated.

2. Low fat.

3. Slow feedings, small amounts at a time.

4. Strict intake and output.

5. Strict calorie control.

6. Supplemental vitamins and iron.

B. Give parental support.

Wilms's Tumor (Nephroblastoma)

Definition: Rapidly developing, malignant solid tumor of the kidneys containing embryonal elements. The incidence is 1 in 10,000 and occurrence is most common in children four to eight years of age.

Signs and Symptoms

A. Presence of a mass on either side of the abdomen with possible pain. (The mass itself should initiate a diagnostic work-up.)

B. Fever and hypertension.

C. Possible weight loss and anemia.

Treatment and Nursing Care

A. Preoperative care.

1. Avoid palpation of the tumor to prevent spreading.

2. Provide emotional support for the family.

3. Observe intake and output with care.

B. Surgical procedure.
1. Tumor can be shrunk with chemotherapy before surgery.
2. Nephrectomy if the nonaffected kidney is functioning.

C. Postoperative care.
1. Observe for toxic reactions to chemotherapy, such as mouth lesions.
2. If radiation therapy is given, provide good skin care.

Cretinism (Congenital Hypothyroidism)

Definition: Deficiency in secretions of thyroid hormones resulting from a rudimental thyroid gland which is either hypoactive or absent. The condition is recognizable when the child is two to three months old.

Signs and Symptoms

A. Body growth is retarded.
B. Eyes are puffy.
C. Tongue protrudes and is thick and large.
D. Hands and feet are short and square.
E. Skin is very dry, pale, and coarse.
F. Hair is very dry and coarse.
G. Frequently, there is an umbilical hernia.
H. Feeding difficulties include choking, lack of interest in food, and sluggishness.
I. Respiratory difficulties include apneic episodes, noisy respirations, and nasal obstructions.

Treatment and Nursing Care

A. Infants given thyroid hormone.
B. Prognosis implies that 50 percent of the children treated before the age of six months will achieve an IQ of 90 or more.

Epilepsy

Definition: Recurrent, transient attacks of disturbed brain function that have a variable symptomatology, characterized by convulsive attacks of unconsciousness or altered consciousness, usually with a series of tonic (stiffening) or clonic (twitching) muscular spasms or other abnormal behavior.

Etiology

A. Idiopathic (the majority of cases do not have an identifiable cause), although a genetic defect in the cerebral metabolism is thought to be responsible.

B. Organic.
1. A group of genetic conditions include epilepsy in their symptomatology, e.g., phenylketonuria and hypoglycemia.
2. Epilepsy can result from cerebral damage acquired in the prenatal, natal, or postnatal period.

Signs and Symptoms of Seizure Types

A. Grand mal.
1. Aura (a sensation of feeling) frequently precedes the onset of this type of seizure.
   a. Sometimes includes twitching or spasm of certain muscle groups; or the sensing of strange odors, visions, or sounds.
   b. Children have difficulty describing the experiences, although parents or caretakers are able to identify headaches, nausea, and irritability as precursors to seizure.
2. Tonic (stiffening) stage.
   a. Onset is abrupt and tonic contractions may occur simultaneously with loss of consciousness.
   b. The child usually pales, pupils dilate, eyes roll upward and to one side, head is thrown backward and to one side, the abdominal and chest muscles are held rigidly, and the limbs are contracted irregularly or are rigid.
   c. The tongue may be bitten as the jaw clamps down in contraction.
   d. Urination and defecation sometimes occur from hard contraction of abdom-

inal muscles.

e. Cyanosis, sometimes severe, may occur with prolonged respiratory cessation.

f. Tonic phase lasts about twenty to forty seconds; then the clonic stage commences.

3. Clonic stage.
   a. Lasts for variable periods of time.
   b. Clonic movements include a quick, jerking, back-and-forth motion of extremities and spasmodic movements of the face.

4. Recovery stage.
   a. The child usually sleeps following the seizure.
   b. May awake with a headache or a feeling of drowsiness or stupor.

5. Nighttime seizures may occur as evidenced by swollen and bitten tongue, blood on the pillow, wet bed, and/or headaches.

6. Status epilepticus exists when seizures are so frequent that they appear constant. It constitutes a medical emergency because of possible brain damage from lack of oxygen.

B. Petit mal.
   1. Transient loss of consciousness.
   2. May be evidenced by eye-rolling, drooping head, and slight quivering of trunk and extremity muscles.
   3. Attacks usually last less than thirty seconds.
   4. Attacks may occur from once or twice a month to several hundred a day.

C. Psychomotor seizures.
   1. Purposeful but inappropriate motor acts which are repetitive.
   2. Frequently a slight aura.
   3. Frequent vasomotor changes such as circumoral pallor.
   4. Usually no tonic or clonic activity.
   5. Following a one-to-five-minute period of unconsciousness, the child may resume normal activity or sleep.

D. Focal or Jacksonian seizures.
   1. Sensory or motor, depending upon the location of the focal area of abnormal neural discharge.
   2. Sometimes preceded by tonic phase.
   3. Usually clonic in nature.
   4. Muscles used in voluntary movement are most frequently involved, such as face and tongue, hand, and sometimes feet and trunk.
   5. Usually begins in one area and spreads in a fixed pattern.
   6. If seizure is localized to one area, loss of consciousness may not occur.
   7. If spread of seizure is extensive and rapid, consciousness is lost and generalized confusion follows, similar to grand mal.

Treatment and Nursing Care

A. Counsel parents.
   ☆ 1. Safety factors.
       a. Protect from hazardous play.
       b. Do not restrain movement of limbs, but protect head with a pillow during seizure.
       c. Use tongue depressor only with physician's orders—use is now controversial.
       d. Design child's environment free of sharp-cornered objects.
       e. Keep medication out of the reach of children.
       f. Reduce stress.
       g. Protect from loud noises and blinking lights.

   2. Medication.
       a. Observe for side effects.
          (1) Dilantin can cause hypertrophy of gums and stomatitis.
          (2) Zarotin can provoke blood dyscrasia.
       b. Observe for signs of toxicity.
       c. Administer dose accurately.
       d. Keep medication out of reach of children.

   3. Emotional factors.
       a. Assist family in understanding the

disease.

   b. Explain how to help child to have as normal a life as possible.

   c. Prevent overprotection.

B. Care of the child in the hospital.

1. Maintain suction equipment in readiness and at bedside.
2. Padded tongue depressor now controversial—may keep at bedside.
3. Observe seizure's progress and note it accurately to aid in the diagnosis of type of seizure.
4. Place the child near nurses' station.
5. Observe the reaction to medication.
6. Make sure crib or bed has side rails.

Infantile Eczema

Definition: Inflammation of the skin which can occur on any area of the body. It is most prevalent before the age of two.

Signs and Symptoms

A. Local redness of the skin (erythema).

B. Papules and vesicles apparent on face, neck, and body folds.

C. Rash characterized by itching, crusting, scaling, and oozing.

Treatment and Nursing Care

A. Treat the symptoms.

B. Provide sedation.

C. Keep infant comfortable.

D. Prevent infections.

E. Provide emotional support.

F. Eliminate the source of allergic sensitivity if known.

The Toddler

Disorders of the Toddler

Cerebral Palsy

Definition: Nonprogressive paralysis resulting from either developmental brain defects or birth trauma—effect is on motor not mental function.

Signs and Symptoms

A. Poor motor development; slow at walking and in other movements.

B. Involuntary movements of extremities and head.

C. Weakness of the extremities.

D. Spasticity of the extremities.

E. One or all of the extremities may be involved.

Nursing Care

A. Care should be individualized to the needs of the specific child.

B. Prevention of contractures of the joints.

C. Good nutrition.

D. Good dental care.

E. Encourage activities of daily living.

F. Encourage normal growth and development.

Croup

Definition: Group of symptoms resulting from obstruction of the larynx. The condition occurs in children under five years of age.

Signs and Symptoms

A. Hoarseness and barking cough.

B. Fever may or may not be present.

C. Inspiratory stridor.

D. Asphyxia.

E. Sudden onset, but recovery usually spontaneous.

Treatment and Nursing Care

A. Observe vital signs with care.
B. Avoid upsetting the child.
C. Provide emotional support for the child and family.
D. Set up mist tent if severe dyspnea experienced.

Pneumonia

Definition: Inflammation of the lung tissue caused primarily by bacteria and viruses.

Signs and Symptoms

A. Cough that is usually nonproductive.
B. Increased pulse and respirations.
C. Fever.
D. Vomiting and diarrhea.
E. Convulsions.
F. Increased white blood count.

Treatment and Nursing Care

A. Treat symptoms.
   1. Control fever.
   2. Position to aid breathing.
B. Urge fluids.
C. Observe vital signs with care.
D. Provide rest.

Bronchitis

Definition: Inflammation of the mucous membrane of bronchial tubes. No obstruction is present.

Signs and Symptoms

A. Usually preceded by an upper respiratory infection.
B. Dry, nonproductive cough.
C. Irritability.
D. Fever.

Nursing Care

A. Provide humidified air.
B. Urge fluids.
C. Provide postural drainage.
D. Observe vital signs with care.

Lead Poisoning

Definition: Poisoning from ingestion of paint or other lead-based materials.

Incidence

A. Occurrence usually between twelve and thirty-six months of age.
B. Death results in 25 percent of the cases of lead encephalopathy.
C. Many neurologic residual problems in survivors.

Signs and Symptoms

A. Gastrointestinal symptoms.
   1. Unexplained, repeated vomiting.
   2. Vague, chronic abdominal pain.
B. Central nervous system symptoms.
   1. Irritability.
   2. Drowsiness.
   3. Ataxia.
   4. Convulsive seizures.

Prevention

A. Inspection of buildings twenty-five years old or older.
B. Covering of areas painted with lead paint with plywood or linoleum.
C. Education of parents in preventive measures.

The Preschooler

Disorders of the Preschool Child

Leukemia

Definition: Unrestrained growth of abnormal, immature white blood cells which causes destruction of the red blood cells. Leukemia is the most common cancer in children.

Signs and Symptoms

A. Increased number of white blood cells which are immature and do not function normally.
B. Anorexia, nausea, and vomiting.
C. Weight loss, fatigue, and weakness.
D. Abdominal pain, joint pain.
E. Fever.
F. Petechiae and bruises.
G. Enlarged liver and spleen.
H. Anemia.
I. Onset is usually rapid.

Treatment and Nursing Care

A. Provide supportive and symptomatic care.
B. Administer antimetabolite drugs.
C. Prevent infection.
D. Handle child gently.
E. Encourage good nutrition.
F. Provide emotional support for the child and the family during therapy.

Hemophilia

Definition: Delayed coagulation of blood due to a hereditary condition involving clot formation. Victims are frequently labeled "bleeders."

Signs and Symptoms

A. Prolonged clotting time so that hemorrhage occurs with the slightest cut.
B. Bruising and swelling of affected or injured areas.

Nursing Care

A. Prevent injury.
B. Educate the child and family.
C. Help to rehabilitate.
D. Provide emotional support.

Acute Glomerulonephritis

Definition: Inflammation of the glomeruli which may be due to an antigen-antibody response to the beta-hemolytic streptococcus which causes changes in the glomerular filtering system.

Signs and Symptoms

A. Onset usually two to three weeks following an infection in site other than kidney.
B. Edema of the face.
C. Grossly bloody urine.
D. Headache and vomiting.
E. Oliguria and anuria.
F. Fatigue.
G. Anemia and malnutrition.
H. Hypertension.
I. Encephalopathy and heart failure.

Treatment and Nursing Care

A. Administer antibiotics.
B. Maintain bed rest.
C. Restrict salt and fluid in diet as necessary.
D. Administer antihypertensive drugs as necessary.
E. Observe vital signs.
F. Observe intake and output.
G. Track weight.
H. Prevent infections.

Nephrotic Syndrome

Definition: Degenerative, noninflammatory disease of the renal tubules with an increase in permeability of the glomerular membrane and necrotic lesions of the tubules.

Signs and Symptoms

A. Gradual development of generalized edema.

B. Malnutrition due to loss of appetite.

C. Anemia.

D. Susceptive to infections.

E. Nephrotic crisis indicated by abdominal pain, fever, and skin eruptions; will subside in a few days with a diuretic.

F. Abnormal laboratory tests.

   1. Urine.

      a. Increased albuminuria.

      b. Increased casts and white blood cells.

      c. Increased lipid granules.

   2. Blood.

      a. Decreased total protein to less than 4 G/100 ml.

      b. Decreased albumin and gamma globulin.

      c. Increased blood lipids and cholesterol.

      d. Increased sedimentation rate.

Treatment and Nursing Care

A. Prevent infections.

B. In treatment of edema, provide good skin care, change position frequently, observe intake and output, and track weight accurately.

C. Prepare for the side effects of medications and be accurate with their dosage.

D. Provide diet high in protein, low in sodium, and high in calories.

Parasitic Worms

Roundworms

A. Life cycle.

   1. Eggs are laid by the worm in the gastrointestinal tract of any host animal and passed out in feces.

   2. After the worms have been ingested, egg batches are laid.

   3. Larvae in the host invade lymphatics and venules of the mesentery and migrate to the liver, the lungs, and the heart.

   4. Larvae from lungs reach the host's epiglottis and are swallowed; once in the gastrointestinal tract, the cycle is repeated—larvae mature and mate, and the female lays eggs.

B. Symptoms.

   1. Atypical pneumonia.

   2. Gastrointestinal symptoms—nausea, vomiting, anorexia, and weight loss.

   3. Insomnia.

   4. Irritability.

   5. Signs of intestinal obstruction.

C. Treatment—piperazine citrate.

D. Nursing management.

   1. Prevention of infection through the use of a sanitary toilet.

   2. Hygiene education of the family.

   3. Careful disposal of infected stools.

Pinworm (Oxyuriasis)

A. Life cycle.

   1. Eggs ingested.

   2. Eggs mature in cecum, then migrate to anus.

   3. Worms exit at night and lay eggs on host's skin.

   4. Itching and reingestion occur.

B. Symptoms.

   1. Acute or subacute appendicitis.

   2. Eczematous areas of skin.

   3. Irritability.

   4. Loss of weight and anorexia.

   5. Insomnia.

   6. Diagnosis by tape test—place transparent adhesive tape over anus and examine tape for evidence of worms.

C. Treatment.

   1. Piperazine hexahydrate.

   2. All infected persons living communally must be treated simultaneously.

D. Nursing management.
1. During treatment, maintain meticulous cleansing of the skin, particularly in the anal region, and the hands and the nails.
2. Bed linens and clothing must be boiled.
3. Use ointment to relieve itching.
4. Teach careful hygiene as a preventative measure.

Hookworm

A. Life cycle.
1. Eggs of the worm are evacuated from the human bowel in feces and left in the soil.
2. Once the larvae are infective (in five to ten days), they invade the host when in contact with the skin—which occurs either by handling the soil or by walking barefoot.
3. The worms live in the upper gastrointestinal tract of the host or suck blood from the intestinal wall for nourishment.

B. Characteristics.
1. Disturbed digestion.
2. Unformed stools containing undigested food.
3. Tarry stool with decomposed blood.
4. Blood loss.
   a. Pallor.
   b. Dull hair.
   c. Anemia.
   d. Increased pulse.
   e. Mental apathy.

C. Treatment.
1. Drug—tetrachloroethylene.
2. Possibly blood transfusions.

D. Nursing management.
1. NPO the evening preceding the treatment.
2. Avoid fats, oils, and alcohol for twelve hours following medication.
3. Prevention of infection.
   a. Hygiene instruction.
   b. Use of shoes in hookworm areas.
4. Careful disposal of stools.

School-Age Child

Disorders of the School-Age Child

Rheumatic Fever

Definition: General systemic disease with damage to the connective tissue (collagen disease) caused by an antigen-antibody reaction to the beta-hemolytic streptococcus.

Signs and Symptoms

A. Migratory or polyarthritis.
B. Abdominal pain.
C. Low-grade fever.
D. Weight loss and anorexia.
E. Myocarditis with a murmur.
F. Increased C-reactive protein in the blood.

Nursing Care

A. Maintain complete bed rest until the symptoms subside.
B. Position legs in good body alignment, and make child comfortable.
C. Provide diversional activities that do not require strenuous effort.
D. Observe vital signs, especially the pulse, with care.
E. Track weight.
F. Provide emotional support.

Nursing of Cardiac Children

General Principles

A. Encourage normal growth and development.
B. Counsel parents to avoid overprotection.
C. Deal with parents' concerns and anxieties.
D. Educate parents about conditions, tests, planned treatments, medications.

E. Assist parents in developing ability to assess child's physical status.

Congestive Heart Failure

Nursing Care

A. Promote rest.
  1. Provide outlets such as drawing, doll play, and reading for the child who may be frustrated by restricted activity.
  2. Organize care to limit time spent disturbing child's rest.
B. Diet supervision.
  1. Provide small frequent feedings.
  2. Make the low sodium diet more palatable through imaginative play and an attractive food arrangement.
  3. Educate parents about diet and its purpose.
C. Medication supervision.
  1. Digoxin.
    a. Monitor vital signs every hour during digitalization.
    b. Observe for digoxin toxicity.
      (1) Nausea, vomiting, diarrhea.
      (2) Anorexia.
      (3) Dizziness and headaches.
      (4) Arrhythmias.
      (5) Muscle weakness.
    c. Always check pulse prior to giving digoxin.
  2. Diuretics.
    a. Observe for electrolyte abnormalities.
    b. Weigh the child daily.

Cardiac Surgery

Preoperative Nursing Care

A. Extensively prepare the child and the parents for the experience—demonstrate tubes and bandages and describe the scar the operation leaves.
B. Teach coughing and deep breathing to the child.
C. Conduct the child and the parents on a tour of the intensive care unit and introduce them to the staff.

D. Observe the child for signs of infection.
E. Make sure all laboratory tests are completed.

Postoperative Nursing Care

A. Maintain adequate pulmonary function.
  1. Keep patent airway.
  2. Patient should deep breathe and cough. Monitor use of IPPB.
  3. Suction if necessary.
  4. Oxygen.
  5. Chest suction for refilling lungs.
  6. Check rate and depth of respirations.
  7. Check water-seal chest drainage.
B. Maintain adequate circulatory functioning.
  1. Check vital signs.
  2. Replace blood where necessary.
  3. Check intake and output every hour.
C. Provide for rest through organized care.
D. Establish adequate hydration and nutrition.
E. Take measures to prevent postoperative complications.
  1. Antibiotic therapy.
  2. Turn patient frequently.
  3. Skin care.
  4. Check extremities for occlusions of major vessels with blood clots: cyanosis, paleness of extremity, or coldness to the touch.
  5. Passive range of motion.
  6. Check dressing for signs of hemorrhage.

Insulin Dependent Diabetes: Type I

Definition: A disorder characterized by metabolic conditions that interfere with the production, availability, or effectiveness of insulin. (Formerly called Juvenile Diabetes.)

Characteristics

A. Pathology.
  1. Interference with the utilization of sugar.
  2. Impaired transportation of glucose across cellular membranes and impaired utilization within the cell.

3. Increased glycogenesis.

4. Diuresis from hyperglycemia, resulting in glucosuria and excessive losses of electrolytes and water.

5. Increased oxidation of fats and proteins, leading to proteinuria and acidosis.

B. Prognosis: degenerative changes associated with diabetes mellitus begin in young adults who have had the disease for ten to twenty years.

1. Arteriosclerosis with hypertension.

2. Retinal changes and cataracts.

3. Nephropathy.

Signs and Symptoms

A. Rapid onset.

B. Loss of weight.

C. Increased thirst and appetite, polydipsia, polyphagia, polyuria, and nocturia.

D. Onset frequently associated with ketoacidosis—an acute, life-threatening condition.

1. Drowsiness.

2. Dryness of skin.

3. Flushed cheeks.

4. Acetone breath.

5. Hyperpnea.

6. Nausea, vomiting, and abdominal pains.

Treatment and Nursing Care

A. Monitor administration of insulin. (Oral hypoglycemic agents generally do not produce satisfactory results because they require some pancreatic function to be effective.)

1. Side effects: hypoglycemia with hunger, irritability, nervousness, headaches, and slurred speech.

2. Insulin treatment.

B. Monitor diet.

1. Diet should be adequate for normal growth and development and regulated according to diabetic needs.

2. The type of diet prescribed is influenced by the philosophy of the physician.

3. Diets vary from free diets to strict dietary control.

Types	Onset (hrs.)	Peak (hrs.)	Total duration (hrs.)
Regular	½ to 1	2 to 3	5 to 10
Semilente	½ to 1	5 to 7	12 to 16
Humulin R	½ to 1	2 to 3	5 to 7
NPH	1 to 1½	8 to 12	24
Lente	1 to 2	7 to 15	24
PZI	4 to 8	10 to 20	36
Ultra	4 to 8	10 to 20	36

C. Provide family and patient education.

1. Signs and symptoms of disease, including acidosis and hypoglycemia.

2. Instruction in insulin injection, sterile technique, and urine testing.

3. Diet control as prescribed by the physician.

4. Prevention of infections through adequate skin and foot care.

5. Knowledge of the effects of increased physical activity and stress on food needs.

6. Patient's responsibility for administering insulin and managing diet.

7. Normal activity and life style appropriate.

D. Provide special counseling because of adolescent's heightened sensitivity to being different and their frequently unusual dietary habits.

Meningitis

Definition: An acute inflammation of the meninges.

Characteristics

A. May be caused by viral or bacterial agents.

B. Diagnosis based on symptoms and culture of C.S.F.

Signs and Symptoms

A. Symptoms of nuchal-spinal rigidity: headache, irritability, nausea, vomiting, fever.

B. Positive Kernig's and Brudzinski's signs.

Nursing Care

A. Isolate child until the causative agent is identified.

B. Administer medications on time.

C. Manage fluids: prevent dehydration and overhydration (causes an increase in cerebral edema).

D. Monitor neurological signs.

E. Maintain bedrest and position child comfortably; most children prefer a side-lying or flat position; sitting up increases pain.

F. Maintain patent airway; administer oxygen if ordered.

G. Provide quiet activities which are age appropriate.

Asthma

Definition: A pulmonary disorder in which physical or chemical irritants cause the release of histamine and other substances which cause edema of the bronchial walls, excess secretion of mucus by the bronchial glands, and constriction of the bronchi.

Characteristics

A. An attack may be provoked by exposure to certain foods, infections, vigorous activity, or emotional excitement.

B. Bronchiolar musculature goes into spasm.

C. Thick tenacious mucus accumulates and causes obstruction of air passages.

D. Trapping of air occurs causing obstructive emphysema.

E. Symptoms include wheezing and rales.

F. Attack may occur slowly or quickly.

G. Child usually coughs continually.

H. Neck veins may distend.

I. Cyanosis may occur.

J. Child appears anxious and upset.

K. Symptoms may become rapidly worse with acute respiratory failure with cyanosis and acidosis.

Nursing Care

A. Identification and removal of suspected allergen.

B. Medication supervision.

1. Epinephrine—acts to reduce congestion and edema.

2. Ephedrine sulfate—reduces congestion and edema.

3. Aminophylline—bronchodilator.

C. Removal and control of secretions.

1. Large fluid intake to liquefy secretions and maintain electrolyte balance.

2. Mist tent.

3. Chest physical therapy and postural drainage.

D. Emotional support for parents and child to reduce anxiety.

E. Child educated to live optimally with chronic problem.

Reye's Syndrome

Definition: Acute encephalopathy with fatty degeneration resulting in marked cerebral edema and enlargement of the liver with marked fatty infiltration.

Characteristics

A. Children from two months to adolescence contact illness; ages 6 and 11 years most often affected.

B. Usually follows a viral infection, especially varicella and influenza B.

Signs and Symptoms

A. Malaise, cough, rhinorrhea, sore throat.

B. Changes in level of consciousness.

C. Temperature changes.

D. Clinical stages of the syndrome.

1. Stage 1: vomiting, lethargy and drowsiness.

2. Stage 2: CNS changes, disorientation, delirium, aggressiveness and combativeness, central neurologic hyperventilation, hyperactive reflexes and stupor.

3. Stage 3: comatose, hyperventilation, decorticate posturing.

4. Stage 4: increasing comatose state, loss of ocular reflexes, fixed, dilated pupils.
5. Stage 5: seizures, loss of deep tendon reflexes, flaccidity and respiratory arrest.

Nursing Care

A. Monitor for signs of increased intracranial pressure.
　1. Major effort is toward recognizing and reducing cerebral edema, as this may lead to death.
　2. Monitor IV mannitol or glycerol when administered to reduce blood osmolarity, thus reducing cerebral edema.
B. Prepare for tracheal intubation and controlled ventilation (to decrease carbon dioxide level).
C. Monitor vital signs frequently and decrease temperature as needed.
D. Monitor closely for signs of seizure activity and utilize seizure precautions.
E. Provide nursing care appropriate for semi-conscious child.
　1. Maintain head elevation at 30 degrees.
　2. Monitor reflexes as indicative of clinical stage of syndrome.
F. Provide adequate fluid balance.
　1. Ensure adequate urinary output of at least 1 ml/1 kg/hr.
　2. Provide and monitor intravenous fluids.
　3. Observe closely for cerebral edema or dehydration.
G. Provide low protein diet.
H. Provide respiratory care; suctioning, ventilation and oxygen as ordered.
I. Provide emotional and supportive care.

Brain Tumor

Definition: Benign or malignant brain mass. In children the tumor is usually located in the cerebellum or the mid-brain.

Characteristics

A. Seventy-five percent of childhood brain tumors are impossible to remove or are so situated as to cause damage if completely removed.
B. Incidence—occur most frequently in the five-to-seven age group.
C. Location—most occur in the posterior fossa.
D. Types most frequently seen in children.
　1. Astrocytoma.
　　a. Located in the cerebellum.
　　b. Insidious onset and slowly progressive course.
　　c. Surgical removal usually possible.
　2. Medulloblastoma.
　　a. Located in the cerebellum.
　　b. Highly malignant.
　　c. Prognosis poor.
　3. Ependymoma.
　　a. Usually there is ventricular blockage, leading to signs of increased intracranial pressure.
　　b. Treated with incomplete internal compression and radiation therapy.
　4. Brain stem gliomas.
　　a. Seventy-five percent of childhood brain tumors.
　　b. Develops slowly with initial symptoms of cranial nerve palsies.

Signs and Symptoms

A. Variety of symptoms depending on location of tumor.
B. Increased intracranial pressure.
　1. Vomiting without nausea; anorexia.
　2. Headache.
　3. Diplopia.
C. Enlargement of the head in children under four years old.
D. Mental change: lethargy, irritability, drowsiness, and stupor.
E. Unsteady gait and muscular uncoordination (ataxia).

Nursing Care

A. Control and relief of symptoms.
B. Seizure precautions.
C. Postoperative care for surgical removal.

1. Maintain child flat in bed on unaffected side.
2. Log roll for change of position.
3. Control fever with hypothermia mattress.
4. Frequently observe vital signs until stable.
5. Reinforce dressing, if wet, with sterile gauze.
6. Notify R.N. of increased wetness of dressing—possible cerebral spinal fluid leakage.

D. Provide emotional support for family and child.

Bone Tumors

Osteogenic Sarcoma

Definition: A malignant tumor originating from osteoblasts (bone-forming cells).

Characteristics

A. Tumor usually located at the end of the long bones (metaphysis).
B. Most frequently seen at the distal end of the femur or the proximal end of the tibia.
C. Primary symptoms are pain at site, swelling, and limitation of movement.
D. Lungs most common site of metastasis.
E. Occurs twice as frequently in boys as in girls.

Treatment and Nursing Care

A. Usually amputation followed by chemotherapy.
B. Administer drugs and monitor for side effects.
   1. Vincristine.
   2. Cytoxan.
   3. Actinomycin D.
C. Provide supportive emotional care.

Ewing's Sarcoma

Definition: A malignant tumor of the bone originating from myeloblasts.

Characteristics

A. Tumor usually located on the shaft of the long bones.

B. Femur, tibia, and humerus common sites.
C. Primary symptoms.
   1. Pain at site.
   2. Swollen area with tenderness.
   3. Fever.
D. Early metastases to lung, lymph nodes, and other bones.
E. Occurs twice as frequently in boys as in girls.

Treatment and Nursing Care

A. Usually radiation, sometimes followed by amputation.
B. Chemotherapy to treat tumor and prevent metastases.
C. Administer drugs and monitor for side effects.
   1. Vincristine.
   2. Cytoxan.
   3. Actinymycin D.
D. Encourage inclusion of patient in discussions of treatment, options, risks and prognosis.
E. Listen to parents, child, and siblings as they work through denial, anger, acceptance—allow them their grieving process.
F. Promote age appropriate activities and group discussions with peers.
G. Assist parents in avoiding overprotection.
H. Treat the side effects of chemotherapy and radiation.

Chemotherapy

Basic Principles

A. Chemotherapeutic agents work on dividing cells.
B. Tumor's location and cell type affect choice of drugs.
C. Most antineoplastic drugs are metabolized in the liver and excreted by the kidneys so they must be in functioning order to prevent toxicity.

Nursing Care

A. Establish baseline data.
   1. Nutritional status.

2. Oral condition.

3. Skin condition.

4. Degree of mobility.

5. Psychological status.

6. Neurological condition.

B. Observe for side effects of cell breakdown.

1. BUN on rise.

2. Stone formation in urinary tract.

C. Observe for side effects on rapidly dividing cells.

1. Gastrointestinal mucosa—diarrhea, nausea, vomiting.

a. Administer antiemetics.

b. Provide mouth care with hydrogen peroxide every 4 hours. No toothbrush or glycerin.

c. Administer anesthetic spray to mouth prior to meals.

d. Provide frequent cold, high calorie beverages.

2. Hair follicles—loss of hair.

a. Prepare patient for loss—suggest wig, scarf.

b. Reassure that it will return in 6 weeks.

c. Apply tourniquet around scalp during chemotherapy plus 2-3 hours following to lessen amount of hair lost.

Common Drugs

A. Prednisone.

1. Side effects.

a. Ravenous appetite.

b. Change in fat distribution.

c. Retention of fluid.

d. Hirsutism.

e. Occasional hypertension.

f. Psychological disturbance.

2. Nursing management—watch blood sugar and tapering of medication.

B. 6-Mercaptopurine.

1. Interrupts the synthesis of purines essential to the structure and function of nucleic acids.

2. Side effects.

a. Produces very little toxicity in children.

b. Increases amount of uric acid that the kidneys must excrete.

3. Nursing management.

a. Observe kidney function.

b. Increase fluid intake.

C. Methotrexate.

1. A folic acid antagonist that suppresses the growth of abnormal cells enough to permit regeneration of normal cells.

2. Side effects.

a. Ulceration of oral mucosa.

b. Nausea, vomiting, diarrhea, and abdominal pain.

3. Nursing management.

a. Observe for ulcerations—drug must be temporarily discontinued at the appearance of ulcers.

b. Observe renal function—drug is excreted.

D. Cytoxan.

1. Alkylating agent that suppresses cellular proliferation; it has greater effect on abnormal than normal cells.

2. Side effects—hemorrhagic cystitis.

3. Nursing management—provide large quantities of fluids preceding and immediately following drug administration to prevent side effects.

E. Vincristine.

1. Alkylating agent.

2. Side effects.

a. Insomnia.

b. Severe constipation.

c. Peripheral neuritis or palsies.

3. Frequently used to induce remissions rapidly, after which the patient is maintained on another, less toxic drug.

Radiation

Basic Principles

A. Radiation affects all cells but is particularly lethal to rapidly developing cells.

B. Radiation can be utilized in conjunction with chemotherapy.

C. Radiation may be used to eradicate the tumor or to relieve pressure.

Nursing Care

A. Treatment of radiation sickness.
  1. Symptoms—nausea, vomiting, malaise.
  2. Offer frequent high caloric feedings (milkshakes with extra protein and vitamins).
  3. Make food trays attractive, palatable.
B. Observe side effects of cell breakdown.
  1. BUN on rise.
  2. Accumulation of uric acid.
  3. Stone formation in urinary tract.
C. Treat side effects of cell breakdown.
  1. Increase fluid intake.
  2. Monitor intake and output.
D. Treat skin breakdown.
  1. Check patient regularly for any redness or irritation at radiation site.
  2. Immediately notify physician.
  3. Usual treatment—apply lotion to area, cover loosely with sterile gauze.
  4. Avoid any irritation to area from clothing, soap or weather extremes.
E. Treat bone marrow depression.
  1. Carefully watch lab values.
  2. Isolate (low leukocytes).
  3. Avoid injections (low platelets).
  4. Antibiotics.

The Adolescent

Disorders of the Adolescent

Obesity

Definition: Excessive accumulation of body fat which is over ten percent of that normal for a young adult with regard to age, height, and body build.

Nursing Care

A. Encourage adolescent to follow proper low caloric diet as prescribed by the physician.
B. Provide emotional support for the adolescent.

Ulcerative Colitis

Definition: Inflammation of the colon and the rectum in which the mucous membrane becomes hyperemic, bleeds easily, and tends to ulcerate.

Etiology

A. Unknown, although the increased incidence within families has given rise to the hypothesis that suggests a hereditary predisposition or an emotional and/or environmental causation.
B. Incidence is highest in young adults and middle-age groups.

Signs and Symptoms

A. Diarrhea.
B. Weight loss.
C. Rectal bleeding.
D. Abdominal pain, nausea, and vomiting.
E. Anemia.
F. Fever and dehydration.
G. Adolescents tend to be passive, pessimistic, fearful, and strongly, though ambivalently, attached to a parent.

Nursing Care

A. Control infection.
  1. Supervise medication regime.
  2. Provide adequate hydration with intravenous therapy and oral fluids as indicated.
B. Provide for rest of intestinal tract.
  1. Observe for type and amount of bowel activity, symptoms of bleeding, and hyperactive peristalsis.
  2. Administer tranquilizers and observe for side effects.

C. Maintain diet therapy.
1. Provide low residue, bland, high protein diet and vitamin therapy.
2. Avoid presenting cold foods because they increase gastric motility.
3. Avoid serving sharp cheeses, highly spiced foods, smoked or salted meats, fried foods, raw fruits, and vegetables.
4. Arrange for attractive environment with opportunities for socialization at mealtimes.
D. Provide counseling.
1. Educate patient about diet, medication, and symptoms of bleeding.
2. Observe for signs of psychological problems; initiate referral if necessary.

Infectious Mononucleosis

Definition: An infectious disease, believed to be viral in origin, that causes an increase in the mononuclear elements of the blood.

Signs and Symptoms

A. Incubation period is around eleven days.
B. Symptoms.
1. Malaise.
2. Sore throat with pharyngitis.
3. Prolonged fever.
4. Enlargement of the lymph nodes.
5. Splenomegaly (enlargement of the spleen).
6. About 10 to 20 percent of the cases exhibit skin rashes that appear between day four and ten. The rash is usually the macular type, occurring primarily on the trunk.

Nursing Care

A. Symptomatic and supportive.
1. Maintain bed rest initially.
2. Increase activity gradually.
3. Administer salicylates for fever, chills, and muscle pain as ordered.
B. No isolation procedures are required.

Hodgkin's Disease

Definition: Malignancy of the lymph system characterized by a large, primitive, reticulum-like, malignant cell. Peak occurrence is between fifteen and twenty-nine years of age.

Signs and Symptoms

A. Enlarged, painless lymph nodes. Nodes are firm and moveable.
B. Lessened sensitivity to specified antigens (anergy).
C. Frequent infections.
D. Prognosis is guarded (over-all five-year survival rate appears to be about 30 percent).

Stages

A. Stage I.
1. Disease restricted to single anatomic site or localized in a group of lymph nodes.
2. Asymptomatic.
B. Stage II.
1. Two or three adjacent lymph nodes in the area on the same side of the diaphragm are affected.
2. Symptoms appear.
C. Stage III.
1. Disease is widely disseminated into the lymph areas and organs.
2. Prognosis poor.

Treatment and Nursing Care

A. Provide for symptomatic relief for the side effects of radiation (used for Stages I, II, and III in an effort to eradicate the disease) and chemotherapy (used in combination is treatment of choice).
B. Counseling.
1. Assist the family and the adolescent to accept the process of treatment.
2. Encourage independence where possible.
C. Observe for pressure from enlargement of the lymph glands on vital organs, particularly for respiratory problems from the compression of the airway.

Juvenile Rheumatoid Arthritis

Definition: Systemic disease with multiple manifestations, arthritis being the most characteristic; etiology unknown.

Pathology

A. Inflammation of joints.
B. Edema and congestion of synovial tissues.
C. As the disease progresses, synovial fluid fills the joint space and causes narrowing, fibrous ankylosis, and bony fusion.
D. Growth centers adjacent to affected joints may undergo either premature closure or accelerated epiphyseal growth.

Signs and Symptoms

A. Involvement of joints.
   1. Arthritis may start slowly with gradual development of joint stiffness, swelling, and loss of motion.
   2. Affects knees, ankles, feet, wrists, and fingers most frequently, although any joint may be involved.
   3. Affected joints are swollen, warm, painful, and stiff.
   4. Young children appear irritable and anxious, guarding their joints.
   5. Weakness and atrophy of muscles appear around affected joints.
   6. Chronically affected joints may become deformed, dislocated, or fused.
B. Systemic involvement.
   1. Frequent occurrence.
   2. Irritability, anorexia, and malaise.
   3. Fever.
   4. Intermittent macular rash on occasion.
   5. Enlarged liver and spleen (hepatosplenomegaly) and generalized lymphadenopathy in 20 percent of the patients.
   6. Anemia is common in active cases of the disease.
   7. Inflammation of eyes with redness, pain, photophobia, decreased visual acuity, and nonreactive pupil.

Treatment and Nursing Care

A. Although there is no specific cure, care can be given to prevent joint destruction and to maintain joint mobility.
   1. Exercise joints.
   2. Provide night splints.
   3. Educate parents in how adolescent should perform exercises, and impress upon them the adolescent's need for physical therapy and night splints.
B. Provide emotional support to the chronically ill adolescent and his family.
C. Administer medications.
   1. Salicylates.
      a. Usually given in large doses.
      b. Observe for signs of toxicity and side effects.
         (1) Ringing in the ear.
         (2) Gastric irritation. (Alleviate by giving drug with milk or antacids.)
         (3) Headaches.
         (4) Disturbances of mental state.
         (5) Hyperventilation and drowsiness.
   2. Gold salts.
      a. Usually given in weekly injections.
      b. Observe for side effects.
         (1) Skin rashes.
         (2) Nephritis with hematuria or albuminuria.
         (3) Thrombocytopenia.
         (4) Neurotoxicity.
      c. Weekly blood and urine tests.
   3. Steroids.
      a. Observe for side effects and toxicity.
         (1) Masked infection.
         (2) Hypertension.
         (3) Vascular disorders.
         (4) Mental disturbances.
         (5) Edema with weight gain.
         (6) Increased appetite.
         (7) Peptic ulcer.
      b. Observe vital signs regularly.
D. Encourage parents to report any signs of eye problems in the adolescent immediately to the physician so that eye damage may be prevented.

Scoliosis

Definition: Lateral curvature of the spine that occurs during the growth spurt at puberty.

Signs and Symptoms

A. One leg shorter in length than the other.

B. One hip or one shoulder higher than the other hip or shoulder.

C. A marked curve in upper part of spine.

Treatment and Nursing Care

A. Preoperative care.
   1. Show patient how to provide for his or her postoperative needs.
   2. Provide emotional support.

B. Surgical procedure.
   1. Bone graft.
   2. Rod insertion.

C. Postoperative care.
   1. Keenly observe for indications of pain, vital signs, and hemorrhage.
   2. Change patient's position by log rolling to prevent injury to the surgical area.
   3. Encourage coughing and deep breathing.
   4. Encourage fluids and food; observe intake and output.
   5. Use the hemovacuum as needed.
   6. Provide emotional support.
   7. Teach parents how to provide home care to adolescent who will be confined to body cast for six to nine months.

Anorexia Nervosa

Definition: A syndrome of self-starvation with underlying emotional disturbance. The psychological aversion to food results in emaciation and physical problems.

Characteristics

A. Almost exclusively female (1 in 100 are males).

B. Most common in adolescent girls and young adults.

C. Often unnoticed in early stages; female "goes on diet to lose weight."

D. Not a disturbance in appetite but distorted body image perceptions: related to disturbance in sense of self, identity, and autonomy.

E. Potentially lethal disease: mortality 15–20 percent.

F. Many anorectics have had a single episode, then recover. Factors associated with positive prognosis include: onset of problem before age 15 and weight gain within two years.

Signs and Symptoms

A. Profound weight loss of 25 percent occurs with this disorder.

B. Delayed sexual development: amenorrhea.

C. Physical symptoms.
   1. Hypotension.
   2. Anemia.
   3. Hypoproteinemia.
   4. Hypothermia.
   5. Slowed heart rate.
   6. Lanugo.

Nursing Care

A. Improve nutritional status (to stabilize medical condition).
   1. Diet.
      a. High protein, high carbohydrate.
      b. Identify foods patient prefers.
      c. Small, nutritious, attractive feedings.
      d. Maintain accurate intake records.
   2. Nasogastric feedings; if patient refuses to eat, administer tube feedings as ordered.

B. Nursing care plan.
   1. Formulate plan that all staff agree on. Do not allow manipulation. Do not engage in power struggle.
   2. Do not focus on food, taste, recipes, etc.
   3. Remain with patient when eating.
   4. Do not accept excuses to leave eating area (to vomit).
   5. Set limits on amount patient must eat. Reward when patient adheres to plan.

6. Ensure that weight is taken same time every day with patient dressed in only a hospital gown.
7. Work with staff on behavior therapy plan.
   a. Set limits with positive and negative reinforcement.
   b. Establish contract that specifies weight-gain privileges, restrictions, etc.
   c. Assist to correct patient's body perceptions and misconceptions about feelings, needs, self-worth, autonomy.

Bulimia

Definition: Eating disorder that involves binge eating, frequently followed by self-induced vomiting.

Characteristics

A. Etiology is unknown but this disorder is often accompanied by an underlying psychopathology.
B. More common in women than men.
C. Begins in adolescence or early adulthood and often follows a chronic course over many years.
D. Generally aware that eating patterns are abnormal (in contrast to anorectics).
E. Typically evidences impaired impulse control, low self-esteem, and depression.

Signs and Symptoms

A. Disruption in life caused by eating disorder.
B. Depression: often due to guilt over eating binges. (New studies suggest link between bulimia and affective disorder.)
C. Weight fluctuation and potential danger of weight loss.

Nursing Care

A. Patient is usually not hospitalized but does require therapy.
B. Behavior-modification and insight-oriented therapy used with limited success.
C. Nursing care plan is similar to anorexia nervosa with focus on interrupting binge/purge cycle and altering attitudes toward food and self.

Special Problems

The Mentally Retarded Child

Definition: Impairment of intelligence that results in a limited capacity to adapt to the environment and to achieve skills necessary for progress on the developmental continuum.

Classifications of Mental Retardation

A. Mild (educable).
   1. Child can acquire simple basic learning skills.
   2. IQ between 50 and 75.
   3. Social and sensorimotor skills can be developed.
   4. Child can learn self-support skills.
B. Moderate (trainable).
   1. Child can acquire simple social skills.
      a. Communication.
      b. Minimal social interaction skills.
   2. IQ between 35 and 50.
   3. Minimal learning ability.
   4. Can be independent with supervision.
C. Severe.
   1. Can benefit from habit-training.
   2. IQ between 20 and 35.
   3. Requires supervision.
   4. Poor communicative, social, and sensorimotor skills.
D. Profound.
   1. Minimal capacity to function.
   2. IQ below 20.
   3. Requires constant supervision (custodial care).

Incidence

A. Approximately 3 percent of the general population is considered to be mentally retarded.
B. Mental retardation occurs in all races and both sexes; there is no differentiation as to socioeconomic status.

C. Incidence of mental retardation according to classification.
1. Educable—75 percent.
2. Trainable—23 percent.
3. Custodial—2 percent.

Nursing Care

A. Treat the child according to developmental age rather than chronological age.
1. Respond to the child on a level he or she can understand. If the developmental age is two years and chronological age is ten, respond to and deal with child as if a two year old.
2. Assessment is often vague and inaccurate so expectations at the developmental age should not be rigid.
B. Provide the child with as much stimulation and love as a normal child.
C. Watch for infections and disease; retarded children are frequently more susceptible.
D. Challenge with behavioral modification, as it frequently works well with these children.
E. Empathize with parents' reaction to the birth of a mentally retarded child.
1. Birth presents a threat to the parents' marital relationship and family dynamics.
2. States of parental reaction.
a. Denial: initial reaction of defense which protects the parents from admitting that this child, this extension of themselves, is not normal.
b. Initial recognition: aware of difference between their child and other children.
c. Active recognition: the parents begin to search for information on their child's problem and are ready to seek professional advice.
F. Work with staff to formulate a plan for dealing with the mentally retarded child if child is to live at home with parents.

Child Abuse

Definition: Physical maltreatment or negligence (not including accidental mishaps) of children that results from an absence of reasonable standards of protection and care by the parents or the child's caretaker.

Incidence

A. Statistics.
1. Among a thousand newborn children, six become battered children.
2. Of all injuries in children under five years of age, as seen in the hospital emergency, about 10 percent are actually caused by parents or are the result of negligence.
B. Distribution.
1. One-third of all abused victims are less than six months old.
2. One-third of them are six months to three years old.
3. One-third of them are over three years old.
4. The risk of becoming a battered child is three times greater for children born prematurely than for those born full-term.
5. Stepchildren have a higher abuse risk than do non-stepchildren.
C. Psychological factors.
1. The abused child usually has demanding behaviors.
2. The abuse usually occurs close in time to a crisis or stressful event.
3. The abuse usually occurs after the parent is provoked to anger.

Clinical Indications of Abuse

A. Account of the injury/ies.
1. The cause given for the injury is implausible.
2. The cause given for the injury is punishment, which is inappropriate considering the age of the child.
3. There are discrepancies in the initial account as presented by neighbors or other family members.
4. There is a delay in seeking medical help for the child.
B. Indications for diagnosis of abuse.
1. Physical examination.

a. Bruises, welts, and scars in various stages of healing.
b. Finger-mark pattern of bruises on the body.
c. Bite, rope, or choke marks in evidence.
d. Cigarette and/or hot water burns are visible.
e. Eye damage, subdural hematoma, and/or intra-abdominal injuries.
f. Radiographic findings of multiple bone injuries at different stages of healing.

2. Other observations.
a. Child perceived as passive, noncommunicative, and/or withdrawn.
b. Child perceived as failing to thrive.

C. Characteristics of abusive parents or caretakers.
1. Abusers usually abused as children.
2. Abusers unable to utilize outside help when angry with their children.
3. Abusers usually are isolated and lonely individuals.
4. Frequently, spouse of abuser does not know how to prevent abuse.
5. Frequently, abusive parents make unreasonable demands of their children.
6. Abusing parents often exhibit certain personality problems such as dependency, low self-esteem, immaturity, and inability to cope with feelings.

D. Legal responsibilities of health team members.
1. Both nurses and doctors have a legal responsibility to report incidences of children who are suspected of being abused to the proper authorities.
2. Designated community authorities have the responsibility to determine further placement of the abused child.

Accidents

Incidence

A. Accidents are the leading cause of childhood deaths.
B. The majority of accidents occur in or near the home.

Classification

A. Automobile accidents.
B. Aspiration of small objects.
C. Accidental falls which result in fractures and serious head injuries.
D. Accidental poisonings.

Treatment and Nursing Care

A. If accidental poisoning occurs, contact local poison control center for pertinent information. Keep the poison container if available.
B. Take children to the nearest emergency room for proper treatment of any type of injuries.
C. Accident prevention is very important; educate both the child and the parents.

Burns

Definition: Destruction of body tissue caused by heat. It is the most frequent accidental injury occurring to infants and children.

Degree of Burns

A. First degree: involves only the epidermis with redness, swelling, and pain.
B. Second degree: involves superficial skin layers with redness, blisters, and pain; scarring may occur.
C. Third degree: involves the epidermis and some of the dermis with charring and destruction of the nerve endings, sweat glands, and hair follicles.

Treatment and Nursing Care

A. Open method (reverse isolation).
B. Pressure dressings.
C. Wet dressings (sterile).
D. Skin grafts.
E. Prevent infection.
F. Observe intake and output.
G. Align body carefully to prevent contractures.
H. Provide a well-balanced diet.

Appendix 1. Nutrition

Nutrition for the Infant

A. Calories.
1. Birth to three months—50 to 55 calories per pound per day.
2. Three months to one year—45 calories per pound per day.

B. Fluids.
1. First six months—two to three ounces per pound per day.
2. Requirements increase in hot weather.

C. Number of feedings.
1. First week—six to ten per day.
2. One week to one month—six to eight per day.
3. One to three months—five to six per day.
4. Three to seven months—four to five per day.
5. Four to nine months—three to four per day.
6. Eight to twelve months—three per day.

D. Vitamins.
1. Breast-fed infants—supplement with vitamins C, D, and A.
2. Formula-fed infants—vitamin supplements depend on type of formula and which vitamins are already included in it.

E. Solid foods—recent trends indicate introduction of solid foods at three to six months of age.
1. Cereal—infants are least allergic to rice; it can be introduced as early as four to six weeks of age.
2. Fruits and vegetables.
   a. New foods should be introduced once a day in small amounts until the infant becomes accustomed to them.
   b. Introduce only one new food per week.
   c. Bananas and applesauce are well tolerated.
   d. Orange juice is usually not well tolerated, initially. It can be introduced, diluted with water, when the infant is two or three months old.
   e. Green and yellow vegetables can be introduced at about four months of age.
3. Eggs.
   a. Introduce after infant is six months old.
   b. Usually yolks are well tolerated, but sometimes there are allergic reactions to egg whites.
4. Meat.
   a. May be introduced at four months.
   b. Usually more palatable if mixed with fruits or vegetables.
5. Starchy foods.
   a. May be introduced after the infant is six months old.
   b. Should not be substituted for green vegetables or fruit.
   c. Chief value is caloric.
   d. Zweiback and other crackers are good for the gumming infant.

F. Diarrhea (temporary).
1. Usually caused by contaminated food.
2. Review feeding preparation and storage of formula with caretaker.
3. Usually corrected by withholding all solids and milk for two or three feedings and giving boiled water or balanced electrolyte solution.

G. Constipation.
1. Increase fluid and sugar intake.
2. In infant three months old or older, increase cereal, fruit, and vegetable intake.
3. On occasion, prune juice (half an ounce) may be given.

Nutrition for the Second Year

A. Rate of growth is slowing down; thus there is a decreased caloric need.
B. Self-selection—children usually select a balanced diet over a period of several days.
C. Child should be feeding self, with some assistance.

Nutrition for the Preschooler

A. Child begins to imitate family's likes and dislikes.

B. Finger foods are popular.

C. Single foods are preferable to a combination of foods.

Nutrition for the School-Age Child

A. Patterns of good eating habits are established at this time.

B. Provide fruits as snacks.

Adolescent Eating Patterns

A. Adolescents often gain weight easily and then resort to fad diets.

B. Girls adapt themselves to fashionable weight goals, some of which may be unhealthy.

C. Eating of nonnutritious foods in a social setting.

Malnutrition

A. Kwashiorkor—caused by a lack of protein.

B. Rickets—caused by a lack of vitamin D.

C. Scurvy—caused by a lack of vitamin C.

Appendix 2. Reflexes in the Newborn

Palmar Grasp

A. Automatic reflex of full-term newborns; elicited by placing finger in infant's palm.

B. Present at birth.

C. Disappears at four months.

Asymmetrical Tonic Neck Reflex

A. Infant assumes fencer's position—when head is turned to one side, arm on that side is extended, and opposite arm is flexed.

B. Present at birth.

C. Disappears at four months.

Moro's Reflex (Startle Reflex)

A. When infant is suddenly jarred or hears a loud noise, the body stiffens, the legs are drawn up, and the arms are brought up, out, and then in front in an embracing position.

B. Present at birth.

C. Disappears at four months.

Reciprocal Kicking

A. Movements of newborns are jerky and usually alternate in the legs.

B. Evolving at birth.

C. Disappears at nine months.

Rooting

A. When infant's cheek is brushed, the head will turn to that side.

B. Present at birth.

C. Rooting while awake disappears at three to four months.

D. Rooting while asleep disappears at seven to eight months.

Sucking

A. Infants make sucking movements when anything touches their lips.

B. Present at birth.

C. Involuntary sucking disappears at or about nine months.

Neck Righting Reflex

A. When the head is turned to one side, the opposite shoulder and trunk will follow.

B. Evolving at four months.

C. Involuntary movement disappears at nine to twelve months.

Babinski's Sign

A. Extension of the great toe on stroking the sole of the foot.

B. Present at birth.

C. Disappears after two years.

Appendix 3. Immunizations

Age	Prevention
2 months	DPT*, TOPV†
4 months	DPT, TOPV
6 months	DPT, TOPV
12 months	Tuberculin test
15 months	MMR‡
1½ years	DPT, TOPV
4 to 6 years	DPT, TOPV
14 to 16 years	TD§, and thereafter every ten years

*DPT—diptheria and tetenus toxoids and pertussis vaccine
†TOPV—trivalent oral polio virus vaccine
‡MMR—measles, mumps, and rubella vaccine; may be combined or separate
§TD—combined tetanus and diptheria toxoids

Appendix 4. Drug Conversion for Children

A. Clark's weight rule for pediatric dosage.

$$\frac{\text{child's weight in pounds}}{150} \times \text{adult dose}$$

$$= \text{approximate dose for child}$$

B. Intravenous microdrip usually has 60 drops/cc.

C. Conversion of administration units.

1 tsp = 5 ml
1 tbl = 15 ml
1 ml = 16 minims
1 grain = 60 mg
1 gm = 1,000 mg
1 oz = 30 ml
1 dram = 4 ml

Appendix 5. Pediatric Communicable Diseases

Disease	Characteristics	Transmission	Nursing Care
Chickenpox (varicella)	Acute viral disease; onset is sudden with high fever; maculopapular rash and vesicular scabs in multiple stages of healing. Incubation is 10 to 21 days.	Spread by droplet or airborne secretions; scabs not infectious.	Isolate. Treat symptoms: Tylenol, fluids for fever. Prevent scratching.
Mumps	Acute viral disease, characterized by fever, swelling, and tenderness of one or more salivary glands. Potential complications, including meningoencephalitis.	Spread by droplet and direct and indirect contact with saliva of infected person. Most infectious 48 hours prior to swelling.	Prevent by vaccination. Isolate. Treat symptoms: ice pack to neck and force fluids. Watch for symptoms of neurological involvement: fever headache vomiting stiff neck.

Disease	Characteristics	Transmission	Nursing Care
Measles (rubeola)	Acute viral disease, characterized by conjunctivitis, bronchitis, Koplik's spots on buccal mucosa, dusky red and splotchy rash 3 to 4 days, and usually photophobia. Complications can be severe in respiratory tract, eye, ear, and nervous system. Incubation is 10 to 12 days.	Spread by droplet or direct contact.	Symptomatic: bed rest until cough and fever subside, force fluids, dim lights in room, tepid baths, lotion to relieve itching.
German measles (rubella)	Viral infection, slight fever, mild coryza, and headache. Discrete pink-red maculopapules that last about three days. Incubation 14 to 21 days. Basically a benign disease.	Spread by direct and indirect contact with droplets. Fetus may contract measles in utero if mother has the disease.	Symptomatic: bed rest until fever subsides.
Diphtheria	Local and systemic manifestations: malaise, fever, cough with stridor. Toxin has affinity for renal, nerve, and cardiac tissue. Incubation 2 to 6 days or longer.	Spread by droplets from respiratory tract or carrier.	Antitoxin and antibiotic therapy to kill toxin. Strict bed rest to prevent exertion. Liquid or soft diet. Observe for respiratory obstruction— suctioning, oxygen, and emergency tracheotomy may be necessary.
Tetanus (lockjaw)	Acute or gradual onset. Muscle rigidity and spasms, headache, fever, and convulsions. Death may result from aspiration, pneumonia, or exhaustion. Incubation 3 to 21 days.	Organisms in soil that enter body through wound. Not communicable man to man.	Toxins must be neutralized. Bed rest during illness in quiet, darkened room. Avoid stimulation that can cause spasms. Observe for complications of laryngospasm and respiratory failure.

Appendix 6. Vital Signs for Children at Different Ages

Vital Sign Chart

Age	Range of Normal Pulse (average)		Average Blood Pressure	Average Respiration
Newborn	70–170	120	80/45	40–90
1 year	80–160	115	96/65	20–40
2 years	80–130	110	99/65	20–30
4 years	80–120	100	99/65	20–25
6 years	75–115	100	100/56	20–25
8 years	70–110	90	105/56	15–20
10 years	70–110	90	110/58	15–20

Pulse

A. Increased rate is significant if maintained during sleep.

B. Body temperature elevation causes an increase of 8 to 10 pulse beats for each degree of elevation.

Appendix 7. Dental Development

Deciduous

	Age at Eruption		Age at Shedding	
	Maxillary	**Mandibular**	**Maxillary**	**Mandibular**
Central incisors	6 to 8 months	5 to 7 months	7 to 8 years	6 to 7 years
Lateral incisors	8 to 11	7 to 10	8 to 9	7 to 8
Cuspids	16 to 20	16 to 20	11 to 12	9 to 11
First molars	10 to 16	10 to 16	10 to 11	10 to 12
Second molars	20 to 30	20 to 30	10 to 12	11 to 13

Permanent Eruption

	Maxillary	**Mandibular**
Central incisors	7 to 8 years	6 to 7 years
Lateral incisors	8 to 9	7 to 8
Cuspids	11 to 12	9 to 11
First molars	6 to 7	6 to 7
Second molars	12 to 13	12 to 13
First premolars	10 to 11	10 to 11
Second premolars	10 to 12	11 to 13
Third molars	17 to 22	17 to 22

Review Questions

1. Mrs. Harrison is the young mother of Susan, a one-month-old infant. Mrs. Harrison is concerned because Susan sleeps so much of the day. You should tell Mrs. Harrison that infants

   A. Sleep all day and stay awake most of the night until they get on a regular routine.
   B. Should have only one nap during the day.
   C. Need at least 12 hours of sleep out of every 24 hours.
   D. Usually sleep about 20 out of every 24 hours.

2. Susan has just received her first DPT shot. Mrs. Harrison asks you what it is for. You tell her that DPT

   A. Immunizes Susan against diphtheria, tetanus, and pertussis.
   B. Is the first poliomyelitis shot.
   C. Is the immunization against all childhood diseases.
   D. Is given to determine Susan's susceptibility to pertussis.

3. By the time Susan is three months old she should be able to

   A. See objects only as shapes and shadows.
   B. Focus her eyes only momentarily.
   C. Distinguish between light and dark only.
   D. Focus her eyes on objects and people.

4. Susan weighed 6 pounds at birth. By the time she is six months old she should weigh about

   A. 21 pounds.
   B. 8 pounds.
   C. 12 pounds.
   D. 26 pounds.

5. At 10 months Susan can stand alone but has not taken any steps. Mrs. Harrison is upset because she has been told by a friend that a lot of babies walk by 10 months of age. You can reassure her by saying

   A. Your friend is exaggerating.
   B. Susan may be slightly retarded.
   C. Perhaps Susan has a mild case of cerebral palsy.
   D. Each child develops at his or her own rate.

6. At the age of exploring, it is most important for Mrs. Harrison to be aware of

   A. Safety hazards, such as poisons and medicine, which are within Susan's reach.
   B. The need for teaching Susan good table manners.
   C. The danger of spoiling the child with too much love and affection.
   D. The possibility that Susan may show extreme jealousy toward others.

7. Which of the following signs and symptoms would be characteristic of a congenital heart defect?

   A. Headaches, increased blood pressure, and high sodium.
   B. Edema, decreased pulse, and severe cough.
   C. Growth retardation, fatigue, and tachycardia.
   D. Bradycardia, dyspnea, and edema.

8. Henry Gibson was admitted soon after birth with a diagnosis of diaphragmatic hernia. It can be defined as

   A. A weakened area of the diaphragm permitting gas to escape.
   B. A hole in the diaphragm permitting abdominal viscera to enter the chest cavity.
   C. An opening between the stomach and the esophagus.
   D. An out-pouching of the pleura causing deflation of one lung.

9. Infantile eczema is

   A. A result of sensitivity to some substance.
   B. Caused by *staphylococcus aureus*.
   C. A parasitic skin disease.
   D. Caused by poor hygiene.

10. The period of negativism begins when the child

    A. Can manipulate his or her parents.
    B. Copies negativistic behavior of siblings.
    C. Is struggling between dependence and independence.
    D. Is learning manual skills.

11. The eating habits of a preschool child are usually

    A. Copied from other members of the family.
    B. Not important.
    C. Well established by two years of age.
    D. Learned from friends.

12. Which one of the following statements best describes the incidence of communicable diseases in children?

    A. Communicable diseases have been eliminated due to immunizations.
    B. Communicable diseases are a necessary part of every child's life.
    C. Communicable diseases are never serious.
    D. Immunizations have reduced the incidence.

13. When providing diversional activities for a child in isolation, it must be remembered that

    A. Any articles brought into the unit should be washable.
    B. These children are always on absolute bed rest.
    C. The room must be darkened to protect the child's eyes.
    D. Most children are satisfied with books.

14. Parents will have fewer conflicts with their adolescent children if they

   A. Formulate a very strict disciplinary code.
   B. Try to remember their own adolescence.
   C. Allow the adolescent to solve some of his or her own problems.
   D. Continuously evaluate the adolescent.

15. Vocational guidance should help adolescents to

   A. Make some decisions about their future.
   B. Realistically assess their assets and limitations.
   C. Get into college.
   D. Find a good job.

16. Many of the fears and fantasies of adolescents can be avoided if

   A. Sex education is accurate and complete.
   B. Religion is respected and valuable to them.
   C. They are kept physically active.
   D. All mixed gatherings are carefully chaperoned.

17. John, a three-year-old, was admitted from the emergency room with a diagnosis of croup. His orders included frequent observations and a croupette with mist. Which of the following facts are true?

   A. The functioning of the croupette should be explained in detail to John.
   B. John should be kept as warm and as dry as possible.
   C. The croupette is used to provide a quiet dark environment for the patient.
   D. All of the above.

18. George has an esophageal atresia. His mother says to the nurse, "I feel as though I've done something wrong to make my child sick." The most appropriate response would be

   A. "Don't be silly. Your child was born with this. You've done the best you can."
   B. "It does no good to feel that way. Your child is sick and needs you. You should spend your time caring for him."
   C. "A lot of mothers feel guilty when their child is ill."
   D. "I can understand your feelings, but remember that this is a congenital defect, which you did not cause."

19. Inez, a premature infant, is visited by her mother. The nurse asks the mother if she would like to feed her. The mother says, "Oh, no, you do it so well. I want my child to be well cared for." The nurse should interpret this as

   A. A compliment to the nurse's ability.
   B. A sign that the mother is still tired from the delivery and is not yet ready to care for the child.

   C. An expression of the mother's sense of inadequacy in caring for her own child.
   D. An admission of the mother's inexperience in dealing with premature infants.

20. The most appropriate response by the nurse to Inez's mother would be

   A. "I'll feed her today. Maybe tomorrow you can try it."
   B. "It's not difficult at all. She is just like a normal baby, only smaller."
   C. "You can learn to feed her as well as I can; I wasn't good when I first fed a premature infant either."
   D. "It's frightening sometimes to feed an infant this small, but I'll stay with you to help."

21. Janet Valdez, a seven-month-old child, is admitted to the pediatric unit for a cardiac catheterization. Mrs. Valdez sees the nurse having difficulty feeding the child cereal and says, "Janet won't take cereal before her bottle, only after." The most appropriate response by the nurse would be

   A. "It's not good to give a bottle first because the infant becomes full and has no desire to eat anything else."
   B. "I think it is time that Janet became used to having her cereal first because that is what she will have to do here."
   C. "Thank you. I'll try it that way and tell the other nurses."
   D. "That's unusual. Most babies like it this way."

22. The surgical procedure used to correct pyloric stenosis is

   A. Mustard.
   B. Fredet-Ramstedt.
   C. Gastrostomy.
   D. Blalock-Taussig.

23. The most important nursing goal prior to surgery for correction of pyloric stenosis is

   A. Prevention of dehydration.
   B. Education of the parents about the procedure.
   C. Provide sensory stimuli for the infant.
   D. Prevention of the development by the infant of a negative attitude toward feeding.

24. The primary problem with esophageal atresia that a nurse should be concerned about is

   A. Aspiration.
   B. Gastric distention.
   C. Poor feeding habits.
   D. Esophageal irritation.

25. The first choice of treatment for intussusception is

   A. Gastric lavage.
   B. Barium enema.
   C. Bowel reduction.
   D. Colostomy.

26. Frequent, watery stools with blood, pus, and mucus are usually found in

   A. Intussusception.
   B. Diarrhea.
   C. Hirschsprung's disease.
   D. Late appendicitis.

27. A child diagnosed as being profoundly retarded would have an IQ that is

   A. Below 20.
   B. Unmeasurable.
   C. Below 50.
   D. Below 75.

28. The type of training that has been found to be very successful with mentally retarded children is

   A. Structured.
   B. Self-pacing.
   C. Behavior modification.
   D. Unstructured.

29. Cretinism is caused by

   A. A malfunctioning pituitary gland.
   B. A hyperactive pancreas.
   C. An inactive or absent thyroid gland.
   D. Amino acid deficiency.

30. While bathing a one-year-old, a nurse feels a large mass in the abdominal area. The nurse thinks it may be a Wilms's tumor. The nurse should

   A. Palpate it to ascertain its exact size and position.
   B. Immediately notify the doctor.
   C. Ask the child if it hurts.
   D. Tell the mother that she should tell the pediatrician about it at the child's next visit.

31. Following a shunting procedure, John Michael, a child with hydrocephalus, has a slightly depressed fontanel. While he is in bed, he should

   A. Be propped in a semi-sitting position.
   B. Be propped with head slightly elevated.
   C. Have his head flat or slightly lowered.
   D. None of the above.

32. A twenty-two-month-old infant is brought to the hospital for treatment of an acute illness. The child's initial adjustment to the hospital will be facilitated if the nurse understands that

   A. It will be beneficial to the child if the mother leaves as soon as the nurse begins the admission procedure.

   B. Participation by the mother in the admission procedure is likely to be beneficial both to her and to the child.
   C. The child's cooperation during the admission procedure will be assured if the mother is allowed to hold the child for a while prior to the procedure.
   D. The mother should be seated at the foot of the crib where the child can see her throughout the admission process.

33. A toddler is hospitalized for surgery. The parents are unable to room in because of other responsibilities at home. The child becomes very quiet and never cries during painful hospital procedures. The nurse should interpret this behavior as evidence that the child

   A. Has given up fighting and has become despondent and hopeless.
   B. Was well prepared by the parents for the separation and hospitalization.
   C. Has been taught not to misbehave in front of strangers.
   D. Does not feel well.

34. A mother of toilet trained fourteen-month-old Calvin expresses concern over her child's bedwetting while hospitalized. The most appropriate response by the nurse would be

   A. "Calvin is a little young to be toilet trained. In a few more months he will be old enough."
   B. "Children get scared in the hospital and frequently wet their beds."
   C. "Hospitalization is so frightening to children that they frequently abandon behaviors that they have recently acquired."
   D. "I'll tell the night nurse to wake Calvin up and take him to the toilet."

35. Which of the following is a cyanotic heart defect?

   A. Ventricular septal defect.
   B. Aortic stenosis.
   C. Tetralogy of Fallot.
   D. Pulmonic stenosis.

36. Which of the following organs has some blood shunted past it in fetal circulation?

   A. Heart.
   B. Lungs.
   C. Brain.
   D. Kidney.

37. What must be present in order for an infant with complete transposition of the great vessels to survive at birth?

    A. Coarctation of the aorta.
    B. Large septal defect.
    C. Pulmonic stenosis.
    D. Mitral stenosis.

38. When a child returns to the pediatric unit following a cardiac catheterization, what nursing activity should immediately follow the taking of vital signs?

    A. Place the child in a warm bed and encourage sleep.
    B. Provide the child with fluids.
    C. Check the peripheral pulses.
    D. Reapply the dressing where the dye was injected.

39. Which of the following activities should a nurse always do prior to administering digoxin?

    A. Obtain an ECG.
    B. Take the blood pressure.
    C. Take the temperature.
    D. Take the pulse.

40. A four-year-old with congestive heart failure is being digitalized. The nurse who is giving the third dose of digoxin observes that the child's temperature is 99.8 and the pulse is 100. The nurse should

    A. Call the physician.
    B. Recognize that these are signs of digoxin toxicity and withhold the dose.
    C. Give the medication.
    D. Give the medication but make a note that the pulse is lower than normal.

41. The best method of feeding an infant with a cleft lip is with a

    A. Gavage tube.
    B. Nipple on the side with the cleft.
    C. Nipple on the side without the cleft.
    D. Rubber-tipped medicine dropper placed on the side without the cleft.

42. The best method of feeding an infant in the first week following the repair of a cleft lip is with a

    A. Gavage tube.
    B. Nipple on the side with the suture.
    C. Nipple on the side without the suture.
    D. Rubber-tipped medicine dropper placed on the side without the suture.

43. What is the most important developmental task you would encourage a mother to teach her child prior to surgery for the repair of cleft palate?

    A. Socializing with peers.
    B. Being comfortable with strangers.
    C. Becoming toilet trained.
    D. Drinking from a cup.

44. Over 50 percent of the children who are abused are

    A. Under one year of age.
    B. Under three years of age.
    C. From three to six years of age.
    D. From six to ten years of age.

45. Which of the following characteristics is least often seen in parents who abuse their children?

    A. They do not want their child.
    B. They are loners.
    C. They expect the child to act older than he or she is.
    D. They were abused as children.

46. Of the following disorders the condition that would indicate use of the drug Dilantin would be

    A. Grand mal seizures.
    B. Psychomotor seizures.
    C. Vascular headache.
    D. All of the above.

47. Tommy, eighteen months old, starts to have a grand mal seizure while the nurse is in the room. Tommy's jaws are clamped, and he is in his crib. What is the most important nursing activity at this time?

    A. Place a padded tongue blade over Tommy's tongue.
    B. Prepare the suction equipment.
    C. Protect the child from harm from the environment.
    D. Restrain the child to prevent injury.

48. During a well-child conference the nurse instructs the mother on the best procedure to follow if her child swallows poison. Which one of the following should the mother do first?

    A. Telephone the local poison control center.
    B. Bring the child to the emergency room.
    C. Give the child some alcohol to drink to induce vomiting.
    D. Ascertain what substance the child drank.

49. The leading cause of accidental deaths in children from one to four years of age is

    A. Motor vehicle.
    B. Fires or burns.
    C. Poisoning.
    D. Drowning.

50. Which of the following are early symptoms of leukemia?

    A. Low-grade fever and lethargy.
    B. Rectal ulcers.
    C. Bruising.
    D. All the above.

51. The test used in the diagnosis of cystic fibrosis is

    A. Sweat chloride.
    B. Blood glucose.
    C. Sputum culture.
    D. Examination of stools for fat content.

52. A child with cystic fibrosis is being discharged from the hospital. The nurse is instructing the mother on the administration of pancreatic enzymes, which the child should take three times a day. Which of the following instructions would be correct?

    A. The child should take them at intervals of eight hours with a large glass of milk.
    B. The medication should be given following breakfast, lunch, and dinner.
    C. The child can take them at any time from six to eight hours apart. The timing should depend on what is most convenient for the family schedule.
    D. The medication should be taken prior to meals.

53. The diet regime usually prescribed for a child with acute glomerulonephritis is

    A. Low sodium, low calorie.
    B. Low potassium, protein free.
    C. Fluid intake of 1000 cc/24 hours.
    D. Low calcium, low potassium.

54. The major objective of nursing a child with meningomyelocele prior to surgery is

    A. Observation of muscle movement below the level of the lesion.
    B. Prevention of infection.
    C. Prevention of contractures.
    D. Maintenance of fluid and electrolyte balance.

55. Credé is a term used for

    A. A type of french catheter.
    B. A surgical procedure for urinary diversion.
    C. A manual method of expelling urine from the bladder.
    D. A method of early toilet training.

56. A controlled diet instituted relatively early after birth may prevent or limit mental retardation in which of these conditions?

    A. Cretinism.
    B. Down's syndrome.
    C. Phenylketonuria.
    D. Tay-Sach's disease.

57. Which of the following reactions would you be most likely to find in a school-age child who is hospitalized?

    A. Fear of abandonment.
    B. Fear of displacement at school.
    C. Concern about body image.
    D. Disruption in identity formation.

58. In preparing a child who is five for a procedure, the nurse should give consideration to the fact that the normal five-year-old

    A. Is beyond the stage of fearing intrusive procedures.
    B. Responds poorly to verbal directions.
    C. Understands simple directions.
    D. Is quiet and shy.

59. When planning activities for school-age children who are in the hospital, it would be appropriate to consider that school-age children

    A. Work well in groups.
    B. Like immediate gratification from projects.
    C. Have a short attention span.
    D. Prefer games that are noncompetitive.

60. A school-age child with a cardiac condition is placed on a low-sodium diet. The most appropriate method of ordering meals would be to

    A. Have the child fill out the menu with the nurse's assistance.
    B. Have the child's mother fill out the menus after the nurse teaches her the diet.
    C. Have the nurse fill out the menu.
    D. Ask the dietician to order the meals.

61. Sharon is diagnosed as having sickle cell anemia. The most accurate description of this disease is

    A. Chronic anemia due to the inability to utilize iron.
    B. Sickle-shaped red blood cells.
    C. Red blood cells that sickle under low oxygen tension.
    D. Anemia due to sickle cells in the blood that combine with the red blood cells and make them less available to the tissues.

62. Sharon is given a blood transfusion. Which of the following signs and symptoms are most characteristic of an allergic reaction to blood?

    A. Fall in blood pressure, distention of neck veins, and rash.
    B. Backache, laryngeal edema, and generalized discomfort.
    C. Wheezing, flushing, and laryngeal edema.
    D. Tachycardia, hives, and flushed skin.

63. If an allergic reaction occurs, the nurse should first

    A. Relieve the symptoms and make the patient comfortable.
    B. Call the physician.
    C. Slow the rate of infusion.
    D. Shut off the transfusion.

64. Which of the following statements about cerebral palsy is not true?

    A. Seventy percent of the children function mentally at a subnormal level.
    B. Cerebral palsy can be the result of difficult labor.
    C. Seventy-five percent of cerebral palsy children have a seizure disorder.
    D. Children with cerebral palsy can exhibit spastic, athetoid, or ataxic movements.

65. Brain tumors are

    A. Rare in children.
    B. Seen primarily in the five to seven age range.
    C. Seen primarily in adolescents.
    D. Seen primarily in infants.

66. The main reason that a high percentage of brain tumors in children cannot be successfully treated is that

    A. By the time the symptoms appear metastasis has occurred.
    B. Most parents refuse to permit brain surgery.
    C. Most tumors are highly malignant.
    D. A large number of tumors are impossible to remove because of their position in the brain.

67. Susan Medieras, fourteen years old, is admitted to the adolescent ward with a tentative diagnosis of juvenile diabetes mellitus. Which of the following fears would you most likely find in Susan?

    A. Fear of being displaced.
    B. Fear of separation.
    C. Fear of loss of independence.
    D. Fear of the unknown.

68. Which of the following symptoms would you expect Susan to exhibit when her insulin injection is delayed?

    A. Thirst, polyuria, and decreased appetite.
    B. Flushed cheeks, acetone breath, and increased thirst.
    C. Nausea, vomiting, and diarrhea.
    D. Gain of weight, acetone breath, and thirst.

69. Her mother is concerned about Susan's future health and her ability to lead a normal life. The most appropriate comment by the nurse would be

    A. "Susan will be able to lead a normal life."
    B. "If Susan follows the correct regime, she will have no problems."
    C. "Juvenile diabetes does not cause a shortened life span."
    D. "Diabetes can have some long term effects on an individual's health; however, how much Susan will be affected is impossible to tell at this time."

70. Susan has been regulated on semilente insulin. When teaching her about its effects, the nurse would tell her that this type of insulin has an onset of

    A. One-half hour.
    B. One hour.
    C. Two hours.
    D. Two and one-half hours.

71. When teaching Susan about regulation of her diabetes at home, which of the following would not be included?

    A. Limitation of vigorous exercise.
    B. Elimination of sugar from diet.
    C. Urine testing for sugar.
    D. Test for acetone.

72. Adolescent diabetics frequently have more difficulty than diabetics in other age groups because

    A. The disease is usually more severe in adolescents than in younger children.
    B. Adolescents as a group have poor eating habits.
    C. Adolescents have a difficult time with long-acting insulin.
    D. Adolescents need table sugar for growth.

73. Which of the following facts about obese adolescents is not true?

    A. They usually have an overweight parent.
    B. They were fat as infants and children.
    C. They frequently have a thyroid disorder.
    D. They are very aware of their excess weight.

74. Karen is fifteen years old and has been admitted to the adolescent ward for scoliosis and insertion of a Harrington rod. Considering the course of therapy with a Harrington rod insertion, which of the following problems would Karen be most likely to exhibit?

    A. Identity crisis.
    B. Body image changes.
    C. Feeling of displacement.
    D. Loss of privacy.

75. The organism responsible for syphilis is

    A. Herpes virus type II.
    B. *Neisseria gonorrhoeae.*
    C. *Treponema pallidum.*
    D. Trichomonas.

76. During a routine physical examination the following reflexes are noted in a nine-month-old child. Which of the following is an abnormal finding?

    A. Parachute reflex.
    B. Neck righting reflex.
    C. Rooting and sucking reflex.
    D. Moro's reflex.

77. Which one of the following toys would be most suitable for a ten-month-old?

    A. Play dough.
    B. A baseball-sized ball.
    C. A box of jacks.
    D. A mobile.

78. At which one of the following ages would finger foods be appropriate for an infant?

    A. Four months.
    B. Six months.
    C. Nine months.
    D. None of the above.

79. In separation anxiety the child may go through all of the following phases except

    A. Protest.
    B. Despair.
    C. Denial.
    D. Adjustment.

80. Following Clark's rule, a child's dosage of a medication would be calculated by which of the procedures listed below?

    A. Adult dose minus child's weight in pounds divided by 150.
    B. Adult dose times child's weight in kilograms divided by 150.
    C. Adult dose times child's weight in pounds divided by 150.
    D. Adult dose times child's weight divided by 100.

81. A child weighs 10 kilograms, and the adult dose of a medication is 10 mg. What would be the closest correct dosage to give the child?

    A. 1.0 mg.
    B. 1.5 mg.
    C. 2.0 mg.
    D. None of the above.

82. In administering medications to children, all the following considerations would be important except

    A. Explain about the medication in words the child can understand.
    B. Mix a distasteful medication with a small amount of appetizing food or syrup.
    C. Tell a child who refuses an oral medication that he or she will have to have an injection.
    D. Indicate by your actions that you expect the child to take the medication.

83. When administering an intramuscular injection to an infant, the appropriate actions by the nurse would include all of the following except

    A. Place the infant in a secure position to prevent movement.
    B. Do not use a needle longer than 2.5 cm.

    C. Use the upper inner quadrant of the thigh.
    D. Hold and cuddle the infant following the injection.

84. When an infant who is nursing is hospitalized, the nurse should encourage the mother to

    A. Accept the fact the baby will need formula while in the hospital.
    B. Continue breast feeding if the baby's condition does not contraindicate it.
    C. Pump her breasts and bring the milk to the hospital.
    D. Breast feed once a day to relieve pressure of milk in the breasts.

85. Brian is six months old and is admitted to the hospital with severe diarrhea. Which one of the following nursing objectives would be *most* important?

    A. Make constant assessment of dehydration level.
    B. Accurately record the number of stools.
    C. Dispose of stools in proper containers.
    D. Monitor electrolyte lab results.

86. Brian continues to have diarrhea in the hospital so it has been decided to feed him via hyperalimentation. The best explanation for this procedure is

    A. A method of providing the necessary fluids and electrolytes to the body.
    B. A method of providing complete nutrition by the intravenous route.
    C. A method of tube feeding that provides necessary nutrients to the body.
    D. A method of blood transfusion.

87. The nurse assigned to Brian is careful to observe for signs of complications resulting from the therapy. Which one of the following signs is *not* considered a possible complication related to the implanted catheter?

    A. Plugging or dislodging of the catheter.
    B. Cardiac arrhythmia.
    C. Catheter in the superior vena cava.
    D. Local skin infection.

88. Which one of the following symptoms would *not* be an indication of the need for oxygen?

    A. Flaring nostrils.
    B. Cyanosis.
    C. Bradycardia.
    D. Deep, regular breathing.

89. If one parent has the sickle cell trait, how many of the children will get the disease?

    A. None.
    B. All of the children.
    C. Half of the children.
    D. Can't tell from the information given.

90. You are assigned to care for Jimmy, a nine-year-old boy who has been hospitalized for a week with cystic fibrosis. He has greatly improved and is about to be discharged. Knowing that cystic fibrosis children often develop pneumonia secondary to colds, which one of the following self-care principles would it be important to teach Jimmy before discharge?

   A. Protein enzymes in his diet will protect him from colds.
   B. Restricted exercise will help to prevent sweating and catching a chill.
   C. Breathing exercises will develop lung potential.
   D. High-protein, high-fat diet will improve nutritional status.

91. A high-protein diet would be prescribed for all of the following childhood conditions *except*

   A. Malabsorption syndrome.
   B. Malnutrition.
   C. Acute leukemia.
   D. Chronic glomerulonephritis.

92. Mrs. Saviana is about to take her one-year-old child home from the hospital. The child was admitted one week previously with a diagnosis of croup. One of the home care techniques you might teach Mrs. Saviana if her child begins to cough and cannot stop is to

   A. Take the child into the bathroom and turn on the shower.
   B. Give the child frequent doses of prescribed cough medicine.
   C. Do not allow the child outside for the cold air will prolong the coughing.
   D. Call the doctor immediately.

93. You are working in a well-baby clinic, and it is one of your responsibilities to take a history on new patients. Mrs. Pala brings her three-year-old in and tells you that she wants a check-up because the child seems small and thin for her age. As you begin to question Mrs. Pala, you learn that the child has frequent nose bleeds and always seems tired. With this information you would suspect that the symptoms might fall into which of the following disease groups?

   A. Heart disease.
   B. Subdural hematoma.
   C. Leukemia.
   D. Hemophilia.

94. Baby Bowden has a diagnosis of T.E. fistula and the doctor has decided to operate. From your knowledge of pediatrics, when is the newborn the best operative risk?

   A. First 24 hours.
   B. Forty-eight to 72 hours.

   C. Three weeks old.
   D. One week old.

95. The responsibility for the care of the mentally retarded is

   A. The parents.
   B. The public schools.
   C. The state.
   D. All of the above.

96. The doctor has ordered a blood transfusion following a tonsillectomy after which the child hemorrhaged. Before the blood transfusion, one important action by the nurse would be to

   A. Check for skin rash or a change in skin color.
   B. Check for restlessness or irritability.
   C. Take the child's temperature.
   D. Check the child for chills or cold sweats.

97. You are assigned to care for a child suffering from third-degree burns on hands and arms. Of the following which one would be an appropriate activity for an eight-year-old child?

   A. Read a story and act out the parts verbally.
   B. Watch a puppet show.
   C. Watch TV.
   D. Listen to the radio.

Answers and Rationale

1. (D)   Most newborns are awake for eating and care only.

2. (A)   The "D" is for diphtheria, the "P" is for pertussis, and the "T" is for tetanus.

3. (D)   At three months an infant is able to recognize people.

4. (C)   Babies should double their birth weight by five to six months.

5. (D)   One of the principles of growth and development is that children develop at different rates.

6. (A)   Children are interested in all things within their reach.

7. (C)   Growth retardation is due to lack of oxygen to the tissues. The heart is working harder to carry more oxygen, causing fatigue and tachycardia.

8. (B)   Hernia is inevitable because of incomplete development of the diaphragm.

9. (A) Poor hygiene or a parasite may make eczema worse but does not cause it.

10. (C) Negativism begins as the child learns to do some things independently and then becomes frustrated by things he or she cannot do.

11. (A) Preschoolers eat at home more than away from home.

12. (D) There are many cases of childhood diseases each year, and they are serious.

13. (A) Things that go into the room will have to be disinfected before they are removed, so they should be washable.

14. (C) Adolescents want to be independent most of all so it is important for them to make their own decisions.

15. (A) At this age it is hard for them to be realistic, but they can make some decisions about the future.

16. (A) They need information about their bodies and what to expect.

17. (B) A three-year-old may not understand a detailed explanation. The tent is clear plastic, letting in the light.

18. (D) The nurse recognizes the mother's feelings, but tries to show that they are not based on fact.

19. (C) This mother is implying that she is not capable of caring for her own child.

20. (D) The nurse, while recognizing and accepting this mother's apprehension, assures her that she will have assistance.

21. (C) The nurse recognizes that the mother knows the child's habits better than anyone else.

22. (B) The Fredet-Ramstedt procedure is used to correct pyloric stenosis.

23. (A) Dehydration from persistent vomiting is the most frequent complication of pyloric stenosis.

24. (A) Aspiration is the most potentially harmful complication of this deformity.

25. (B) Most physicians will attempt to reduce the bowel with a barium enema. If this is not successful, a bowel reduction is done.

26. (B) Usually Hirschsprung's disease and appendicitis cause constipation. Intussusception can cause

stools with blood, pus, and mucus, but the stools are usually infrequent.

27. (A) Profound is the most severe category of mental retardation.

28. (C) Behavior modification with its immediate reward system is best understood by slow children.

29. (C) The first two answers deal with other glandular disorders; cretinism is caused by hypofunction of the thyroid gland.

30. (B) A suspected Wilms's tumor should never be palpated more than necessary because of the potential for metastasis.

31. (B) If cerebral spinal fluid is allowed to drain out too quickly, the ventricles may collapse.

32. (B) The mother is accepted as an important participant in the child's care, and the child does not feel deserted by the mother.

33. (A) A toddler who passively accepts aggressive painful intrusions into his or her life has usually given up any sense of hope.

34. (C) The nurse explains the principle of regression.

35. (C) In cyanotic heart defects there is a right-to-left shunt which permits unoxygenated blood to move into the systemic circulation.

36. (B) The ductus arteriosus and foramen ovale permit the shunting of blood past the lungs in the fetus.

37. (B) Since complete transposition results in two closed blood systems, the child can survive only if there is an opening between the two, such as a septal defect.

38. (C) The nurse must ensure that the peripheral circulation is intact. The other activities are done but are not first.

39. (D) The nurse should always check the pulse prior to administering digoxin because of its slowing effect on the heart.

40. (C) A normal pulse for a four-year-old is 100; elevated temperature is not a sign of digoxin toxicity.

41. (C) A nurse should use a soft or regular nipple with a slightly enlarged hole and feed on the side opposite the cleft.

42. (C) Following surgery the nurse must prevent any pressure on or trauma to the suture line.

43. (D) It is imperative that a child know how to drink from a cup since that is the only way the child can drink following surgery.

44. (B) The highest number of abused children are under three years old.

45. (A) Abused children are usually wanted by the parents. It is after the arrival of the child that the parents experience anger and frustration that leads to abuse.

46. (D) Dilantin is used not only for relief of seizures but also for vascular conditions such as migraine headaches.

47. (C) The best way to protect a child from injury during a seizure is to remove all objects from his or her environment.

48. (D) It is important that the mother know what the child drank since the emergency treatment will depend on the type of substance consumed.

49. (A) It is important for the nurse to know the leading causes of accidents and deaths so that he or she can teach appropriate preventive measures.

50. (D) All these are early signs of leukemia.

51. (A) Cystic fibrosis children produce abnormally high levels of sodium chloride in their sweat. Although C and D might be used during the diagnostic workup, they do not definitely diagnose the disease.

52. (D) The purpose of the enzymes is to replace the enzymes in the child's system that assist with the digestion of fats; therefore, they should be taken prior to the ingestion of food.

53. (B) A diet restricted from potassium and protein is necessary for children who demonstrate some degree of renal failure.

54. (B) Although the other objectives are important, infection represents the greatest threat to this child prior to surgery.

55. (C) Credé is never used on a child with normal nerve functioning.

56. (C) A strictly controlled diet for PKU children will prevent or limit mental retardation.

57. (B) A school-age child's concern is primarily present oriented.

58. (C) A preschooler can understand simple directions. Although a five-year-old may be quiet and shy, these qualities are not applicable to this situation.

59. (A) This age group benefits from association and interaction with peers in a group setting.

60. (A) Ordering meals in this manner allows the child some independence and control and at the same time provides an excellent teaching opportunity.

61. (C) The patient's red blood cells are not always sickled but become this way under certain conditions.

62. (C) All other symptoms listed are a combination of allergic and transfusion reactions.

63. (D) If the nurse suspects an allergic reaction, the blood should be shut off immediately, and then the physician should be notified.

64. (A) Approximately 50 percent of cerebral palsy children function mentally at a subnormal level.

65. (B) School-age children have the highest incidence of brain tumors in children.

66. (D) Many tumors are so placed that to remove them would involve brain damage.

67. (C) Adolescents, having recently achieved some measure of independence, have a fear of losing it.

68. (B) All the other choices have one wrong answer. Decreased appetite (A), diarrhea (C), and weight gain (D), are symptoms not usually associated with this condition.

69. (D) The best response is to be honest with Susan's mother.

70. (A) Semilente insulin has an onset of one-half hour, peaks at two to four hours, and has a duration of ten to twelve hours.

71. (A) If a patient is in good health and understands the increased glucose needs of the body following exercise, there is no reason to restrict activities.

72. (B) As young adults start spending more time with their peer groups, they frequently adopt eating habits of this group which are often not appropriate for diabetics.

73. (C) The great majority of obese adolescents are overweight due to a poor eating pattern.

74. (B) This question is difficult. The body casting that follows Harrington rod insertion does create some privacy problems; however, Karen's changed body image is likely to cause more difficulty.

75. (C) All of the answers are the cause of venereal disease; however, syphilis is specifically caused by *Treponema pallidum.*

76. (D) Moro's reflex begins to fade at the third or fourth month.

77. (B) Play dough is more appropriate for a toddler and older children. Jacks will go right into the mouth of infants. A ten-month-old might reach and grab a mobile.

78. (C) Nine months is an appropriate age to introduce finger foods.

79. (D) Denial may be mistaken for a happy adjustment.

80. (C) The adult dose is multiplied by the child's weight in pounds and then is divided by 150.

81. (B) To calculate this problem, translate the child's weight into pounds and then apply Clark's rule.

82. (C) Never threaten a child with an injection if the child refuses an oral medication.

83. (C) The upper outer quadrant of the thigh is the appropriate site for IM injections.

84. (B) If possible, it is more therapeutic for both mother and baby to continue breast feeding.

85. (A) While all the objectives listed in the answers are important, assessment of dehydration level and acidosis are the most crucial, for this condition can be life-threatening.

86. (B) This is a method that involves infusion of a solution of protein, glucose, electrolytes, vitamins, and minerals—complete nutrition by the intravenous route.

87. (C) This is not a complication, but the actual site of insertion of the indwelling catheter.

88. (D) Shallow and irregular breathing indicate the need for oxygen.

89. (A) No children will get sickle cell anemia if both parents do not have at least recessive genes. One parent can pass the gene on so that the children may be carriers.

90. (C) Children with cystic fibrosis typically evidence shallow breathing, which does not utilize lung potential and may contribute to frequent infections.

91. (D) In renal disease with a demonstrated degree of renal failure the protein would be restricted.

92. (A) Warm, moist air reduces epiglottic edema and helps to relieve coughing.

93. (A) The child manifests symptoms common to heart disease; other symptoms might be cyanosis and slow weight gain.

94. (A) During the first 24 hours the newborn is the best risk as he or she still has the extra blood volume, placenta hormones, and nourishment from the mother.

95. (D) The responsibility is the combination of all three groups.

96. (C) It is important to take the child's temperature before administration of blood. A reaction to the blood would be indicated if the temperature rises after the transfusion.

97. (A) This activity involves the child so that he or she is actively, if not physically, participating in play.

Mental Health Nursing

Mental Health Continuum

Mental Illness

Definition: Mental illness is the general term that is used for a variety of behavioral reactions to life stresses that range from severe personality disorganization to the milder forms of temporary inability to cope with daily stress. Mental health, according to the World Health Organization, is "the presence of physical and emotional well-being."

Characteristics

A. Mental illness is a major health problem in the United States. One out of three individuals experiences some form of mental illness during a period of his or her life.
B. There has been an ever increasing number of clients admitted to mental hospitals or special units in private hospitals.
C. The criteria of mental illness might be said to be the extent to which problems are not dealt with through rational decisions.

Community Mental Health Movement

A. National Mental Health Act placed emphasis on the quality of care hospitalized mentally ill clients received.
B. It also emphasized the level of skills necessary to deliver higher quality care and lower rate of chronic hospitalized clients.
C. Object of act was to alter the state hospital model which was linked to chronicity and severity of disease.
D. Primary objectives were stated as preventing mental illness, coping with symptoms of illness, and returning the client to community as soon as possible.

Anxiety

Definition: Anxiety is an affective state that is subjectively experienced as a response to stress. It is experienced as painful vague uneasiness, tension, or diffuse apprehension. It is a form of energy whose presence is inferred from its effect on attention, behavior, learning, and perception.

Characteristics

A. Anxiety is subjectively perceived by the conscious portion of the personality.
B. It can occur as a result of conflicts between the personality and the environment or between different aspects within the personality.
C. It may be a reaction to threats of deprivation of something vital to the person, biologically or emotionally.
D. The individual may be unaware of the conflicts.
E. The degree of anxiety is in relation to its effect on the individual.
F. Level of anxiety is influenced by:
   1. The extent to which the self feels threatened.
   2. The extent to which behavior reduces anxiety.
G. Varying levels of anxiety are common to all individuals at one time or another.
H. Anxiety can be transmitted from individual to individual.
I. Realistic anxiety can be constructive.
J. Anxiety may be placed on a continuum of degrees.
   1. Absent (ataraxia).
      a. Uncommon.
      b. Apparent in the person who takes drugs.
      c. Indicator of a low level of motivation.
   2. Mild.
      a. Senses are alert.
      b. Attentiveness is heightened.
      c. Motivation is increased.
   3. Moderate.
      a. Selective inattention because it narrows perception.
      b. Point at which it becomes pathological depends on individual.
      c. May be seen as behaviors that are complaining, arguing, teasing.

d. Can convert to physical symptoms, such as headache, low back pain, nausea, diarrhea.

4. Severe.
   a. Extremely painful psychologically.
   b. Nursing intervention always indicated.
   c. No longer useful to client.
   d. Drains energy.
   e. Defense mechanisms may be used to "solve" underlying problem.
   f. Behavior becomes automatic.
   g. All senses are gravely affected.

5. Panic.
   a. Individual is overwhelmed.
   b. Personality may disintegrate.
   c. Condition is now pathological.
   d. Anxiety cannot be tolerated very long.
      (1) Individual cannot control his behavior.
      (2) Individual feels helpless.
      (3) Individual is briefly psychotic.
   e. Observed behavior.
      (1) Ineffective.
      (2) Wild and desperate, causing possible bodily harm to self and others.
   f. Needs immediate intervention.
      (1) Physical restraint.
      (2) Constant presence of attendant.
      (3) Tranquilizers.
      (4) Nonstimulating environment.

K. Neurotic anxiety.
   1. Disproportionate to the danger.
   2. Involves repression and dissociation.
   3. Behavior is relatively ineffective and is inflexible.

L. Anxiety is always present in emotional disorders.

M. Physiological reactions to anxiety.
   1. Increased heart rate.
   2. Increased or decreased appetite.
   3. Increased blood supply to skeletal muscles.
   4. Tendency to void.
   5. Dry mouth.
   6. "Butterflies" in stomach, nausea, vomiting, cramps, diarrhea.
   7. "Flight" or "fight" response.

Nursing Care

A. Intervene when client unable to cope with anxiety or is ineffective in reducing it.
B. Be aware of own anxiety.
C. Maintain positive attitudes toward client.
   1. Acceptance.
   2. Matter-of-fact approach.
   3. Willingness to listen and help.
   4. Calmness and support.
D. Recognize anxiety-produced behavior.
E. Provide activities that decrease anxiety and provide an outlet for energy.
F. Establish person-to-person relationship.
   1. Allow client to express feelings.
   2. Proceed at client's pace.
   3. Avoid forcing client to express feelings.
   4. Assist client in identifying anxiety.
   5. Assist client in learning new ways of dealing with anxiety.
G. Provide appropriate physical environment.
   1. Nonstimulating.
   2. Structured.
   3. Arrange to prevent physical exhaustion or self-harm.
H. Administer medication as directed and, after assessment, as needed.

Crisis Intervention

Definition: Crisis intervention is the form of therapy aimed at immediate intervention into an acute episode or crisis that the individual is unable to cope with alone.

Profile of a Crisis Situation

A. The individual is typically in a state of equilibrium (homeostatic balance).
   1. State is maintained by behavioral patterns that govern interchange between the individual and the environment.
   2. The individual uses learned coping techniques to deal with simple problems as they arise.

B. A crisis situation develops when a problem (triggering event) becomes too complex to be handled by previously learned coping techniques.

   1. Functioning modes become grossly disorganized.

   2. The individual is more amenable to intervention in circumstances of inability to resolve crisis.

   3. The potential for problem resolution as a result of intervention is positive.

C. Precipitant factors of a crisis.

   1. Threat to one's sense of security.

      a. Situational crisis: may include an actual or potential loss of job, friend, or mate.

      b. Developmental crisis: may include any change in role as occurs in marriage or birth of a child.

      c. The concurrence of two or more severe problems.

   2. Precipitants typically occur within two weeks after onset of disorganization.

Characteristics

A. Crisis is self-limiting, acute, and lasts one to six weeks.

B. Crisis is initiated by a triggering event (death, loss, etc.); usual coping mechanisms are inadequate for the situation.

C. Situation is dangerous to the person; he or she may harm self or others.

D. Individual will return to a state that is better, worse, or the same as before the crisis; therefore, intervention by the therapist is important.

E. Person is totally involved—hurts all over.

F. At this time the individual is most open for intervention; therefore, major changes can take place and the crisis can be the turning point for the person.

Stages of Crisis Development

A. Initial perception and comprehension of scope of problem.

B. Rise in tension and anxiety which instigates the usual coping mechanisms.

C. Consultation with the usual supportive contacts.

D. Familiar methods prove unsuccessful and tension increases.

E. Seeks new problem-solving methods; if unsuccessful, the problem remains and interferes with individual's life.

   1. Functioning becomes disorganized.

   2. Extreme anxiety is likely to be experienced.

   3. Perception is narrowed.

   4. Coping ability is further impaired.

   5. Situation may cause self-harm or harm to others.

   6. Individual totally involved and hurts all over.

F. Resolution will occur within six weeks with or without intervention.

Assessment of Crisis

A. Determine period of disorganization.

   1. Extent of disorganization.

   2. Length of time situation existed.

   3. Level of functioning.

B. Evaluate percipitant event.

   1. The nature of the event that triggered crisis.

   2. The significance of the event to the individual.

C. Examine effectiveness of coping mechanisms.

   1. History in experiencing similar situations.

   2. History in coping with similar situations.

D. Identify situational supports.

   1. Significant others.

   2. Agencies.

E. Suggest alternative coping modes.

   1. New coping alternatives.

   2. Situational supports.

Principles of Crisis Intervention

A. Goal is the return of client to pre-crisis level and maintainance of functioning.

B. Intervene immediately because it is important that intervention occur within the six week time limit.

C. Assess problem accurately and keep focus on this problem with reality-oriented therapy ("here and now" focus).

D. Set limits.

E. Remain with client or have significant person available as necessary.

F. Explore coping mechanisms available to client.
   1. Develop strengths and capitalize on them.
   2. Do not focus on weakness or pathology.
   3. Help explore the available situational supports.

G. Help the client to understand the problem and to integrate the events in his or her life.

H. Determine if continuing therapy with a professional may be needed for future support.

☆ Nursing Care

A. Focus on immediate problem.

B. Use reality-oriented approach.

C. Stay with "here and now" focus.

D. Set limits.

E. Stay with patient or have significant persons available if necessary.

F. Explore available coping mechanisms.
   1. Develop strengths and capitalize on them.
   2. Do not focus on weakness or pathology.
   3. Help explore the available situational supports.

G. Clarify the problem and help the individual understand the problem and integrate the events in his life.

H. When the above steps are completed, some plans for future spport should be worked out by the therapist and the patient.

Defense Mechanisms

Definition: Defense mechanisms, or adjustive techniques, are methods that are assumed by an individual to relieve or decrease anxieties produced by an uncomfortable situation that threatens self-esteem.

Characteristics

A. The purpose of adjustive techniques is to attempt reduction of anxiety and reestablishment of equilibrium.

B. An individual's adjustment depends on the ability to vary responses so that anxiety is decreased.

C. Individuals use essentially the same techniques, which may vary in form.

D. The exercise of a defense mechanism may be a conscious process, but it is usually generated at the unconscious level.

E. Adjustive techniques are compromise solutions that include many forms (see Appendix 1— Defense Mechanisms).

F. Healthy adjustment to life forces.
   1. A healthy adjustment is characterized by:
      a. The infrequent need to use unconscious adjustive techniques.
      b. The ability to form new responses.
      c. The ability to change the external environment.
      d. The ability to modify one's own needs.
   2. Healthy adjustment mechanisms may include rationalization, sublimation, compensation, and suppression.

G. Unhealthy adjustment to life forces.
   1. An unhealthy adjustment is characterized by:
      a. The inability or loss of ability to vary responses.
      b. The individual's retreat from the problem or from reality.
      c. Continual use, which may interfere with maintenance of self-image.
   2. Unhealthy adjustment mechanisms may include regression, repression, denial, projection, and isolation.

Nursing Care

A. Be aware of your own behavior and the use of adjustive techniques.

B. Avoid criticizing the client's behavior and use of adjustive techniques.

C. Assist the client in learning new or alternative adjustment techniques for healthier adaptation.

D. Use techniques to help alleviate the client's anxiety.

E. Do not attempt to arbitrarily eliminate adjustive techniques without replacement for they serve a purpose for the client.

Affective Disorders

Bipolar Disorders

Manic-Depressive Illness—Manic Episode

Definition: One manifestation of an affective disorder that involves mood swings of elation, euphoria, and grandiose behavior with or without a history of depression. Cyclothymic disorder is the second category of bipolar disorder and refers to a milder form of the same illness.

Characteristics

A. Specific etiology is unknown. May be related to a genetic predisposition to illness or to increased levels of dopamine in the brain. Attempts are now being made to discover why lithium is therapeutic in hopes of solving the mystery of manic illness.

B. Women experience this illness slightly more frequently than men. The lifetime risk of developing this illness is 1–2 percent of the population.

C. The first manic episode usually occurs before age 30 and, interestingly, is more common in the higher socio-economic group.

D. Mania refers to a pronounced, elated, high mood that is evidenced by a high level of activity and general demeanor of cheerfulness.

Signs and Symptoms

A. Mood is one of euphoria which can lead to grandiose behavior and delusions.

B. Individual overresponds to stimuli.
  1. Rapid talk, with play on words and flight of ideas.
  2. Increased motor activity.
  3. Increased thought processes.

C. Individual exercises poor judgment, i.e., spends money foolishly, runs up charge accounts, etc.

D. Individual's attitude is narcissistic and will not tolerate guidance or criticism.

E. Individual gives little attention to physical health.
  1. Poor sleep habits with no apparent fatigue.
  2. Poor nutrition.
  3. Poor, or even bizarre, habits of grooming.

F. Behavior varies from delightful and playful to restless, irritable, sarcastic, and even antagonistic and combative.

G. If behavior is not controlled, the individual will become incoherent, overtly aggressive, and hostile.

Nursing Care

A. Maintain safe environment.
  1. Reduce external stimuli such as noise, people, and motion.
  2. Eliminate client's participation in competitive activities.
  3. Redirect client's energy into brief but useful activities.

B. Establish one-to-one relationship.
  1. Maintain an accepting and nonjudgmental attitude.
  2. Create conditions favorable to the development of mutual trust.
  3. Avoid entering into client's playful, joking activity if it appears to be a manic reaction.
  4. Allow the client to verbalize his or her feelings, especially hostility.

C. Set realistic limits on behavior.
  1. Set scope and limitations to behavior to provide for a sense of security.
  2. Restrain destructive behavior.

3. Be firm and consistent.

D. Give attention to physical needs.
   1. Provide a diet that is high in calories, vitamins, and fluids.
   2. Ensure adequate rest and sleep.
   3. Protect client from inadvertent self-harm.

Major Depressive Episode

Definition: A unipolar condition in which the feeling state of the individual is abnormal and manifests itself by a complex of symptoms. The symptoms may be mild and only slightly debilitating or pathological, implying overwhelming intensity and long duration.

Characteristics

A. The most common of all psychiatric illnesses, depression is a symptom probably experienced by 15 out of 100 adults in our society.

B. One cause is now thought to involve a genetic link; other possible causes are personality traits such as low self-esteem, neuro-chemical imbalances, and other biological factors.

C. Most acute depressive episodes are self-limiting and last from a few weeks (with treatment) to a few months.

D. More than half of those persons who experience a first episode go on to suffer a recurrence.

E. About 20–25 percent never return to their premorbid state of mental health.

Signs and Symptoms

A. The distinguishing quality of depression is mood; affect is one of sadness or gloom.

B. Behavior is slowed down with purposeful movement nearly diminished.

C. Personal appearance is neglected.

D. Thought processes are slowed down until there is paucity of thinking.

E. Attitudes are pessimistic and self-denigrating, and focus is on the problems and uselessness of life. The individual lacks inner resources and strengths to cope effectively.

F. Physical symptoms usually reflect a preoccupation with body and poor health. Weight loss, insomnia, and general malaise are typically in evidence.

G. Social interaction is reduced and inappropriate. The depressed client feels isolated but cannot resolve that condition because he or she cannot contribute to a relationship.

H. A common outcome of depression is possible suicide (refer to section on suicide).

Major Depressive Episode Subtypes

A. Depression with melancholia.
   1. Predisposing factors appear to be dissatisfaction with accomplishments in life and loss of pleasure in the usual activities.
   2. Emphasis is on the vegetative signs and variation in mood (often called involutional melancholia).
   3. Common symptoms that accompany this disorder are a general depressed mood that is worse in the morning, psychomotor retardation, or agitation and anorexia which may result in weight loss.

B. Depression with psychotic symptoms.
   1. This subtype of depression is accompanied by an inability to test reality: delusions, hallucinations, and confusion.
      a. May also have severe impairment of personal and social functioning.
      b. May be severely withdrawn.
   2. Approximately 10 percent of those depressed have psychotic symptoms.
   3. Psychotic depressions are considered to be biologically based.

Dysthymic Disorder (Depressive Neurosis)

A. Symptoms of depression fluctuate and are less severe than with the major depressive disorder.
   1. Mild symptoms are present for at least two years.
   2. Depression may be episodic or constant.

B. Psychosis is not present.

C. Several of the following symptoms are usually present with this diagnosis.
1. Low energy level.
2. Loss of interest in pleasurable activities.
3. Pessimistic attitude toward the future; thoughts of suicide.
4. Tearful, crying demeanor.
5. Feelings of low self-esteem.
6. Decreased ability to concentrate.

Table 1. Affective Illness

Depression Type	Distinguishing Feature

Bipolar
  Manic-depressive
    disorder
  Cyclothymic
    disorder
	History of elation episodes with or without depression

Unipolar
  Major depressive
    disorder
  Depression with
    melancholia
  Depression with
    psychotic
    features
  Dysthymic disorder
	History of depression without any history of elation

Nursing Care

A. Provide a safe milieu, and protect the client from self-injury (prevent suicide).
B. Provide a structured environment to mobilize the patient.
1. Encourage daily activities, and allow time for them.
2. Provide stimulation for occupational and recreational activity.
3. Reactivate interests outside of the client's present concerns.
4. Motivate client for treatment.
5. Encourage psychotherapy and occupational therapy activities.

C. Build trust through one-to-one relationship.
1. Employ a supportive and unchallenging approach.
2. Project behaviors and attitudes that are accepting and nonjudgmental.
3. Show interest. Listen and give positive reinforcement.
4. Redirect the client's monologue away from painful and depressing thoughts.
5. Focus on the client's underlying anger, and encourage its expression.
D. Help build the self-esteem of the client.
1. Encourage simple tasks that invite successful experiences.
2. Limit decision-making with the severely depressed.
3. Support use of defenses to alleviate suffering.
E. Be attentive to the client's physical needs: provide adequate nutrition and opportunity for sleep and exercise.

Suicide

Definition: The act of killing oneself intentionally.

Characteristics

A. Suicide is the seventh most common cause of death in the United States today.
B. Suicide statistics.
1. Suicide ranks fourth as the cause of death in the fifteen to forty age group.
2. For every successful suicide, it is believed that there are five to ten attempted suicides.
3. Women make more suicide attempts than men.
4. Suicide is more common in the elderly age group.
5. Adolescent suicide is increasing.
6. Suicides are incurred by means of auto accidents; because they are not reported as such, statistics remain low.
C. Causes of suicide attempts.
1. Depression is the primary cause.

2. The secondary cause is alcohol.

3. Inability to cope with problems in living.

4. Attempts to control others.

D. Depressed individuals, when severely ill, rarely commit suicide.

   1. They do not have the drive and energy to make a plan and follow it through when severely depressed.

   2. Danger period is when depression begins to lift.

E. Eight out of ten known suicide cases give warnings or messages through direct or indirect means.

F. Danger symptoms range from depression, disorientation, and defiance to intense dependence on another.

Nursing Care

A. Provide safe environment to protect client from self-destruction.

B. Observe closely at all times, especially when depression is lifting.

C. Establish supportive relationship, letting the client know you are concerned for his welfare.

D. Encourage expression of feelings, especially anger.

☆E. Determine client's capacity to entertain suicide ideas.

   1. Ask questions such as, "Are you thinking of suicide?" "Did you think you might do something about it?" "What?" "Have you taken any steps to prepare?" "What are they?"

   2. Important to recognize a continued desire to commit suicide.

F. Focus on strengths and successful experiences that can enhance self-esteem.

G. Follow a structured schedule, and involve the client in activities with others.

H. Help structure a plan for coping when client next experiences ideas of suicide.

I. Help the client plan for continued professional support after discharge.

Somatoform Disorders

Definition: Somatoform disorders (also called psychosomatic disorders) are physical diseases that may involve any organ system, and whose etiologies are in part related to emotional factors.

Characteristics

A. An individual must adapt and adjust to stresses in life.

   1. The way a person adapts depends on individual characteristics and extent of inner stability.

   2. Emotional stress may exacerbate or percipitate an illness.

B. Psychosocial stress or anxiety is an important factor in symptom formation.

   1. If stress or anxiety cannot be expressed through verbalization, it finds expression through particular organ symptoms.

   2. Exact relationship between stress and illness is unknown.

   3. It is thought that somatic symptoms occur in individuals who have never had to resolve dependent-independent struggles of childhood; dependent needs not met.

   4. Illness provides focus for individual away from original anxiety; it provides secondary gains of sympathy and attention from others.

C. Structural changes in body systems may occur and pose a life-threatening situation.

   1. Individual not faking illness; it is real and requires direct medical attention.

   2. Correcting physical illness may not alter the underlying cause of anxiety.

D. There can be synergistic reaction from repressed feelings and overexcited organs.

E. Psychosomatic illness provides individual with coping mechanisms.

   1. Means to handle anxiety and stress.

   2. Ways to gain socially acceptable attention.

   3. Rationalization for failures.

   4. Means for adjusting to dependency needs.

5. Ways to handle anger and aggression.

6. Ways to punish self and others.

F. Kinds of adjustive techniques used (see Appendix 1—Defense Mechanisms).

   1. Repression.
   2. Denial.
   3. Projection.
   4. Conversion.

G. A psychosomatic disorder may involve any body system.

   1. Gastrointestinal system.
      a. Peptic ulcer.
      b. Colic.
      c. Ulcerative colitis.
   2. Cardiovascular system.
      a. Hypertension.
      b. Tachycardia.
      c. Migraine headaches.
   3. Respiratory system.
      a. Asthma.
      b. Hay fever.
      c. Hiccoughs.
   4. Skin (most expressive organ of emotion).
      a. Blushing.
      b. Flushing, perspiring.
      c. Dermatitis.
   5. Nervous system.
      a. Chronic general fatigue.
      b. Exhaustion.
   6. Endocrine.
      a. Dysmenorrhea.
      b. Hyperthyroidism.
   7. Musculoskeletal system.
      a. Cramps.
      b. Rheumatoid arthritis.
   8. Other associated disorders.
      a. Diabetes mellitus.
      b. Obesity.
      c. Sexual dysfunctions.
      d. Hyperemesis gravidarum.
      e. Accident proneness.

Nursing Care

A. Observe closely and assess client's condition.

   1. Collect data about the physical illness, psychosocial adjustment, life situations, natural stresses, strengths, etc.

   2. Report the kinds of things that aggravate or release the symptom.

B. Attend to the whole person, physically and emotionally.

C. Reduce demands on the client.

D. Develop nurse-client relationship.

   1. Respect the client and acknowledge his or her problems.
   2. Assist the client to express his or her feelings.
   3. Help the client to release anxiety and explore new coping mechanisms.
   4. Allow the client to meet dependency needs.
   5. Allow the client to feel in control of his or her life.

E. Encourage the client to work through problems and to learn new methods of responding to stress.

F. Provide safe and nonthreatening environment.

   1. Balance therapy and recreation.
   2. Decrease distracting stimuli.
   3. Provide activities that can deemphasize or help to alleviate the client's physical symptoms.

Conversion Reaction

A. Anxiety that results from an unconscious conflict is converted into physical symptoms for which there is no organic explanation.

B. Specific nursing approaches.

   1. Understand that client's lack of concern or indifferent attitude is at the same time a symptom of the illness.
   2. Recognize that illness is frequently used for primary gains, i.e., solving conflict by not solving it and removing the source of stress. Illness used as secondary gains provide client with sympathy and attention to physical handicap.
   3. Do not confront the client with his or her illness.
   4. Divert client's attention from symptoms.

Do not respond to client's secondary gains.

5. Reduce pressure or demands on client.
6. Create positive relationship.
7. Use a matter-of-fact approach.
8. Provide client with recreational and socializing activities.
9. Teach necessities of daily living, and give assistance as needed, i.e., if client is blind, help and show how to feed self.

Hypochondriasis

A. A severe, morbid preoccupation with one's own body; abnormal anxiety about one's health.
B. Specific nursing approaches.
   1. Accept the client and his or her complaints.
   2. Provide diversional activities in which the client can succeed.
   3. Use friendly, supportive approach.
   4. Provide for client's physical needs.
   5. Assist client to refocus interest.

Anxiety Disorders

Definition: A mild to moderately severe psychologic disorder that affects thought and feeling processes. The individual suppresses and represses unpleasant thoughts and/or feelings to alleviate the discomfort of the resulting anxiety. The consequent conflicts are handled by means of anxiety reaction, phobias, obsessive-compulsive reaction, dissociation, hypochondriasis, and neurasthenia.

Characteristics

A. No apparent physiologic basis for symptoms.
B. Threats to ego cause anxiety, and ego protects the person by developing defenses, the neurotic behavior.
C. A neurosis is an attempt to deal with anxiety.
D. Individuals have little difficulty talking, but conversation may be vague and unrevealing.
E. Individual is generally unaware of his or her behavior patterns.

F. Individual becomes more dependent as time goes on.
G. Secondary gains from neurosis become associated problems.
   1. These are the fringe benefits that client receives from symptoms.
   2. Secondary gains reinforce neurotic behavior.
H. Common defense mechanisms include repression and projection.
I. Evidence of low self-esteem is observable.
J. No gross distortion of reality.
K. Personality is not grossly disorganized.
L. The martyr syndrome is common.
M. Individual is highly suggestible.

Nursing Care

A. Nurse needs to understand and recognize own feelings and attitudes in dealing with neurotics.
B. Convey an attitude of acceptance and understanding of client's symptoms because client relies on them to control anxiety.
C. Plan nonthreatening activities that will reduce anxiety and enhance self-esteem.
D. Do not make unreasonable demands upon the client.
E. Remain with extremely anxious client.
F. Avoid using labels for client's behaviors.
G. Provide a safe, supportive environment.
H. Be alert to the specific needs of clients as demonstrated by their behavior.

Anxiety Reaction

A. Anxiety is diffuse (free-floating).
B. Anxiety cannot be controlled by means of defense mechanisms.
C. Psychological symptoms.
   1. Cannot concentrate on work.
   2. Feels depressed and guilty.
   3. Harbors fears of sudden death or insanity.
   4. Dreads being alone.
   5. Confused.
   6. Tense.

7. Agitated and restless.

D. Physiological symptoms.
1. Tremors.
2. Dyspnea.
3. Palpitations.
4. Tachycardia.
5. Numbness of extremities.

E. Specific nursing approaches.
1. Calm, serene approach with recognition of own anxiety.
2. Nonverbal reassurance.
3. Listen.
4. Provide physical outlet for anxiety.
5. Remain with client.
6. Decrease environmental stimuli.

Phobic Reactions

A. By means of displacement, anxiety is transferred from the original source to a symbolic idea or situation.
B. Phobic disorders are classified into three types.
1. Agoraphobia
   a. Marked fear of and avoidance of being alone or in public places where escape might be difficult or help not available in case of sudden incapacitation.
   b. Increasing constriction of normal activities until fear dominates the individual's life.
2. Social phobia
   a. A persistent irrational fear and compelling desire to avoid a situation in which the individual is exposed to scrutiny by others.
   b. Fear of acting in a way that may be humiliating or embarrassing.
   c. Distress about disturbance and feelings.
3. Simple phobia
   a. A persistent irrational fear and compelling desire to avoid an object or a situation other than agoraphobia or social.
   b. Fear of heights, closed spaces, or animals.
   c. Distress about symptoms.
C. Specific nursing approaches.
1. Slowly develop a trusting relationship with the client.

2. Do not force client into feared situations.
3. Divert client's attention from the phobia.
4. Direct client's focus to awareness of self.
5. Encourage but do not force client to discuss fears and feelings.
6. Support client during program of phobic desensitization.

Obsessive-Compulsive Reaction

A. Anxiety is associated with the persistence of undesired ideas or impulses; repetitive ritualistic actions alleviate anxiety.
B. Specific nursing approaches.
1. Avoid punishment or criticism for compulsive repetition of acts.
2. Set limits to protect client from harmful acts.
3. Provide climate of acceptance and understanding.
4. Orient nursing care around client's need to perform rituals.
5. Provide for client's physical needs.

Schizophrenic Disorders

Definition: Schizophrenia is a syndrome that carries with it varied etiology, psychodynamics, and psychopathology. The clinical course of the illness varies from patient to patient, so the nurse should view the disease as a syndrome with varying clinical entities.

Characteristics

A. Schizophrenia may be the result of many variables: genetic constellation, individual adaptive patterns, poor family relationships, lack of ego strength, earlier traumatic experiences, or distorted cognition.
B. Regression and repression are regarded as the primary mechanisms of schizophrenia.
C. Major maladaptive disturbances: impaired interpersonal relationships, ineffective mental and emotional processes, and disturbances in overt behavior patterns.

D. Individuals generally demonstrate personality disorganization and coping difficulty.

E. Schizophrenic reactions may become acute and/or chronic.

Primary Disturbances

A. Thoughts are confused and disorganized so that ability to communicate clearly is limited.

B. Feelings (affect) may be expressed in an inappropriate manner.

C. Behavior may be bizarre or lack purposeful direction.

D. Close and trusting interpersonal relationships are difficult to establish.

Clinical Signs and Symptoms

A. The four "A's."
1. *Affect*—feelings or subjective aspect of emotions are minimal, i.e., "flat affect"; apathetic, inappropriate expression of moods and responses.
2. *Associative looseness*—no connection between thoughts and expressed ideas; difficulty in discerning logical from illogical thought.
3. *Autistic thinking*—thoughts are self-serving and focus inward, i.e., client uses neologisms or invented words and lives in a world of inner fantasy.
4. *Ambivalence*—two equally strong feelings, such as love and hate, neutralize each other and immobilize client.

B. Other important clinical signs.
1. *Reality testing* difficulty—objective facts cannot be distinguished from wishes or imagination.
2. *Delusions*—fixed misinterpretation of reality. False beliefs maintained despite evidence to the contrary.
3. *Hallucinations*—sensory input (smell, taste, sound, touch, sight) that has no basis in the real world. One "hears" voices, "sees" visions, etc.
4. *Withdrawal*—behavior that signifies the client's desire to regress into more satisfying world of own making (autism).

5. The above signs may manifest themselves in singular or combined forms.

Nursing Care

A. General approaches.
1. Establish nurse-client relationship.
   a. Develop positive and trusting relationship.
   b. Provide a safe and secure environment.
2. Stress situational reality.
   a. Help client to reality-test and come out of fantasy world.
   b. Involve the client in reality-oriented activities.
   c. Help the client to find satisfaction in the external environment.
3. Accept the client as he or she is.
   a. Do not invalidate disturbed thoughts or fantasies.
   b. Do not invalidate the client's sense of self by your inappropriate responses.
4. Use only therapeutic communication techniques.
   a. Encourage client to express negative and/or positive emotions.
   b. Encourage client to express thoughts, fears, and problems.
   c. Match your nonverbal with your verbal communications.
   d. Communicate clearly with the client.
5. Do not foster a dependency relationship.
6. Avoid stressful situations that can increase the client's anxiety.

B. Approaches to specific behaviors.
1. Working with delusions.
   a. Help the client to recognize distorted views of reality.
   b. Focus on client's strengths.
   c. Provide a safe, nonthreatening milieu.
   d. Divert focus from delusional material to reality.
   e. Provide situations that can create successful experiences for the client.
   f. Specific nursing responses:
      (1) Avoid confirming or feeding into delusion.

470

(2) Stress reality by denying you believe the client's delusion.

(3) Respond to client's feelings, i.e., validate his or her feelings by saying, "I sense you are afraid. Is this true?"

2. Working with withdrawn behavior.
   a. Assist client in developing a satisfying relationship with you.
      (1) Initiate interaction.
      (2) Show sincerity for a trusting relationship by being consistent in keeping appointments, in attitudes, and in nursing practice.
      (3) Be honest and direct in what you say and do.
      (4) Deal with your feelings incurred by client's hostility or rejection.
   b. Help client to modify self-perception.
      (1) Structure situations in which client will succeed.
      (2) Focus on client's assets or strengths to enhance self-esteem.
      (3) Relieve client from making choices until able to make decisions.
   c. Teach client how to restore social skills.
      (1) Gradually increase opportunities for social contacts with staff and other clients.
      (2) Increase opportunities for social contact with significant others (family) as appropriate.
   d. Focus on reality situations.
      (1) Use nonthreatening approach.
      (2) Provide safe nonthreatening milieu.
   e. Attend to physical needs of nutrition, sleep, exercise, occupational therapy.

Schizophrenic Subtypes

A. Catatonic type.
   1. Secondary symptoms of motor involvement are present.
      a. Underactivity results in bizarre posturing.
      b. Overactivity leads to agitation.
   2. Negativism: doing the opposite of what is asked.
      a. Rigidity is the simplest form of negativism.
      b. Mute behavior is another form of negativism.
B. Disorganized type.
   1. Inappropriate affect: giggling and silly laughter (formerly labeled hebephrenia).
   2. Disorganization of speech.
   3. Regression.
   4. Absence of systematized delusions.
C. Undifferentiated type.
   1. This type is characterized by a combination of symptoms, none of which discriminates a specific type of disorder.
   2. Flat affect and/or autism is usually present.
   3. Association disorders and thought disturbance, such as delusions or hallucinations, are usually present.
   4. This condition includes other behavioral maladaptations that cannot be otherwise classified.
D. Paranoid schizophrenia.
   1. A type of schizophrenic reaction that manifests delusions of persecution and other maladaptive behavior.
   2. Characteristics.
      a. Individual is extremely suspicious and withdraws from emotional contact with others.
      b. The onset is gradual and usually occurs between the ages of thirty and forty.
      c. Certain stressful events in the individual's life may precipitate onset of paranoid reaction.
         (1) Real or imaginary loss of a loved one.
         (2) Experiences of failure with subsequent loss of self-esteem.
      d. Individual expresses abnormal concern with health (hypochondriasis).
         (1) Complains of insomnia and weakness.

(2) Complains of strange bodily sensations.

(3) Complains of other somatic disturbances.

e. Individual projects common paranoic delusional thoughts.

    (1) Feels persecuted, i.e., individual fears that people are out to harm, injure, or destroy him or her.

    (2) Behaves as if in a state of grandeur.

    (3) Expresses jealousy.

f. Paranoic reactions can occur in organic, senile, alcoholic, and other mental illnesses.

3. Clinical signs and symptoms.

    a. Extreme suspiciousness and mistrust of others.

    b. Hostility toward others.

    c. Delusions of persecution or grandeur.

    d. Chronic insecurity, inadequate self-concept, low self-esteem.

    e. Chronic high anxiety level.

    f. Client denies delusional role.

    g. Hypochrondriasis.

4. Nursing care.

    a. Establish a trusting relationship.

        (1) Be consistent and friendly despite client's hostility.

        (2) Avoid talking and laughing when the client can see but not hear you.

        (3) If client is very suspicious, relate one-to-one and not in a group situation.

        (4) Involve the client in the treatment plan.

        (5) Give nonpunitive support.

    b. Reduce anxiety associated with interpersonal interactions.

        (1) Avoid power struggles, i.e., do not argue with the client because it increases anxiety and hostility.

        (2) Proceed with nursing therapy slowly because a paranoid client is suspicious and often mistrustful of others.

        (3) Show consistency and honesty.

c. Help client differentiate delusion from reality (refer to section on delusions).

    (1) Do not explain away imagined thoughts for they are real to the client.

    (2) Use reality-testing whenever possible.

    (3) Focus on reality situations in the environment.

Table 2. Profile Differentiation

Schizophrenic	Non-Schizophrenic
Major ego impairment. Includes faulty reality testing, delusions, hallucinations (especially auditory).	No grave impairment of reality testing. No hallucinations or delusions.
Serious impairment of client's life, including social, vocational, and sexual.	Difficulty in relating, but interaction with others not prevented. Personality usually remains organized.
Little insight into problems and behavior. Client generally does not recognize he or she is ill.	Some awareness into problems. Keenly feels subjective suffering. Often unconsiously fights any changes in status (getting well).
Severe personality disorganization, e.g., poor judgment, memory, and perceptions.	Less severe disorganization. Can function but with decreased efficiency.
May be caused by both physiological or psychological factors.	Always a functional disorder; not organic in origin.
Usually requires hospitalization and long-term treatment.	Usually does not require hospitalization. May require long-term treatment.
Maladaptive adjustment mechanisms used in rigid, fixed way. May be seen as severe regression.	Suppression and repression used to handle internal conflicts; defenses are largely symbolic.
No secondary gain received.	Symptoms generally exploited for secondary gain.

Paranoid Disorders

Definition: Diagnosis of paranoid disorder is made when paranoid features dominate the personality. Other symptoms of maladaptive behavior may be absent.

Characteristics

A. Paranoia is characterized by extreme suspiciousness and withdrawal from all emotional contact with others.
B. The onset is usually gradual.
C. The onset of paranoid reactions may be precipitated by certain stressful events in client's life.
   1. Real or imaginary loss of a love object.
   2. Experiences of failure with subsequent loss of self-esteem.

Signs and Symptoms

A. Intense focus on hypochondriasis.
B. Complaints of insomnia and weakness.
C. Complaints of strange bodily sensations.
D. The more common paranoid psychosis is manifested by delusional thoughts:
   1. The most common delusions are of persecution (people are out to harm, injure, or destroy).
   2. Other delusions may center around grandeur, somatic complaints, or delusions of jealousy.
E. Suspiciousness and mistrust of others.
F. Hostility toward others.

Dissociative Disorders

Definition: This disorder is a sudden temporary alteration in the integrative functions of consciousness, identity, or motor behavior.

Characteristics

A. Client attempts to deal with anxiety through various disturbances of by walling off certain areas of the mind from consciousness.

B. Client remains in contact with reality.
C. Repression is used.

Signs and Symptoms

A. Amnesia: circumscribed, selective, generalized and continuous.
B. Fugue or physical flight.
C. Interference in lifestyle and interpersonal relationships.
D. Accompanying symptoms such as depression, suicide ideation, etc.

Nursing Care

A. Support therapeutic modality as established by treatment team.
B. Reduce anxiety-producing stimuli.
C. Redirect client's attention away from self.
D. Avoid sympathizing with client.
E. Increase socialization activities.

Personality Disorders

Definition: An individual with a personality disorder adjusts to life situations with difficulty and interacts with others in an unsatisfactory manner. Behavioral problems rather than symptoms are exhibited. This individual is known as a psychopathic or sociopathic personality.

Characteristics

A. Experiences difficulty in developing warm interpersonal relationships.
   1. Affective responses are shallow.
   2. Relationships tend to be superficial.
B. Responds poorly to intellectual and emotional demands made of them.
C. Aggressive and sexual impulses are expressed overtly.
D. Tolerance for anxiety is low so that the person will go to any length to avoid situations that provoke anxiety.
   1. The attempts to gain relief from anxiety produce inappropriate behavior.

2. Individual is unaware that behavior is contrary to social expectations.

E. Exhibits poor impulse control and poor judgment; rejects all authority.

F. Social assets include intelligence and charm; skilled in manipulation.

G. Behavior often perceived as direct or indirect attack on laws and mores of society.

H. Personality profiles.

1. Antisocial (dissocial) personality.
   a. Lies, cheats, and steals (a pathologic diagnosis common in prisons).
   b. Shows evidence of emotional immaturity.
   c. Indicates little or no capacity for good judgment.
   d. Rationalizes behavior so that it appears justified; lacks a moral conscience.
   e. Is the typical "con artist."

2. Inadequate personality.
   a. Responds to intellectual and emotional demands ineffectively.
   b. Does not learn from experience or punishment, indicating poor judgment.
   c. Is socially unstable.
   d. Lacks ability to adapt.

3. "Social deviate" personality types.
   a. Sadist—inflicts pain on another.
   b. Masochist—inflicts pain on self.
   c. Voyeur—enjoys "peeping Tom" behavior.
   d. Exhibitionist—exposes own body for pleasure.

4. Addictive personality (see section on addiction).

5. Schizoid personality.
   a. Lacks close interpersonal relationships.
   b. Is shy and behavior is withdrawn.
   c. Projects eccentric behavior patterns.
   d. Unable to express hostility; affect is flat.

6. Paranoid personality.
   a. Suspects intentions of others.
   b. Unable to sustain interpersonal relationships because of inability to trust.
   c. Experiences jealousy and envy in relating to others.

General Nursing Care

A. Participate in planning a therapeutic nurse-client relationship that focuses on reinforcement of positive behavior.

1. Accept the client for what and where he or she is (in terms of abilities).
   a. Set realistic expectations.
   b. Assess capabilities realistically so that excessive expectations will not reinforce failure.

2. Maintain control, and protect other clients from antisocial behavior.

3. Allow expression of frustration and hostility.

4. Assist client to tolerate frustration and postpone satisfaction.

5. Explore new alternatives for client's living patterns that are socially acceptable.

6. Be aware of your own negative attitudes that may arise in working with these clients.

B. Set limitations firmly and with consistency.

1. Avoid falling into the client's charming and manipulative ways.

2. Understand that the client's anxiety will increase if manipulative behavior is ineffective.

C. Recognize that punishment does not resolve problems or change behavior.

1. Confront behavior but do not demean the client.

2. Plan a supportive environment.
   a. Provide the patient with a sense of security.
   b. Provide opportunities for client to learn how to cope with impulses.

D. Help client to formulate realistic future plans.

E. Set specific guidelines for working with sociopathic and/or psychopathic behavior.

1. Attempt to develop a trusting relationship; it is difficult because the client usually does not want help.

2. Follow the total care plan as determined

by the physician. This is important because therapy is oriented toward reconstruction of personality.

3. Focus on reality, and do not allow client to manipulate.

4. Give approval only for acceptable behavior.

Nursing Approaches to Maladaptive Behavior

Aggressive or Combative Behavior

A. Observe sharply for clues that the client is getting out of control.
   1. Note rising anger from client's verbal and nonverbal behavior.
   2. Note erratic or unpredictable responses to staff or other clients.

B. Intervene immediately when aware that client's loss of control is imminent.

C. Approach the client in a nonthreatening manner.

D. Set firm limits on unacceptable behavior.

E. Maintain calm demeanor, and do not show fear.

F. Avoid engaging in an argument or provoking the client.

G. Summon assistance only when indicated: sudden involvement of many people will increase the client's agitation.

H. Remove the client from a threatening situation as soon as possible.

I. Use seclusion and/or restraints only if necessary.

J. Attempt to calm the client so that control can be regained.

K. Be supportive and remain with the client.

L. Use a problem-solving focus following outburst of aggressive or combative behavior.
   1. Encourage discussion of feelings surrounding incident.
   2. Attempt to discuss causal factors of the behavior.

3. Examine the client's initial response to stimulus, and explore alternative responses.

4. Point out consequences of aggressive behavior.

5. Discuss the client's role in taking responsibility for his aggressive behavior.

Verbally Abusive Behavior

A. Do not respond in kind to abusive comments.

B. Try not to take abuse personally.

C. Interact with the client on a therapeutic basis.
   1. Help the client examine own feelings.
   2. Do not reject the client.
   3. Give client feedback concerning your reactions to abusive comments.
   4. Teach alternative ways to express feelings.

D. Maintain a calm, accepting approach to client.

Demanding Behavior

A. Do not ignore demands; they will only increase in intensity.

B. Attempt to determine causal factors of behavior, e.g., high anxiety level.

C. Set limits to your own response patterns when client is demanding.

D. Control own feelings of anger and irritation.

E. Teach alternative means for getting needs met.

F. Plan nursing care to include frequent contacts that are initiated by the nurse.

G. Alert the staff to try to give client needed reassurance.

Rape Intervention

Definition: Rape is a sexual assault on a person that is basically an act of violence; only secondarily considered a sex act.

Characteristics

A. Recognize that the assault of rape is a humiliating and violent experience and that the victim is experiencing severe psychological trauma.

B. Accept the fact that the victim was indeed raped and that the victim is to be supported, not treated as the "accused."

C. Understand that the victim's behavior might vary from hysterical crying and/or laughing to very calm and controlled.

D. Crisis response
   1. Acute: shock, crying, high anxiety, hysterical, incoherent, agitated, fearful, volatile, poor problem-solving ability.
   2. Beginning to cope: denial, appears calm and controlled, withdrawn, fearful, begins to talk about feelings, expresses anger, makes decisions.
   3. Resolution: realistic attitudes, able to express feelings, controlled anger, acceptance of facts.

Nursing Care

A. Treatment focus.
   1. Emotional: crisis counseling and call Women Against Rape.
      a. Degree of emotional trauma.
      b. Presence of symptoms.
   2. Medical: immediate medical care: assess assault and degree of trauma.
      a. Assist with a complete physical examination.
      b. Carefully assess and document all physical damage: injuries; signs of physical entry.
   3. Legal: do not bathe, douche, or change clothes; gather evidence.

B. Interventions
   1. Provide immediate privacy for examination.
   2. Choose a staff member of the same sex to be with the victim.
   3. Remain with the victim.
   4. Administer physical care.
      a. Do not allow client to wash genital area

or void before examination; these actions will remove any existing evidence such as semen.
      b. Keep client warm.
      c. Prepare client for complete physical examination to be completed by physician (same sex as client if possible).
      d. Physical exam includes:
         (1) Head-to-toe exam.
         (2) Pap smear.
         (3) Saline suspension to test for presence of sperm.
         (4) Acid-phosphatase to determine recency of attack.
      e. Physical treatment may include:
         (1) Prophylactic antibiotics.
         (2) Tranquilizers.
   5. Provide emotional support.
      a. Demonstrate a nonjudgmental and supportive attitude.
      b. Express warmth, support, and empathy in relating to the victim.
      c. Listen to what the victim says and document all information.
      d. Encourage the victim to relate what happened, having her tell you in her own words if it appears that she would like to talk about the experience.
      e. Do not insist if client chooses not to talk; allow the victim to cope in her own way.
      f. During the interview, continue to be sensitive to the victim's feelings and degree of control. If, in relating the attack, she becomes hysterical, do not continue questioning at this time.
   6. Termination of crisis relationship.
      a. Counsel client to receive repeat test for sexually transmitted diseases in three weeks or sooner if symptoms appear.
      b. Help reestablish contact with significant people.
      c. Refer to appropriate community resource for follow-up care.
      d. Keep accurate records, as they may be important in future legal proceedings.

Substance Abuse

Definition: Substance abuse includes any process by which an individual ingests any mind-altering, non-prescribed chemical that produces physiological and/or psychological dependence. Withdrawal symptoms are usually manifest when substance is not taken.

Characteristics

A. Psychological dependence: emotional dependence, desire, or compulsion to continue taking the substance or drug.
B. Tolerance: the gradual increase of the amount required to obtain the desired effect.
C. Physical dependence: physical need for the substance manifested by appearance of withdrawal symptoms when substance is withheld.

Alcoholism

Definition: The abuse of any alcoholic substance combined with physical and psychological addiction.

Characteristics

A. Alcohol consumption is permitted by law and supported by most people in our society as a recreational activity.
B. A fine line exists between the social drinker and the addicted or problem drinker.
C. The greatest difference involves the degree of compulsion to drink and the inability to survive the trials of everyday living without the ingestion of alcohol.
D. Alcoholism, the third largest health problem in the United States (heart disease and cancer rank first and second), affects 10 million people.
E. Alcoholism is involved in about 30,000 deaths and one-half million injuries (auto accidents) every year.
F. Alcoholism decreases life span 10 to 12 years.
G. Loss to industry caused by alcoholism is estimated at 15 billion dollars a year (affecting primarily the 35 to 55 age group).
H. Major U.S. social concern is the dramatic rise in teenage alcoholism, (estimated to affect 3 million adolescents).

Dynamics of Alcoholism

A. Alcoholic disease implies the consumption of alcohol to the point where it interferes with the individual's physical, emotional, and social functioning.
   1. The syndrome consists of two phases: problem drinking and alcohol addiction.
   2. Dependence on other drugs is very common.
B. No hereditary or organic basis for alcoholism has been proven to date.
C. Alcohol blocks synaptic transmission, depresses the central nervous system (CNS), and releases inhibitions. It acts initially as a stimulant but is actually a depressant.
   1. Chronic excessive use can lead to brain damage (sedative effect on CNS).
   2. High blood levels may cause malfunctions in cardiovascular and respiratory systems.
D. Blood level of 0.15% or more of alcohol is considered the level of intoxication.
E. Psychological effects of alcohol appear to be the gratification of oral impulses and the reduction of superego forces; abuse leads to shame and guilt and impaired ego function.
F. Alcohol may be said to b a defense against anxiety; therefore, the client needs to work on problems causing his or her anxiety.
G. Illnesses associated with alcoholism.
   1. Korsakoff's syndrome.
   2. Delirium tremens.
   3. Chronic gastritis.
   4. Poor nutritional intake resulting in beriberi, pellagra, cerebellar degeneration, and anemia.
   5. Laënnec's cirrhosis and hepatitis.
   6. Peripheral neuropathy.
   7. Osteoporosis.
   8. Individual is prone to infection.

Characteristics of an Alcoholic

A. Dependent personality but resents authority.

B. Sets high self-expectations but has a low tolerance for frustration.

C. Inclined toward patterns of failure.

D. Uses alcohol to gain a false sense of success, power, confidence, and self-worth.

E. Uses alcohol to ease suffering, reduce anxiety, and to help cope with life stresses.

F. Functions with less intellectual, emotional, and social ability as need for alcohol increases.

Nursing Care

A. Help reestablish the client's healthy physical condition.
   1. Provide adequate nutrition with fluids and a high vitamin, high calorie, and high protein diet.
   2. Promote adequate rest and sleep.
   3. Observe client for symptoms of impending delirium tremens.

B. Maintain a controlled and structured environment until the client is able to manage his or her own circumstances.
   1. Set behavior limits, and confront the manipulative client.
   2. Suggest group interaction for lonely clients.
   3. Remember that the client needs support, firmness, and a reality-oriented approach.

C. Treatment techniques.
   1. Client must first go through detoxification—intensive care to prevent the toxic state and then the return to a nonalcoholic state.
   2. Stress need for a change in attitudes.
      a. To accept fact that alcoholism is an illness.
      b. To accept fact that life must be managed without the support of alcohol.
   3. Promote psychotherapy techniques of group and family therapy; establish positive nurse-client relationship therapy.
      a. Therapy goals.
         (1) Focus on the underlying emotional problems.
         (2) Offer assistance in handling anxiety.
         (3) Focus on relief of inferiority feelings and low self-esteem.
      b. Advantages of group therapy.
         (1) Client receives support from peers.
         (2) Client can receive negative feedback from peers without feeling threatened.
         (3) Client can be supported in efforts to change by nonprofessional groups (AA), but change will not occur unless client wants to be helped.
   4. Encourage rehabilitation or long-term supportive care.
      a. Continued psychotherapy on an outpatient basis.
      b. Referral to Alcoholics Anonymous.
      c. Medication such as Antabuse (alcohol sensitizing drug that causes vomiting and cardiovascular symptoms if the client drinks after taking drug).
      d. Referral to social or vocational rehabilitation community program.

D. Nursing attitudes.
   1. Maintain a nonjudgmental attitude toward the alcoholic.
   2. Approach client with firmness and consistency.
   3. Accept the individual but not his deviant behavior.
   4. Support client's attempts to change life patterns.

Drug Addiction

Definition: Drug addiction is the dependency on drugs other than alcohol or tobacco that alter perception and/or mood.

Characteristics of Narcotic Addiction

A. The most common narcotics are heroin and morphine.

B. Emotional dependence on the drug (to alter

mood) is followed by physical dependence on the drug.

C. Narcotics have a sedative effect on the CNS.

D. As tolerance level increases, greater amounts of the drug are necessary to produce pleasurable effects.

E. Addiction tends to be chronic; the rate of relapse is high.

F. Withdrawal symptoms.

   1. Anxiety.

   2. Nausea and vomiting.

   3. Sneezing, yawning, and watery eyes.

   4. Tremor and profuse perspiration.

   5. Stomach cramps and dehydration.

   6. Convulsions and coma.

G. Characteristics of the narcotic addict personality.

   1. Emotionally immature with feelings of inadequacy and inferiority.

   2. Difficulty in establishing interpersonal relationships; untruthful and insecure.

   3. Poor judgment and inability to tolerate frustration.

Characteristics of Barbiturate Addiction

A. The most common barbiturates are Seconal and Sodium Amytal.

B. Barbiturates have a sedative effect on the CNS.

C. Danger of death from overdose.

D. Emotional dependence on the drug is followed by physical dependence on the drug.

E. Originally may have been taken to relieve pain or sleeplessness.

F. Addicts usually have emotional problems and an anxious temperament.

Characteristics of Other Common Drug Addictions

A. Amphetamines.

   1. The most common amphetamines are Benzedrine and Dexedrine.

   2. They are CNS stimulants so that overuse may result in brain damage.

   3. They have the effect of producing a "high."

   4. Large doses produce a hyperactive and agitated state.

   5. They produce an emotional addiction, especially for persons who feel insecure and inadequate.

   6. They reduce appetite and awareness of bodily needs so that the person's physical condition suffers.

B. LSD, or "Acid."

   1. A hallucinogenic drug that mimics hallucinations seen in psychoses.

   2. Produces changes in perception and logical thought processes.

   3. Not considered addictive per se, but individual may become emotionally dependent on the drug.

   4. Experiences following LSD ingestion range from ectasy to terror; the consequences are unpredictable.

C. Marijuana.

   1. The abuse potential is minimal because it produces neither tolerance nor physical dependence.

   2. Produces "dreamy" state and feelings of euphoria, hilarity, and well-being.

   3. Moods vary according to environmental stimuli.

   4. Changes in perception of space and time seem to distort and extend.

   5. High dosage may produce hallucinations and delusions.

D. Cocaine.

   1. Classified as a stimulant.

   2. Usually sniffed or used intravenously.

   3. Strong psychological dependence may occur.

   4. Does not develop a physical dependence or tolerance.

E. PCP—"crystal," "elephant tranquilizer."

   1. Usually smoked with marijuana. May also be ingested or injected.

   2. Reactions vary from sense of well-being to total disorientation and hallucinations.

3. Considered an extremely dangerous street drug.

4. Psychological dependence may occur.

5. Cerebral cellular destruction and atrophy may occur with even small amounts.

6. Overdoses or "bad trips" are characterized by erratic and unpredictable behavior, withdrawal, disorientation, self-mutilation, and self-destructive behaviors.

7. Overdoses are treated with sedatives, with a decrease of environmental stimuli, and with protection of the client from self-harm and harm of others.

Nursing Care

A. General nursing approaches and attitudes are similar to those enumerated for alcoholism.

B. Special approaches to drug addiction.

1. First step is withdrawal treatment; accomplished abruptly ("cold turkey") or gradually over a period of days.

2. The substitute drug methadone is used to reduce the physical reaction to withdrawal.

3. Extended medical and psychiatric treatment for physical and emotional deterioration must be part of convalescence.

4. Resocialization process of client needs supportive treatment from professional and/or community resources.

5. Rehabilitation programs must be directed toward helping the person reenter the mainstream of society.

   a. Many organizations operated by ex-addicts offer help in rehabilitation.

   b. Therapeutic communities and group therapy programs also assist with rehabilitation

6. Specific guidelines.

   a. Provide a structured environment, and set consistent and strict limits.

   b. Identify client's attempts to manipulate; maintain control.

   c. When client distorts reality, affirm the situational facts.

   d. Give equal concern to client's physical, social, and emotional needs.

Adjunct Therapies

Psychotropic Drugs

Definition: Psychotropic drugs are those used in psychiatry in conjunction with other forms of therapy to temporarily modify behavior. They control symptoms but do not cure disorder.

Characteristics

A. Psychotropic drugs affect both the central and autonomic nervous systems.

B. These drugs affect behavior indirectly by chemically interacting with other chemicals, enzymes, or enzyme substrates.

1. Changes in cellular, tissue, and organ functions occur.

2. Drug effects vary from cellular activity to psychosocial interaction.

Antipsychotic Drugs

A. These drugs are also known as ataractic, neuroleptic, or major tranquilizers.

B. Introduced about 1953.

C. Most common drugs are phenothiazine derivatives (Thorazine, Stelazine, Trilafon, Vesprin, and Prolixin).

D. Antipsychotic drugs control hallucinations, delusions and bizarre behavior and can calm an excited client without producing a marked impairment of motor function or sleep.

E. Side effects.

1. Blood dyscrasias.

   a. Agranulocytosis occurs in first 3–5 weeks of treatment. *Symptoms:* fever, sore throat.

   b. Leukopenia, preceded by altered white blood count.

2. Extrapyramidal effects occur in 30 percent of clients, affecting the voluntary movements and skeletal muscles.

   a. Parkinsonism: symptoms occur 1–4 weeks; signs are similar to classic parkinsonism: rigidity, shuffling gait, pillrolling hand movement, tremors, dyskinesia, and mask-like face.

  b. Akathisia: very common; occurs 1-6 weeks; uncontrolled motor restlessness, foot-tapping, agitation, pacing.

  c. Dystonia: occurs early, 1-2 days; limb and neck spasms; uncoordinated, jerky movements; difficulty in speaking and swallowing, and rigidity and spasms of muscles.

  d. Tardive dyskinesia: develops late in treatment; estimated to occur in up to 50 percent of chronic schizophrenics. Antiparkinson drugs are of no help in decreasing symptoms. This is a permanent side effect; symptoms are shuffling gait, drooling, and general dystonic symptoms.

3. Hypotension: orthostatic hypotension may occur. Monitor closely when client is elderly. Keep client supine for 1 hour and advise to change positions slowly.

4. Anticholinergic effects: dry mouth, blurred vision, tachycardia, nasal congestion and constipation. Treat symptomatically.

5. Potentiate CNS depressant, especially alcohol.

6. Antacids reduce absorption.

F. Another common antipsychotic drug is derived from butyrophenone (Haldol).

  1. These drugs are less sedative than phenothiazines.

  2. High incidence of severe extrapyramidal reactions.

  3. Side effects include leukocytosis, blurred vision, dry mouth, urinary retention.

  4. Avoid alcohol.

G. The most common drugs of the thioxanthene classification are Taractan and Navane.

Antianxiety Drugs

A. These drugs induce sedation, relax muscles, and inhibit convulsions; major use to reduce anxiety.

B. These drugs are the most frequently prescribed drugs in medicine; demand is great for relief from anxiety and they are safer than sedative-hypnotics.

C. They potentiate drug abuse. Greatest harm occurs when combined with alcohol and other CNS depressants.

D. They are prescribed in neuroses, psychosomatic disorders, or functional psychiatric disorders, but do not modify psychotic behavior.

E. Drugs from two major classes. Benzodiazepines: safer and more common (Librium, Valium, Centrax, Serax, and Xanax—being tested for use in depression and panic disorders). Nonbenzodiazepines: Vistaril, Equanil, and Miltown.

F. Side effects.

  1. Drowsiness (avoid driving or working around equipment).

  2. Blurred vision, constipation, dermatitis, mental confusion, anorexia, polyuria, menstrual irregularities, and edema.

  3. Habituation and increased tolerance.

  4. Pancytopenia, thrombocytopenia, and agranulcytopenia.

Antidepressant Drugs

A. The tricyclics, the most commonly used antidepressants, include Elavil, Norpramin, Tofranil, Aventyl, and Vivactil.

  1. Anticholinergic: take 1-3 weeks to be effective. Produce antagonism of the parasympathetic system.

  2. Clients with morbid fantasies do not respond well to these drugs.

  3. Side effects.

    a. Anticholinergic effects: dry mouth, blurred vision, constipation, postural hypotension.

    b. CNS effects: tremor, agitation, angry states, mania.

    c. Cardiovascular effects: palpitations. Exert a quinidine-like effect on the heart so assess any patient with history of myocardial infarction.

  4. If client is switched from a tricyclic drug to an MAO inhibitor, a period of 1-3 weeks must elaspe.

B. The monoamine oxidase inhibitors include

Marplan, Niamid, Nardil, and Parnate.

1. MAO inhibitors are toxic, potent, and produce many side effects.
2. They should not be the first antidepressant drug used; effect is at best equal to a tricyclic and side effects more dangerous.
3. Side effects.
   a. Most dangerous is hypertensive crisis.
   b. Drug interactions can cause severe hypertension, hypotension, or CNS depression.
   c. Postural hypotension, headaches, constipation, anorexia, diarrhea, and chills.
   d. Tachycardia, edema, impotence, dizziness, insomnia, and restlessness.
   e. Manic episodes and anxiety.
4. All clients must be warned not to eat foods with high tyramine content (aged cheese, wine, beer, chicken liver, yeast), drink alcohol, or take other drugs, especially sympathomimetic drugs (amphetamines, L-Dopa, epinephrine).
5. MAO inhibitors must not be used in combination with tricyclics.

C. Hypertensive crisis.

1. Severe symptoms: headache, confusion, drowsiness, vomiting.
2. Monitor for potential complications: encephalopathy, heart failure.
3. Treatment.
   a. Drug of choice: Regitine, IV 5 mg with close monitoring; antihypertensive.
   b. Monitor vital signs, EKG and neurological signs; BP q5min.
   c. Norepinephrine is administered for severe hypotension.

D. Trazodone is a new class of antidepressant drugs released in 1981.

1. Inhibits the re-uptake of serotonin.
2. Well-tolerated with minimal side effects (sedation and dizziness).

Antimanic Drugs

A. These drugs control mood disorders, especially the manic phase.

B. Before lithium therapy is begun, baseline studies of renal, cardiac and thyroid status obtained.

C. The most common form of drug is lithium carbonate, a naturally occurring metallic salt.

D. Drug must reach certain blood level before it is effective.

1. Stabilizing concentration occurs in 5–7 days; therapeutic effects 7–10 days.
2. Serum level can be simply and reliably measured in mEq/liter of blood.

E. Lithium is metabolized by the kidney.

1. Deficiency of sodium results in more lithium being reabsorbed thus increasing risk of toxicity.
2. Excessive sodium causes more lithium to be excreted and may lower level to a nontherapeutic range.
3. Normal dietary intake of sodium with adequate fluids to prevent dehydration.
4. Serum levels measured 2–3 times weekly (12 hours after last dose) in beginning of therapy; for long term maintenance therapy, every 2–3 months.

F. Drug concentration and side effects.

1. Therapeutic range of serum levels is 0.8–1.2 mEq/liter; for acute manic state, 1.2–1.5 mEq/liter.
2. Side effects occur at upper ranges, usually about 1.5 mEq/liter.
3. Gastrointestinal disturbances, metallic taste in mouth, muscle weakness, fatigue, thirst, polyuria, and fine hand tremors.
4. Hypothyroidism.

G. Lithium toxicity.

1. Appears when blood level exceeds 1.5–2.0 mEq/liter. Many appear sooner depending on individual client.
2. Central nervous system is the chief target.
3. Initial symptoms include nausea, vomiting, drowsiness, tremors, slurred speech, blurred vision.
4. If drug is continued, coma, convulsions, and death may result.
5. Treatment for toxicity: gastric lavage, correction of fluid balance, drug (Mannitol) to increase urine excretion.

Antiparkinson Drugs

A. The term "extrapyramidal disease" refers to motor disorders often associated with pathologic dysfunction in the basal ganglia.
   1. Clinical symptoms of the disease include abnormal involuntary movement, changes in tone of the skeletal muscles, and a reduction of automatic associated movements.
   2. Reversible extrapyramidal reactions may follow the use of certain drugs.
   3. The most common drugs are the phenothiazine derivatives.
B. Antiparkinson drugs act on the extrapyramidal system to reduce disturbing symptoms.
   1. They are usually given in conjunction with antipsychotic drugs.
   2. Two of the most common drugs are Artane and Cogentin.
   3. Side effects are dizziness, gastrointestinal disturbance, headaches, urinary hesitancy, and memory impairment.

☆ Drug Administration in a Psychiatric Setting

A. Give correct *drug* and *dose* at correct *time* to correct *client* according to physician's orders.
B. Learn the specific actions and uses of drugs.
C. Become familiar with the side effects and precautions associated with major drug groups.
D. Observe client carefully for side effects.
E. Be familiar with the drug groups that are not compatible.
F. Refer to psychotropic drug classification chart in Appendix 2.

Other Forms of Therapy

Electroshock Therapy

A. Passing of electric current through brain to induce seizures as treatment for depression; breaks up behavior patterns by causing temporary amnesia.
B. In several weeks, as memory returns, most of the self-depreciation and sadness will have dissipated.
C. Provide support by listening to the client's expression of fear concerning the procedure.
D. Assure client that she or he will not be alone during or after treatment.
E. Remove client's dentures (if present), and give nothing by mouth prior to treatment. Assist physician during treatment.
F. Reorientate client following procedure, and explain feelings of confusion.
G. Observe and record client's response to treatments.

Insulin Coma Therapy

A. Used infrequently in treatment of schizophrenia.
B. Carefully observe client for signs and symptoms of insulin shock following treatment.

Socialization or Motivational Therapy

A. Intended to motivate and get client moving again.
B. Client can socialize and be motivated by means of group therapy, occupational therapy, environmental therapy.
C. Encourage client's participation in therapy.
D. Support client's efforts to share feelings.

Appendix 1. Defense Mechanisms

Compensation
Covering up a lack or weakness by emphasizing a desirable trait, or making up for a frustration in one area by overemphasis in another area. Learned early in childhood and may be recognized in adult behavior, for example, the physically handicapped individual who is an outstanding scholar.

Denial
Refusal to face reality. The ego protects itself from unpleasant pain or conflict by rejecting obvious facts or truth. Example, a person not seeing a doctor because he does not want to know the truth. Individual who avoids reality by becoming ill.

Displacement
Discharging pent-up feelings from one object to a less dangerous object. Example, your supervisor yells at you and you yell at your husband.

Fantasy
Gratification by imaginary achievements and wishful thinking. Example, children's play.

Fixation
Persistence into later life of interests and behavior patterns appropriate to an earlier age.

Identification
Assumption of desirable personality attributes of one admired. Satisfaction can be derived from assuming the success or the experience of others. Example, nurse who feels sick watching a traumatic procedure on her patient.

Insulation
Passive withdrawal. Inaccessible to avoid further threatening circumstances. Sometimes the person appears cold and indifferent to his surroundings. Insulation is usually harmless, but can become very serious if it prevents interaction with others.

Isolation
Walling off of certain ideas, attitudes, or feelings. Isolation is separating the feelings from the intellect, by putting our emotions concerning a specific traumatic event into a lock-tight compartment. Example, the individual talks about a significant situation such as an accident or death without a display of feelings. This pattern can be positive if used temporarily to keep the ego from being overwhelmed.

Projection
Attribution of one's own undesirable traits to someone else. Example, the child who says to a parent, "You hate me," after the parent has spanked the child. In an adult this technique may be a predominant indicator of paranoia.

Rationalization
The attempt that is almost universally employed to prove or justify behavior. It is face saving to give a reason that is acceptable rather than the real reason, as in remarks such as, "It wasn't worth it anyway" "It's all for the best." This mechanism relieves anxiety temporarily and helps the person avoid facing reality.

Reaction-Formation
Prevention of dangerous feelings and desires from being expressed by exaggerating the opposite attitude—a kind of denial. The overly

neat, polite, conscientious individual may have an unconscious desire to be untidy and carefree. The behavior becomes pathological when it interferes with tasks or produces anxiety and frustration.

Regression	Resorting to an earlier developmental level in order to deal with reality. Regression is an immature way of responding, and is frequently seen during a physical illness. It is sometimes used to an extreme degree by the mentally ill, who may regress all the way back to infancy.
Repression	The unconscious process in which undesirable and unacceptable thoughts are kept from entering the conscious. This repressed material may be the motivation for some of our behavior. The superego is largely responsible for repression; the stronger, more punitive the superego, the more emotion will be repressed. The child who is frustrated and downtrodden by a parent may rebel in later life against authority.
Sublimation	The mechanism by which a primitive or unacceptable tendency is redirected into socially constructive channels. This adjustment pattern is at least partly responsible for many artistic and cultural achievements, such as painting and poetry.
Suppression	The act of keeping unpleasant feelings and experiences from awareness.
Symbolization	An idea or object used by the conscious mind to represent an actual event or object. Sometimes the meaning is not clear because the symbol may be representative of something unconscious. Children use symbolization in this way and have to learn to distinguish between the symbol and the thing being symbolized. Examples include obsessive thoughts or behavior (hand washing, cleansing) and the incoherent speech of the schizophrenic (by the time the painful thoughts reach the surface, they are so jumbled that they lose their painfulness).
Undoing	A specific action is performed that is considered to be the opposite of a previously unacceptable action. This action is felt to neutralize or "undo" the original action. Example, Lady MacBeth rubbing and washing her hands.

Appendix 2. Drug Classification Chart

Common Psychotropic Drugs

Major Tranquilizers

Drug	Method of Administration	Daily Dose
Thorazine	Tablets, concentrate, syrup, I.M., I.V., suppositories	25–1500 mg.
Sparine	Tablets, concentrate, syrup, capsules, I.M., I.V.	50–100 mg.
Mellaril	Tablets, concentrate	100–800 mg.
Serentil	Tablets, concentrate, I.M.	30–400 mg.
Trilafon	Tablets, concentrate, syrup, I.M., suppositories	6–64 mg.
Prolixin, Permitil	Tablets, concentrate, I.M.	0.5–20 mg.
Stelazine	Tablets, concentrate, I.M.	2–50 mg.
Quide	Tablets	10–180 mg.
Compazine	Tablets, capsules, syrup, concentrate, I.M., I.V., suppositories	15–150 mg.
Taractan	Tablets, concentrate, I.M.	30–600 mg.
Navane	Capsules, concentrate, I.M.	6–60 mg.
Haldol	Tablets, concentrate, I.M.	2–40 mg.

Minor Tranquilizers (Antianxiety)

Drug	Method of Administration	Daily Dose
Atarax	Tablets, syrup	50–400 mg.
Vistaril	Capsules, suspension, I.M. only	50–400 mg. 50–100 mg.
Librium, Librax	Tablets, capsules, I.M., I.V.	10–100 mg.
Valium	Tablets, I.M., I.V.	2–40 mg.
Serax	Capsules, tablets	30–120 mg.
Equanil	Tablets, capsules, suspension	400–1200 mg.
Miltown	Tablets	400–1200 mg.

Antidepressants (Mood Elevators)

MAO Inhibitors

Drug	Method of Administration	Daily Dose
Marplan	Tablets	10–30 mg.
Niamid	Tablets	125–200 mg.
Nardil	Tablets	15–75 mg.
Parnate	Tablets	20–30 mg.

Tricyclics		
Tofranil	Tablets, I.M.	75–300 mg.
Elavil	Tablets, I.M.	50–200 mg.
Norpramin	Tablets	75–150 mg.
Aventyl	Capsules, liquid	20–100 mg.
Vivactil	Tablets	15–60 mg.
Sinequan	Capsules	25–300 mg.

Antimanic		
Lithium carbonate, Lithane, Litho-Tabs, Lithonate	Tablets, capsules	600–1800 mg.

Antiparkinson		
Cogentin	Tablets, I.M.	1–6 mg.
Artane	Tablets, elixir, capsules	1–10 mg.
Akineton	Tablets, I.M., I.V.	1–8 mg.
Kemadrin	Tablets	6–15 mg.

Appendix 3. Glossary

Acting out Expression of unconscious emotional conflicts of hostility or love in actions that the person does not consciously know are related to such conflicts of feelings.

Affect Generalized feeling, tone, or mood.

Aggression Any verbal/nonverbal activity that may be forceful abuse of self, another person, or thing.

Ambivalence The simultaneous existence of contradictory and contrasting emotions toward a person or object at the same time, that is, love and hate.

Amnesia A condition where the individual experiences a loss of memory because of physical or emotional trauma.

Anxiety A persistent feeling of tension and apprehension arising from within the individual. Response to vague, unspecific danger that may be real or imagined.

Apathy Pathological indifference.

Autism Detachment from reality when self-preoccupation and involvement predominate.

Compulsion An irresistible urge to repeat an act that must be carried out to avoid anxiety.

Conflict A struggle between two or more opposing forces.

Covert Hidden, below the surface.

Cyclothymia Alternations in mood from high to low.

Defense mechanism Originally identified by Anna Freud, an activity of the ego which defends itself by not allowing unacceptable thoughts or feelings to come into awareness to cause anxiety.

Delusion A false belief maintained in spite of facts or evidence to the contrary.

Depression An unshakable feeling of sadness accompanied by feelings of hopefulness, worthlessness, and the feeling of a bleak future.

Disorientation A condition where the individual manifests loss of ability to recognize or locate himself in respect to time, place, or other persons.

Echolalia A condition where the individual constantly repeats what is heard.

Echopraxia A condition where the individual mimics what is done.

Ego A Freudian term denoting that aspect of the psyche which is conscious and most in touch with external reality; the "I" part of the person. Also, that part of the personality that makes decisions, is conscious, and represents the thinking-feeling part of a person.

Electroshock A medical procedure of applying electric current to certain areas in the brain. Used in the treatment of certain psychiatric disorders (especially depression).

Etiology The cause or causes of disease.

Euphoria A feeling of elation or joy.

Fear Response to an actual person or situation of external danger.

Fixation A stage in development when there is an abnormal attachment; inability to move on to later developmental tasks.

Frustration A feeling that may contain elements of anger, hopelessness, or defeat, which results when goals set by perceived needs are blocked.

Fugue A condition experienced as a transient disorientation—patient is unaware that he or she has physically escaped or run to another place.

Functional Used in psychiatry to denote mental illness existing without known physical causes or structural changes.

Hypochondriasis A state of morbid concern about one's body or health for which there is no physical evidence.

Hysteric Involves elements of both conscious and unconscious exaggerated reaction, often in a dramatic manner, to some stimuli situation.

Id A Freudian term denoting a division of the psyche from which come blind, instinctual impulses that lead to immediate gratification of primitive needs, dominated by the pleasure principle.

Ideas of reference A distortion of reality where a person believes that activities of others have a personal reference to one's self.

Illusion Distorted perceptual experience where the individual misinterprets actual data from the environment. Examples: a mirage on the desert; seeing a lake when it is only light refraction.

Insight An individual's understanding of the origin and mechanisms of his or her attitudes and behavior.

Interpersonal Existing between two or more persons.

Intrapersonal Existing within one person.

Labile Refers to rapid shifts in emotions from high to low.

Manipulation The process by which one individual influences another individual to function in accordance with his needs without regard to the other's needs or goals.

Mental retardation A term for mental deficiency or lack of normal development of intelligence.

Milieu The total environment, emotional as well as physical.

Narcissistic Loving one's self excessively in a childish or an infantile fashion.

Negativism A strong resistance to suggestions coming from others.

Neologism A term that refers to the coining of a new word, as seen in schizophrenia.

Obsession A persistent repetitive and unwanted thought.

Organic Based on structural alterations, gross or microscopic.

Overt Discernible; out in the open.

Parataxic A term coined by Sullivan to mean distorted perception.

Phobia The dread of an object, an act, or a situation that is not realistically dangerous but that has come to represent a danger.

Premorbid personality The status of an individual's personality (conflicts, defenses, strengths, weaknesses) before the onset of clinical illness.

Psyche A term meaning the mind or the mental and emotional "self."

Psychogenic   Originating within the psyche or mind. Sometimes used to describe physical disorders that are believed to stem from the emotions.

Rapport   A component of a relationship where one feels harmony or empathy with another.

Regression   Reverting to types of behavior characteristic of an earlier level of development.

Resistance   A mechanism an individual employs to avoid certain ideas or feelings coming into consciousness.

Schizoid   A term used to describe a form of personality disorder characterized by an unsocial, withdrawn, shy type of personality.

Seclusive   A term describing persons who are unsociable, reserved, secretive, and adverse to interacting with people.

Soma   A term meaning body.

Superego   A Freudian term referring to a system within the total psyche that is developed by incorporating parental standards such as moral values; the two components of superego are *conscience* and *ego ideal*.

Unconscious   A term coined by Freud to refer to that part of the mind where mental activity is always going on, but not on a conscious level.

Undoing   A defense mechanism aimed at the removal of a painful memory.

Waxy flexibility   A condition associated with catatonic schizophrenia, where a posture is maintained for long periods of time.

Appendix 4. Mental Assessment Summary

General appearance, manner, and attitude

Assess *physical appearance.*

Note *grooming,* mode of dress, and *personal hygiene.*

Note *posture.*

Note speed, pressure, pace, quantity, volume, and diction of *speech.*

Note relevance, content, and organization of *responses.*

Expressive aspects of behavior

Note *general motor activity.*

Assess *purposeful movements* and gestures.

Assess style of *gait.*

Consciousness

Assess level of *consciousness.*

Thought processes and perception

Assess coherency, logic, and relevance of *thought processes.*

Assess *reality orientation:* time, place, and person.

Assess *perceptions* and reactions to stimuli.

Thought content and mental trend

Ask questions to determine general themes that identify *degree of anxiety.*

Assess *ideation* and *concentration.*

Mood or affect

Assess prevailing or variability in mood by observing behavior and asking questions such as "How are you feeling right now?" Check for presence of abnormal *euphoria.*

If you suspect *depression,* continue questioning to determine depth.

Memory

Assess *past and present memory* and *retention* (ability to listen).

Assess *recall* (recent and remote).

Judgment

Assess *judgment* and interpretations.

Insight

Assess *insight,* the ability to understand.

Intelligence and fund of information

Assess *intelligence.*

Assess *fund of information.*

Sensory ability

Assess the five *senses.*

Developmental level

Assess patient's *developmental level.*

Addictive patterns

Identify *addictive patterns.*

Coping devices and defense mechanisms

Identify *defense-coping mechanisms* and their effect.

Review Questions

1. Which one of the following drugs is an antidepressant?

   A. Mellaril (thioridazine).
   B. Tofranil (imipramine).
   C. Librium (chlordiazepoxide).
   D. Cogentin (benztropine mesylate).

2. Electrotherapy is a possible method of treating severe depression, especially if other methods have failed. All of the following are potential side effects of ECT *except*

   A. Fractures.
   B. Degeneration of brain cells.
   C. Cardiac arrest.
   D. Anxiety and loss of recent memory.

3. The two main drugs (a curare-like drug and a barbiturate) given to clients before ECT are aimed at reducing which of the following side effects?

   A. Cardiac arrest and loss of memory.
   B. Convulsions and fractures.
   C. Fractures and anxiety.
   D. Anxiety and loss of memory.

4. Mrs. Jones, admitted to a psychiatric unit two days previously with a diagnosis of acute depression, made a suicide attempt on the evening shift. The staff intervened in time to prevent Mrs. Jones from harming herself. What would be the most important rationale for the staff to use in discussing this situation after the fact?

   A. They need to reenact the attempt so that they understand exactly what happened.
   B. The staff needs to file an accident report so that the hospital administration is kept informed.
   C. The staff needs to discuss the client's behavior prior to the attempt to determine what cues in her behavior might have warned them that she was contemplating suicide.
   D. Because Mrs. Jones made one suicide attempt, there is a high probability she will make a second attempt in the immediate future.

5. There is a major difference between affective disorders and thought disorders for people who are emotionally disturbed. The major difference in nursing approaches to dealing with these two categories would be

   A. In thought disorders a nursing approach emphasis would be on reality orientation.
   B. Thought disorders imply a fundamental problem with the client's intellectual development; thus, the nurse focuses on the thinking process.

   C. There is no difference in the nursing approaches for the two categories.
   D. In affective disorders the nursing emphasis is on teaching control of feelings.

6. All of the following characteristics distinguish neurotic depression from manic-depressive or involutional depression *except*

   A. Neurotic depression is milder than either manic-depressive or involutional depression.
   B. Neurotic depression is more variable in mood by day.
   C. Neurotic depression is not easily influenced by outside events.
   D. Neurotic depression characteristically is accompanied by evening insomnia.

7. Patti, age fourteen, was admitted to the pediatric unit with complaints of lower limb paralysis. She seemed to have little or no anxiety about her paralysis. She was the only child at home and had a very domineering mother. Her two older sisters had run away from home. Medical tests revealed no physical cause for her paralysis. In utilizing an effective plan of care for Patti, the nurse needs to have an understanding of psychodynamic principles related to conversion reactions. Which one of the following reactions is *not* a correct principle?

   A. Conversion symptoms tend to reflect the patient's concept of disease and her cultural background.
   B. Conversion symptoms actually serve an unconscious purpose and are responsible for the relative lack of distress toward the symptoms (la belle indifference).
   C. Conversion is a strong emotional conflict that either is expressed or is converted to physical symptoms.
   D. The client is consciously aware of the cause of her symptoms.

8. Patti's *primary* gain is to

   A. Get attention.
   B. Handle her anxiety.
   C. Manipulate her mother.
   D. Avoid her responsibilities at home.

9. The most effective nursing approach would be to

   A. Focus on the symptom—try to make Patti walk.
   B. Develop a warm, open approach to the client.
   C. Tell the client she is just "faking" and that she could walk if she wanted to.
   D. Plan activities that would encourage Patti to use her legs.

10. Mr. Chew, fifty-two years old, has begun a daily ritual for the past five weeks of washing and straightening everything in his room before he can participate in his planned activities for the day. The first week he missed breakfast because of his compulsive behavior. Now the nursing staff is unable to get him to attend morning psychotherapy at 11:00 A.M. An assessment-and-intervention team meeting was held in order to discuss Mr. Chew's behavior and possible interventions. The psychotherapy team should be aware that Mr. Chew's compulsive room cleaning is probably an attempt to

A. Keep his room cleaner than the rooms of the other patients on the ward.
B. Avoid going to psychotherapy.
C. Reduce his anxiety.
D. Manipulate the team members.

11. In planning nursing care for Mr. Chew, which concept or principle is incorrect and should *not* form the foundation of a nursing care plan?

A. The obsessive individual is involved in a conflict between obedience and defiance.
B. Unbearable tension is momentarily relieved through compulsive behavior.
C. Ritualistic behavior provides a way for the individual to remain detached and isolated from his own emotions and relationships with others.
D. Usually the client no longer needs ritualistic behavior if tension has been relieved by performing the compulsive act.

12. To assist the client and reduce his anxiety the nurse could

A. Manipulate the environment to minimize any anxiety-provoking stimuli and to increase self-esteem.
B. Initiate a close interpersonal relationship with the client.
C. Set definite limits on the client's behavior.
D. Use humor to help the client realize how maladaptive his behavior is.

13. Jane failed her psychology final exam and spent the entire evening berating the teacher and the course. This behavior is an example of

A. Reaction-formation.
B. Compensation.
C. Projection.
D. Acting out.

14. One defense mechanism used by psychiatric clients is regression. Which of the following best describes this mechanism?

A. Regression is an immature way of responding.
B. It works most effectively to eliminate anxiety.
C. It fosters dependence.
D. It provides security through child-like behavior.

15. A terminally ill twenty-four-year-old woman says to the nurse, "I don't know why you are all so concerned; I'm not that sick." She is using which adjustment mechanism?

A. Denial.
B. Rationalization.
C. Projection.
D. Regression.

16. Isolation can best be described as

A. An idea or thought used by the conscious mind to represent an idea or object.
B. A withdrawal into passivity.
C. The discharge of pent-up emotions on a less dangerous object.
D. A walling-up of certain ideas, attitudes, or feelings.

17. Persons with overly suspicious behavior patterns tend to use projection. What is the purpose of this mechanism?

A. To handle feelings of inadequacy and low self-esteem.
B. To manipulate others.
C. To avoid reality.
D. To prevent painful memories.

18. Doug, a new client on the psychiatric ward where you work, has just spent 20 minutes telling you his sad history. He told you that he had been wounded in Vietnam, his wife had left him, and his friends had deserted him. After checking his chart, you learned that all these stories were untrue. You would suspect which one of the following diagnoses?

A. Depressive personality.
B. Paranoid personality.
C. Sociopathic personality.
D. Neurotic personality.

19. Doug has been certified for 14 days on the locked unit. While there he becomes friendly with a very disturbed young woman and convinces her to escape with him when a visitor comes through the locked door. This is an example of impairment in which one of the following areas?

A. Judgment.
B. Emotional response to others.
C. Unconscious processes.
D. Intellectual development.

20. Doug is constantly trying to manipulate the staff as a way of getting his needs met. Which response to Doug would indicate that the nurse understands the psychodynamic principle behind manipulation?

A. "Doug, I won't allow you to manipulate me."
B. "Doug, I won't be able to do as you ask, but I will stay with you and talk."

C. "Doug, if this behavior doesn't stop, I shall have to tell your doctor."

D. "Doug, let's focus on your anxiety so we can deal with all this manipulation."

21. While persons convicted of felonies are usually put in prisons, many of them have underlying emotional problems. Probably the most common diagnosis seen in prisons is

A. Psychotic personality.
B. Antisocial personality.
C. Paranoid personality.
D. Adolescent adjustment.

22. Ellen, a nineteen-year-old medical student, is brought into the hospital by her roommate, who is worried about Ellen's lack of interest in anything, loss of weight, somatic complaints, and constant tiredness. Ellen says that her major problem is her indecision about continuing to pursue her medical career or changing fields entirely. You are the nurse assigned to care for her. In light of her presenting symptoms, how would you expect Ellen to answer the question, "How does the future look to you"?

A. "It looks pretty bleak and miserable."
B. Noncommital.
C. "Oh, I'm sure I'll be able to make a decision soon."
D. A tangential response, since ambivalence has an immobilizing effect.

23. Of the following categories, which is the one most likely not to be associated with suicidal potential?

A. Depression.
B. Chronic alcoholism.
C. Organic brain disease.
D. Psychoneurotic syndrome.

24. Antidepressive drugs act on the brain's chemistry; therefore, they would be more useful in which form of depression?

A. Endogenous.
B. Exogenous.
C. Reactive.
D. Secondary.

25. Which one of the following drugs is used to reduce the extrapyramidal side effects that are common with use of the phenothiazines?

A. Cogentin.
B. Niamid.
C. Ritalin.
D. Miltown.

26. In providing nursing care for the individual with a psychosomatic illness, the nurse needs to know which of the following general concepts?

A. The nurse must incorporate concepts of adaptation, stress, body image, and anxiety.
B. The area of symptom formation may be symbolic to the patient.
C. Psychosomatic illnesses may be life threatening.
D. All of the above concepts are important.

27. Gerry, an eighteen-year-old unemployed male laborer, was admitted to the hospital vomiting red blood. A tentative diagnosis of a peptic ulcer was made. Gerry is married and has twin eighteen-month-old sons. He continually refuses the ulcer diet and criticizes the nursing staff. What might Gerry's behavior indicate?

A. He is not interested in getting well.
B. He does not understand what is expected of him.
C. He is concerned about his family and his economic problems that have been complicated by his illness.
D. He needs some attention and to be able to trust and rely on the nursing staff.

28. Gerry becomes very agitated one day while his mother is visiting and asks her to leave. This behavior may indicate

A. An emotional conflict between his role as an independent adult and his need to be dependent.
B. Gerry is allowing his hostility to become conscious and is handling it in a more effective manner.
C. Gerry's behavior has become worse.
D. A conflict exists, and there is a need for clarification and exploration.

29. Which would be the most effective nursing approach to Gerry's behavior?

A. Restrict his mother from visiting.
B. Approach Gerry in a warm, supportive manner and assist him in exploring his feelings.
C. Confront Gerry with his rudeness to his mother.
D. Ask Gerry if he would like his prn sedative.

30. Gerry's family is making plans for his discharge. What will have the greatest effect on his further recovery?

A. His wife's clear understanding of Gerry's dietary needs.
B. The amount of emotional support he receives from his family.
C. His understanding of the cause and treatment of his illness.
D. His expectations of himself to assume his share of responsibility in his family.

31. Gerry is primarily using which of the following defense mechanisms?

    A. Repression.
    B. Reaction formation.
    C. Sublimation.
    D. Projection.

32. Mrs. Rain is a client who never discusses her problems or her illness. Occasionally, the nurse observes Mrs. Rain's crying as she passes the door. A response using an effective communication technique would be

    A. Ignore the crying as you realize she wants to let down alone.
    B. As you pass the door, acknowledge her by saying, "Good morning, Mrs. Rain."
    C. Go in the room and ask her to tell you why she is crying.
    D. Go in the room, sit down, and stay quietly with her.

33. Phobic reactions differ from obsessive compulsive reactions in which of the following ways?

    A. Phobias are beyond voluntary control and cannot adequately or logically be explained by the client.
    B. With phobic reactions, the client's behavior is directed toward reducing tension and anxiety.
    C. Phobias interfere with the client's everyday life.
    D. Phobias may be associated with an unreasonable fear of specific objects or situations.

34. Mrs. Kelly, age forty-seven, was referred to the community mental health center by her family physician. In the past seven years she has been examined by numerous physicians for vague complaints of abdominal pains and chronic constipation. Mrs. Kelly spends a great deal of time reading and collecting articles on possible causes for her complaint. Gradually, the amount of time she spends being ill has increased, which has interfered with her family life. Finally, her husband has convinced her to keep her initial appointment at the mental health center. Which of the following would be the most effective approach to Mrs. Kelly?

    A. Sympathize with her physical complaints.
    B. Involve her in activities at which she can succeed.
    C. Convince her that her complaints have no physical basis.
    D. Use a matter-of-fact but unempathic approach.

35. Which one of the following psychodynamic concepts does the nurse need to know in order to provide care for Mrs. Kelly?

    A. Physical complaints are used to create interest and attention.
    B. Specific symptom choice is not symbolic but directly related to the client's faulty identification with a parent.
    C. Regression is the primary coping mechanism.
    D. The client's symptoms are faked and are used to gain sympathy.

36. Which one of the following behaviors may indicate that the individual who uses psychoneurotic behavior patterns is dealing more effectively with his problems?

    A. Verbalizes thoughts and feelings rather than demonstrating them through physiological symptoms or maladaptive behavior.
    B. Openly expresses hostility.
    C. Freely chooses activities that include other people.
    D. Initiates contact with others.

37. The neurotic client generally demonstrates

    A. A grossly disorganized personality.
    B. A distortion of external reality.
    C. The symptom of anxiety in some form.
    D. Odd, unexplained, impulsive behavior.

38. Mr. Allen, seventy-two years old, has been hospitalized in a long-term nursing care facility for the past six months. He is confused and disoriented most of the time. His behavior alternates between calling for his deceased wife and screaming and sobbing uncontrollably. Mr. Allen shuffles up to the station, crying and screaming, "Nobody cares if I live or die! You all hate me! You all hate me!" Which response by the nurse would be most therapeutic?

    A. "Mr. Allen, what makes you think we hate you?"
    B. "Pete, you are always saying that and you know we all love you."
    C. "Pete, here is a cigarette. Now go in the dayroom and watch TV."
    D. "Mr. Allen, you seem very upset. Let's take a walk and we can talk."

39. In planning Mr. Allen's daily schedule, it is important for the nurse to understand which one of the following principles?

    A. The client may have moderate to severe memory impairment and short periods of concentration.
    B. The more rigid his daily schedule, the more comfortable he will be.
    C. The client is more likely to be able to remember current experiences than past ones.
    D. The client can usually be trusted to be responsible for his daily care needs.

40. Mrs. Maring was brought to the locked unit of the county medical center by the police. She was found wandering around the streets, incoherent, and her behavior appeared to be inappropriate. She was tentatively diagnosed as schizophrenic and held in the hospital for a three-day evaluation. Miss James, an LPN/LVN on the locked unit, is assigned to Mrs. Maring. The nurse knows that a diagnosis of schizophrenia implies that a client would manifest which one of the following behaviors?

    A. Inability to concentrate.
    B. Loss of contact with reality.
    C. Guilt feelings.
    D. Feelings of worthlessness.

41. Mrs. Maring says that the voices are telling her to do things and she can't stop listening. The best response from the nurse would be

    A. "Never mind the voices; let's just concentrate on the game."
    B. "The voices will go away soon."
    C. "I don't hear any voices. I think the voices are part of your illness. Try to listen to what I'm saying."
    D. "Just stop listening to what is in your head and they will go away."

42. On the second day of Mrs. Maring's stay in the hospital, she appears withdrawn and spends most of her time alone in her room staring at the wall. The nurse recognizes that this behavior is a symptom of schizophrenia known as

    A. Social withdrawal.
    B. Autism.
    C. Loose associations.
    D. Stress.

43. Mrs. Maring, after a two-week stay, appears much better. She is in contact with reality and is able to interact with others in an appropriate way. The doctor is sending her home with medication. The most common medications given for schizophrenia are

    A. ECT.
    B. Phenothiazines.
    C. MAO inhibitors.
    D. Antidepressants.

44. The nursing staff is planning an all-day outing for a group of clients. All the clients are on large doses of phenothiazines. Which precautionary measure is most important for the nursing staff to enforce?

    A. All clients should be kept in the shade as much as possible and should wear clothing or hats to protect exposed skin areas.
    B. Avoid excessive stimuli.
    C. Take along a first-aid kit, because psychiatric clients are accident prone.

    D. Avoid foods such as cheese, coke, coffee, or wine that are high in tyramine.

45. Drug addiction is a major social problem in our society. Aside from the physical deterioration of the individual and the subculture participation that may lead to crime, a further result of the addiction may be

    A. The development of psychosis.
    B. The disintegration of family relationships.
    C. Addiction to other substances such as alcohol.
    D. Intellectual dependence on the drug.

46. The treatment for delirium tremens may include all of the following *except*

    A. High calorie, vitamin, and fluid diet.
    B. Tranquilization.
    C. Restraints to prevent self-injury.
    D. Morphine to induce rest.

47. Paranoid symptoms can be observed as secondary symptoms to schizophrenia. In which of the following disorders would you also be apt to observe paranoid symptoms?

    A. Organic syndromes.
    B. Involutional melancholia.
    C. Alcoholism.
    D. All of the above.

48. Mr. Davis has been admitted to your hospital unit with a tentative diagnosis of paranoid schizophrenia. He tells you that he was walking down the corridor at work and saw two friends talking and laughing. He assumed they were talking about him, but was willing to consider other reasons for their conversation. Mr. Davis has expressed a symptom known as

    A. Delusion of reference.
    B. Idea of reference.
    C. Illusion.
    D. Suspicious response.

49. Mr. Davis continues to be suspicious toward others in his immediate environment. His ideas of reference become fixed, and he manifests symptoms of paranoid schizophrenia known as delusions. The most common delusions associated with this illness are

    A. Delusions of grandeur.
    B. Delusions of persecution.
    C. Delusions of jealousy.
    D. Delusions of sexual preference.

50. The nurse may expect Mr. Davis to exhibit all of the following characteristics along with his paranoid ideation *except*

    A. Jealousy.
    B. Tendency to violence.
    C. Tendency to flight.
    D. Alcoholism.

51. In order for Mr. Davis to return to society, the nurse knows that

    A. His paranoid ideas must be completely absent.
    B. As long as Mr. Davis can keep his paranoid ideas to himself, he can be discharged.
    C. The family must have therapy, because the family is the source of his paranoid ideation.
    D. The paranoid ideas have to be investigated to ensure that there is no truth in them.

52. An important nursing goal in planning care for the individual with chronic brain syndrome is

    A. To allow the client to function as independently as therapeutically possible.
    B. To continually orient the client to reality.
    C. To provide a safe, structured environment with appropriate recreational activities.
    D. All of the above.

53. Which of the following best describes the general characteristics of the individual with chronic brain syndrome?

    A. Is ritualistic about daily activities.
    B. Shows impaired judgment.
    C. Shows impairment in all areas of the personality and mental functioning.
    D. Uses confabulation to compensate for memory impairment.

54. The aged, senile individual should be

    A. Allowed to be responsible for his own nutritional needs.
    B. Kept active through plenty of exercise.
    C. Kept in his room to avoid potentially unsafe situations.
    D. Given opportunities to be useful.

55. The mental health of the aged is most influenced by

    A. Basic personality structure and make-up.
    B. Philosophical point of view and attitudes about life and death.
    C. Family attitudes toward the aged.
    D. Cultural and environmental factors.

56. Which of the following is *not* a possible cause for organic brain syndrome?

    A. Senility.
    B. Arteriosclerosis.
    C. Trauma.
    D. Intoxication.

57. Confabulation is a symptom frequently seen in Korsakoff's psychosis, a syndrome of chronic alcoholism. Confabulation can best be defined as

    A. Amnesia of recent events.
    B. A defense mechanism to control anxiety.
    C. The falsifying of facts to fill in memory gaps.
    D. A mechanism to raise self-esteem.

58. Mr. Meteress has been admitted to an alcohol detoxification unit. He sits dejected in a corner, and when approached by the nurse, he says, "I'm really no good. I drink and don't take care of my family, and I'm a rotten father." A response by the nurse using an effective communication technique would be

    A. "But now you are doing something about your problem, Mr. Meteress."
    B. "Sounds as though you are feeling pretty guilty about drinking."
    C. "I'm sure that you are a good father, Mr. Meteress."
    D. "What makes you think you are no good?"

59. Alcoholics who have been heavy drinkers for a number of years are prone to experience all of the following *except*

    A. Some brain cell destruction.
    B. Esophageal varices.
    C. Malnutrition.
    D. Serum hepatitis.

60. Mrs. Jones has been a client on the oncology unit for two months. She has become a favorite with the staff, and although her condition is deteriorating, she remains cheerful and pleasant. One day she says to you, "Well, I've given up all hope. I know I'm going to die soon." What would be the most therapeutic response you could make?

    A. "Now, Mrs. Jones, one should never give up all hope. We are finding new cures every day."
    B. "Mrs. Jones, would you like to talk about dying?"
    C. "You've given up all hope?"
    D. "You know, your doctor will be here soon. Why don't you talk to him about your feelings and giving up all hope?"

61. Mrs. Jones's condition is critical, and you are assigned to care for her. Of the following tasks, which one would have lowest priority?

    A. Attending to her physical needs and assessing the situation for changes.
    B. Supporting the family and giving them needed encouragement.
    C. Encouraging Mrs. Jones to express and talk about her fears of dying.
    D. Contacting her lawyer so she can tie up loose ends.

62. One year ago Mrs. Brown lost her husband to whom she had been married for ten years. They had had a stormy marriage, punctuated by frequent disagreements and several separations. Mrs. Brown is experiencing intense grief, which she seems

unable to work through. To understand this behavior, the nurse should be familiar with which of the following principles?

A. The longer the marriage, the more intense the grief.
B. The more dependent the relationship, the more difficult the grief process.
C. The more ambivalent the relationship, the more intense the grief.
D. It is too soon to expect Mrs. Brown to have worked through the grief process.

63. Abnormal patterns of behavior include all of the following *except*

A. Withdrawal.
B. Aggression.
C. Use of ritualistic behavior.
D. Integration.

64. Symptoms of mental disorders include all of the following *except*

A. Perception.
B. Thinking.
C. Affect.
D. Stress.

65. Susan, a twenty-year-old female, comes into the crisis clinic, and you are assigned to interview her. From your knowledge of crisis theory, you know that success of crisis therapy would be most influenced by which of the following factors?

A. Past history of the client's illness.
B. Availability of support systems.
C. Previous unsatisfactory relationships.
D. Financial resources available.

66. Sadness of brief duration that follows an obvious loss should be termed

A. Crisis.
B. Grief.
C. Melancholia.
D. Neurotic depression.

67. Group therapy has been an accepted method of treatment for psychiatric clients for several years. The best rationale for this form of treatment is

A. It is the most economical—one staff member can treat many clients.
B. The format of the therapy is not psycho-analytically based and does not deal with unconscious material.
C. It enables clients to become aware that others have problems and that they are not alone in their suffering.
D. It provides a social milieu similar to society in general, where the client can relate to others and validate perceptions in realistic settings.

68. Mrs. Smith, a client who is known to be very withdrawn, suddenly screams at you, "You are all stupid! Can't even make a bed right! Get out of my room!" As a nurse, your response should be

A. "Don't scream at me. I'm only human."
B. "Not all of us are stupid, Mrs. Smith."
C. "You sound angry, Mrs. Smith."
D. Ignore Mrs. Smith's remarks.

69. A seclusion room or quiet area is sometimes needed for the aggressive client to prevent

A. Physical exhaustion of the client.
B. Harm to the staff.
C. Others from hearing and seeing a hostile client.
D. Other clients from copying the aggressive behavior.

70. A very attractive young man with whom you have a nurse-patient relationship continues to make sexual advances toward you that make you very uncomfortable. The best approach would be to

A. Ignore the advances and hope he will stop.
B. Don't reject the young man, for you know this will reinforce his negative self-image.
C. Be direct in communicating your discomfort with his advances and set limits on his behavior.
D. Tell his doctor, who should be informed of his inappropriate behavior.

71. During the initial phase of the nurse-client relationship, it is most important that the nurse understand which of the following concepts?

A. The focus is on mutual attempts to know each other and help the client become oriented to his environment.
B. Identifying expectations is important to accomplish before the relationship begins.
C. Recognizing and testing attitudes of the nursing staff.
D. The relationship is effected by the degree of comfort the nurse feels.

72. For the best therapeutic care of the psychiatric client, the nurse must

A. Like every client for whom she is responsible.
B. Accept the client as a person of worth and reject the maladaptive behavior.
C. Sympathize with the client's problems and circumstances.
D. Maintain a distant, professional attitude.

73. Mr. Perls, a fifty-four-year-old alcoholic, has been admitted to the ward for detoxification and treatment. Which of the following statements by him may be a barrier to the development of a therapeutic relationship?

A. "Nurse, you said I reminded you of your alcoholic father."
B. "You want to spend some time talking with me. Won't you just be wasting your time?"

C. "I bet you love to see us old drunks come in!"

D. "How many children do you have, nurse?"

74. A basic prerequisite for understanding the therapeutic relationship is

A. All the needs of the emotionally disturbed client are at times common to all human beings.

B. All behavior has meaning and purpose.

C. To assist others, the nurse must understand his or herself.

D. Behavior is directed toward the elimination of threat with the greatest conservation of energy.

75. Which of the following is *not* a behavior that is evoked by anxiety?

A. Anger.

B. Withdrawal.

C. Crying.

D. Perspiring.

76. Mr. Oliver is unable to sleep. He is pacing the floor, head down, and wringing his hands. The nurse recognizes that he is anxious. In which way would the nurse intervene?

A. Help the client talk about his behavior.

B. Give him his prn sleeping medicine.

C. Let the client know the nurse is interested, is willing to listen, and wants to assist him.

D. Explore with him alternatives to his problem.

77. Of the four levels of anxiety—mild, moderate, severe, and panic—which of the following statements is characteristic of severe anxiety?

A. The senses become more alert.

B. Experience inflicts pain that is difficult to bear.

C. Perception narrows; person is unaware of peripheral activities (selective inattention).

D. Sense of being overpowered and disintegrating control.

78. A client of yours has just been told that her father was in a serious automobile accident and is critically ill in the hospital. Her response is a smile and to ask what time lunch is served. This is an example of

A. Lack of affect.

B. Inappropriate affect.

C. Disturbed association of ideas.

D. Primary disturbance.

79. Which of the following is *not* a type of schizophrenia?

A. Paranoid.

B. Regressive.

C. Catatonic.

D. Hebephrenic.

80. The purpose or function of adjustment (defense) mechanisms is to

A. Increase self-esteem.

B. Decrease anxiety.

C. Conserve energy.

D. Cope with internal conflicts in an efficient manner.

81. Defense mechanisms can reduce anxiety by

A. Moving away from anxiety (flight).

B. Moving against anxiety (fight).

C. Moving toward anxiety (problem solving).

D. All of the above.

82. The most common adjustment mechanism used is

A. Rationalization.

B. Undoing.

C. Sublimation.

D. Projection.

83. Jennifer, a thirty-year-old mother of two, was brought to the hospital by her husband. He complained that Jennifer could not manage the house, was easily distracted, and was constantly in motion. The nurse noticed that Jennifer was unable to converse rationally and changed the subject frequently. This is most clearly an example of

A. Delusions.

B. Associative looseness.

C. Flight of ideas.

D. Echolalia.

84. Jennifer's diagnosis is manic-depressive-manic illness. She manifests an excess of energy and cannot sit still. The most useful activity that the nurse might suggest for Jennifer would be to

A. Play volleyball outside.

B. Engage in group exercises (occupational therapy).

C. Play table tennis in the day room.

D. Deliver linen to the rooms.

85. Jennifer's disruptive behavior on the ward has been extremely annoying to the other clients. One approach by the nurse might be to

A. Tell Jennifer she is bothering others and confine her to her room.

B. Ignore her behavior, realizing it is consistent with her illness.

C. Set limits on her behavior and be consistent in approach.

D. Make a rigid, structured plan that Jennifer will have to follow.

86. Jennifer frequently exhibits bizarre and inappropriate behavior. Such behavior may be best explained by all of the following *except*

A. One purpose of the behavior is to attract attention.

B. Jennifer has little or no control over her impulsive behavior.

C. Her behavior is a method of expressing herself in a symbolic way.

D. Her behavior is caused by a genetic imbalance.

87. Mrs. Long, age thirty-four, has been on 5 mg tid chlordiazepoxide (Librium) for the past six months. Which of the following is *not* an appropriate statement about antianxiety drugs?

A. Antianxiety drugs may become habitual as the patient acquires an increased tolerance.

B. Mrs. Long may experience extrapyramidal side effects.

C. Librium is one of the most widely abused drugs because the public sees it as "aspirin for nervousness."

D. Sudden, abrupt drug withdrawal may create marked changes in behavior with physiological complications.

88. Lithium carbonate is used to treat manic-type behavior disorders. Which of the following symptoms is *not* a common side effect?

A. Gastrointestinal disturbances (nausea, vomiting, diarrhea, abdominal pain).

B. Muscle weakness.

C. A sluggish, dazed feeling.

D. Anuria.

89. Mr. Braner, a sixty-year-old retired tool-and-die maker, has been admitted to your ward, a short-term acute center for the care and treatment of psychiatric disorders. His symptoms are fatigue, an inability to concentrate, and an inability to complete everyday tasks. Mr. Braner refuses to care for himself, does not eat, and prefers to sleep all day. Mr. Braner has been in the hospital a week, and you notice a sudden improvement in his state of depression. He says that things are beginning to fall into place and he feels better. Your understanding of the syndrome of depression leads you to which one of the following conclusions?

A. Mr. Braner is finally coming out of the depression, and you can begin to consider discharge plans.

B. Mr. Braner may be planning to commit suicide so he should be watched carefully.

C. Now that Mr. Braner feels better, you should begin to discuss the source of his depression.

D. You should notify his wife so that family therapy sessions can begin.

90. Depressed persons exhibit which of the following overt expressions of depressed affect?

A. Unable to concentrate.

B. Sad and hopeless.

C. Unable to complete everyday tasks.

D. Guilty and agitated.

Answers and Rationale

1. (B) Elavil, Triavil, Aventyl, Vivactil, and Sinequan are also antidepressant drugs. Answer A (Mellaril) is an antipsychotic drug. Answer C is an antianxiety drug. Answer D is an antiparkinson agent used in conjunction with the antipsychotic drugs.

2. (B) As far as is known, the electric current (75 to 150 volts, 60 cycle) does not destroy brain cells. All of the other answers are side effects.

3. (C) The curare-like drug lessens strong muscular contraction during the convulsion, and the barbiturate is given to reduce anxiety by putting the patient to sleep for 5 to 10 minutes.

4. (C) Even though all of the reasons are important and should not be ignored, the most important task is that the staff should learn to assess the client's behavior and to identify cues that might indicate an impending suicide attempt.

5. (A) With thought disorders the individual has difficulty in keeping in touch with reality, which is not usually a problem with people experiencing problems in the affective area.

6. (C) A main characteristic of neurotic depression is that it is easily influenced by events in the outside world. The word used to describe this condition is "exogenous" depression.

7. (D) Neurosis is an unconscious process. The client is aware he has a problem but is not conscious of its cause.

8. (B) The symptom is formed to alleviate a high level of anxiety. Selections A, C, and D are secondary gains.

9. (B) An observant, warm, nonthreatening approach is more effective. A is incorrect because focusing on the symptom will only increase the anxiety level. C and D are incorrect because the client is actually experiencing the symptom in conversion reactions even though there are no physiological reasons for the problem.

10. (C) Symptom formation is to avoid the anxiety and its discomfort.

11. (D) Ritualistic behavior does not disappear until the underlying basic conflict is resolved. Through the behavior, the anxiety is *temporarily* relieved, but the cause is not resolved.

12. (A) The nurse needs to keep environmental stimuli nonthreatening. B is incorrect because close intimate contact increases the client's anxiety. He wants and needs the contact but is afraid as it is a source of "hurt" and "disappointment" for him. C is incorrect. Rigidly defended limits again increase this obsessive-compulsive anxiety level. D is incorrect. Humor is inappropriate and may be misinterpreted by the client as an attack on his already low self-esteem.

13. (C) Jane is placing blame on others and not taking responsibility for her own behavior.

14. (B) Regression is a way to reduce anxiety and cope with different situations by going back to a time that was more safe and comfortable.

15. (A) The client simply refuses to accept her terminal illness to protect herself from the unpleasant reality of death.

16. (D) A is symbolization. B is insulation. C is displacement.

17. (A) The main goal of an adjustment mechanism is to protect the self-image.

18. (C) Characteristics such as pathological lying, manipulation, and deception are common to sociopathic character disorders.

19. (A) Psychopathic personalities evidence poor judgment, poor superego control, as well as poor emotional responses to others. The only area unimpaired is the intellect.

20. (B) It is important to set limits but not to reinforce low self-esteem, so staying with Doug would be therapeutic.

21. (B) These persons exercise poor judgment and do not learn from experience.

22. (A) Ellen's symptoms are indicative of depression, and typically these patients feel the future is bleak and hopeless.

23. (D) While all patients who are impulsive may be potentially suicidal, the least likely category is neurosis.

24. (A) Endogenous depression is more related to internal chemical changes than depressions influenced by external events.

25. (A) The others are incorrect—Niamid and Ritalin are antidepressant drugs, and Miltown is an antianxiety drug.

26. (D) Psychosomatic illnesses focus on the "holism" of the individual.

27. (D) It is more basic and includes selections B and C.

28. (D) Selections A, B, and C are drawing conclusions without validation. Selection D provides the validation intervention.

29. (B) This approach would help decrease Gerry's anxiety and assist him in gaining insights. Selection A and D deny the problem, whereas C may increase his anxiety and prolong his illness.

30. (B) Selections A, C, and D are important, but the emotional support of his family is vital. Intellectual understanding may not effect an improvement in his condition, inasmuch as it may be used to avoid the underlying feelings and conflicts.

31. (A) The client is keeping his undesirable and painful thoughts and feelings on an unconscious level and is handling them through his body.

32. (D) The most effective communication technique in this case would be silence; support the client nonverbally, accept her, and open up the opportunity for an expression of feeling.

33. (D) Phobias involve unreasonable fears of specific objects or situations. Obsessions are recurring thoughts that create discomfort. Both involve a high level of anxiety.

34. (B) The hypochondriac has a severe, morbid preoccupation with the state of his own body. Approaches and activities that increase self-esteem and direct the client's attention outward are therapeutic.

35. (C) Hypochondriasis is the rarest and most serious of the psychoneuroses. Narcissistic body preoccupation and severe regression are common.

36. (A) The verbalization of thoughts and feelings is indicative of effectively dealing with problems. This answer encompasses the other selections.

37. (C) The cardinal symptom of psychoneurotic behavior is anxiety.

38. (D) The nurse acknowledges the client and his feelings without focusing directly on them. A asks for an analysis of feelings. B is making light of the client's feelings. C is ignoring the problem.

39. (A) It is important to remember that clients usually have some memory and concentration impairment. The degree depends upon the individual and is influenced by the basic personality structure

and the cause of the problem.

40. (B) Loss of contact with reality is a symptom of schizophrenia. All of the other symptoms are indicative of depression.

41. (C) It is the best answer, for it helps the client cope with reality by validating that another person does not hear them, as well as directing the client to focus on reality content.

42. (B) Autistic behavior is the basic social isolation of schizophrenics when they withdraw into their own inner world.

43. (B) Tranquilizers help clients to cope with reality by modifying their symptoms.

44. (A) One of the major side effects of the phenothiazine drug group is photosensitivity. Skin burns and irritations may be caused by even short exposure to direct sunlight. B is correct, but is not the most important precaution. C is incorrect in that psychiatric clients are no more accident prone than the general population; however, it would be appropriate to include a first-aid kit. D is incorrect because avoidance of those foods is important when using MAO inhibitors.

45. (B) Family relationships generally suffer or cease entirely when a person becomes addicted to hard drugs.

46. (D) Morphine, a CNS depressant, would be contraindicated.

47. (D) Paranoid symptoms can accompany all of the disorders, but not necessarily.

48. (B) A delusion of reference (A) refers to a fixed belief when no amount of evidence can alter the belief.

49. (B) Feelings of persecution or extreme suspicion or mistrust are the most common manifestation of the paranoid position.

50. (D) Alcoholism may be accompanied by paranoid delusions, but alcoholism per se is not a characteristic of paranoid conditions.

51. (B) Even though his paranoid ideas have not disappeared, if they are localized to a small area of his life and kept to himself, Mr. Davis can return and continue to function in society.

52. (D) Each answer is important in providing care for the client.

53. (C) All the other answers are correct, but C includes them and is therefore more comprehensive.

54. (D) This allows the client to function at an optimum level for as long as possible and also assists in maintaining his self-esteem. The other answers are incorrect.

55. (A) It broadly encompasses the other answers.

56. (A) Senility is not a cause but a label for behaviors associated with organic brain syndrome. B, C, and D are a few of the common causes of organic brain syndrome.

57. (C) As the client experiences memory gaps, he fills them in with stories unsubstantiated by facts to preserve his self-esteem.

58. (B) The nurse paraphrases the client's comments to give feedback, to show she understands what he has said, and to encourage him to continue expressing his feelings.

59. (D) Serum hepatitis is caused by the use of unsterile instruments used in injections and would be a more common result of heroin addiction.

60. (C) This reflective response will open up communication and enable the client to express whatever concerns or feelings she has without confining her to a discussion of dying (answer B).

61. (D) Supporting the family is part of your role as a nurse, but contacting the lawyer is not your responsibility.

62. (C) When both positive and negative feelings are felt toward the deceased, the grief process is more difficult to resolve because of guilt arising from the negative feelings.

63. (D) Integration is a healthy pattern of behavior.

64. (D) Stress affects all humans and is not a symptom of a mental disorder.

65. (B) The more supports the client has available during a crisis period, the more easily she may develop coping mechanisms to handle the crisis.

66. (B) Grief occurs following an obvious loss, is a normal reaction to the loss, and is of short duration, while the other depressed states are abnormal reactions to loss.

67. (D) Since many people's problems occur in an interpersonal framework, the group setting is a way to correct faulty perceptions as well as to work on more effective ways of relating to others.

68. (C) Reflection of the feeling should cause the client to continue to verbalize.

69. (A) A client may need to be removed physically from an environment that is too stimulating.

70. (C) This client needs direct feedback and clear delineation of limits to the relationship.

71. (A) Both the nurse and the client need to become comfortable with each other in the initial phase before the working phase can begin.

72. (B) While the behavior is maladaptive, the client must feel that the nurse sees him as a worthwhile individual. Most of the time, clients have low self-esteem. Answer A is incorrect because the nurse must realize that she is a human being with her own point of view and prejudices; therefore, she cannot like everyone. She must be aware of her feelings so that they do not interfere and block the client's treatments. Sympathizing with the client meets the nurse's needs, not the client's. The nurse must maintain a therapeutic, professional attitude but allow her humanness to show; it is important to be able to relate as one human being to another.

73. (A) The nurse's unresolved attitudes and feelings toward her father may spill over and influence her relationship with the client. If the nurse is not aware of her attitudes, she may lose her objectivity.

74. (B) It encompasses the other answers and is more fundamental.

75. (D) Perspiring is not a behavior but a physiological reaction to anxiety. A, B, and C are behaviors that may be seen as a result of moderate to severe anxiety.

76. (C) It includes the other three answers. Sleeping medicine should be avoided if at all possible or unless absolutely necessary, because it helps suppress the client's feelings only temporarily.

77. (B) Severe anxiety cannot be used to serve the client and requires nursing intervention to lower it. As this anxiety becomes more unbearable, an adjustment mechanism will likely be used. A is mild anxiety; C is moderate anxiety; and D is panic.

78. (B) The response is inappropriate to the situation. This is an example of one of the two forms of abnormal affect. The other form is lack of affect, where no response (including facial expression) would be present.

79. (B) While schizophrenics may exhibit regressive behavior, it is a symptom, not a classification.

80. (D) All of the choices are true, but D includes the basic idea of the others and is more comprehensive.

81. (D) The mind is set up to handle threats to the self (anxiety) by moving away or toward or against the threat.

82. (A) Undoing and projection are fairly ineffective ways of adjusting to anxiety and if used repeatedly may indicate problems. Sublimation is also a common mechanism but not as common as rationalization.

83. (C) The symptom is a characteristic flow of ideas in which one idea rapidly triggers another.

84. (D) This activity would channel her energy, but would not increase external stimuli as group activities would do.

85. (C) Setting limits is important to avoid the client's being rejected by others, with subsequent lowering of self-esteem.

86. (D) That mania is caused by a chemical imbalance and is transmitted through the genes is only a theory.

87. (B) Extrapyramidal side effects are associated with the antipsychotic drugs. The other answers are important to be aware of when monitoring the use of antianxiety drugs.

88. (D) The usual side effect is polyuria, not anuria.

89. (B) When depression lifts, the client has enough energy to commit suicide. Satisfaction may well indicate a well-formulated plan.

90. (B) The other answers do not refer to depressed affect (feelings), but rather to behavior—also characteristic of a depressed person.

Legal Issues in Nursing

Nurse Practice Act

Composition

A. A series of statutes enacted by each state's legislature to regulate the practice of nursing in that state.
B. Establishment of scope of nursing practice for which the registered nurse and/or the vocational/practical nurse is held legally responsible by a particular state.

Provisions

A. Definition of nursing to include functions, responsibilities, and personal qualifications.
B. Authorization to practice (licensure).
C. Educational requirements.
D. Implementation and reinforcement of act by State Board of Nursing.
E. Proceedings and penalties of professional misconduct.

Scope of LPN/LVN Functions

A. Administer nursing care, utilizing basic scientific knowledge and understanding, under the direction and supervision of a registered nurse, or licensed physician.
B. Assist the registered nurse or licensed physician with patients who require more complex medical care.

State Board of Nursing

Composition

A. A group invested with authority by a state to administer its Nurse Practice Act.
B. Members of a board are appointed from among the nursing profession and interested public.

Responsibilities

A. Accredits schools of nursing which meet preestablished standards.
   1. Withholds accreditation from schools which do not meet standards.
   2. Withdraws accreditation from the schools which do not conform to standards.
B. Provides guidelines and minimum standards for nursing curriculum.
C. Governs all aspects of licensing.
   1. Administers the official nursing examinations.
   2. Grants licenses to authorized applicants.
   3. Takes necessary legal action required for denial, revocation, and suspension of license.
D. Conducts investigations and hearings on violations of established standards, laws, and regulations.

Licensure

A. Licensure is granted to individuals who have met predetermined standards.
   1. One main reason for licensure is protection of the public from unqualified practitioners.
   2. It is the responsibility of the LVN or LPN to be familiar with the laws of the state in which he or she will practice.
B. Requirements for practice.
   1. A license to practice is mandatory requirement in some states.
      a. Without license, titles of LVN or LPN may not be used.
      b. Without license, compensation for service as LVN or LPN cannot be received.
   2. Some states have a permissive law that allows one to practice without a license.
C. Methods of obtaining a license.
   1. Application reviewed by State Board of Nursing.
   2. Attain established educational and personal standards and pass licensing examination.

3. If licensed in another state, some states will recognize that license and grant a license by *reciprocity* or *endorsement*.

D. Bases for disciplinary action.
  1. Obtaining a license fraudulently.
  2. Practicing nursing during period of revocation or suspension of license.
  3. Permitting or aiding unlicensed person to perform those nursing activities requiring a license.
  4. Performing duties beyond scope of nursing practice.
  5. Practicing in a manner that is judged to be incompetent and/or negligent.
  6. Practicing when functional ability is impaired by drugs, alcohol, or other disability.

The Nurse and Patient

Patient's Rights

A. A violation of a patient's right, or claim to a right, may be established by a court of law.
B. A nurse should be totally familiar with all aspects of a patient's rights when those rights are associated with health care.
C. Basic rights are guaranteed by the United States Constitution.
  1. Freedom of expression.
  2. Due process of law.
  3. Freedom from cruel and inhumane treatment.
  4. Equal protection for all citizens.

Consent to Receive Health Services

A. Consent is the approval by a patient, or those authorized to give consent, to have his or her body touched by health services personnel (e.g., physician, nurse, or other allied health personnel).
B. Factors in consent-giving process.
  1. Consent may be implied or expressed in either written or verbal form.

2. Consent must be *informed consent*.
  a. Patient must be fully informed regarding the mode and extent of tests, surgery, and varieties of treatment to be administered.
  b. Patient must understand that intended results may not be accomplished.
  c. Patient must understand that unintended, potentially harmful consequences may result.
  d. Does not mean a patient can insist on having whatever he wants.
  e. The patient has the right to make choices between "acceptable options."
  f. To make decisions, the patient must have the emotional/mental/legal capacity to do so.
3. A prior consent may be rescinded in either verbal or written form.

C. Individuals authorized to give consent for health services.
  1. Mentally competent adult patients.
  2. Parents or legal guardians of minors.
  3. Court-approved individuals responsible for the mentally incompetent patient.
  4. Holders of durable power of attorney.

D. Emergency situations requiring immediate life-preserving action require no prior consent.
  1. Serious injury and extreme body dysfunction (e.g., cardiac or respiratory arrest).
  2. Imminent death from other causes.

E. Liabilities of a nurse regarding consent.
  1. Nurse is liable if he or she requests signature of patient on a consent form when he or she knows (or *should have known*) patient had not been informed by either the physician or authorized hospital staff regarding potential harmful consequences of treatment, procedures, or surgery.
  2. Nurse is liable if he or she does not respect rights of a mentally competent adult patient to refuse health care.

Medical Records

A. A medical record is a complete and accurate written account of a patient's medical history which includes past and present medical conditions, a recording of all tests, surgeries, procedures, medications, and other relevant data.

B. A medical record functions as a tool of communication within a hospital, clinic, or physician's office for allied health personnel.

1. Provides continuity of health care given and to be given to patient.
2. Provides data for purposes of research.
3. Provides data necessary for assessing quality care by hospital committees.

C. Nurse's legal and ethical obligations.

1. Help to maintain complete and timely records.
2. Sign or countersign only those entries which are accurate and complete.

Public Law and the Nurse

The Law

A. Binding rules and standards of an extended community which are formally recognized, obeyed, and enforced by authority.

B. The purpose of the law is the preservation of order and the promotion of safety.

C. Obligations of a nurse to the law are no different than that required of other citizens.

1. An individual is responsible for his or her own behavior unless that individual is mentally incompetent.
2. An individual is responsible to know the law and its ramifications.
3. Punitive action may be taken against the individual who fails to abide by the law.

Nursing Contracts

A. A contract is a binding agreement (usually in printed form) between two or more individuals that gives evidence to specified terms and conditions expected of both parties to the agreement.

B. A contract entered into by a nurse and employer may be in the form of either a written or verbal agreement.

C. Conditions of the agreement.

1. The nurse is required to perform all nursing duties with skill and knowledge.
2. Performance is to be in accordance with the standards of care established by the Nurse Practice Act for licensure.
3. The employer is required to issue fair compensation for services given.

D. Breach of the agreement (contract) occurs when one or more parties to the agreement fail to fulfill the obligations stipulated within it.

Civil Torts

A. Wrongful act committed by one person against another.

B. Types of litigation (lawsuit).

1. *Negligence* is failure to perform the extent of care a reasonable and prudent person would exercise.
   a. *Malpractice* is negligent performance by a physician, RN, LVN, LPN, or other allied health personnel.
   b. *Respondeat superior* is the legal doctrine that holds an employer responsible for negligent acts of employees in course and scope of employment. (A nurse continues to be liable for negligent performance.)
2. *Invasion of privacy* is the interference by one individual of another individual's right to privacy. (Refers only to nonpublic individuals.)
   a. Make an individual's private affairs public.
   b. Exhibit an individual's likeness publicly.
3. *Defamation of character* is the harm of an individual's reputation or the disgrace of character by a second individual.
   a. *Libel* is a written or published defamation.
   b. *Slander* is an oral defamation.

Criminal Law

A. *Crime* is an offense against the public for which the state prosecutes and seeks punishment.

B. *Felony* is a serious crime punishable by imprisonment or death.

C. Felonious acts.

   1. *Assault* is the threat or attempt to do harm or come into physical contact with another individual without consent.

   2. *Battery* is actual use of force or contact with another individual without consent.

   3. *Euthanasia* is the act of killing a hopelessly ill or injured individual for reasons of mercy.

   4. *False imprisonment* is the intentional restraint of an individual against his or her will without legal justification.

D. *Misdemeanor* is a crime less serious than a felony.

Professional Organizations

Purposes

A. Maintain and improve nursing standards.

B. Provide a vehicle for continuing education.

   1. Workshops.

   2. Publications.

   3. National and state conventions.

C. Provide opportunity to share professional interests.

D. Enhance an individual's sense of belonging.

National Associations

A. National Association for Practical Nurse Education and Service, Inc. (NAPNES).

   1. Membership—extended to any individual with an interest in education of practical nurse and/or other aspects of practical nursing.

   2. Publication—*The Journal of Practical Nursing.*

B. National Federation of Licensed Practical Nurses (NFLPN).

   1. Membership—limited to licensed practical or vocational nurses.

   2. Publication—*Journal of Nursing Care.*

C. National League for Nurses (NLN).

   1. Membership—extended to any individual with an interest in nursing.

   2. Publication—*Nursing and Health Care, Nursing Research* and professional directories.

   3. Functions.

      a. Prepare and score selection and achievement tests.

      b. Conduct workshops.

      c. Nationally accredit schools of registered nursing.

D. American Nurses' Association (ANA).

   1. Membership—limited to registered nurses, students of vocational/practical nursing.

   2. Publication—the *American Journal of Nursing.*

Vocational Ethics

A. Ethics is a study that deals with issues of good and bad, moral duty and obligation.

B. Issues are frequently translated into principles of conduct that govern individual or group behavior.

Characteristics of a Set of Principles

A. Principles are generally predetermined and set down by the same group of individuals whose conduct will be guided by them.

B. The group will abide by these principles voluntarily.

C. The moral duties and obligations governing nursing care practice are embodied in the set of guiding principles.

D. The principles clarify desirable attitudes that ought to be basic to a nurse's performance.

NAPNES Code of Ethics

A. The licensed practical/vocational nurse shall:

1. Consider as a basic obligation the conservation of life and the prevention of disease.

2. Promote and protect the physical, mental, emotional, and spiritual health of the patient and his or her family.

3. Fulfill all duties faithfully and efficiently.

4. Function within established legal guidelines.

5. Accept personal responsibility (for his acts) and seek to merit the respect and confidence of all members of the health team.

6. Hold in confidence all matters coming to his knowledge, in the practice of his profession, and in no way and at no time violate this confidence.

7. Give conscientious service, and charge just remuneration.

8. Learn and respect the religious and cultural beliefs of his or her patient and of all people.

9. Meet his or her obligation to patients by keeping abreast of current trends in health care through reading and continuing education.

10. As a citizen of the United States of America, uphold the laws of the land and seek to promote legislation which shall meet the health needs of its people.

B. The code of ethics provides principles to guide the performance of licensed practical/vocational nurses.

Appendix 1. Directory of Boards of Nursing

Executive Officer
Board of Nursing
500 Eastern Blvd.
Montgomery, Alabama 36117

Executive Secretary
Alaska Board of Nursing
360 "C" St., Suite 722
Anchorage, Alaska 99503

Executive Secretary
Arizona State Board of Nursing
5050 W. 19th Ave., Suite 103
Phoenix, Arizona 85015

Executive Director
Arkansas State Board of Nursing
4120 W. Markham, Suite 308
Little Rock, Arkansas 72205

Executive Secretary
Board of Vocational Nursing and
    Psychiatric Technical Examiners
1020 N Street, Room 406
Sacramento, California 95814

Program Administrator
Colorado State Board of Nursing
1525 Sherman Street, Room 132
Denver, Colorado 80203

Executive Secretary, Nursing
    Department of Health Services
150 Washington St.
Hartford, Connecticut 06106

Executive Director
Delaware Board of Nursing
O'Neill Bldg., PO Box 1401
Dover, Delaware 19901

President
District of Columbia Board of
    Practical Nursing
614 H Street NW, Room 923
Washington, DC 20001

Executive Director
Florida State Board of Nursing
111 E. Coastline Dr.
Jacksonville, Florida 33202

Executive Director
Georgia Board of Examiners of
    Lic. Practical Nurses
166 Pryor Street, S.W.
Atlanta, Georgia 30303

Chairman
Guam Board of Nurse Examiners
PO Box 2816
Agana, Guam 96910

Executive Secretary
Hawaii Board of Nursing
Box 3469
Honolulu, Hawaii 96801

Executive Director
Idaho State Board of Nursing
700 West State St.
Boise, Idaho 83702

Nursing Education Coordinator
Department of Registration and Education
320 W. Washington St.
Springfield, Illinois 62786

Executive Secretary
State Board of Nurses Registration and Nursing
    Education
964 N. Pennsylvania St.
Indianapolis, Indiana 46204

Executive Director
Iowa Board of Nursing
1223 E. Court Ave.
Des Moines, Iowa 50319

Executive Administrator
Kansas State Board of Nursing
503 Kansas, Box 1098, Suite 330
Topeka, Kansas 66601

Executive Director
Kentucky Board of Nursing
4010 Dupont Cir., Suite 430
Louisville, Kentucky 40207

Executive Director
Louisiana State Board of
    Practical Nurse Examiners
4201½ Canal St.
New Orleans, Louisiana 70119

Executive Director
Maine State Board of Nursing
105 Water Street
Augusta, Maine 04330

Executive Director
State Board of Examiners of Nurses
201 West Preston Street
Baltimore, Maryland 21201

Supervisor
Board of Registration in Nursing
100 Cambridge Street, Room 150
Boston, Massachusetts 02202

Board Secretary
Michigan Board of Nursing
PO Box 30018
Lansing, Michigan 48909

Executive Secretary
Minnesota Board of Nursing
717 Delaware Street, S.E.
Minneapolis, Minnesota 55414

State Supervisor
Health Occupations Education
Division of Vocational Education
State Department of Education
Jackson, Mississippi 39205

Executive Director
Missouri State Board of Nursing
3523 N. Ten Mile Drive
Jefferson City, Missouri 65101

Executive Secretary
Montana State Board of Nursing
1424 Ninth Avenue
Helena, Montana 59620

Executive Director
State Board of Nursing
State House Station, Box 95065
Lincoln, Nebraska 68509

Executive Director
Nevada State Board of Nursing
1135 Terminal Way, Room 209
Reno, Nevada 89502

Executive Director
State Board of Nursing
105 Loudon Road
Concord, New Hampshire 03301

Executive Director
New Jersey Board of Nursing
1100 Raymond Boulevard, Room 319
Newark, New Jersey 07102

Executive Director
New Mexico Board of Nursing
5031 Central N.E., Suite 905
Albuquerque, New Mexico 87108

Executive Secretary
New York State Board of Nursing
The Cultural Center, Room 3013
Albany, New 12230

Executive Director
Board of Nursing
320 W. Jones St.
Raleigh, North Carolina 27602

Executive Director
North Dakota Board of Nursing
418 E. Rosser
Bismarck, North Dakota 58501

Executive Secretary
State Board of Nursing Education and
    Nurse Registration
65 S. Front St., Room 509
Columbus, Ohio 43215

Executive Director
Board of Nurse Registration and
    Nursing Education
4001 N. Lincoln Blvd., Room 400
Oklahoma City, Oklahoma 73105

Executive Director
Oregon State Board of Nursing
1400 South West 5th Avenue, Room 904
Portland, Oregon 97201

Secretary
Pennsylvania State Board of Nurse Examiners
Trans & Safety Bldg., 6th Floor
Harrisburg, Pennsylvania 17120

Director
Commonwealth Board for Vocational-Technical
    Education
Box 759
Hato Rey, Puerto Rico 00919

Director
Board of Nurse Registration
75 Davis Street, Room 104
Providence, Rhode Island 02908

Executive Director
State Board of Nursing for South Carolina
1777 St. Julian Place, Suite 102
Columbia, South Carolina 29204

Executive Secretary
South Dakota Board of Nursing
304 W. Phillips Avenue, Suite 205
Sioux Falls, South Dakota 57102

Executive Director
TDPH State Office Building
383 Plus Park
Nashville, Tennessee 37219

Executive Director
Board of Vocational Nurse Examiners
1300 E. Anderson Lane, Bldg. C-225
Austin, Texas 78752

Executive Secretary
Utah State Board of Nursing
Room 5257, State Office Bldg.
Salt Lake City, Utah 84114

Executive Director
Vermont Board of Nursing
Licensing and Registration Division
109 State Street
Montpelier, Vermont 05602

Executive Secretary
Virgin Islands Board of
    Nurse Licensure
PO Box 7309
St. Thomas, Virgin Islands 00801

Executive Secretary
Virginia State Board of Nursing
517 W. Grace St., PO Box 27708
Richmond, Virginia 23230

Executive Secretary
State Board of Practical Nursing
Business and Profession Administration
Professional Division
Olympia, Washington, 98504

Executive Secretary
Board of Examiners for LPN's
922 Quarrier Street, Suite 506
Charleston, West Virginia 25301

Administrator
Wisconsin State Bureau of Nursing
1400 East Washington Avenue
Madison, Wisconsin 53702

Executive Director
State of Wyoming Board of Nursing
2223 Warren Ave., Suite One
Cheyenne, Wyoming 82002

Review Questions

1. The function of the State Board of Nursing is to

   A. Establish certain nursing procedures in the hospitals.
   B. Execute laws pertaining to nursing.
   C. Operate schools of nursing in the state.
   D. Establish in-service programs in the hospital.

2. Mandatory licensing of practical/vocational nurses means that

   A. Only those practicing in hospitals need to be licensed.
   B. The practical/vocational nurse can decide when to obtain a license.
   C. The practical/vocational nurse can register by waiver.
   D. All practicing practical/vocational nurses are required by law to be licensed.

3. To practice in a particular state, nurses must meet the legal requirement for registration in the state in which they

   A. Are intending to practice.
   B. Were born.
   C. Were married.
   D. Took their training.

4. In practicing nursing, the practical/vocational nurse does *not* need to have legal knowledge of

   A. Licensing laws.
   B. Drug Abuse Prevention and Control Act.
   C. Contracts.
   D. Hill-Burton Act.

5. The practical/vocational nurse has legal obligations toward patients. She may be held legally responsible if she

   A. Fails to perform certain acts expected of a practical/vocational nurse.
   B. Causes injury to a patient by negligence or ignorance of procedures she would be expected to perform as a practical nurse.
   C. Does not refuse to perform certain acts that are considered to be above the level of practical/vocational nursing.
   D. All of these.

6. Malpractice suits may result from

   A. A patient falling out of bed when side rail was let down.
   B. Giving the wrong medication.
   C. Improper use of the patient's personal belongings.
   D. All of these.

7. A legitimate reason for revoking a nurse's license is

   A. Failure to arrive on duty at the prescribed time.
   B. Too many sick days.
   C. Addiction to drugs.
   D. Inability to work with others in a given situation.

8. A practical/vocational nurse is told by a professional nurse to instill a medication into a patient's bladder. The practical/vocational nurse goes ahead with the procedure even though she had never performed or been instructed in this procedure before. Injury to the patient results. Who is *primarily* responsible?

   A. The professional nurse who gave the order.
   B. The practical/vocational nurse who carried out the order.
   C. The patient's doctor who is responsible for the original order.
   D. The patient for allowing the nurse to perform the procedure.

9. If a licensed practical/vocational nurse performs duties resulting in injury to people or property, she is described as being

   A. Emotionally incapable.
   B. Negligent.
   C. Malicious.
   D. Illegal.

10. The most important quality that all practical/vocational nurses should have is

    A. Knowledge of their limitations.
    B. Pride to prevent them from asking questions.
    C. Ability to carry out procedures that they have learned even against hospital regulations.
    D. Ability to report directly to the physician in hospital nursing.

11. Which of these organizations would most likely formulate a code of ethics for the licensed practical/vocational nurse?

    A. National League for Nurses.
    B. National Federation of Licensed Practical Nurses.
    C. American Nurses' Association.
    D. National Association for Practical Nurse Education and Service.

12. Which of these groups nationally accredits all levels of schools of nursing?

    A. National League for Nurses.
    B. National Association for Practical/Professional Nurse Education.
    C. State Boards of Nursing.
    D. American Nurses' Association.

13. A licensed practical/vocational nurse may not belong to

   A. National League for Nurses.
   B. National Federation of Licensed Practical Nurses.
   C. American Nurses' Association.
   D. National Association for Practical Nurse Education and Service.

14. A licensed practical/vocational nurse should join a local or state nursing organization

   A. To make it easier to find a job.
   B. To facilitate collective bargaining.
   C. To obtain lower enrollment fees in educational courses.
   D. To keep abreast of possible changes in the nursing profession.

Answers and Rationale

1. (B)   A State Board of Nursing implements the laws governing the practice of nursing. The boards do not operate schools of nursing or establish procedures or programs in hospitals.

2. (D)   Mandatory licensure means that a license is necessary in order to practice for compensation anywhere in that particular state.

3. (A)   The Nurse Practice Act of each state defines the licensing requirements. The practical/vocational nurse is responsible for meeting the requirements of the state in which she intends to practice.

4. (D)   Nurses are responsible for their own acts. It is the obligation of the nurse to have knowledge of laws pertaining to the practice of nursing. The Hill-Burton Act was established to provide funds for creating new health care institutions or upgrading established facilities.

5. (D)   The practical/vocational nurse is legally responsible to perform within the scope of practice as defined by the state in which she is employed. Duties may not be performed that are determined to be beyond the scope of such practice.

6. (D)   All are state Nurse Practice Act grounds for disciplinary action.

7. (C)   The other options are not state Nurse Practice Act grounds for disciplinary action.

8. (B)   Nurses are responsible for their own acts.

9. (B)   Negligent conduct is when a person acts or does not act in a reasonable or prudent manner and thus does harm to another.

10. (A)   Nurses are responsible for their own acts. The practical/vocational nurse is held responsible to perform those duties for which she is employed.

11. (B)   Since a code of ethics should be prepared by the group to which the ethics pertain, NFLPN is the best answer because the organization's membership is limited to LPN/LVN's. It would be possible for a group of LPN/LVN's, working within a larger group, to prepare such a code; for example, LPN/LVN's with membership in NLN or NAPNES.

12. (A)   NLN nationally accredits all levels of nursing schools. Some VN/PN schools are accredited by NAPNES on a national level. State Boards simply accredit on a state level.

13. (C)   ANA membership is limited to registered nurses.

14. (D)   Active membership in an organization is often the easiest and/or only way to keep up-to-date with latest developments. Some organizations are involved in collective bargaining.

Bibliography

Abrams, Anne Collins. *Clinical Drug Therapy*. Philadelphia: J.B. Lippincott Company, 1983.

Adams, Catherine G., and Macione, Alberta. *Handbook of Psychiatric-Mental Health Nursing*. New York: John Wiley & Sons, Inc., 1983.

American Heart Association and National Academy of Sciences-National Research Council. "Standards and Guidelines for Cardiopulmonary Resuscitation (CPR) and Emergency Cardiac Care (ECC)." *JAMA* 244(5): 453-509, 1980.

American National Red Cross. *Standard First Aid and Personal Safety*. 2nd ed. Garden City: Doubleday, 1980.

Anderson, Betty Ann, et al. *The Childbearing Family*, Vol. I, *Pregnancy and Family Health*. 2nd ed. New York: McGraw-Hill Book Company, 1984.

Anthony, Catherine P., and Gary A. Thibodeau. *Structure and Function of the Body*. 7th ed. St. Louis: The C.V. Mosby Company, 1984.

Arieti, Silvano, ed. *American Handbook of Psychiatry*, Vols. I, II, and III. New York: Basic Books, Inc., Publishers, 1974.

Armstrong, Margaret, et al. *McGraw-Hill Handbook of Clinical Nursing*. New York: McGraw-Hill Book Company, 1979.

Asperheim, Mary K., and Eisenhauer, Laurel A. *The Pharmacologic Basis of Patient Care*. 5th ed. Philadelphia: W.B. Saunders Company, 1985.

Barber, Janet and Susan Budassi, *Mosby's Manual of Emergency Care*. St. Louis: The C.V. Mosby Company, 1984.

Barnard, Martha U., et al. *Human Sexuality for Health Professionals*. Philadelphia: W.B. Saunders Company, 1978.

Barry, Jean. *Emergency Nursing*. New York: McGraw-Hill Book Company, 1978.

Bates, Barbara. *A Guide to Physical Examination*. 3rd ed. Philadelphia: J.B. Lippincott Company, 1984.

Beck, Cornelia, et al. *Mental Health-Psychiatric Nursing*. St. Louis: The C.V. Mosby Company, 1984.

Beland, Irene, and Passos, Joyce. *Clinical Nursing*. 4th ed. New York: Macmillan Publishing Company, 1981.

Bergersen, Betty S. *Pharmacology in Nursing*. 15th ed. St. Louis: The C.V. Mosby Company, 1982.

Bethea, Doris C. *Introductory Maternity Nursing*. 4th ed. Philadelphia: J.B. Lippincott Company, 1984.

Birchenall, Joan, and Streight, Mary Eileen. *Care of the Older Adult*. 2nd ed. Philadelphia: J.B. Lippincott Company, 1982.

Bleir, Inge J. *Workbook in Bedside Maternity Nursing*. 3rd ed. Philadelphia: W.B. Saunders Company, 1982.

Bloom, B. S. ed. *Taxonomy of Educational Objectives, Handbook I: Cognitive Domain*. New York: David McKay Co., 1956.

Bordick, Katherine. *Patterns of Shock Implications for Nursing Care*. New York: Macmillan Publishing Company, 1965.

Brill, Ester L. *Foundations for Nursing*. 2nd ed. New York: Appleton-Century-Crofts, 1986.

Brink, Pamela J., ed. *Transcultural Nursing*. Englewood Cliffs, NJ: Prentice-Hall, Inc., 1976.

Broadribb, Violet. *Introductory Pediatric Nursing*. 3rd ed. Philadelphia: J.B. Lippincott Company, 1982.

Brooks, Stewart. *Basic Facts of Body Water and Ions*. New York: Springer Publishing Company, Inc., 1973.

Brunner, Lillian Sholtis, and Suddarth, Doris Smith. *The Lippincott Manual of Nursing Practice*. 4th ed. Philadelphia: J.B. Lippincott Company, 1986.

Brunner, Lillian Sholtis, and Suddarth, Doris Smith. *Textbook of Medical-Surgical Nursing*. 5th ed. Philadelphia: J.B. Lippincott Company, 1984.

Budassi, Susan, and Barber, Janet. *Emergency Nursing: Principles and Practice*. 2nd ed. St. Louis: The C.V. Mosby Company, 1985.

Buckley, Kathleen, and Kulb, Nancy. *Handbook of Maternal-Newborn Nursing*. New York: John Wiley & Sons, Inc., 1983.

Bullough, Bonnie. *The Law and the Expanding Nursing Role*. 2nd ed. New York: Appleton-Century-Croft, 1980.

Burgess, Ann Wolbert, and Lazare, Aaron. *Psychiatric Nursing in the Hospital and the Community*. 4th ed. Englewood Cliffs, NJ: Prentice-Hall, Inc. 1984.

Burnside, Irene Mortenson and Ethel Percy Andrus. *Nursing and the Aged*. 3rd ed. New York: McGraw-Hill Book Company, 1981.

Burrow,, G. N., and Ferris, T. F. *Medical Complications During Pregnancy*, 2nd ed. Philadelphia: W.B. Saunders Company, 1982.

Carnevali, Doris, and Patrick, Maxine. *Nursing Management for the Elderly*. 2nd ed. Philadelphia: J.B. Lippincott Company, 1986.

Cataldo, C. B., and Smith, L. "Tube Feedings: Clinical Applications." Ross Laboratories, 1980.

Cazalas, Mary W. *Nursing and the Law*. Germantown, MD: Aspen Systems Corporation, 1979.

Chaffee, Ellen, and Lytle, Ivan. *Basic Physiology and Anatomy*. 4th ed. Philadelphia: J.B. Lippincott Company, 1980.

Cherniack, R. M., et al. *Respiration in Health and Disease*. Philadelphia: W. B. Saunders Company, 1972.

Chinn, Peggy L. *Child Health Maintenance: Concepts in Family Centered Care*. St. Louis: The C.V. Mosby Company, 1979.

Clark, Ann, and Affonso, Dyanne. *Childbearing: A Nursing Perspective*. 2nd ed. Philadelphia: F.A. Davis Company, 1979.

Cohen, Stephen. "Nursing Care of a Patient in Traction." *Americal Journal of Nursing*, October 1979.

Conway, Barbara. *Carini and Owens' Neurological and Neurosurgical Nursing*. 8th ed. St. Louis: The C.V. Mosby Company, 1982.

Cosgriff, James, and Anderson, Diann. *The Practice of Emergency Nursing*. 2nd ed. Philadelphia: J.B. Lippincott Company, 1984.

Crawford, Annie Lauri, and Virginia C. Kilander. *Mental Health and Psychiatric Nursing*. 6th ed. Philadelphia: F.A. Davis Company, 1985

Creighton, Helen. *Law Every Nurse Should Know*. 5th ed. W.B. Saunders Company, 1985.

Culver, Vivian M. *Modern Bedside Nursing*. 8th ed. W.B. Saunders Company, 1975.

Dickason, Elizabeth J., and Schultz, Martha Olsen. *Maternal and Infant Care*. 2nd ed. New York: McGraw-Hill Book Company, 1979.

Dunphy, J. Englebert, and Way, Lawrence L. *Current Surgical Diagnosis and Treatment*. 5th ed. Los Altos, CA: Lange Medical Publications, 1983.

Engle, George L. "Grief and Grieving." *American Journal of Nursing*, September 1964.

Erikson, Erik H. *Childhood and Society*. New York: W.W. Norton and Company, Inc. 1963.

Ferholt, Deborah. *Clinical Assessment of Children: A Comprehensive Approach to Primary Pediatric Care*. Philadelphia: J.B. Lippincott Company, 1980.

Fischbach, Frances. *A Manual of Laboratory Diagnostic Tests*. 2nd ed. Philadelphia: J.B. Lippincott Company, 1984.

Food and Nutrition Board, National Research Council, National Academy of Sciences. *Recommended Dietary Allowances*. Washington, DC: 1979

French, Ruth. *Guide to Diagnostic Procedures*. 5th ed. New York: McGraw-Hill Book Company, 1980.

Gardner, Ernest, et al. *Anatomy: A Regional Study of Human Structure*. 4th ed. Philadelphia: W.B. Saunders Company, 1980.

Gillies, Dee Ann, and Alyn, Irene Barrett. *Saunders Tests for Self-Evaluation of Nursing Competence*. 3rd ed. Philadelphia: W. B. Saunders Company, 1980.

Govoni, Laura E., and Hayes, Janice E. *Drugs and Nursing Implications*. 5th ed. Appleton-Century-Crofts, 1985.

Grant, Harvey, and Murray, Robert. *Emergency Care*. 3rd ed. Bowie, MD: Robert J. Brady Company, 1982.

Guthrie, Helen Andrews. *Introductory Nutrition*. 5th ed. St. Louis: The C.V. Mosby Company, 1983.

Guyton, Arthur C. *Textbook of Medical Physiology*. 6th ed. Philadelphia: W. B. Saunders Company, 1981.

Haber, Judith, et al. *Comprehensive Psychiatric Nursing*. 2nd ed. New York: McGraw-Hill Book Company, 1982.

Hall, Joanne E., and Weaver, Barbara. *Nursing of Families in Crisis*. Philadelphia: J.B. Lippincott Company, 1974.

Hamilton, Persis. *Basic Maternity Nursing*. 5th ed. St. Louis: The C.V. Mosby Company, 1984.

Hamilton, Persis. *Basic Pediatric Nursing*. 4th ed. St. Louis: The C.V. Mosby Company, 1982.

Hayman, Laura, and Sporing, Eileen. *Handbook of Pediatric Nursing*. John Wiley & Sons, Inc., 1985.

Hemelt, Mary D., and Mackert, Mary E. *Dynamics of Law in Nursing and Health Care*. 2nd ed. Reston: Reston Pub. Co., 1982.

Holloway, Nancy M. *Nursing the Critically Ill Adult*. 2nd ed. Menlo Park, CA: Addison-Wesley Publishing Company, 1984.

Howe, Jeanne, et al. *The Handbook of Nursing*. John Wiley & Sons, Inc., 1984.

Hudak, Carolyn M., et al. *Critical Care Nursing*. 4th ed. Philadelphia: J.B. Lippincott Company, 1986.

Ingalls, A. Joy, and Salerno, M. Constance. *Maternal and Child Nursing*. 5th ed. St. Louis: The C.V. Mosby Company, 1983.

Jacob, Stanley, Francone, Clarice, and Lossow, Walter J. *Structure and Function in Man*. 5th ed. Philadelphia: W.B. Saunders Company, 1982.

Jensen, Margaret, et al. *Maternity and Gynecologic Care: The Nurse and the Family*. 3rd ed. St. Louis: The C.V. Mosby Company, 1985.

Juneau, Patricia. *Essentials of Maternity Nursing*. New York: Macmillan Publishing Company, 1985.

Kalkman, Marion, and Davis, Ann. *New Dimensions in Mental-Health Psychiatric Nursing*. 5th ed. New York: McGraw-Hill Book Company, 1980.

Karones, Shelton B. *High-Risk Newborn Infants*. St. Louis: The C.V. Mosby Company, 1981.

Keane, Clare B. *Essentials of Medical-Surgical Nursing*. 2nd ed. Philadelphia: W.B. Saunders Company, 1985.

Kinney, M. R., et al. *AACN's Clinical Reference for Critical-Care Nursing*. New York: McGraw-Hill Book Company, 1981.

Kozier, Barbara, and Erb, Glenora L. *Fundamentals of Nursing: Concepts and Procedures*. 2nd ed. Menlo Park, CA: Addison-Wesley Publishing Company, 1983.

Krupp, Marcus A., and Chatton, Milton J. *Current Medical Diagnosis and Treatment*. Los Altos, CA: Lange Medical Publications, 1985.

Krupp, Marcus, et al. *Physician's Handbook*. 20th ed. Los Altos, CA: Lange Medical Publications, 1982.

Kubler-Ross, Elisabeth. *On Death and Dying*. New York: Macmillan Publishing Company, 1969.

Langley, L. L., et al. *Dynamic Anatomy and Physiology*. 5th ed. New York: McGraw-Hill Book Company, 1980.

Leifer, Gloria. *Principles and Techniques in Pediatric Nursing*. 4th ed. Philadelphia: W.B. Saunders Company, 1982.

Luckmann, Joan, and Sorensen, Karen Creason. *Medical-Surgical Nursing: A Psychophysiologic Approach*. 3rd ed. Philadelphia: W.B. Saunders Company, 1984.

Malasanos, Lois, et al. *Health Assessment*. 3rd ed. St. Louis: The C.V. Mosby Company, 1985.

Marlow, D. R. *Textbook of Pediatric Nursing*. Philadelphia: W.B. Saunders Company, 1979.

Marram, Gwen D. *The Group Approach in Nursing Practice*. St. Louis: The C.V. Mosby Company, 1979.

Mason, Mildred. *Basic Medical-Surgical Nursing*. 5th ed. New York: Macmillan Publishing Company, 1984.

McCaffery, Margo. *Nursing Management of the Patient with Pain*. 2nd ed. Philadelphia: J.B. Lippincott Company, 1979.

Mead, Johnson. *Dialogues in Nutrition. Nutritional Care of the Critically Ill Patient: Selection of Appropriate Feeding Modalities*. Vol. 3, No. 2, 1979.

Meeks, Dorothy, et al. *Practical Nursing*. 5th ed. St. Louis: The C.V. Mosby Company, 1974.

Memmler, Ruth, and Wood, Dena Lin. *The Human Body in Health and Disease*. 5th ed. Philadelphia: J.B. Lippincott Company, 1983.

Memmler, Ruth, and Wood, Dena Lin. *Structure and Function of the Human Body*. 4th ed. Philadelphia: J.B. Lippincott Company, 1983.

Metheny, Norma M., and Snively, W. D. *Nurses' Handbook of Fluid Balance*. 4th ed. Philadelphia: J.B. Lippincott Company, 1983.

Millar, Sally. *Methods in Critical Care: The AACN Manual*. Philadelphia: W.B. Saunders Company, 1980.

Murchison, Irene, et al. *Legal Accountability in the Nursing Process*. 2nd ed. St. Louis: The C.V. Mosby Company, 1982.

Narrow, Barbara W. *Patient Teaching in Nursing Practice, A Patient and Family-Centered Approach*. New York: John Wiley & Sons, Inc., 1979.

Neeson, Jean D., and Stockdale, Connie R. *The Practitioner's Handbook of Ambulatory Obstetrics and Gynecology*. New York: John Wiley and Sons, Inc., 1981.

Olds, Sharon, et al. *Obstetric Nursing*. 2nd ed. Menlo Park: Addison-Wesley Publishing Company, 1985.

Parcel, Guy. *Basic Emergency Care of the Sick and Injured*. 2nd ed. The C.V. Mosby Company, 1982.

Pellitteri, Adele. *Nursing Care of the Growing Family: A Child Health Text*. Boston: Little, Brown & Company, 1981.

Perry, Anne, and Potter, Patricia. *Clinical Nursing Skills and Techniques*. St. Louis: The C.V. Mosby Company, 1986.

Petrillo, M., and Sanger, S. *Emotional Care of Hospitalized Children*. 2nd ed. Philadelphia: J.B. Lippincott Company, 1980.

Petty, Thomas, L. *Intensive and Rehabilitative Respiratory Care*. 3rd ed. Philadelphia: Lea and Febiger, 1982.

Physician's Desk Reference to Pharmaceutical Specialties and Biologicals. Oradell, NJ: Medical Economics, Inc. 1984.

Phipps, Wilma, et al. *Medical-Surgical Nursing*. 2nd ed. St. Louis: The C.V. Mosby Company, 1983.

Potter, Patricia, and Perry, Anne. *Fundamentals of Nursing*. St. Louis: The C.V. Mosby Company, 1985.

Pritchard, Jack A., and MacDonald, Paul C. *Williams Obstetrics*. 16th ed. New York: Appleton-Century-Crofts, 1980.

Redman, Barbara Klug. *The Process of Patient Teaching in Nursing*. 4th ed. St. Louis: The C.V. Mosby Company, 1980.

Reeder, Sharon, et al. *Maternity Nursing*. 15th ed. Philadelphia: J.B. Lippincott Company, 1983.

Rodman, Morton. *Clinical Pharmacology in Nursing*. 2nd ed. Philadelphia: J.B. Lippincott Company, 1984.

Rodman, Morton J., and Smith, Dorothy. *Pharmacology and Drug Therapy in Nursing*. 3rd ed. Philadelphia: J.B. Lippincott Company, 1984.

Rosdahl, Caroline Bunker. *Textbook of Basic Nursing*. 4th ed. Philadelphia: J.B. Lippincott Company, 1985.

Ross, Carmen. *Personal and Vocational Relationships in Practical Nursing*. 5th ed. Philadelphia: J.B. Lippincott, 1981.

Sanderson, Richard. *The Cardiac Patient, a Comprehensive Approach*. 2nd ed. Philadelphia: W.B. Saunders Company, 1981.

Saxton, Dolores, et al. *The Addison-Wesley Manual of Nursing Practice*. Menlo Park: Addison-Wesley Publishing Company, 1983.

Saxton, Dolores, and Haring, Phyllis. *Care of Patients With Emotional Problems*. 4th ed. St. Louis: The C.V. Mosby Company, 1984.

Saxton, Dolores, and Hyland, Patricia. *Planning and Implementing Nursing Intervention*. 2nd ed. St. Louis: The C.V. Mosby Company, 1979.

Scherer, Jeanne, C. *Introductory Clinical Pharmacology*. 3rd ed. Philadelphia: J.B. Lippincott Company, 1986.

Scherer, Jeanne. *Introductory Medical-Surgical Nursing*. 4th ed. Philadelphia: J.B. Lippincott Company, 1986.

Scipien, Gladys, et al. *Comprehensive Pediatric Nursing*. 2nd ed. New York: McGraw-Hill Book Company, 1983.

Selye, Hans. *The Stress of Life*. New York: McGraw-Hill Book Company, 1965.

Shafer, Kathleen Newton, et al. *Medical Surgical Nursing*. 6th ed. St. Louis: The C.V. Mosby Company, 1979.

Silver, H. K., et al. *Handbook of Pediatrics*. 14th ed. Los Altos, CA: Lange Medical Publications, 1983.

Smith, Sandra, and Duell, Donna. *Clinical Nursing Skills*. Los Altos, CA: National Nursing Review, Inc., 1985.

Smith, Sandra. *Sandra Smith's Review for NCLEX-RN*. 4th ed. Los Altos, CA: National Nursing Review, Inc., 1986.

Solnick, Robert L., ed. *Sexuality and Aging*. Los Angeles: Ethel Percy Andrus Gerontology Center, 1978.

Sorenson, Karen, and Luckman, Joan. *Basic Nursing*. 2nd ed. Philadelphia: W.B. Saunders Company, 1986.

Squire, J. E., and Welch, J. M. *Basic Pharmacology for Nurses*. 6th ed. St. Louis: The C.V. Mosby Company, 1977.

Stroot, Violet R., et al. *Fluids and Electrolytes: A Practical Approach*. Philadelphia: F.A. Davis Company, 1977.

Suitor, Carl W., and Hunter, Merilly F. *Nutrition: Principles and Application in Health Promotion*. 2nd ed. Philadelphia: J.B. Lippincott Company, 1984.

Taylor, Cecelia. *Mereness' Essentials of Psychiatric Nursing*. 12th ed. St. Louis: The C.V. Mosby Company, 1986.

Thompson, Eleanor Dumont. *Pediatric Nursing: An Introductory Text*. 4th ed. Philadelphia: W.B. Saunders Company, 1981.

Thompson, June, et al. *Clinical Nursing*. St. Louis: The C.V. Mosby Company, 1986.

Travelbee, Joyce. *Intervention in Psychiatric Nursing. Process in the One-to-One Relationship*. 2nd ed. Philadelphia: F.A. Davis Company, 1979.

Tucker, Susan Martin, et al. *Patient Care Standards*. 3rd ed. St. Louis: The C.V. Mosby Company, 1983.

Turner, Jeffrey S., and Helms, Donald B. *Contemporary Adulthood*. Philadelphia: W.B. Saunders Company, 1979.

U.S. Department of Agriculture, *A Daily Food Guide: The Basic Four*. Rev. ed. Washington, DC: Government Printing Office, 1979.

Vaughan, Victor C. R., et al. *Nelson Textbook of Pediatrics*. 11th ed. Philadelphia: W.B. Saunders Company, 1979.

Wade, Jacqueline. *Respiratory Nursing Care: Physiology and Techniques*. 3rd ed. St. Louis: The C.V. Mosby Company, 1982.

Waechter, Eugenia, et al. *Nursing Care of Children*. 10th ed. Philadelphia: J.B. Lippincott Company, 1985.

Wasserman, Edward, and Slobody, Laurence B. *Survey of Clinical Pediatrics*. 7th ed. New York: McGraw-Hill Book Company, 1981.

Wiener, Matthew B., et al. *Clinical Pharmacology and Therapeutics in Nursing*. New York: McGraw-Hill Book Company, 1980.

Williams, Sue Rodwell. *Essentials of Nutrition and Diet Therapy*. 5th ed. St. Louis: The C.V. Mosby Company, 1982.

Wilson, Holly Skodal, Kneisl, Carol Ren. *Psychiatric Nursing*. 2nd ed. Menlo Park, CA: Addison-Wesley Publishing Company, 1983.

Wolff, Lu Verne, Weitzel, Marlene, and Fuerst, Elinor. *Fundamentals of Nursing*. 7th ed. Philadelphia: J.B. Lippincott, 1983.

Wood, Lucile A., ed. *Nursing Skills for Allied Health Services*. 2nd ed. Philadelphia: W.B. Saunders Company, 1980.

Woods, Nancy Fugate. *Human Sexuality in Health and Illness*. 2nd ed. St. Louis: The C.V. Mosby Company, 1983.

Yura, Helen, and Walsh, Mary B. *The Nursing Process; Assessing, Planning, Implementing, Evaluating*. 4th ed. New York: Appleton-Century-Crofts, 1983.

Ziegel, Erna, and Cranley, Mecca. *Obstetric Nursing*. 8th ed. New York: Macmillan Publishing Company, 1984.